MEDICAL RADIOLOGY
Diagnostic Imaging

Editors:
A. L. Baert, Leuven
M. Knauth, Göttingen
K. Sartor, Heidelberg

Dear Akira,

I wish all the best for your journey in NY and the MSK world.

Hope to see you back here.

Best regards —

Ali

6/24/09

A. Gangi · S. Guth · A. Guermazi (Eds.)

Imaging in Percutaneous Musculoskeletal Interventions

With Contributions by

R.S. Adler · G. Bierry · X. Buy · A. Chevrot · M. Court-Payen · J.-L. Dietemann · J.-L. Drapé
J. Dubois · A. Feydy · K.C. Finzel · A. Gangi · L. Garel · D. Godefroy · T. Gross · A. Guermazi
S. Guth · L. Hacein-Bey · B. Hamze · J.C. Hodge · R. Huegli · J.-P. Imbert · F. Irani · A.L. Jacob
P. Klurfan · J.-D. Laredo · G. Levin · J.S. Luchs · D. Malfair · K. Mattila · P. Messmer
P.L. Munk · A.O. Ortiz · C. Parlier-Cuau · P. Peetrons · W.C.G. Peh · M.E. Simons · K. Tan
K.G. TerBrugge · M. Wybier

Series Editor's Foreword by

A. L. Baert

Forewords by

H. K. Genant and G. Y. El-Khoury

With 370 Figures in 980 Separate Illustrations, 200 in Color and 7 Tables

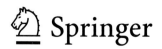 Springer

Afshin Gangi, MD, PhD
Professor of Radiology
Department of Radiology B
University Hospital of Strasbourg
Pavillon Clovis Vincent BP 426
67091 Strasbourg
France

Ali Guermazi, MD
Associate Professor of Radiology
Department of Radiology
Section Chief, Musculoskeletal
Boston University School of Medicine
820 Harrison Avenue, FGH Building, 3rd Floor
Boston, MA 02118
USA

Stéphane Guth, MD
Senior Radiologist
Department of Radiology B
University Hospital of Strasbourg
Pavillon Clovis Vincent BP 426
67091 Strasbourg
France

Medical Radiology · Diagnostic Imaging and Radiation Oncology
Series Editors:
A. L. Baert · L. W. Brady · H.-P. Heilmann · M. Knauth · M. Molls · C. Nieder · K. Sartor

Continuation of Handbuch der medizinischen Radiologie
Encyclopedia of Medical Radiology

ISBN 978-3-540-22097-8   eISBN 978-3-540-49929-9

DOI 10.107/978-3-540-49929-9

Medical Radiology · Diagnostic Imaging and Radiation Oncology ISSN 0942-5373

Library of Congress Control Number: 2006935018

© 2009, Springer-Verlag Berlin Heidelberg

Cover design and Layout: PublishingServices Teichmann, 69256 Mauer, Germany

Printed on acid-free paper

9 8 7 6 5 4 3 2 1 0

springer.com

Series Editor's Foreword

Image guided percutaneous musculoskeletal interventions are a rapidly developing and specialized area in the large field of interventional radiology. They require special skills, knowledge and insights from those performing these procedures.

This book offers a comprehensive overview of basic procedures, as well as highly specialised techniques in percutaneous musculoskeletal interventions, that have been developed over the past few years and have now matured and been incorporated in daily radiological practice. They apply both to percutaneous diagnostic techniques as well as to more therapeutic oriented interventions.

Dr. A. Gangi is internationally renowned for his pioneering role and extensive clinical experience in this area of interventional radiology. Together with his two co-editors, S. Guth and A. Guermazi, both also very experienced interventional musculoskeletal radiologists, and supported by a large group of internationally well-known experts, he has produced this remarkable volume, one of the first books available on these new techniques. The book is exquisitely illustrated with many high quality cases studies.

I am very much indebted to editors and authors for preparing this outstanding volume.

It is highly recommended to interventional as well as musculoskeletal and general radiologists as a guide and an update of their knowledge. However, it will also be of interest to orthopaedic surgeons and rheumatologists to assist them for a better therapeutic management of their patients.

I am convinced that this volume, which nicely complements the list of topics dealt with in our series, will meet with the appropriate interest and success among our readership.

Leuven   ALBERT L. BAERT

Foreword

Percutaneous musculoskeletal interventions have shown continual and substantial improvements over the past two decades. Interventional radiologists have lead the considerable effort in improving the execution of these interventions, and also in introducing new interventional techniques, i.e. kyphoplasty, cryoablation, radiofrequency ablation, and others like these, all for the benefit of patients. In this remarkable evolution, cross-sectional imaging has played an important role in better visualizing the anatomy, permitting a safer choice of paths, and allowing better overall performance of the interventions. Furthermore, these advances have been achieved with only rare complications.

As a radiologist and scientist who has spent his entire career investigating the diagnosis and management of musculoskeletal disorders, especially osteoporosis, I believe that percutaneous intervention aimed at osteoporotic vertebral fractures represents a major advance in this field. In the 1970s, there were no diagnostic tools for osteoporosis, and no treatments were available. Nowadays, several imaging and biomarker surrogates are available for early diagnosis of osteoporosis. Nevertheless, osteoporotic fractures represent a burden to society, with increased morbidity and mortality. Pain and disability are common features of osteoporotic vertebral fractures and contribute substantially to morbidity and consequent costs, borne by society. Percutaneous kyphoplasty and vertebroplasty represent major advances in medical care, consolidating and strengthening the affected vertebra and hence decreasing pain and disability. These two techniques are described comprehensively. All important aspects of the techniques are described, i.e. materials used, single and dual guidance, cement preparation and injection, as well as normal and abnormal results. Attention is also drawn to the occasional complications, how to prevent their occurrence and how to manage them if they do occur. Other chapters describe the basic procedures and different guidance techniques, ranging from biopsy and joint injection to management of pain and tumors. This volume is thoroughly researched and carefully written and illustrated. It abounds with excellent images. All chapters are written by international experts, most of whom I know as fellow members of the Interantional Skeletal Society.

Drs. Gangi, Guth, and Guermazi are widely recognized interventional radiologists, who impart a deep understanding of imaging and minimally-invasive treatment of serious and life-threatening disorders. These editors have undertaken the challenge of compiling a comprehensive reference textbook, describing percutaneous imaging in musculoskeletal interventions. To this end, they have enlisted the aid of an international group of acclaimed radiologists, making this book the most current and comprehensive available on the subject. This work will be of great interest to interventional radiologists, as well as to musculoskeletal and general radiologists.

San Francisco

HARRY K. GENANT
Professor Emeritus of Radiology, Medicine and Orthopaedic Surgery
University of California, San Francisco
President, International Skeletal Society, 2004–2006

Foreword

Upon reviewing this book I was reminded of the history of musculoskeletal radiology. It is a relatively young subspecialty, that started to thrive independently only in the mid 1980s. Most of my musculoskeletal colleagues who started their careers in the 1970s or earlier believe that the driving force behind the emergence of musculoskeletal radiology was the advent of MRI. In my opinion, another factor also propelled our subspecialty to the forefront. It was the proliferation of interventional musculoskeletal procedures. These procedures require additional training and expertise over and above what is typically available in residency training programs.

If we were to examine the current literature, we would find a plethora of articles and books dedicated to the imaging of musculoskeletal disorders. This is not the case with interventional procedures. If I were to perform a transoral needle biopsy of the C_2 vertebral body or perform a steroid injection of the facet joint of the occiput-C_1 or C_1-C_2 facet joint, I would fret since there is hardly any literature to guide me in performing such procedures.

I congratulate the editors for having the insight and determination to fill this glaring gap in our literature. The book is comprehensive; each procedure is thoroughly discussed and beautifully illustrated. Each chapter begins with an outline which serves as a guide to the contents of the chapter. This book will be a valuable addition to my reference shelf. I will definitely be using this book in my practice, and it will be a "must read" for my fellows.

My gratitude and admiration go to all the authors who contributed to the creation of such an outstanding book.

Iowa City

GEORGES Y. EL-KHOURY
Professor of Radiology and Orthopaedics
Director, Musculoskeletal Radiology Section
University of Iowa College of Medicine

Preface

Although there are already a few books on percutaneous musculoskeletal interventions on the market, that did not stop us from writing another. We took the task of clearly and succinctly describing all that is known on the topic as a challenge. Our goal was to render these complex interventions as simple procedures, easy to imagine and hopefully also easy to execute. Some chapters are written almost like recipes for beginners, so that novices will have a clear idea of the interventions described and can begin to use them immediately, to the benefit of their patients. We also introduce some new techniques and "tricks" that experienced readers will find useful.

To make the book as interesting and informative as possible, we chose the best internationally renowned authors. Without exception, they have provided chapters that are clear, concise and extremely informative.

Many people have helped us to bring this project to fruition; without their assistance, which we gratefully acknowledge, this book would never have been published. We would especially like to thank Professor Albert Baert, who supported our idea and made its realization possible. We would like to express our sincere and special thanks and recognition to Dr. Xavier Buy who, even though he came a little late to this project, has done fabulous work and brought unprecedented energy and enthusiasm to the team.

We are also grateful to the authors who have made working on this volume really enjoyable. We should apologize to them for the delay caused by the complexity of the subjects. We should not forget David Breazeale for his unconditional editorial assistance, Ursula Davis for her support and endless patience, and Christian Kauff for his excellent art work.

Finally, we would like to thank our wives for their patience and the weekends they spent alone while we were preparing and editing this volume. We would like to dedicate this volume to our dearest children for all the love they gave during the time we spent working on the book.

Strasbourg   Afshin gangi
Strasbourg   Stéphane guth
Boston   Ali Guermazi

"The best style is the clearest, the style that needs no explication and no notes, that conforms to the subject expressed, neither exceeding it nor falling short."

Abu 'Uthman 'Amr Ibn Bahr Al-Basri Al-Jahiz 776–868

"A physician should always try to convince his patient of improvement and hope in the effectiveness of treatment, for the psychological state of the patient has a great effect on his physical condition."

Abu Bakr Muhammad Ibn Zakariya Al-Razi (Rhazes) 864–930

"Things should be made as simple as possible, but not any simpler."

Albert Einstein 1879–1955

Contents

1 Procedure Basics and Technique Guidance
STÉPHANE GUTH, XAVIER BUY, ALI GUERMAZI, and AFSHIN GANGI 1

2 Percutaneous Biopsy of Soft Tissues and Muscular Lesions
JACQUELINE C. HODGE and KIMMO MATTILA 15

3 Percutaneous Bone Biopsy
GUILLAUME BIERRY, XAVIER BUY, STÉPHANE GUTH, ALI GUERMAZI,
and AFSHIN GANGI 37

4 Percutaneous Spinal Facet and Sacroiliac Joint Injection
GALINA LEVIN, JONATHAN S. LUCHS, and A. ORLANDO ORTIZ 73

5 Percutaneous Infiltration of the Craniovertebral Region
ALAIN CHEVROT, JEAN-LUC DRAPÉ, DIDIER GODEFROY, and ANTOINE FEYDY 83

6 Percutaneous Treatment of Intervertebral Disc Herniation
XAVIER BUY, AFSHIN GANGI, STÉPHANE GUTH, and ALI GUERMAZI 93

7 Provocative Discography
WILFRED C. G. PEH 119

8 Percutaneous Joint Injections
KATHLEEN C. FINZEL and RONALD S. ADLER 143

9 Percutaneous Treatment of Chronic Low Back Pain
XAVIER BUY, AFSHIN GANGI, and ALI GUERMAZI 157

10 Percutaneous Interventions in the Management of Soft Tissue Conditions
DAVID MALFAIR and PETER L. MUNK 179

11 Percutaneous Cementoplasty
AFSHIN GANGI, XAVIER BUY, FARAH IRANI, STÉPHANE GUTH, ALI GUERMAZI,
JEAN-PIERRE IMBERT, and JEAN-LOUIS DIETEMANN 197

12 Percutaneous Kyphoplasty in Vertebral Compression Fractures
LOTFI HACEIN-BEY and ALI GUERMAZI 259

13 Percutaneous Intraosseous Cyst Management
JOSÉE DUBOIS and LAURENT GAREL 283

14 Percutaneous Bone Tumors Management
AFSHIN GANGI and XAVIER BUY 301

15 Percutaneous Management of Painful Shoulder
Caroline Parlier-Cuau, Marc Wybier, Bassam Hamze,
and Jean-Denis Laredo 329

16 Closed Reduction and Percutaneous Fixation of Pelvic Fractures
Rolf Huegli, Thomas Gross, Augustinus L. Jacob, and Peter Messmer. 343

17 Interventional Vascular Radiology in Musculoskeletal Lesions
Paula Klurfan, Karel G. TerBrugge, Kongteng Tan,
and Martin E. Simons 367

18 Ultrasound-Guided Musculoskeletal Interventional Procedures
Philippe Peetrons and Michel Court-Payen. 385

Subject Index. 399

List of Contributors 411

Procedure Basics and Technique Guidance

1

Stéphane Guth, Xavier Buy, Ali Guermazi, and Afshin Gangi

CONTENTS

1.1 Introduction *1*

1.2 Prevention of Infection *1*

1.3 Pathogenesis *2*

1.4 Risk Prevention *2*
1.4.1 Patient Characteristics *2*
1.4.2 Operative Characteristics *2*
1.4.2.1 Preoperative Antiseptic Showering *2*
1.4.2.2 Preoperative Hair Removal *2*
1.4.2.3 Patient Skin Preparation in the
Operating Room *3*
1.4.2.4 Preoperative Hand/Forearm Antisepsis for
the Operating Team *3*
1.4.2.5 Antimicrobial Prophylaxis *5*
1.4.3 Intraoperative Issues *5*
1.4.3.1 Ventilation of the Operating Room *5*
1.4.3.2 Environmental Surfaces *6*
1.4.3.3 Sterilization of Instruments *6*
1.4.3.4 Surgical Clothing and Drapes *6*
1.4.4 Postoperative Issues *7*

1.5 Guidance Technique *7*
1.5.1 Imaging Techniques *7*
1.5.2 Puncture Techniques *9*
1.5.3 Guidance Technique *10*

1.6 Conclusion *13*

References *13*

S. Guth, MD, Senior Radiologist
X. Buy, MD, Senior Radiologist
A. Gangi, MD, PhD, Professor of Radiology
Department of Radiology B, University Hospital of Strasbourg, Pavillon Clovis Vincent BP 426, 67091 Strasbourg, France
A. Guermazi, MD, Associate Professor of Radiology
Department of Radiology, Section Chief, Musculoskeletal, Boston University School of Medicine, 88 East Newton Street, Boston, MA 02118, USA

Introduction

Musculoskeletal interventional radiology procedures, in common with all interventional procedures, require some basic knowledge: prevention of infections, guidance techniques and needle manipulation techniques.

Prevention of Infection

The Centers for Disease Control and Prevention (CDC) and National Nosocomial Infections Surveillance (NNIS) system monitor reported trends in nosocomial infections in United States acute care hospitals. According to NNIS system reports, intervention site infections (ISI) are the third most frequently reported nosocomial infection, accounting for 14–16% of all nosocomial infections among hospitalized patients (unpublished data) (Mangram et al. 1999). In 1980, Cruse and Foord estimated that an ISI increased a patient's hospital stay by approximately 10 days and cost an additional $2,000. A 1992 analysis showed that each ISI resulted in 7.3 additional postoperative hospital days, adding $3,152 in extra charges. Despite advances in infection control, ISIs remain a substantial cause of morbidity and mortality. Of course, all musculoskeletal procedures require strict adherence to standards of sterility. With bone procedures especially, a single mistake can lead to complications like osteitis or osteoarthritis. These are major complications of bone interventional procedures and they must absolutely be avoided. Strict adherence to the following asepsis rules is always mandatory.

1.3
Pathogenesis

Microbial contamination of the intervention site is the precursor of ISI. The risk of ISI can be summarized as (ALTEMEIER and CULBERTSON 1965; CRUSE 1992): Dose of bacterial contamination × virulence / resistance of the host patient = risk of ISI.

Quantitatively, it has been shown that if an intervention site is contaminated with >10^5 microorganisms per gram of tissue, the risk of ISI is markedly increased (KRIZEK and ROBSON 1975). However, the dose of contaminating microorganisms required to produce infection may be much lower when foreign material is present at the site (i.e. 100 staphylococci per gram of tissue introduced on silk sutures) (ELEK and CONEN 1957; JAMES and MacLEOD 1961).

For most ISIs, the source of pathogens is the endogenous flora of the patient's skin or mucous membranes. When mucous membranes or skin are incised, the exposed tissues are at risk for contamination.

Exogenous sources of ISI pathogens include surgical personnel, especially members of the operating team (CALIA et al. 1969; LETTS and DOERMER 1983), the operating room environment (including air), as well as all tools, instruments and materials brought to the sterile field during the procedure.

Endogenous and exogenous flora pathogens responsible for infections in interventional bone procedure are the same as in orthopedic surgery:
● Staphylococcus aureus
● Coagulase-negative Staphylococci
● Gram-negative bacilli

1.4
Risk Prevention

1.4.1
Patient Characteristics

Patient characteristics associated with an increased risk of an ISI include:
● Coincident remote site infections or colonization (BRUUN 1970; EDWARDS 1976; VALENTINE et al. 1986; PERL and GOLUB 1998; MANGRAM et al. 1999)
● Diabetes (GIL-EGEA et al. 1987; MANGRAM et al. 1999)

● Cigarette smoking (MANGRAM et al. 1999)
● Systemic steroid use (GIL-EGEA et al. 1987; MANGRAM et al. 1999)
● Obesity (>20% ideal body weight) (MANGRAM et al. 1999)
● Extremes of age (CRUSE and FOORD 1973; DOIG and WILKINSON 1976; SHARMA and SHARMA 1986; MISHRIKI et al. 1990; MANGRAM et al. 1999)
● Poor nutritional status (CRUSE and FOORD 1973; MANGRAM et al. 1999)
● Perioperative transfusion of certain blood products (VAMVAKAS and CARVEN 1998; MANGRAM et al. 1999)
● Preoperative nares colonization with *Staphylococcus aureus*
● Altered immune response
● Length of preoperative stay

The following recommendations are important in preventing ISIs:
● All infections remote from the surgical site must be identified before intervention
● The intervention must be postponed on patients with remote site infections until the infection has resolved
● Blood serum glucose levels must be controlled in all diabetic patients and perioperative hyperglycemia particularly must be avoided

1.4.2
Operative Characteristics

1.4.2.1
Preoperative Antiseptic Showering

A preoperative antiseptic shower or bath decreases skin microbial colony counts. In a study of 700 patients, chlorhexidine reduced bacterial colony counts nine-fold, while povidone-iodine or triclocarban-medicated soap reduced colony counts by 1.3- and 1.9-fold, respectively (GARIBALDI 1988). Patients should be required to shower or bathe with an antiseptic agent at least the night before the operative day (MANGRAM et al. 1999).

1.4.2.2
Preoperative Hair Removal

Preoperative shaving of the surgical site the night before an operation is associated with a significantly higher ISI risk than either the use of depilatory agents or no hair removal (SEROPIAN and REYNOLDS 1971; HAMILTON et al. 1977; CRUSE and FOORD 1980; ALEXANDER et al. 1983; OLSON et al. 1986; MISHRIKI et al. 1990; MANGRAM et al. 1999). The increased ISI risk associated with shaving has been attributed to microscopic cuts in the skin that later serve as foci for bacterial multiplication. Shaving immediately before the operation compared to shaving within 24 h preoperatively was associated with a lower ISI risk (3.1% vs 7.1%); if shaving was performed more than 24 h prior to operation, the ISI rate exceeded 20% (SEROPIAN and REYNOLDS 1971).

1.4.2.3
Patient Skin Preparation in the Operating Room

Skin preparation is a three phase process:
1. Skin should be assessed before preparation, and the presence of moles, warts, rashes, or other skin conditions at the surgical site should be noted. The skin around the surgical site should be free of soil and debris. Removal of superficial soil, debris and transient microbes before applying the antiseptic agent(s) reduces the risk of wound contamination by decreasing the organic debris on the skin. Therefore, the skin at and around the incision site should be thoroughly washed and cleaned to remove gross contamination before performing antiseptic skin preparation (MANGRAM et al. 1999). This can be done by washing the surgical site immediately before applying the antiseptic agent in the operating room. This skin washing is best done with an antiseptic scrub.
2. After washing, the scrub is removed by applying sterile water or sterile saline. Sterile towels should be used for drying the skin (ASSOCIATION of OPERATING ROOM NURSES 2002; ASSOCIATION of periOPERATIVE REGISTERED NURSES RECOMMENDED PRACTICES COMMITTEE 2004).
3. The patient's skin is prepared by applying an antiseptic in concentric circles, beginning in the area of the proposed incision. The prepared area should be large enough to extend or modify the incision site. Antiseptic agents used for skin preparation should be applied using sterile supplies. Infection can occur due to a high microbial count at the incision site; therefore, skin preparation should progress from the incision site to the periphery using a sponge/applicator, which should be discarded after the periphery has been reached (MANGRAM et al. 1999; ASSOCIATION OF

OPERATING ROOM NURSES 2002; ASSOCIATION OF periOPERATIVE REGISTERED NURSES RECOMMENDED PRACTICES COMMITTEE 2004).

Friction during the cleansing process and application of antimicrobial agents are the primary methods for removing soil and transient organisms. Several antiseptic agents are available for preoperative preparation of skin at the incision site. The iodophors (povidone-iodine), alcohol-containing products, and chlorhexidine gluconate are the most commonly used agents. No studies have adequately assessed the comparative effects of these preoperative skin antiseptics on ISI risk under well-controlled, operation-specific conditions.

Data from current research, manufacturers' literature, and recommendations from the Association for Professionals in Infection Control and Epidemiology, the CDC and the U.S. Food and Drug Administration should be consulted when selecting an antiseptic agent for skin preparation.

Products for skin antisepsis should be chosen carefully according to the patient's condition. Antiseptic agents used on the skin of patients with known hypersensitivity reactions may cause adverse outcomes (rashes).

1.4.2.4
Preoperative Hand/Forearm Antisepsis for the Operating Team

Operating team personnel with draining skin lesions must be excluded from duty until infection has been ruled out or they have received adequate therapy and the infection has resolved. Finger nails of the operating team personnel should be kept short and artificial nails, hand or arm jewelry should be prohibited (MANGRAM et al. 1999).

Members of the team who have direct contact with the sterile operating field or sterile instruments or supplies used in the field wash their hands and forearms by performing a traditional procedure known as scrubbing (the surgical scrub) immediately before donning sterile gowns and gloves. Preoperative surgical scrubs should be performed for at least 2–5 min using an appropriate antiseptic (Table 1.1). Scrub the hands and forearms up to the elbows (MANGRAM et al. 1999).The first scrub of the day should include a thorough cleaning under fingernails, usually with a brush (COMMITTEE ON CONTROL OF SURGICAL INFECTIONS OF THE COMMITTEE ON PRE AND POSTOPERATIVE CARE 1984; LARSON

1995; Association of Operating Room Nurses 2002; Association of periOperative Registered Nurses Recommended Practices Committee 2004). Antiseptic agents for surgical scrubbing commercially available in the United States for this purpose contain alcohol, chlorhexidine, iodine/iodophors, para-chloro-meta-xylenol (PCMX), or triclosan (Table 1.1) (Larson 1988, 1995; Mayhall 1993; Hardin and Nichols 1997).

Alcohol is considered the gold standard for surgical hand preparation in several European countries (Lowbury et al. 1974; Lilly et al. 1979). Alcoholic compounds used as hand rub kill 3.2–5.8 $\log_{10}$ cfu, compared to 1.8–2.8 $\log_{10}$ cfu in 30 s removed with medicated soap (Ayliffe et al. 1978; Rotter 1999; Widmer 2000). The "European Norm 1500" describes the standard by which a hand disinfectant must demonstrate efficacy before it can be marketed in Europe (Borneff et al. 1981). The compound should be as effective as propan-2-ol 60 vol.%, the reference alcohol. Alcohol-containing products are used less frequently in the United States than in Europe, and the procedure for hand/forearm antisepsis is different in Europe. The use of a hand rub for routine hand hygiene is microbiologically more effective in vitro and in vivo, it saves time, and preliminary data demonstrate better compliance than with hand washing. Hand rubs are also highly effective against mycobacteria, the bacteria most resistant to any disinfection process (Widmer et al. 1999). Multiple in vitro studies and in vivo experiments indicate significantly better killing with hand disinfectants than with hand washing (Wewalka et al. 1977). These conclusions have been validated in a randomized crossover clinical trial of preoperative hand scrubs (Ayliffe et al. 1978). Therefore, in most European countries, use of a hand rub is the standard for hand hygiene. A two phase procedure is recommended for optimal antisepsis:

- First the hand/forearm are scrubbed with a conventional scrub for at least 2 min The first scrub of the day should include a thorough cleaning under fingernails, usually with a brush. Towels can be used for drying the skin.
- Then the hands are rubbed with a waterless alcohol-based compound (Rotter 1984) (e.g., ethanol, *n*-propanol, or isopropanol). This type of hand hygiene is fundamentally different from the washing procedures. Approximately 3 mL of the alcoholic compound is taken from a dispenser onto dry hands and rubbed in for 30 s to 2 min or until the alcohol evaporates (Fig. 1.1).

After performing the surgical scrub, hands should be kept up and away from the body (elbows in flexed position) so that water runs from the tips of the fingers toward the elbows. Sterile towels should be used for drying the hands and forearms before donning a sterile gown and gloves (Association of Operating Room Nurses 2002; Association of periOperative Registered Nurses Recommended Practices Committee 2004).

Table 1.1. Mechanism and spectrum of activity of antiseptic agents commonly used for preoperative skin preparation and surgical scrubs. (From Larson 1988; Mangram et al. 1999)

Agent	Mechanism of Action	Gram+ bacteria	Gram− bacteria	Mtb	Fungi	Virus	Rapidity of action	Residual activity	Toxicity	Uses
Alcohol	Denature proteins	E	E	G	G	G	Most rapid	None	Drying, volatile	SP, SS
Chlorhexidine	Disrupt cell membrane	E	G	P	F	G	Intermediate	E	Ototoxicity, keratitis	SP, SS
Iodine/iodophors	Oxidation/substitution by free iodine	E	G	G	G	G	Intermediate	Minimal	Absorption from skin with possible toxicity, skin irritation	SP, SS
PCMX	Disrupt cell wall	G	F	F	F	F	Intermediate	G	More data needed	SS
triclosan	Disrupt cell wall	G	G	G	P	U	Intermediate	E	More data needed	SS

E=excellent, F=fair, G=good, P=poor, Mtb=*Mycobacterium tuberculosis*, PCMX=para-chloro-meta-xylenol, SP=skin preparation, SS=surgical scrubs, U=unknown

Fig. 1.1. The standard hands rub procedure. Pour appropriate volume of hand rub product into the cupped dry hands and rub hands for 30 s in accordance with the standard hand rub illustrated above to ensure total coverage of the hands. Each step is repeated five times before proceeding to the next step. After concluding step *F*, recommence the series of steps as appropriate to complete the washing time of 5 min. Step *A*: Palm to palm. Step *B*: Right palm over left dorsum and left palm over right dorsum. Step *C*: Palm to palm with fingers interlaced. Step *D*: Backs of fingers to opposing palms with fingers interlocked. Step *E*: Rotational rubbing of right thumb clasped in left palm and vice versa. Step *F*: Rotational rubbing, backwards and forwards with clasped fingers of right hand in left palm and vice versa

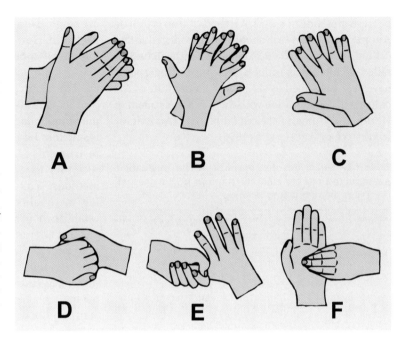

1.4.2.5
Antimicrobial Prophylaxis

Surgical antimicrobial prophylaxis (AMP) refers to a brief course of an antimicrobial agent initiated just before an operation begins. Its aim is to reduce the microbial burden of intraoperative contamination to a level that cannot overwhelm host defenses. Intravenous infusion is the mode of AMP delivery used most often in practice (DiPiro et al. 1986; Page et al. 1993; Nooyen et al. 1994).

The infusion of the initial dose of antimicrobial agent has to be timed so that a bactericidal concentration of the drug is established in serum and tissues by the time the skin is incised (Classen et al. 1992). The therapeutic levels of the antimicrobial agent in both serum and tissues must be maintained throughout the operation and until, at most, a few hours after the procedure (Nichols 1989, 1995; Mayhall 1993; Trilla and Mensa 1993; McDonald et al. 1998).

Cephalosporins are the most thoroughly studied AMP agents. These drugs are effective against many Gram-positive and Gram-negative microorganisms. They also share the features of demonstrated safety, acceptable pharmacokinetics, and a reasonable cost per dose. Cefazolin provides adequate coverage for musculoskeletal procedures (Nichols 1989).

1.4.3
Intraoperative Issues

1.4.3.1
Ventilation of the Operating Room

Intervention room air may contain microbe-laden dust. The microbial level in operating room air is directly proportional to the number of people moving about in the room (Ayliffe 1991).Efforts should be made to minimize personnel traffic during operations. The number of personnel entering the operating room must be limited to necessary personnel. Operating room doors should be kept closed except as needed for passage of equipment, personnel, and the patient.

Intervention rooms should be maintained at positive pressure with respect to corridors and adjacent areas (Lidwell 1986). Positive pressure prevents airflow from less clean areas into more clean areas.

All ventilation or air conditioning systems in hospitals, including those in operating or intervention rooms, should have two filter beds in series, with the efficiency of the first filter bed being >30% and that of the second being >90% (American Institute of Architects 1996).Conventional operating room ventilation systems produce a minimum of about 15 air changes of filtered air per hour, 3 (20%) of which must be fresh air (NICHOLS 1992; AMERICAN INSTITUTE OF ARCHITECTS 1996). Air should be introduced at the ceiling and extracted via exhausts near the floor. Detailed ventilation parameters for operating rooms have been published by the American Institute of Architects in collaboration with the U.S. Department of Health and Human Services (Table 1.2) (AMERICAN INSTITUTE OF ARCHITECTS 1996).

Table 1.2. Parameters for operating room ventilation, American Institute of Architects (NICHOLS 1992; AMERICAN INSTITUTE OF ARCHITECTS 1996)

Temperature	20–24 °C, depending on normal ambient temperatures
Relative humidity	30–60%
Air movement	From "clean to less clean" areas
Air changes	Minimum 15 total air changes per hour. Minimum 3 air changes of outdoor air per hour

1.4.3.2
Environmental Surfaces

It is important to perform routine cleaning of environmental surfaces in the intervention room (e.g., CT table, tables, floors, walls, ceilings, lights) to reestablish a clean environment after each procedure (COMMITTEE ON CONTROL OF SURGICAL INFECTIONS OF THE COMMITTEE ON PRE AND POSTOPERATIVE CARE 1984; NICHOLS 1992). When visible soiling or contamination with blood or other body fluids of surfaces or equipment occurs during an operation or even in routine cleaning, an Environmental Protection Agency (EPA)-approved hospital disinfectant should be used to decontaminate the affected areas before the next operation.

Wet-vacuuming of the floor with an EPA-approved hospital disinfectant should be performed routinely after the last operation of the day or night (COMMITTEE ON CONTROL OF SURGICAL INFECTIONS OF THE COMMITTEE ON PRE AND POSTOPERATIVE CARE 1984; NICHOLS 1992).

Very septic interventions like drainages of abscesses should be done last.

1.4.3.3
Sterilization of Instruments

Most of the instruments (needles, drills) used for interventional procedures in interventional radiology

are single use and already sterilized and adequately packaged. However some multiple use materials like hammers, spoons, pressure guns, special needles and drills must be sterilized and adequately packaged for surgical use.

Adequate sterilization of surgical instruments is mandatory; lack of adherence to sterilization has resulted in ISI outbreaks (SOTO et al. 1991). Surgical instruments can be sterilized by steam under pressure, dry heat, ethylene oxide, or other approved methods. The importance of routinely monitoring the quality of sterilization procedures is well established (COMMITTEE ON CONTROL OF SURGICAL INFECTIONS OF THE COMMITTEE ON PRE AND POSTOPERATIVE CARE 1984; GARNER 1986; AMERICAN INSTITUTE OF ARCHITECTS 1996; ASSOCIATION OF OPERATING ROOM NURSES 2002; ASSOCIATION OF periOPERATIVE REGISTERED NURSES RECOMMENDED PRACTICES COMMITTEE 2004). Detailed recommendations for sterilization of surgical instruments have been published (FAVERO and BOND 1991; ASSOCIATION OF OPERATING ROOM NURSES 2002; MANGRAM et al. 1999; ASSOCIATION OF periOPERATIVE REGISTERED NURSES RECOMMENDED PRACTICES COMMITTEE 2004). All surgical instruments must be sterilized according to published guidelines (FAVERO and BOND 1991; AMERICAN INSTITUTE OF ARCHITECTS 1996).

Flash sterilization should be used only as an exceptional procedure for patient care items that will be used immediately (for example to reprocess an accidentally dropped instrument). Flash sterilization is not recommended as a routine sterilization method (MANGRAM et al. 1999).

1.4.3.4
Surgical Clothing and Drapes

Surgical clothing consists of scrub suits, caps/hoods, shoe covers, masks, gloves, and gowns. The use of these barriers is prudent to minimize a patient's exposure to the skin, mucous membranes or hair of surgical team members, as well as to protect the surgical team from contamination.

Surgical team members usually wear a uniform called a "scrub suit" that consists of pants and a shirt. The Association of Operating Room Nurses recommends that scrub suits be changed after they become soiled and that they be laundered only in an approved and monitored laundry facility.

All personnel in the intervention room must wear a surgical mask that fully covers the mouth and nose when entering the operating room if an operation is about to begin or already under way, or if sterile instruments are exposed. This mask must be worn throughout the operation.

All personnel in the intervention room must wear a cap or hood to cover fully hair on the head and face when entering the intervention room.

All members of the operating team must wear sterile gloves. Sterile gloves are put on after surgical scrubbing and donning sterile gowns. Wearing two pairs of gloves (double-gloving) has been shown to reduce hand contact with patients' blood and body fluids when compared to wearing only a single pair (SHORT and BELL 1993; TOKARS et al. 1995; MANGRAM et al. 1999).

Drapes are carefully placed all over the patient respecting aseptic principles and delineating the intervention field. This operating field must be as small as possible. The skin of that operating field is previously prepared as explained above. Gowns and drapes can be disposable (single use) or reusable (multiple use) but they should be impermeable to liquids (MANGRAM et al. 1999).

1.4.4
Postoperative Issues

At the end of the interventional radiology procedure the incision or needle entry point on the skin must be covered with a sterile dressing for 48 h (MANGRAM et al. 1999). During this time if an incision dressing has to be changed, a sterile technique, i.e. with sterile gloves and equipment, must be used.

In current practice, many patients are discharged soon after the procedure (immediately or the next day usually), before incisions have fully healed. The patient and family must be educated before discharge regarding proper incision care, symptoms of ISI, the need to report such symptoms, and whom to contact to report any problems. It must be made clear to the patient that baths and swimming pools are prohibited until incisions have fully healed.

Two studies have shown that most ISIs become evident within 21 days after the procedure (WEIGELT et al. 1992; SANDS et al. 1996), which is why post-discharge surveillance is so important. Surveillance can be done either by direct examination of the patients' wounds during follow-up visits or by mail or telephone.

1.5
Guidance Technique

1.5.1
Imaging Techniques

The guidance technique used for percutaneous interventions should provide both precision and safety. It has to be minimally invasive, while delivering the minimum possible dosage of radiation to the operator and patient. The choice of technique depends on the patient and the nature of the intervention.

Ultrasound is an excellent guidance technique especially for superficial interventions on soft tissues or in the pediatric population. It has the advantages of multi-planar as well as real time imaging, but it is operator-dependent and ineffective with bone and air-filled structures.

Fluoroscopy can provide real time information for guidance on bone procedures. It is less precise than CT fluoroscopy but delivers less radiation and allows a three-dimensional view, which is important in procedures like vertebroplasty. Bi-plane fluoroscopic equipment allows multiplanar, real time visualization, and rapid alternation between imaging planes is possible without complex equipment movement or projection realignment. Vertebroplasty and nucleotomy can be done with fluoroscopy alone.

CT can provide very precise control in bone as well as in soft tissues (Fig. 1.2). Conventional CT guidance does not provide real time surveillance but this can be achieved by a dual guidance technique

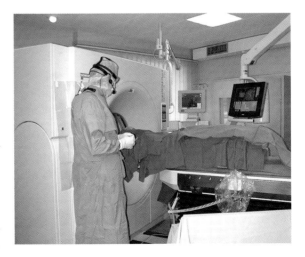

Fig. 1.2. The CT interventional room during an interventional procedure

combining CT and a C-arm or bi-plane fluoroscopy device, or with CT fluoroscopy.

The dual guidance technique (Fig. 1.3) using CT and C-arm fluoroscopy is particularly relevant for percutaneous cementoplasty. A mobile C-arm is used, positioned in front of the CT gantry. By using a rotating fluoroscope and CT, the structure to be punctured can be visualized three-dimensionally and with exact differentiation of anatomic structures, which in many cases is not possible with fluoroscopy alone. Two mobile monitors are placed in front of the physician, displaying the last stored image and the fluoroscopic image. The operator can switch from CT to fluoroscopy and vice versa at any time. In percutaneous vertebroplasty, the intervention begins with CT and is followed by fluoroscopy. The needle is placed precisely and safely under CT guidance. The injection of cement in vertebroplasty requires real time imaging and is therefore performed under fluoroscopic control. Dual guidance is the safest guidance method for vertebroplasty, periradicular infiltrations, bone biopsy, nucleoplasty, tumor management and treatment of osteoid osteomas.

CT fluoroscopy can provide real time imaging but only in a thin plane that is defined by collimation (usually 1–10 mm). Unlike fluoroscopy, CT fluoroscopy can not provide adequate three-dimensional real time surveillance of cement distribution in a 4 cm high vertebra during cement injection. Moreover the radiation dosage of CT fluoroscopy is very high compared to conventional fluoroscopy when time is taken into account. Therefore we recommend the use of the dual guidance technique for vertebroplasty and other bone interventions. CT fluoroscopy

can however be used in a few difficult cases. Using the dual technique the operator can switch from fluoroscopy to CT fluoroscopy if necessary. The use of a needle holder has been described to reduce the radiation dose provided to the operator's hand during CT fluoroscopy but such devices also reduce the operator's tactile sensation (IRIE et al. 2001).

MR guidance may be the future of interventional guidance techniques (Fig. 1.4). MR imaging is devoid of ionizing radiation and allows successful needle placement for musculoskeletal use in clinical practice. MR guidance can deliver a very precise three-dimensional real time image. T1-weighted or even fast or turbo spin echo T2-weighted MR imaging sequences with asymmetric low matrix resolutions are used for guidance. This requires MR imaging-compatible needles (needles using non-ferromagnetic materials like titanium, carbon). The main problem however lies in both the high costs and limited availability of adapted interventional MR equipment (open MR magnets) and interventional material (non-ferromagnetic biopsy devices). Moreover, MR guided procedures are time consuming. However, MR guidance and ultrasound are the only possible methods for performing a biopsy during pregnancy. Closed MR units can be used as well. In addition, MR imaging-guided interventional procedures have the potential to allow temperature monitoring, which introduces new opportunities for treatment such as thermal ablation procedures. With improvements in interventional MR systems, MR imaging may become the modality of choice for guidance of certain musculoskeletal interventional procedures (Fig. 1.5).

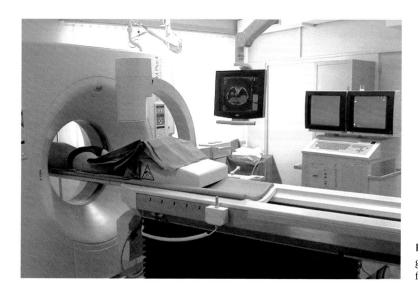

Fig. 1.3. Dual CT and fluoroscopy guidance. The C-arm is positioned in front of the CT-gantry

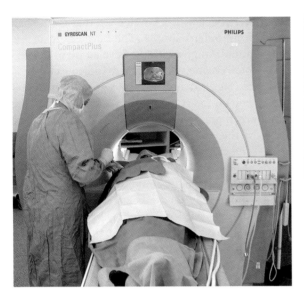

Fig. 1.4. The MR imaging room during an interventional procedure

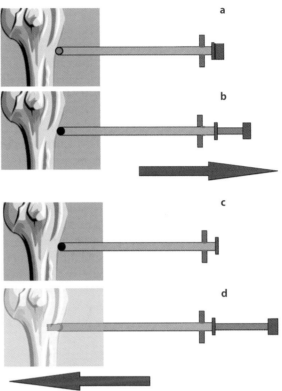

Fig. 1.6a–d. Drawings showing the coaxial technique. **a** The needle tip is in the designated place. **b,c** The stylet is removed. **d** The larger outer cannula is used to introduce another smaller needle, for example a drill

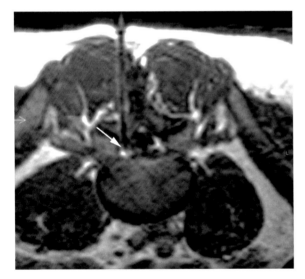

Fig. 1.5. Periradicular steroid injection under MR imaging control in a 32-year-old woman. Axial T1-weighted MR image with patient in prone position shows the needle placed in the right periradicular region (*arrow*) during steroid injection

1.5.2
Puncture Techniques

Two puncture techniques are used to produce a puncture pathway in our procedures: the coaxial technique (Fig. 1.6) and the tandem technique (Fig. 1.7). These techniques allow safe and precise pathway guidance.

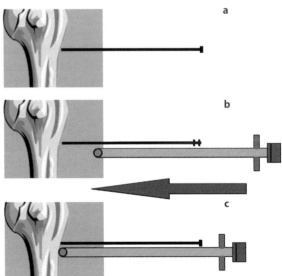

Fig. 1.7a–c. Drawings showing the tandem technique. **a** A small 22-gauge needle is placed first for local anesthesia. **b,c** Once in the correct site the needle tip is used under fluoroscopy to guide another needle

The needles used in the coaxial technique usually have two components: an outer cannula through which a smaller needle is inserted in a coaxial fashion and an inner stylet that seals the cannula. The stylet of these needles should always remain entirely within the cannula when the needle is taken forward; failure to do so can damage the needle especially when approaching dense bone structures. The stylet can be removed when the needle tip is in the designated place; it should not be moved any further forward. The principle of the coaxial technique is then to use the large outer cannula to introduce smaller needles for biopsy or other procedures. The coaxial technique provides excellent control of the needle's path and limits damage to soft tissues.

The tandem technique is used under fluoroscopic guidance. A small 22-gauge needle is placed first for local anesthesia. The pathway and correct position of the needle is checked on fluoroscopy and CT. Once in the right place, the needle tip is used under fluoroscopy to guide another needle. This second needle is placed under fluoroscopic guidance in contact and parallel to the first fine needle. The tandem technique allows quick and safe placement of the second needle under fluoroscopy guidance alone.

1.5.3
Guidance Technique

One of the keys to success for interventional procedures is proper needle placement. It is imperative to know which pathway to use and how to modify the course of the needle to reach the desired location. The aim of needle manipulation techniques is to permit needle course correction during bone puncture. There are three ways to change the course of the needle (GANGI and DIETEMANN 1994; FENTON and CZERVIONKE 2003): at the entry point, after cortical perforation, and with a modified needle.

At the entry point, with a stiff needle, the pathway can be corrected only by directly changing the angulation (Fig. 1.8). However, this is difficult after deep penetration. Therefore the needle direction should only be adjusted by changing the angulation before deep bone penetration.

After cortical perforation, and once deep inside the bone, it is usually not possible to change the path of the needle directly. We prefer beveled needles for this reason. Bone vertebroplasty needles (Fig. 1.9) (Cemento-RE, OptiMed, Ettlingen, Germany), for example, normally have two components: a remov-

able inner stylet with a beveled tip that is inserted through an outer cannula. The beveled tip of the outer cannula aligns with the beveled tip of the stylet. A notch on one side of the hub indicates the beveled face (Fig. 1.5) and corresponds to a tiny metal protrusion on the stylet. When the cannula and the stylet are aligned they can be locked together. The stylet of the needle should always remain locked within the cannula when the needle is moved forward; otherwise the needle can be damaged as it is advanced, especially in dense bone. Once in the bone, the needle bevel can be used to adjust slightly the direction of the needle. Because the beveled needle tip is an asymmetrical wedge, the course of the needle will be deflected away from the beveled face. For example, if the bevel face and notch are cephalad the needle will be forced caudally. Careful use of this technique allows optimal placement of the vertebroplasty needle (Fig. 1.10), even when the needle is deep inside the vertebral body. Even cement distribution in the vertebral body can be modified by rotating the bevel face during injection. We recommend the use of bevelled needles for vertebroplasty procedures specifically for this reason. This technique does not work with diamond tip needles.

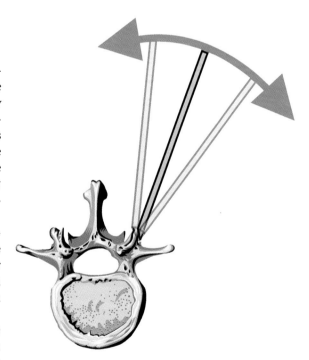

Fig. 1.8. Drawing showing needle positioning before penetration of the cortical bone. Once the sharp tip of the needle is inserted in the periosteum, the needle direction can be modified by changing the angulation at the entry point

Fig. 1.9. Percutaneous cementoplasty needle. Cemento-RE, 10-gauge needle, has convenient metal wings for easy insertion/ removal and rotation of the needle, and a special beveled edge (*arrow* 2). Notch indicating the bevel face (*arrows* 3, 6 and 7). Metal protrusion to fix the stylet (*arrow* 4) on the hub (*arrow* 5). The outer cannula (*arrow* 1). The bevel face (*arrow* 8)

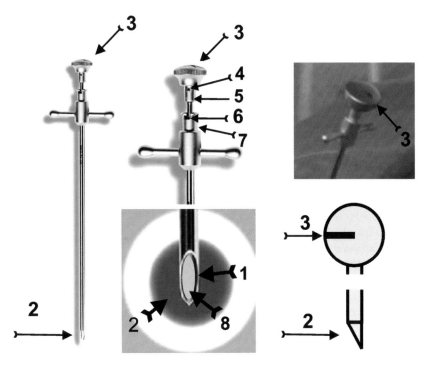

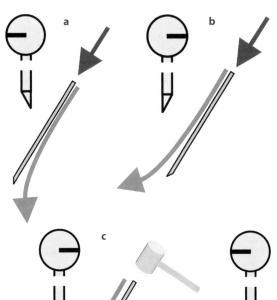

Fig. 1.10a–e. Drawings showing the different stages of a transpedicular puncture during vertebroplasty. The use of a beveled needle is described. **a** The hub notch in medial position and bevel tip in medial position leading the course of the needle to the side (*blue arrow*). **b** The hub notch in side position, bevel tip in lateral position leading the course of the needle medially (*blue arrow*). **c** The hub notch in side position, bevel face in lateral position leading the course of the needle medially (*blue arrow*). The needle is in contact with the spinal canal, and should be corrected. **d** Changing the bevel face direction by turning the connector 180°. The hub notch in medial position, bevel face in medial position leading the course of the needle to the side (*blue arrow*). **e** Hammering, needle course correction

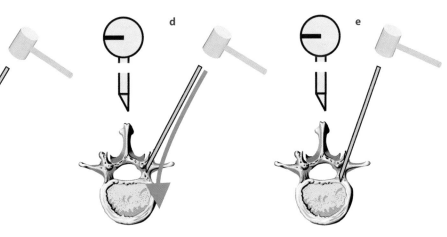

The third way to modify the needle course is to modify the needle. Stiff needles can be bent manually. Placing a 10–20° curve in such a needle 2–3 cm below the tip will allow a curved pathway. However, curved needles are difficult to control and require some experience. Further, it is difficult to traverse a straight line through a large amount of tissue without rotating the needle tip, which can cause tissue damage or hematoma. Curved needles are, therefore, not generally advisable in routine practice. Still, they can be useful when a straight pathway is not possible. For example, disc puncture at the L5-S1 level is obstructed by the iliac bone and a straight pathway is impossible. A straight outer cannula with a bent central stylet enables both straight and curved pathways; this technique is used in nucleotomy procedures (Figs. 1.11 and 1.12). Bent needles can only be used in soft tissues, not in bone.

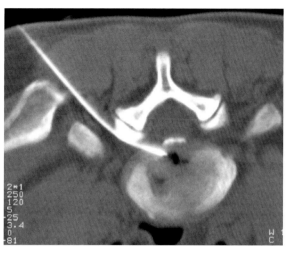

Fig. 1.12. Disc puncture at L5-S1 level. Nucleotomy in a 29-year-old man with disk herniation. Axial CT scan with patient in prone position shows a disc puncture at L5-S1 level with a bent needle. A straight pathway is not possible

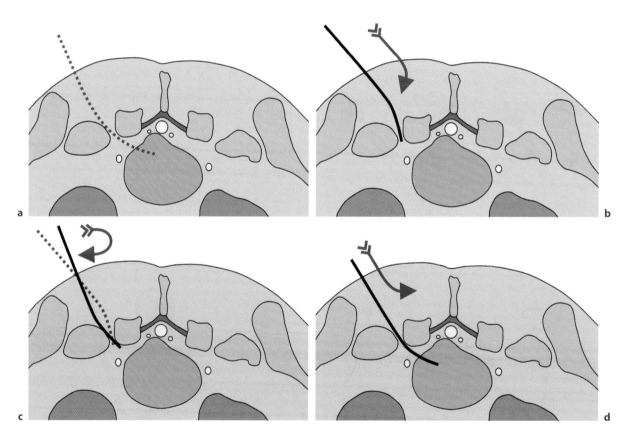

Fig. 1.11a–d. Drawings showing the different stages of needle insertion for a percutaneous nucleotomy at L5-S1 level. **a** Disc puncture at L5-S1 level; the iliac bone does not permit a direct straight pathway and only a curved pathway is possible. **b** Disc puncture at L5-S1 level with a bent needle, the needle tip systematically goes in the opposite direction. **c** Disc puncture at L5-S1 level with a bent needle, rotating the needle tip to achieve the curve pathway. **d** Disc puncture at L5-S1 level with a bent needle, curved pathway, needle in right end position inside the posterior nucleus

1.6
Conclusion

Minimally invasive procedures are, slowly but surely, replacing open surgery. It is now possible to perform many invasive musculoskeletal procedures without open surgery. To perform these procedures successfully, a clear understanding of the techniques for imaging and needle guidance is essential. Constant and strict adherence to the rules of asepsis for bone interventional procedures is very important, as the consequences of infection in the bones can be severe. Septic complications must absolutely be avoided.

References

Alexander JW, Fischer JE, Boyajian M, Palmquist J, Morris MJ (1983) The influence of hair-removal methods on wound infections. Arch Surg 118:347–352

Altemeier WA, Culbertson WR (1965) Surgical infection. In: Moyer CA, Rhoads J, Allen JG, Harkins HN (eds) Surgery, principles and practice. Lippincott Philadelphia, pp 51–77

American Institute of Architects (1996) Guidelines for design and construction of hospital and health care facilities. American Institute of Architects Press, Washington, DC

Association of Operating Room Nurses (2002) Recommended practices for skin preparation of patients. AORN J 75:184–187

Association of periOperative Registered Nurses Recommended Practices Committee (2004) Recommended practices for surgical hand antisepsis/hand scrubs. AORN J 79:416–418, 421–426, 429–431

Ayliffe GA (1991) Role of the environment of the operating suite in surgical wound infection. Rev Infect Dis 13:800–804

Ayliffe GA, Babb JR, Quoraishi AH (1978) A test for hygienic hand disinfection. J Clin Pathol 31:923–928

Borneff J, Eggers HJ, Grun L, Gundermann KO, Kuwert E, Lammers T, Primavesi CA, Rotter M, Schmidt-Lorenz W, Schubert R, Sonntag HG, Spicher G, Teuber M, Thofern E, Weinhold E, Werner HP (1981) Directives for the testing and evaluation of chemical disinfection methods – 1st part (1.1.1981). I. In vitro tests. II. Tests under medical practice conditions. 1. Hygienic hand disinfection. 2. Surgical hand disinfection. Zentralbl Bakteriol Mikrobiol Hyg [B] 172:534–562

Bruun JN (1970) Post-operative wound infection. Predisposing factors and the effect of a reduction in the dissemination of staphylococci. Acta Med Scand Suppl 514:3–89

Calia FM, Wolinsky EM, Abrams JS, Rammelkamp CJ (1969) Importance of the carrier state as a source of Staphylococcus aureus in wound sepsis. J Hyg (Lond) 67:49–57

Classen DC, Evans RS, Pestotnik SL, Horn SD, Menlove RL, Burke JP (1992) The timing of prophylactic administration of antibiotics and the risk of surgical-wound infection. N Engl J Med 326:281–286

Committee on Control of Surgical Infections of the Committee on Pre and Postoperative Care ACoS (1984) Manual on control of infection in surgical patients. Lippincott, Philadelphia

Cruse PJ (1992) Surgical wound infection. In: Wonsiewicz MJ (ed) Infectious diseases. Saunders, Philadelphia, pp 758–764

Cruse PJ, Foord R (1973) A five-year prospective study of 23,649 surgical wounds. Arch Surg 107:206–210

Cruse PJ, Foord R (1980) The epidemiology of wound infection. A 10-year prospective study of 62,939 wounds. Surg Clin North Am 60:27–40

DiPiro JT, Cheung RP, Bowden TA, Mansberger JA (1986) Single dose systemic antibiotic prophylaxis of surgical wound infections. Am J Surg 152:552–559

Doig CM, Wilkinson AW (1976) Wound infection in a children's hospital. Br J Surg 63:647–650

Edwards LD (1976) The epidemiology of 2056 remote site infections and 1966 surgical wound infections occurring in 1865 patients: a four year study of 40,923 operations at Rush-Presbyterian-St. Luke's Hospital, Chicago. Ann Surg 184:758–766

Elek SD, Conen PE (1957) The virulence of Staphylococcus pyogenes for man: a study of problems with wound infection. Br J Exp Pathol 38:573–586

Favero MS, Bond W (1991) Sterilization, disinfection, and antisepsis in the hospital. In: Balows A HWJ, Herrmann KL, Isenberg HD, Shadomy HJ (eds) Manual of clinical microbiology. American Society of Microbiology, Washington, DC, pp 183–200

Fenton DS, Czervionke LF (2003) Basic needle manipulation techniques. In: Fenton DS, Czervionke LF (eds) Image-guided spine intervention. Saunders, Philadelphia, pp 1–7

Gangi A, Dietemann JL (1994) Techniques de guidage. In: Gangi A, Dietmann JL (eds) Tomodensitometrie interventionnelle. Vigot, Paris, pp 17–29

Garibaldi RA (1988) Prevention of intraoperative wound contamination with chlorhexidine shower and scrub. J Hosp Infect 11(Suppl B):5–9

Garner JS (1986) CDC guideline for prevention of surgical wound infections, 1985. Supersedes guideline for prevention of surgical wound infections published in 1982. (Originally published in November 1985). Revised. Infect Control 7(3):193–200

Gil-Egea MJ, Pi-Sunyer MT, Verdaguer A, Sanz F, Sitges-Serra A, Eleizegui LT (1987) Surgical wound infections: prospective study of 4,486 clean wounds. Infect Control 8:277–280

Hamilton HW, Hamilton KR, Lone FJ (1977) Preoperative hair removal. Can J Surg 20:269–271, 274–275

Hardin WD, Nichols RL (1997) Handwashing and patient skin preparation. In: Malangoni MA (ed) Critical issues in operating room management. Lippincott-Raven, Philadelphia, pp 133–149

Irie T, Kajitani M, Itai Y (2001) CT fluoroscopy-guided intervention: marked reduction of scattered radiation dose to the physician's hand by use of a lead plate and an improved I-I device. J Vasc Interv Radiol 12:1417–1421

James RC, MacLeod CJ (1961) Induction of staphylococcal infections in mice with small inocula introduced on sutures. Br J Exp Pathol 42:266–277

Krizek TJ, Robson MC (1975) Evolution of quantitative bacteriology in wound management. Am J Surg 130:579–584

Larson E (1988) Guideline for use of topical antimicrobial agents. Am J Infect Control 16:253–266

Larson EL (1995) APIC guideline for handwashing and hand antisepsis in health care settings. Am J Infect Control 23:251–269

Letts RM, Doermer E (1983) Conversation in the operating theater as a cause of airborne bacterial contamination. J Bone Joint Surg Am 65:357–362

Lidwell OM (1986) Clean air at operation and subsequent sepsis in the joint. Clin Orthop 211:91–102

Lilly HA, Lowbury EJ, Wilkins MD, Zaggy A (1979) Delayed antimicrobial effects of skin disinfection by alcohol. J Hyg (Lond) 82:497–500

Lowbury EJ, Lilly HA, Ayliffe GA (1974) Preoperative disinfection of surgeons hands: use of alcoholic solutions and effects of gloves on skin flora. Br Med J 4:369–372

Mangram AJ, Horan TC, Pearson ML, Silver LC, Jarvis WR (1999) Guideline for prevention of surgical site infection. Infection control and hospital epidemiology 20:250–264

Mayhall CG (1993) Surgical infections including burns. In: Wenzel RP (ed) Prevention and control of nosocomial infections. Williams & Wilkins, Baltimore, pp 614–664

McDonald M, Grabsch E, Marshall C, Forbes A (1998) Single versus multiple-dose antimicrobial prophylaxis for major surgery: a systematic review. Aust N Z J Surg 68:388–396

Mishriki SF, Law DJ, Jeffery PJ (1990) Factors affecting the incidence of postoperative wound infection. J Hosp Infect 16:223–230

Nichols RL (1989) Antibiotic prophylaxis in surgery. J Chemother 1:170–178

Nichols RL (1992) The operating room. In: Bennett JV, Brachman PS (eds) Hospital infections. Little Brown, Boston, pp 461–473

Nichols RL (1995) Surgical antibiotic prophylaxis. Med Clin North Am 79:509–522

Nooyen SM, Overbeek BP, Brutel de la Riviere A, Storm AJ, Langemeyer JM (1994) Prospective randomised comparison of single-dose versus multiple-dose cefuroxime for prophylaxis in coronary artery bypass grafting. Eur J Clin Microbiol Infect Dis 13:1033–1037

Olson MM, MacCallum J, McQuarrie DG (1986) Preoperative hair removal with clippers does not increase infection rate in clean surgical wounds. Surg Gynecol Obstet 162:181–182

Page CP, Bohnen JM, Fletcher JR, McManus AT, Solomkin JS, Wittmann DH (1993) Antimicrobial prophylaxis for surgical wounds guidelines for clinical care. Arch Surg 128:79–88

Perl TM, Golub JE (1998) New approaches to reduce Staphylococcus aureus nosocomial infection rates: treating S. aureus nasal carriage. Ann Pharmacother 32:S7–S16

Rotter M (1999) Hand washing and hand disinfection. In: Mayhall CG (ed) Hospital epidemiology and infection control. Williams & Wilkins, Baltimore, pp 1339–1355

Rotter ML (1984) Hygienic hand disinfection. Infect Control 5:18–22

Sands K, Vineyard G, Platt R (1996) Surgical site infections occurring after hospital discharge. J Infect Dis 173:963–970

Seropian R, Reynolds BM (1971) Wound infections after preoperative depilatory versus razor preparation. Am J Surg 121:251–254

Sharma LK, Sharma PK (1986) Postoperative wound infection in a pediatric surgical service. J Pediatr Surg 21:889–891

Short LJ, Bell DM (1993) Risk of occupational infection with blood-borne pathogens in operating and delivery room settings. Am J Infect Control 21:343–350

Soto LE, Bobadilla M, Villalobos Y, Sifuentes J, Avelar J, Arrieta M (1991) Post-surgical nasal cellulitis outbreak due to Mycobacterium chelonae. J Hosp Infect 19:99–106

Tokars JI, Culver DH, Mendelson MH, Sloan EP, Farber BF, Fligner DJ (1995) Skin and mucous membrane contacts with blood during surgical procedures: risk and prevention. Infect Control Hosp Epidemiol 16:703–711

Trilla A, Mensa J (1993) Perioperative antibiotic prophylaxis. In: Wenzel RP (ed) Prevention and control of nosocomial infections. Williams & Wilkins, Baltimore, pp 665–682

Valentine RJ, Weigelt JA, Dryer D, Rodgers C (1986) Effect of remote infections on clean wound infection rates. Am J Infect Control 14:64–67

Vamvakas EC, Carven JH (1998) Transfusion of white-cell-containing allogeneic blood components and postoperative wound infection: effect of confounding factors. Transfus Med 8:29–36

Weigelt JA, Dryer D, Haley RW (1992) The necessity and efficiency of wound surveillance after discharge. Arch Surg 127:77–82

Wewalka G, Rotter M, Koller W (1977) Comparison of efficacy of 14 procedures for the hygienic disinfection of hands. Zentralbl Bakteriol 165:242–249

Widmer AF (2000) Replace hand washing with use of a waterless alcohol hand rub? Clin Infect Dis 31:136–143

Widmer AF, Shah D, Frei R (1999) Efficacy of 4 hand disinfectants against Mycobacterium terrae. Infect Control Hosp Epidemiol 20:286

Percutaneous Biopsy of Soft Tissues and Muscular Lesions

Jacqueline C. Hodge and Kimmo Mattila

CONTENTS

2.1 Introduction   15
2.2 Modality Selection   15
2.3 Biopsy Planning   18
2.4 Biopsy Execution   35
2.5 Conclusion   35
    References   36

2.1
Introduction

The twentieth century has seen the development of many medical techniques, including the closed biopsy. Prior to this development, a biopsy was a major undertaking, requiring general or local anesthesia and hospitalization. Thanks to the remarkable advances in musculoskeletal imaging, particularly ultrasound, computed tomography (CT) and magnetic resonance (MR) imaging, the open biopsy has been largely replaced by the imaging-guided biopsy. Although there are still indications for open biopsy, whether incisional or excisional, these now comprise a relatively small percentage of all biopsies performed. Moreover, because of the pathognomonic imaging characteristics of certain tumors, the overall need to perform any sort of biopsy, for the sole purpose of diagnosis, has been greatly reduced. Thus, it is with these recently acquired tools that the

J. C. Hodge, MD
Attending Radiologist, Department of Radiology, Lenox Hill Hospital, 100 E 77th Street, New York, NY 10021, USA
K. Mattila, MD, PhD
Section Chief, Musculoskeletal Radiology, Department of Diagnostic Radiology, Turku University Hospital, Kiinamyllynkatu 4–8, 20520 Turku, Finland

imager approaches the soft tissue mass, determining first if the lesion requires biopsy for diagnosis and, if so, which modality is most appropriate.

2.2
Modality Selection

Percutaneous biopsy of soft tissue lesions can be easily, accurately and safely performed under CT guidance in the overwhelming majority of cases (Hodge 1999; Yao et al. 1999). On occasion, fluoroscopic or ultrasound-guided percutaneous biopsy may be quicker and/or more practical, particularly for superficial lesions. The main advantage of fluoroscopy is economic; in centers with limited resources and equipment, use of fluoroscopy for biopsy guidance reserves the CT scanner for more complicated cases. Additional benefits of fluoroscopy-guided biopsy are its relatively low cost, and its real-time capabilities, which allows for continuous observation of the needle during its placement into the lesion of interest.

Although ultrasound-guided biopsy is most often used for biopsy of breast and thyroid lesions, high-frequency megahertz transducers provide improved detail of the extremities so that ultrasound-guided biopsy of these areas is easier than ever. Despite this fact, ultrasound-guidance is probably most often used for ganglion cyst aspiration, with or without injection of corticosteroids. Provided that ultrasound can visualize the lesion, it is the modality of choice when biopsy of a pregnant woman in the first or second trimester is requested, due to its lack of ionizing radiation. Moreover, as with fluoroscopy, ultrasound offers real-time capability and is relatively inexpensive.

Alternatively, percutaneous biopsy may be performed under MR guidance. Despite a lack of ionizing radiation and a high sensitivity for lesion detection, this technique has limited clinical utility in today's practice. It is expensive, relatively time-consuming, and, according to some authors, less accurate than CT or ultrasound-guided biopsy (GENANT et al. 2002; PARKKOLA et al. 2001). It should be noted that case selection, which can have a substantial effect on tissue sampling success rates, was not accounted for in these comparisons. In one paper (GENANT et al. 2002) the success rates for MR-guided core biopsies was 100%, while the lower overall 92% success rate was based on nondiagnostic fine needle samples. Thus, MR-guided biopsy, for clinical purposes, is advised in a setting where the lesion, or the neurovascular structures along with the needle trajectory, are poorly or not at all visualized under CT or ultrasound (Fig. 2.1). Additional considerations for MR-guided biopsy include MR compatible instruments, as well as an open-bore or C-arm design magnet to allow the radiologist access to the patient.

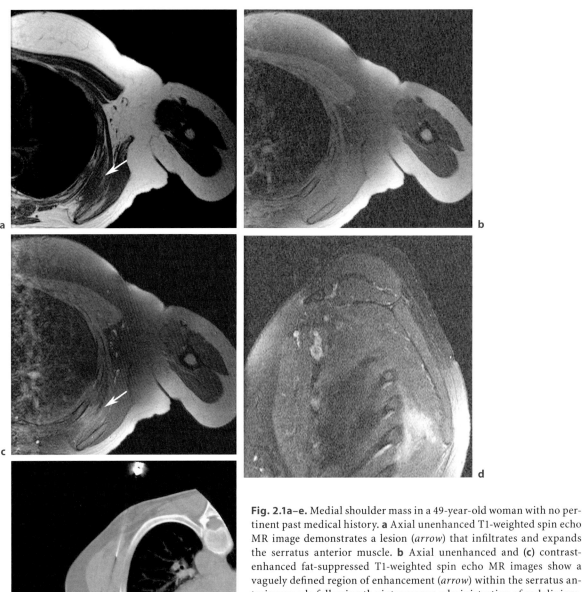

Fig. 2.1a–e. Medial shoulder mass in a 49-year-old woman with no pertinent past medical history. **a** Axial unenhanced T1-weighted spin echo MR image demonstrates a lesion (*arrow*) that infiltrates and expands the serratus anterior muscle. **b** Axial unenhanced and (**c**) contrast-enhanced fat-suppressed T1-weighted spin echo MR images show a vaguely defined region of enhancement (*arrow*) within the serratus anterior muscle following the intravenous administration of gadolinium. **d** Sagittal contrast-enhanced fat-suppressed T1-weighted spin echo MR image confirms the presence of this ill-defined lesion. **e** Biopsy had to be performed under CT guidance, although the lesion is poorly visualized, because of the closed nature and relatively high field strength of the 1.5 T MR scanner. The diagnosis of elastofibroma dorsi was confirmed at the time of surgical excision

Once these minimum criteria have been met, the radiologist must then consider: (a) how to achieve satisfactory image quality when the quality has been compromised by going from the relatively high field strength closed-bore magnet to the lower field strength open-bore or C-arm design magnets, and (b) how best to visualize the biopsy device.

Experience has demonstrated that fast spin echo (FSE) sequences tend to give better lesion visibility, whereas spoiled gradient echo (SGE) sequences give more favorable needle visibility. If more tissue-specific imaging is required for the biopsy, the three-point Dixon technique has successfully allowed low field strength magnets to reproduce fat-selective and/or water-selective sequences that previously could only be generated on high field strength magnets.

As for needle visibility, MR imaging shares some characteristics with ultrasound. Like ultrasound, real-time or nearly real-time MR imaging can be achieved with C-arm magnets. Moreover, as with ultrasound, needle trajectory is critical to needle visualization. For accurate needle tip localization under MR imaging, the needle trajectory usually should not be parallel to the magnetic field, unlike ultrasound; with ultrasound, the needle is better visualized the more parallel it is to the surface of the transducer that is in direct contact with the skin.

With regard to MR imaging, diligent use of susceptibility artifacts enables instrument visualization. Disadvantages are the dependence of visualization of the needle on the orientation of the magnetic field, and that the size of the artifact is dependent on pulse sequence, or is even uncontrollable (Fig. 2.2). However, triangulation systems have been designed for use in optical tracking systems that allow virtual reality visualization of the needle. The technique

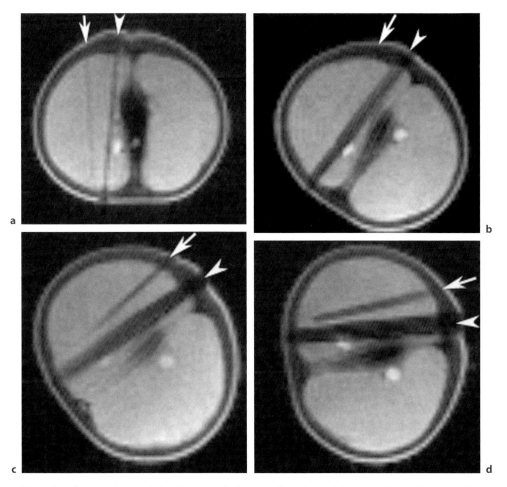

Fig. 2.2a–d. Dependence of visualization of a fine-needle and core-biopsy needle on the orientation in the magnetic field. Needles inserted (*arrow* and *arrowhead*) in an orange, with the orientation altered between images. **a–d** Images obtained using an open C-arm 0.23 T imager. The main magnetic field is vertical. The artefact is smallest when the needle is parallel to the B0

identifies a holder with a light emitting diode in its 3D position in the MR imaging space. The direction and tip of a straight tool mounted on this holder can be extrapolated when its length is known. This reduces the dependence of real (passive) needle visualization on orientation, or on the pulse sequence (SCHWARTZ et al. 1999).

An additional consideration with regard to MR-guided biopsy is that MR is superior to CT and ultrasound in its ability to depict the neurovascular structures, making it much easier to avoid them. Dynamic contrast-enhanced imaging, performed at regular intervals (for example, every few seconds), provides direct visualization of the vessels within or adjacent to the tumor.

MR-guided biopsy is contraindicated in patients with MR-incompatible devices, such as pacemakers. However, once the patient has successfully passed the preliminary MR questionnaire and undergone a diagnostic three-plane MR imaging on a high field strength magnet, the patient can be scheduled for MR-guided biopsy on any of the access-friendly magnets discussed above.

2.3
Biopsy Planning

Before beginning a percutaneous biopsy, the radiologist should determine: (a) whether the lesion can or should be biopsied, (b) the ideal approach to the lesion (Figs. 2.3–2.5), and (c) what specimens are necessary.

The location of the lesion relative to important anatomic structures, and the risk of damaging those structures, determine the feasibility of the percutaneous biopsy. If the benefits of the biopsy do not outweigh the risks, open biopsy should be considered. Other lesions, although easily accessible, may be pathognomonic based upon their imaging features and thus require no further intervention for diagnosis (e.g. lipoma) (Figs. 2.6, 2.7) (SIEGEL 2001; NISHIMURA et al. 2001; SANDERS and PARSONS 2001). Likewise, additional history may sometimes elucidate the nature of the soft tissue mass, eliminating the need for percutaneous biopsy or any further intervention (Fig. 2.8).

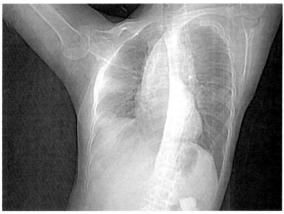
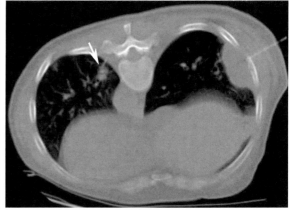

a   b

Fig. 2.3a,b. Right chest wall mass in a 48-year-old woman with known tongue carcinoma. Biopsy was requested to determine whether the chest wall lesion was a metastasis or second primary malignancy. **a** Topogram from CT-guided biopsy shows both arms have been raised over her head. By elevating the scapula, the lesion becomes accessible from the due lateral position rather than postero- or antero-laterally, which would require passing through a lung. A peripheral soft tissue mass sits beside the right posterolateral third and fourth ribs. A fracture of the third rib is apparent. **b** Axial CT scan shows the patient placed prone oblique, rather than prone, to avoid contamination of the needle while moving the patient in and out of the gantry to check needle position. It is now clear that the epicenter of the lesion is the rib, as a soft tissue mass projects both within and external to the rib cage. A 20-gauge 9.5 cm spinal needle was advanced into the lesion. Note that a left lower lobe pulmonary nodule (*arrow*) is also present. As the risks of biopsy of that lesion would be greater, the right rib was preferable for biopsy. The final tissue diagnosis was squamous cell carcinoma, which could be either metastatic from the head and neck tumor or from the pulmonary nodule

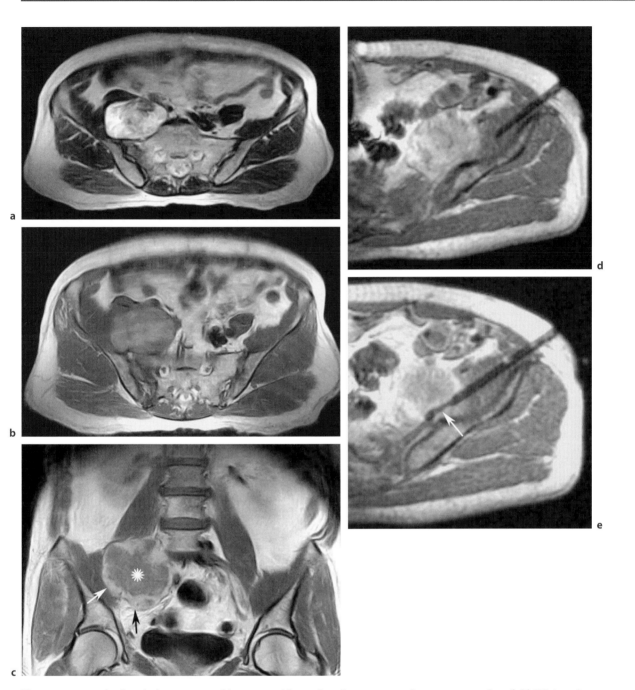

Fig. 2.4a–e. Low back pain in a 72-year-old woman with previous hysterectomy due to sarcoma. Low field MR imaging (0.23 T) of the pelvis was requested to evaluate the patient's back pain. **a** Axial T2-weighted fast spin echo MR image shows a large soft tissue lesion within the right hemipelvis, abutting the anterior cortex of the sacrum. The tumor has high signal intensity at its periphery, with heterogeneous intermediate signal intensity tissue centrally. **b** Axial T1-weighted spin echo MR image shows the lesion homogeneously intermediate in signal intensity. **c** Coronal contrast-enhanced T1-weighted spin echo MR image demonstrates peripheral enhancement (*arrows*), which probably represents a viable tumor, while the central unenhanced region (*star*) is probably necrotic fluid. **d** Axial contrast-enhanced T1-weighted MR image during antero-lateral approach MR-guided biopsy using coaxial system shows the needle traversing the iliacus muscle. **e** The inner stylet has been advanced to the periphery of the tumor (*arrow*) immediately before the semi-automated biopsy gun is fired to capture the specimen. Histopathologic examination revealed a metastasis from a sarcoma

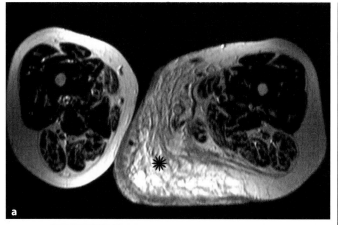

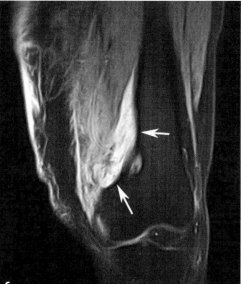

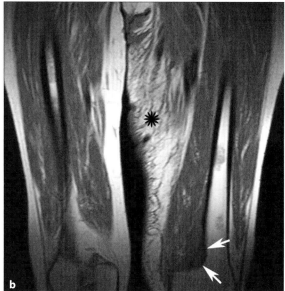

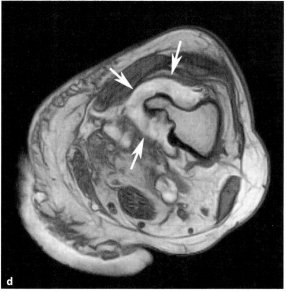

Fig. 2.5a–e. Indolent ill-defined large tumor of the medial subcutaneous tissues of the left thigh in a 64-year-old man with known neurofibromatosis. **a** Axial-T2 weighted and **b** coronal T1-weighted spin echo MR images show the large plexiform neurofibromas (*star*), interspersed with areas of edema within the subcutaneous fat, which causes an elephantiasis neurofibromatosa type thigh. Scalloping and erosion of the medial aspect of the distal left femoral metaphysis has been caused by the pressure of this chronic adjacent soft tissue tumor (*arrows*) on (**c**) coronal T1-weighted spin echo and STIR MR images. **d** Rapid enhancement of this suspected plexiform neurofibroma (*arrows*) subsequent to intravenous gadolinium administration caused concern that it might be malignant. Thus MR-guided biopsy was requested. **e** Axial contrast-enhanced T1-weighted spin echo MR image shows the biopsy gun has traversed the vastus medialis and has been advanced to the soft tissue mass that abuts the distal femoral cortex; the inner stylet (*arrow*) was extruded from the outer cannula immediately before the specimen was obtained. No sign of malignant transformation of the neurofibroma was detected on histopathology

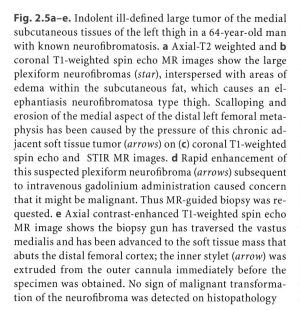

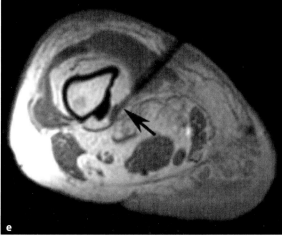

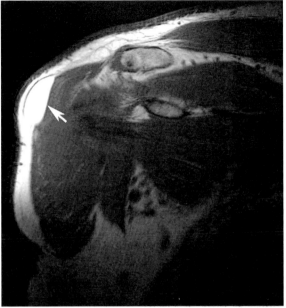

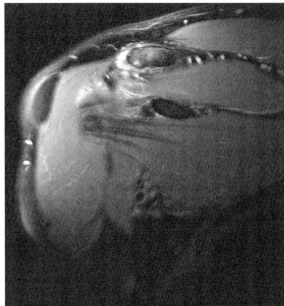

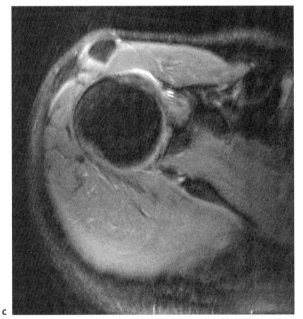

Fig. 2.6a–c. Pea-sized superficial nodule on the right shoulder in a 67-year-old man. **a** Coronal oblique T1-weighted spin echo MR image demonstrates a $3 \times 1.3 \times 1$ cm discrete mass (*arrow*), isointense to subcutaneous fat. Visualization of the coracoid process and subscapularis tendon indicate that the mass is relatively anterior. **b** Coronal oblique fat-suppressed proton density-weighted fast spin echo MR image shows that the lesion follows the signal intensity of yellow marrow and subcutaneous soft tissues, confirming that it is fat-containing. Degenerative changes at the acromioclavicular joint, with mild impingement upon the supraspinatous tendon, are noted. **c** Axial fat-suppressed proton density-weighted fast spin echo MR image confirms the anterior location of this uniformly fatty lesion within the deltoid muscle

The diagnosis of other lesions can be suspected with great certainty, based on their anatomic location and/or continuity with a neighboring joint or tendon sheath (Figs. 2.9, 2.10). Although ganglion cysts and bursae usually demonstrate imaging characteristics suggestive of their homogenous fluid content (i.e. anechoic on US, density < 20 HU on CT and/or low signal intensity on T1-weighted spin echo sequence and high signal intensity on T2-weighted spin echo sequence on MR imaging), they may appear slightly heterogeneous due either to volume averaging or internal debris such as joint mice, blood clots or inflammation (Fig. 2.11). However, in the overwhelming majority of cases, the imager can confidently arrive at the correct diagnosis on the strength of the anatomic location and enhancement patterns on CT or MR imaging, thus eliminating the need for percutaneous biopsy (Fig. 2.12).

Biopsy of some lesions may cause more confusion than clarity in the diagnostic workup; such lesions should either not be biopsied or the biopsy should be postponed until a suitable time. The clas-

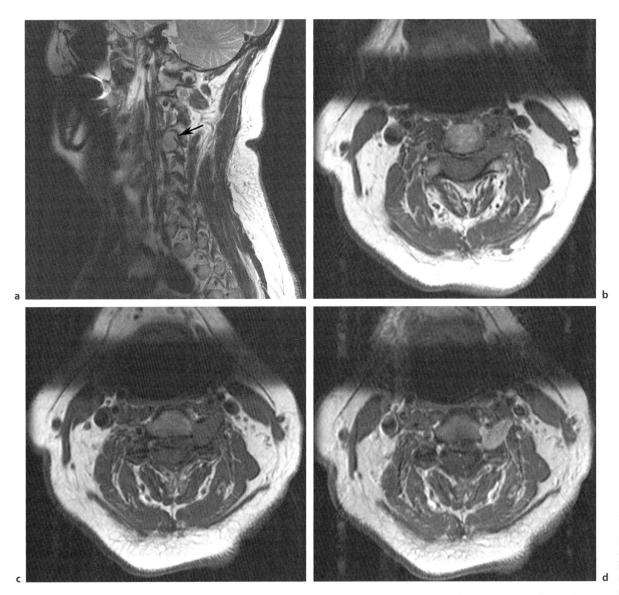

Fig. 2.7a–d. Diminished arm strength without neck or arm pain in an 81-year-old man. MR imaging requested to evaluate for spinal stenosis. **a** Sagittal T2-weighted fast spin echo MR image demonstrates a 1.8 × 1.2 cm well-circumscribed mass (*arrow*) sitting within the left C3–4 neural foramina. The lesion is isointense to brain parenchyma. Axial unenhanced T1-weighted spin echo MR images show (**b**) a left oblong isointense encapsulated mass originating from the spinal canal, (**c**) coursing through the neural foramina, anteriorly displacing and compressing the vertebral artery. Moderate spinal stenosis, incidentally noted, is due to a large disc bulge. **d** Axial contrast-enhanced T1-weighted spin echo MR image shows marked, nearly uniform enhancement of the lesion, typical for a neurinoma

sic example of the latter is a suspected hematoma, which is often confused with a sarcoma prior to its complete liquefaction (Figs. 2.13, 2.14) (Gomez and Morcuende 2004; Nakanishi et al. 2003). Biopsy at the time of presentation of the lesion interferes with the natural course of the hematoma, delaying its resolution, which is normally expected in approximately 6–12 weeks from its initial appearance

(Bush 2000). Without percutaneous intervention, the vast majority of hematomas will continue to decrease in size over time. Any increase in size, without a history of re-injury to the extremity, should suggest that the lesion may in fact represent a sarcoma, and appropriate steps to make the diagnosis should be performed at this stage. Although there have been a few reports of expanding hematomas,

Fig. 2.8. Plain radiograph of both knees in a 64-year-old man. Anteroposterior plain radiograph of the knees demonstrates two discrete soft tissue densities, much larger laterally than medially, within the proximal right calf. No history was given. When the referring physician was notified of this unexpected finding, she stated that the patient had had trauma 3 years previously for which a gastrocnemius muscle flap had been performed as part of reconstructive surgery. No further imaging was required given this information. Incidentally, there is severe right knee tricompartmental osteoarthritis, right medial distal thigh clips and two screws within the left medial femoral condyle for presumed ORIF

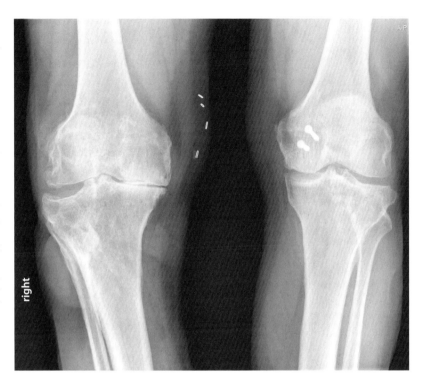

they are the exception rather than the rule (OKADA et al. 2001). If the lesion is in fact a sarcoma, the delay in biopsy by a matter of weeks –from the sarcoma's time of presentation to the time of biopsy – is a relatively small percentage of the time that the lesion has likely been present and is thus unlikely to alter the clinical outcome.

Other lesions that may cause diagnostic confusion, particularly if the diagnosis is based solely on their MR imaging appearance, are myositis ossificans and diabetic muscle infarction (KRANSDORF et al. 1991; SHIRKHODA et al. 1995; LAFFORGUE et al. 1999). Although there may be a history of trauma with myositis ossificans, frequently the patient can not recall any such event. Once ossification begins to take place at the periphery of the lesion, CT and plain radiography are certainly superior to MR in their ability to suggest the diagnosis. However, biopsy during the early stages of myositis ossificans is known to be misleading, as pathologic tissue often resembles a sarcoma due to the large amount of mitotic activity during the early stages of this benign entity. Thus, if myositis ossificans is even a remote possibility, it is prudent to delay biopsy for 4–6 weeks, at which time a CT scan may demonstrate early ossification of the lesion's periphery.

MR imaging is by far the most sensitive modality for detecting diabetic muscle infarction. The vague ill-defined area of soft tissue edema, readily seen on MR imaging, is often completely normal in appearance on CT or ultrasound in its incipient stages (Fig. 2.15). The lack of specificity with MR imaging can make it difficult to distinguish this lesion from an aggressive neoplastic process (MOULTON et al. 1995). The clinical history should make one cautious of prematurely diagnosing sarcoma. Signs of infection in a diabetic patient, without any antecedent trauma, are indicative of diabetic muscle infarction, an entity that is self-limited, resolving within a few weeks with rest and supportive therapy. Thus, patience is needed to wait for diabetic muscle infarction to resolve, rather than embarking on an extensive workup that will often include percutaneous biopsy for exclusion of tumor and/or infection.

The last group of lesions that require caution are those that are highly vascular; for example, metastases from renal cell tumors. Extra prudence is required to select a lesion that, should it bleed profusely, will not cause an accumulation of blood in restricted spaces, such as the spinal canal or an anatomic compartment. In the latter instance, a compartment syndrome can develop.

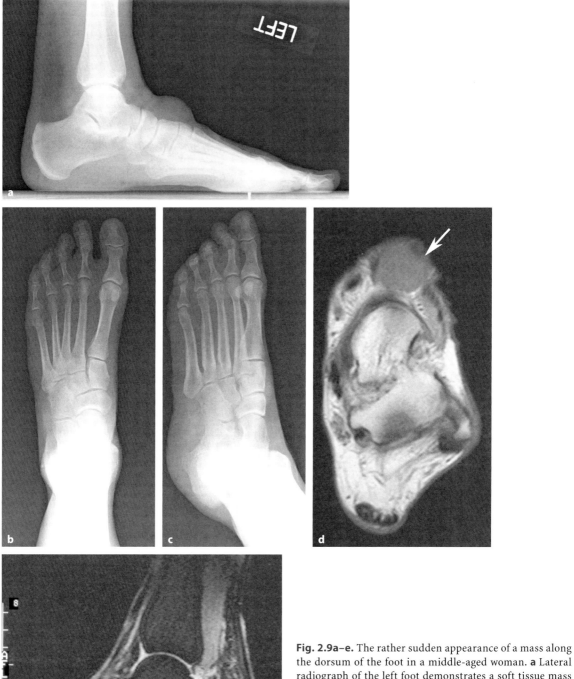

Fig. 2.9a–e. The rather sudden appearance of a mass along the dorsum of the foot in a middle-aged woman. **a** Lateral radiograph of the left foot demonstrates a soft tissue mass along the dorsum of the foot. No bony destruction detected. **b** Anteroposterior and (**c**) internal oblique radiographs do not offer any additional information. **d** Axial T1-weighted spin echo MR images show a 1.5 × 1.5 cm well-defined mass (*arrow*) with intermediate signal intensity, arising either from one of the lateral extensor tendons and/or tendon sheaths, most likely the extensor digitorum communis. **e** Sagittal STIR MR image shows a parasagittal 3 × 1.5 cm mass (*arrow*), isointense to fluid, which appears to be deep to the extensor tendon. Findings are consistent with a ganglion cyst

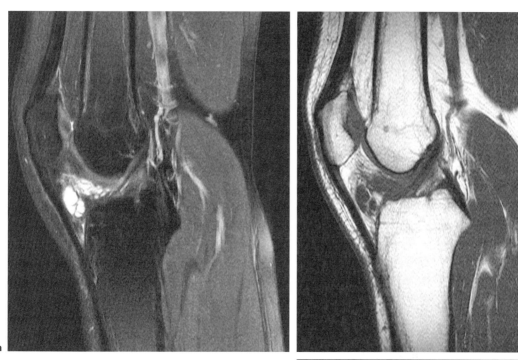

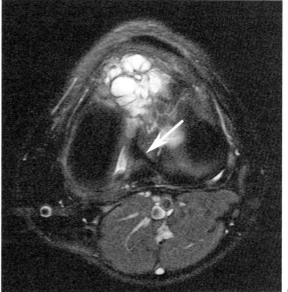

Fig. 2.10a–c. Persistent knee pain and a palpable mass within the anterior soft tissues of the knee in a 27-year-old woman. MR imaging performed for further evaluation. Ganglion cyst confirmed at arthroscopy. **a** Sagittal fat-suppressed T2-weighted fast spin echo MR image shows a multiloculated hyperintense mass within Hoffa's fat pad. A possible connection with the anterior cruciate ligament is suspected. **b** Sagittal T1-weighted spin echo MR image demonstrates an intermediate signal intensity mass. Residual fat between the mass and the patellar ligament indicates that the lesion is distinct from this ligament. **c** Axial fat-suppressed T2-weighted fast spin echo MR image shows a cystic lesion anteriorly. A transverse view of the anterior cruciate ligament (*arrow*) is noted within the intercondylar notch

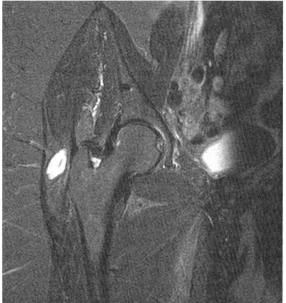

a

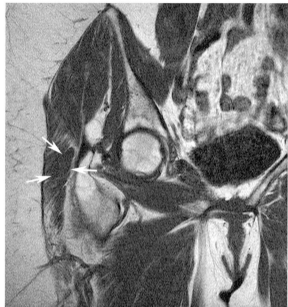

b

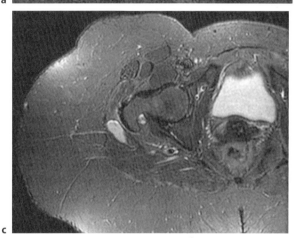

c

Fig. 2.11a–c. Right hip pain in a 59-year-old man. **a** Coronal fast STIR MR image shows a 3×3×1.5 cm discrete lesion with signal intensity identical to fluid. **b** Coronal T1-weighted spin echo image shows an ovoid intermediate signal intensity collection noted between subcutaneous fat and that of gluteal muscles (*arrows*). **c** Axial fast STIR MR image shows that the fluid collection lies adjacent to the greater trochanter, most likely representing the trochanteric bursa

Once it has been determined that the lesion warrants percutaneous biopsy, a short list of diagnostic possibilities should be formulated. If malignancy is a possibility, the surgeon should be consulted to avoid tracking the tumor into any compartment(s) that will be left behind (Fig. 2.16). With adequate knowledge of the anatomy and the surgeon's plan, the radiologist should direct the needle into the lesion via the compartment that is to be resected. Of course, with amputation, such careful planning is unnecessary. However, careful pre-biopsy planning is imperative if limb-salvage surgery is a possibility (Anderson et al. 1999).

Once the radiologist has selected a biopsy site and chosen the appropriate needle type (aspiration or soft core-biopsy needle), there is one last item to consider: the specimen. Any aspirates should be sent to cytology, and soft tissue cores to pathology. Several studies have shown that cytology is equal to pathology in its ability to provide the correct diagnosis from percutaneously obtained specimens (Fig. 2.17) (Hodge 1999). Furthermore, if lymphoma or any other round cell tumor is a strong consideration, the extra tissue should be taken if possible. Lymphoma, in particular, often requires special stains and cell blocks for diagnosis, and thus more tissue is required than for diagnosis of non round cell lesions (Fig. 2.18). Finally, if there is even a remote possibility that the lesion in question could be an infection, a specimen, preferably the first so as to minimize contaminants, should be submitted to microbiology (Fig. 2.19).

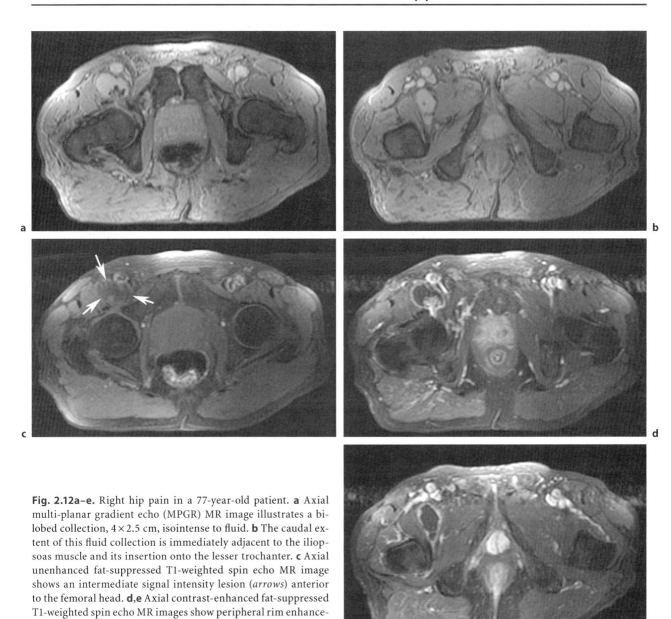

Fig. 2.12a–e. Right hip pain in a 77-year-old patient. **a** Axial multi-planar gradient echo (MPGR) MR image illustrates a bi-lobed collection, 4 × 2.5 cm, isointense to fluid. **b** The caudal extent of this fluid collection is immediately adjacent to the iliopsoas muscle and its insertion onto the lesser trochanter. **c** Axial unenhanced fat-suppressed T1-weighted spin echo MR image shows an intermediate signal intensity lesion (*arrows*) anterior to the femoral head. **d,e** Axial contrast-enhanced fat-suppressed T1-weighted spin echo MR images show peripheral rim enhancement of the lesion. Its direct communication with the hip joint confirms the diagnosis of an iliopsoas bursa

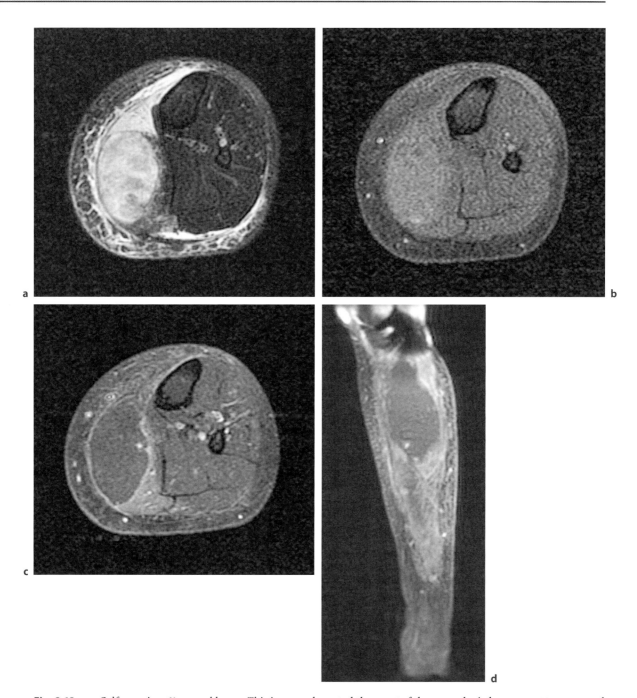

Fig. 2.13a–g. Calf mass in a 61-year-old man. This jogger, who noted the onset of the mass, denied any recent trauma. **a–d** Images were obtained at the time of presentation to his family physician. **e–g** Images were made 12 weeks later. **a** Axial fat-suppressed T2-weighted fast spin echo MR image shows a 8×4 cm posteromedial encapsulated inhomogeneous right calf mass within the medial head of the gastrocnemius muscle. There is circumferential skin thickening and mild subcutaneous   ▷▷

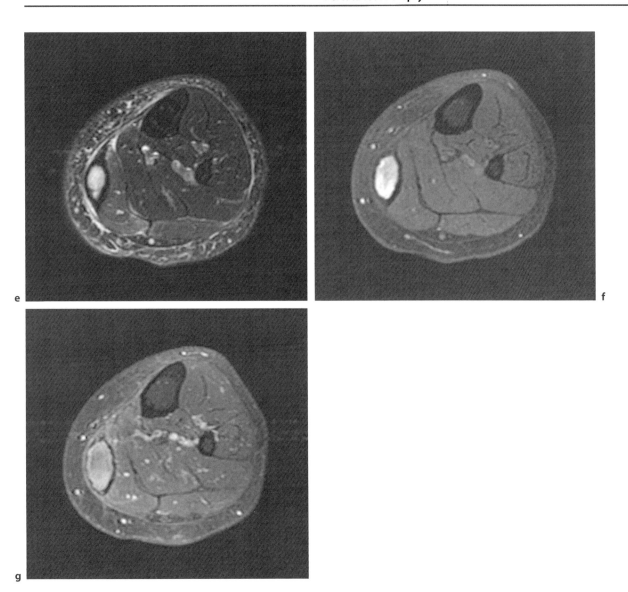

edema, but no bone contusion or fracture. Axial (**b**) unenhanced and (**c**) contrast-enhanced fat-suppressed T1-weighted spin echo MR images show faint peripheral enhancement of the lesion, which was essentially isointense with surrounding musculature. The lack of central enhancement suggests the presence of fluid, i.e. either blood or necrosis. The mean on pre- and post-contrast images was 138 and 142, respectively. **d** Sagittal contrast-enhanced fat-suppressed T1-weighted MR image illustrates rim enhancement of the mass. **e** Axial fat-suppressed T2-weighted fast spin echo MR image shows interim perceived thickening of the very low signal intensity capsule due to the presence of both fibrous tissue and hemosiderin, the latter giving rise to blooming. The lesion is now much smaller, measuring 2 × 1 cm. There is residual edema within the medial and lateral heads of the gastrocnemius muscle and within the subcutaneous tissues. Axial (**f**) unenhanced and (**g**) contrast-enhanced fat-suppressed T1-weighted spin echo MR images demonstrate a lack of enhancement in the predominantly bright encapsulated lesion. The mean on pre- and post-contrast images was 317 and 306, respectively; i.e. statistically insignificant. The high signal is most likely attributed to methemoglobin, a by-product found in the resolving hematoma

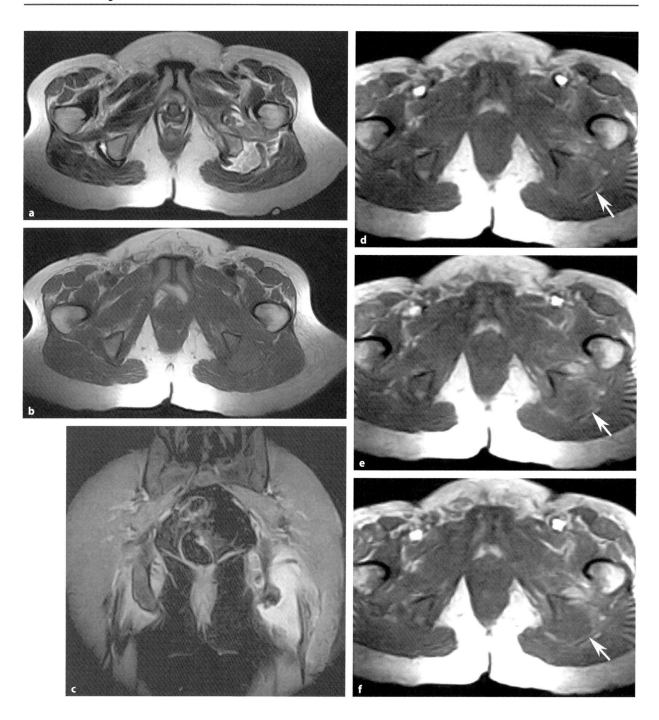

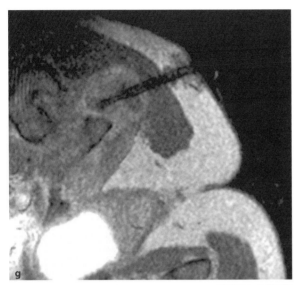

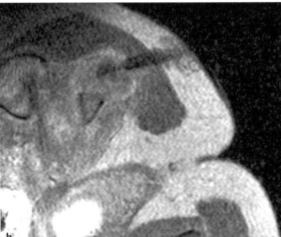

Fig. 2.14a–h. Suspicion of a malignant tumor surrounding the left ischial tuberosity in a 74-year-old woman who was referred from another hospital for MR-guided biopsy. MR images taken elsewhere were remarkable for bilateral common hamstring origin tears: partial on the right, complete on the left on (**a**) axial T2-weighted spin echo image, (**b**) axial T1-weighted spin echo image, and (**c**) coronal STIR image. **d–f** Dynamic contrast-enhanced MR images obtained at 16, 20 and 24 sec, respectively, demonstrate slow peripheral enhancement (*arrow*) thought to represent a seroma and/or bursa. However, the tumor surgeon requested biopsy of the lesion because there was no history of antecedent trauma to explain the hamstring tears. **g** Axial contrast-enhanced T1-weighted field echo MR image with patient in the prone position shows central nonenhancing part of the lesion was first aspirated. Samples were submitted to cytology. **h** Subsequent soft tissue core biopsy specimens, obtained from the periphery of the lesion, were sent to pathology. No sign of a neoplasm was detected in either specimen. The pathologist noted inflammatory cells and synovial tissue, probably representing the wall of a bursa

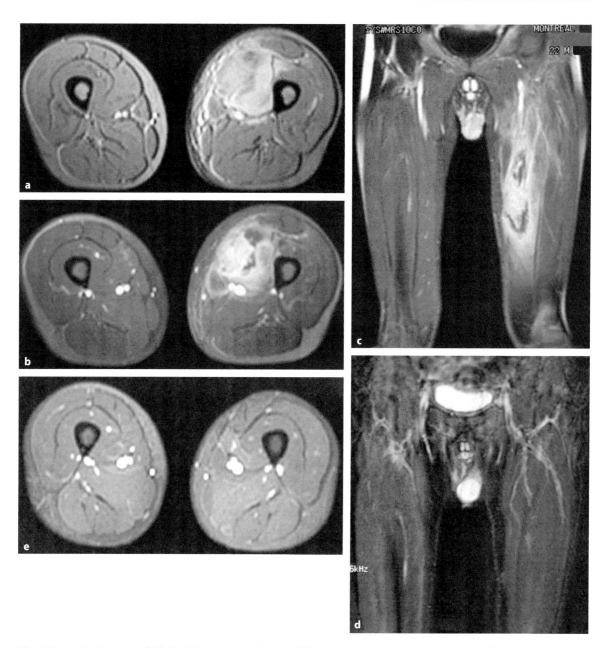

Fig. 2.15a–e. Indolent painful left thigh mass in a 22-year-old diabetic man. **a–c** Images were obtained at the time of initial presentation. **d,e** Images at 12 month follow-up. Axial (**a**) unenhanced and (**b**) contrast-enhanced fat-suppressed T1-weighted spin echo MR images demonstrate mild enhancement of the heterogeneous lesion predominantly involving the vastus medialis muscle. There is no involvement of the neurovascular bundle or the adjacent bone marrow. **c** Coronal contrast-enhanced fat-suppressed T1-weighted spin echo MR image shows vague, heterogeneous enhancement of this $10 \times 4 \times 4$ cm lesion. **d** Coronal STIR MR image shows normal signal intensity of the vastus medialis muscle. **e** Axial T1-weighted fat suppressed spin echo MR image shows normal signal of the soft tissues, neurovascular bundle and bone marrow. There is no enhancement

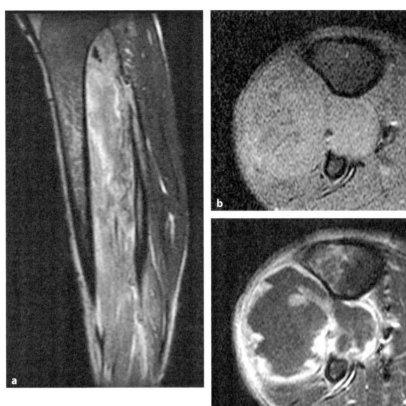

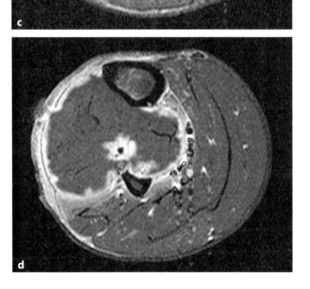

Fig. 2.16a–d. Redness of the right lower extremity in a 33-year-old HIV-positive man. Incision and drainage specimens were positive for *E. coli*, thus the patient was started on ciprofloxacin. MR imaging was performed 3 weeks later for worsening cellulitis. Because of the ominous-looking enhancement pattern of the mass on MR imaging, the patient was taken for surgical debridement and open biopsy. Multiple specimens were obtained, all of which were negative for tumor. The final pathology was necrotizing muscle. **a** Sagittal STIR MR image shows poorly defined heterogeneous 26 cm lesion extending for almost the entire length of the calf. Axial (**b**) unenhanced and (**c**) contrast-enhanced fat-suppressed T1-weighted MR images show peripheral frond-like enhancement of the bilobed lesion, which measures 6×5 cm. Minimal tibial enhancement is felt to be due to reactive edema, rather than osteomyelitis. **d** Axial contrast-enhanced fat-suppressed T1-weighted MR image shows two skin ulcers laterally, in addition to enhancement of the subcutaneous tissues and periphery of the lesion. The sinus tract opening to the skin is highly suggestive of infectious etiology

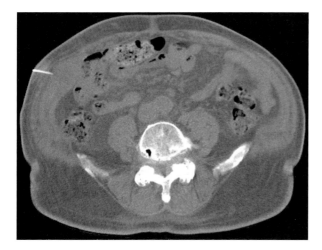

Fig. 2.17. Lateral abdominal wall mass in an otherwise healthy 82-year-old man. Axial CT scan demonstrates asymmetric enlargement of the right external oblique muscle with loss of the fat planes separating the internal and external oblique muscles. None of the four passes performed with a 19-gauge 1.5-inch needle yielded aspirates. No soft tissue core was obtained. Cytologic diagnosis was positive for anaplastic carcinoma

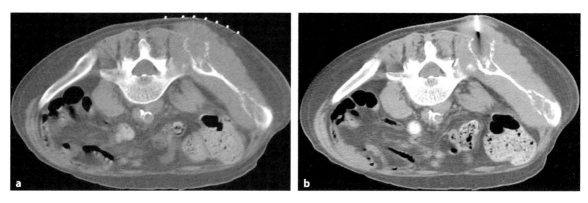

Fig. 2.18a,b. Right buttock mass in a 78-year-old man with no pertinent past medical history. **a** Axial CT scan with the patient placed prone shows that the lesion almost certainly originates from the right ilium, as the soft tissue extension of the lesion is involved with both the iliacus and gluteus medius/minimus muscles. **b** Axial CT scan with the patient placed in the prone position to provide the easiest access to the lesion shows the osteolytic destruction of the entire ilium. A perpendicular approach provides the shortest distance to the lesion and is also the most secure with regard to needle placement, since a needle is least likely to glide off the surface of a lesion to which it is perpendicular. Biopsy resulted in a diagnosis of B-cell type non-Hodgkin lymphoma

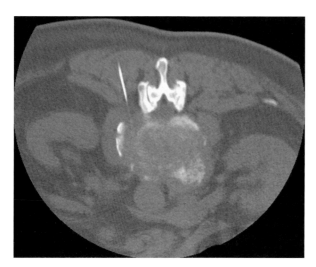

Fig. 2.19. Suspected discitis on MR imaging in a 77-year-old woman. Axial CT scan with the patient placed in the prone position to gain access to the L1–2 disc space shows 20-gauge 3.5-inch spinal needle is introduced into the disc space via a posterolateral approach. Due to the degree of lumbar lordosis, a pillow was placed beneath the patient's abdomen to improve access to the disc space, a technique often used during discography

2.4
Biopsy Execution

From this point, percutaneous biopsy of soft tissue lesions is relatively straightforward, and is generally similar to the technique used to approach osseous lesions, except that specimen removal requires much less physical strength. As with any percutaneous biopsy, there is the risk that, despite having obtained seemingly excellent specimens, tissue that is either not representative of the larger mass or that is necrotic may have been harvested. Whether a sampling error (as in the former case) or an inadequate number of cells, either problem may preclude establishment of a diagnosis. To avoid biopsy of necrotic areas in neoplasms with different components, dynamic contrast-enhanced MR imaging can be used to determine the best site for biopsy within a lesion. The fastest enhancing intratumoral site probably represents the viable tumor. Alternatively, correlation with PET images, if available, will indicate the most active and viable parts of the tumor.

It is not sufficient to confirm that the PT, PTT and INR are normal. Indeed, these lab values may be normal in the setting of some blood dyscrasias and are unaffected by antiplatelet drugs (e.g. Plavix). In this latter group, it is advised to avoid the use of core biopsy needles to reduce the risk of blood loss associated with the biopsy. In the course of obtaining written consent, it should be explained to the patient that, in addition to the more serious possible complications (pneumothorax, tumor seeding, infection, neural damage, bleeding), it is also possible that the biopsy will be non diagnostic.

Whatever the modality selected for guidance during the biopsy, patient positioning is critical (Fig. 2.3). The patient should be positioned appropriately for the planned biopsy route (compartment anatomy). The route to the lesion should also keep the trajectory of the needle as far as possible from any nearby structures that could be injured. It is also important that the patient be able to maintain this position for the duration of the biopsy.

Following localization of the lesion, the access area should be prepped and draped in the usual sterile fashion. In our experience, a cocktail of Versed and/or Fentanyl provides excellent sedation; these drugs are quite short-lived and their effects are almost transparent by the completion of the procedure, thus minimizing the post-biopsy observation period.

Needle selection is determined by the appearance of the tissue at the biopsy site and user preference. A predominantly fluid lesion should be approached with an aspiration-type needle, such as a spinal needle or Chiba, whereas either a cutting (Tru-cut, Vacu-cut or Percu-cut) or aspiration-type needle can be used with a solid lesion. If the lesion is deep, or if one suspects that several passes will be required to obtain adequate tissue, a coaxial system should be considered – that is, placing an outer sheath through which another needle can be passed down to the lesion. A dedicated coaxial system can either be bought or it can be improvised by using an 18- or 20-gauge needle as the stationary outer sheath with a larger gauge needle placed through its bore. If the biopsy is to be performed under MR-guidance, all instruments must be fully MR compatible, significantly limiting the choice of biopsy equipment. Specimens to be submitted to cytology should be in alcohol, and those submitted to pathology should be in formalin. Microbiology specimens should be placed in culture bottles, if provided; otherwise, submit them, without additives, in a specimen container. Ideally, the biopsy site should be tattooed on the skin with ink to facilitate surgical excision of the entire trajectory should the lesion prove to be a malignant neoplasm.

The length of post-biopsy observation is dependent upon the complications, if any, and the patient's response to the sedation. In a routine, uncomplicated case, patients may leave the department within 30 min, provided they have a companion to escort them home. As a precaution, they should be advised not to drive for the remainder of the day.

No post-biopsy care is required if no skin incision has been made. If a small incision was necessary, a bandage may be placed at the conclusion of the biopsy and changed as necessary. Since there is no increased fracture risk, as with bone biopsies, patients may resume their normal activities on the day of the exam.

2.5
Conclusion

Although the literature is replete with reports on the success and diagnostic accuracy of the percutaneous image-guided biopsy, the reader should keep in mind that there is some variation with regard to outcome, depending on: (a) the experience of the individual carrying out the biopsy with the modality used to guide the procedure, and (b) the tumor type, i.e. carcinoma versus sarcoma. Because sarcomas tend to have a relatively heterogeneous content, imaging characteristics play a more significant role in selecting the particular site of biopsy within a lesion. Finally, in doing good, it is important to do no harm. It does not help to spare the patient an open biopsy if the biopsy is performed in such a manner that limb-salvage surgery is made more difficult. Pre-biopsy consultation with the surgeon planning the resection of the tumor will guide you to select the most appropriate biopsy route, thus optimizing the likelihood of a successful outcome.

Acknowledgements

Dr. J. C. Hodge would like to thank Lenox Hill Hospital Radiology Associates and Radiology Department at McGill University Health Centre for allowing her to use some of the case material from their facilities.

References

Anderson MW, Temple HT, Dussault RG, Kaplan PA (1999) Compartmental anatomy: relevance to staging and biopsy of musculoskeletal tumors. AJR Am J Roentgenol 173:1663–1671

Bush CH (2000) The magnetic resonance imaging of musculoskeletal hemorrhage. Skeletal Radiol 29:1–9

Genant JW, Vandevenne JE, Bergman AG, Beaulieu CF, Kee ST, Norbash AM, Lang P (2002) Interventional musculoskeletal procedures performed by using MR imaging guidance with a vertically open MR unit: assessment of techniques and applicability. Radiology 223:127–136

Gomez P, Morcuende J (2004) High-grade sarcomas mimicking traumatic intramuscular hematomas: a report of three cases. Iowa Orthop J 24:106–110

Hodge JC (2003) Bone biopsies. In: Hodge JC (Ed) Musculoskeletal Procedures: Diagnostic and Therapeutic, TX, Landes Bioscience, Ch. 13, pp175–188

Hodge JC (1999) Percutaneous biopsy of the musculoskeletal system: A review of 77 cases. Can Assoc Radiol J 50:121–125

Kransdorf MJ, Meis JM, Jelinek JS (1991) Myositis ossificans: MR appearance with radiologic-pathologic correlation. AJR Am J Roentgenol 157:1243–1248

Lafforgue P, Janand-Delenne B, Lassman-Vague V, Daumen-Legre V, Pham T, Vague P (1999) Painful swelling of the thigh in a diabetic patient: diabetic muscle infarction. Diabetes Metab 25:255–260

Moulton JS, Blebea JS, Dunco DM, Braley SE, Bisset GS 3rd, Emery KH (1995) MR imaging of soft-tissue masses: diagnostic efficacy and value of distinguishing between benign and malignant lesions. AJR Am J Roentgenol 164:1191–1199

Nakanishi H, Araki N, Sawai Y, Kudawara I, Mano M, Ishiguro S, Ueda T, Yoshikawa H (2003) Cystic synovial sarcomas: imaging features with clinical and histopathologic correlation. Skeletal Radiol 32:701–707

Nishimura H, Zhang Y, Ohkuma K, Uchida M, Hayabuchi N, Sun S (2001) MR imaging of soft-tissue masses of the extraperitoneal spaces. Radiographics 21:1141–1154

Okada K, Sugiyama T, Kato H, Tani T (2001) Chronic expanding hematoma mimicking soft tissue neoplasm. J Clin Oncol 19:2971–2972

Parkkola RK, Mattila KT, Heikkila JT, Ekfors TO, Komu ME, Vaara T, Aro HT (2001) MR-guided core biopsies of soft tissue tumours on an open 0.23 T imager. Acta Radiol 42:302–305

Sanders TG, Parsons TW 3rd (2001) Radiographic imaging of musculoskeletal neoplasia. Cancer Control 8:221–231

Schwartz RB, Hsu L, Wong TZ, Kacher DF, Zamani AA, Black PM, Alexander E 3rd, Stieg PE, Moriarty TM, Martin CA, Kikinis R, Jolesz FA (1999) Intraoperative MR imaging guidance for intracranial neurosurgery: experience with the first 200 cases. Radiology 211:477–488

Shirkhoda A, Armin AR, Bis KG, Makris J, Irwin RB, Shetty AN (1995) MR imaging of myositis ossificans: variable patterns at different stages. J Magn Reson Imaging 5:287–292

Siegel MJ (2001) Magnetic resonance imaging of musculoskeletal soft tissue masses. Radiol Clin North Am 39:701–720

Yao L, Nelson SD, Seeger LL, Eckardt JJ, Eilber FR (1999) Primary musculoskeletal neoplasms: effectiveness of core-needle biopsy. Radiology 212:682–686

Percutaneous Bone Biopsy

Guillaume Bierry, Xavier Buy, Stéphane Guth, Ali Guermazi, and
Afshin Gangi

CONTENTS

3.1   Introduction   37

3.2   Indications   38

3.3   Contraindications   38
3.3.1   General Contraindications   38
3.3.2   Specific Contraindications   38

3.4   Bone Biopsy Techniques   39
3.4.1   Coaxial Technique   39
3.4.2   Tandem Technique   39
3.4.3   Bone Penetration   40
3.4.4   Value of Dual Guidance   40
3.4.5   Interest and Specificity of
       MR Guidance   42

3.5   Procedure   42
3.5.1   Material   42
3.5.2   Medications   43
3.5.3   Needles   43
3.5.3.1   Ostycut Biopsy Needle   43
3.5.3.2   Bonopty Penetration Set   44
3.5.3.3   Laredo Needle Set   45
3.5.3.4   Surgical Biopsy Set   45
3.5.3.5   Temno Biopsy Device   47

3.6   Patient Preparation and Positioning   48

3.7   Needle Biopsy Technique   48

3.8   Examination of Tissue Samples   49

3.9   Spine Biopsy   49
3.9.1   Lumbar Spine Biopsy   49
3.9.1.1   Bone Biopsy   49
3.9.1.2   Paraspinal Mass Biopsy   52
3.9.1.3   Posterior Structures Biopsy   53
3.9.1.4   Disc Biopsy   53

3.9.2   Thoracic Spine Biopsy   55
3.9.2.1   Bone Biopsy   55
3.9.2.2   Paraspinal and Posterior Structures
       Biopsy   58
3.9.2.3   Disc Biopsy   58
3.9.3   Cervical Spine Biopsy   60
3.9.3.1   Vertebral and Disc Biopsy   60
3.9.3.2   Posterior Arch   60

3.10   Appendicular Skeleton Biopsy   61
3.10.1   Flat Bones   61
3.10.2   Pelvis   62
3.10.3   Upper and Lower Limbs   64
3.10.3.1   Compartmental Anatomy and
        Consequences   64
3.10.3.2   Classical Approaches   64

3.11   Results   68
3.11.1   General Results   68
3.11.2   Specific Results   70
3.11.3   Complications   70
3.11.3.1   General Complications   70
3.11.3.2   Local Complications   70

3.12   Post-Procedure Management   71

3.13   Conclusion   71

       References   71

G. Bierry, MD, PhD, Fellow
X. Buy, MD, Senior Radiologist
S. Guth, MD, Senior Radiologist
A. Gangi, MD, PhD, Professor of Radiology
Department of Radiology B, University Hospital of Strasbourg, Pavillon Clovis Vincent BP 426, 67091 Strasbourg, France
A. Guermazi, MD
Associate Professor of Radiology, Department of Radiology, Section Chief, Musculoskeletal, Boston University School of Medicine, 88 East Newton Street, Boston, MA 02118, USA

3.1
Introduction

As musculoskeletal lesions rarely have a pathognomonic radiographic appearance, histological or bacteriological examinations are required for a precise diagnosis. Biopsy is necessary, either traditional surgical biopsy or percutaneous musculoskeletal biopsy (PMSB). Since the initial descriptions of core needle biopsy or fine needle aspiration (FNA) by Martin and Ellis (1930) and Coley et al. (1931), the technology of needle design and imaging have improved to the point that PMSB is often preferred when a biopsy is necessary. Percutaneous biopsy has many advantages over surgical biopsy: bone structure is not weakened through surgical removal, avoiding immobilization or osteosynthesis; there is minimal soft-tissue injury and no scar; general anesthesia is unnecessary and the patient can be sent home without hospitalization; and reduced cost.

The efficacy of PMSB for spinal lesions has diminished the role of surgical spine biopsy. CT and fluoroscopy allow precise visual guidance of the needle to almost every part of the axial and appendicular skeleton. The great majority of bone and soft tissue lesions can be approached percutaneously and samples acquired without damaging the surrounding tissues, i.e. nerves, vessels, viscera. PMSB is less traumatic (Logan et al. 1996) and less expensive (Fraser-Hill and Renfrew 1992; Fraser-Hill et al. 1992; Ruhs et al. 1996) than surgical biopsy in secondary lesions, bony localizations of hemopathy, infectious diseases and some primary bone tumors.

Thorough knowledge of the relevant anatomy (entry points and pathways, compartmental anatomy) and of the needle and guidance technology (CT, fluoroscopy, MR imaging, ultrasound) is required for a successful procedure. A complete radiologic evaluation, including plain films, CT, MR imaging and/or bone scan, is necessary. Extension to surrounding soft tissue or to articulation must be noted. Each procedure should be performed after careful estimation of the lesion type; primary tumors and metabolic disease may require different approaches. The biopsy route should be discussed with orthopedic surgeons before the procedure to ensure that the needle tract can be excised at the time of surgical resection. The whole medical team in charge of the patient including orthopedic pathologists, medical oncologists, radiation oncologists and orthopedic surgeons must be aware of the limits of such diagnostic technique, especially if insufficient material is aspirated. Every member of the team should be able to discuss the biopsy results in case of clinical or radiological mismatches.

3.2
Indications

The general purpose of PMSB is to obtain a sufficient amount of tissue for characterization of the lesion by histologic, cytological, and bacteriological analysis (Ayala and Zornosa 1983; Faugere and Malluche 1983). PMSB is also effective for osseous lesions that do not require immediate surgery. Thus, PMSB has many uses:

- Characterization of vertebral collapse: benign (osteoporotic, post traumatic) or pathologic (metabolic, neoplastic) fractures
- Confirmation of tumoral involvement in the vertebral body, paraspinal soft mass and epidural space for spinal lesions; bone, surrounding soft tissues and joint for peripheral lesions
- Characterization of histological type of vertebral metastases in patients with multiple primary neoplasms
- Immunohistochemical and ultrastructural analysis for diagnosis and staging of primary neoplasms
- Confirmation of osteomyelitis, spondylodiscitis, discitis or facet joint infection and bacteriological characterization (Gram stain, culture, sensitivity)
- Assessment of local recurrence or additional lesions in patients with known disease
- Contribution to the assessment of tumor effects in patients receiving chemotherapy or radiotherapy
- Histological proof when integrity of the overlapping tissues must be maintained for the final surgical therapy (limb-salvage procedure)

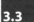
3.3
Contraindications

3.3.1
General Contraindications

- Hemostasis abnormalities: INR >1.5, prothrombin time >1.5 times control, platelets <50,000/mm^3
- Skin infection at the puncture site
- Systemic infection
- Allergy to any medication required for the procedure
- Pregnancy, because of radiation (although MR guidance should be considered as an alternative)

3.3.2
Specific Contraindications

- Spinal cord compression at the puncture level because of potential creation or aggravation of a myelopathy.

- Epidural involvement within the spinal canal due to the extensive bleeding risk with possible spinal cord compression. This is a relative contraindication; in this case the best pathway is usually to pass only through healthy bone structures (by using a transpedicular or costovertebral pathway) thus avoiding any risk of bleeding inside the spinal canal.

tions on coaxial needles but they are all based on the same principle. A larger first needle (10- to 19-gauge) with two parts, an outer cannula and an inner stylet is placed into the lesion. This outer cannula has to be large enough to hold a significant amount of material. The smaller needle is introduced inside the larger one after the inner stylet is removed (Fig. 3.1). Of course, the second needle has to be longer and smaller than the outer cannula. The coaxial technique is quite flexible. It allows several aspirations or core biopsies, drilling, or spring loaded needle biopsy of a soft tissue tumor through a single incision.

3.4
Bone Biopsy Techniques

3.4.1
Coaxial Technique

The coaxial technique can be used under CT or fluoroscopic control. The main principle is to introduce a smaller needle inside a bigger one. The coaxial technique limits the risk of tumoral or infectious dissemination and reduces damage to the surrounding normal tissue. There are many varia-

3.4.2
Tandem Technique

This technique can be performed under fluoroscopic or CT guidance. A 20- to 22-gauge needle is placed in the periphery of the lesion where it is used to deliver local anesthesia to the periosteum and to the subcutaneous layers along the needle route. The biopsy needle is then progressively introduced, as

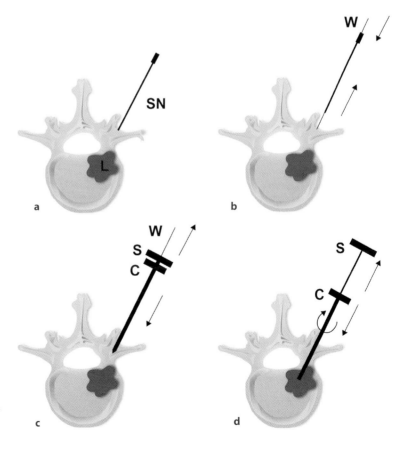

Fig. 3.1a–d. Coaxial needle technique. Example of a Laredo set. **a** The first step is the insertion of a 22- or 20-gauge spinal needle (*SN*) next to the lesion (*L*). **b** Once the position of this first needle is correct, a metallic wire (*W*) is passed into the spinal needle which can be removed. **c** The biopsy needle, composed of an outer cannula (*C*) and an inner stylet (*S*), is passed over the metallic wire (*W*) and inserted in the lesion. Once this needle is correctly placed, the metallic wire is retrieved. **d** The stylet (*S*) is removed and the cannula (*C*) is forced into the lesion by rotation and pressure. The inner biopsy needle can be passed through the outer cannula several times to obtain as many samples as necessary

close to and as parallel as possible to the 22-gauge needle which serves as a guide (Fig. 3.2). The correct position of the final biopsy needle should be regularly checked by CT or fluoroscopy; when the desired location is achieved, the 22-gauge needle can be removed. The coaxial technique is more appropriate for spring loaded needle biopsy of a soft tissue tumor, in which several needle passes are required to ensure a sampling of different regions of the tumors.

3.4.3
Bone Penetration

When there is mild ossification or cortical material surrounding the lesion, penetration by direct percussion with a surgical hammer is necessary, using for example a 14-gauge Ostycut bone biopsy needle. A surgical hammer can ease cortical penetration (Fig. 3.3a).

When there is dense ossification, or dense cortical bone surrounding the lesion, percussion will not work. Direct percussion could damage the needle

tip, and a bent needle, or worse, a broken tip can be very difficult to extract. In these cases penetration by drilling is safer and very elegant (Fig. 3.3b,c). Several drilling systems, usually based on the coaxial principle, are used. We use a Bonopty penetration set, a Laredo set or the Aesculap 2-mm diameter trephine hand drill.

An orthogonal approach to the bone cortex reduces the risk of the needle slipping. Drilling devices, especially when they are eccentric, often slip at the cortical entry point; we usually do a shallow cortical perforation (1–2 mm) with a hammer before drilling. The coaxial technique makes this relatively simple.

3.4.4
Value of Dual Guidance

Bone biopsy is usually performed with a single imaging technique, either fluoroscopy or CT, both of which have advantages and disadvantages.

Fluoroscopy offers multiple planes and direct imaging with real time needle visualization. Its

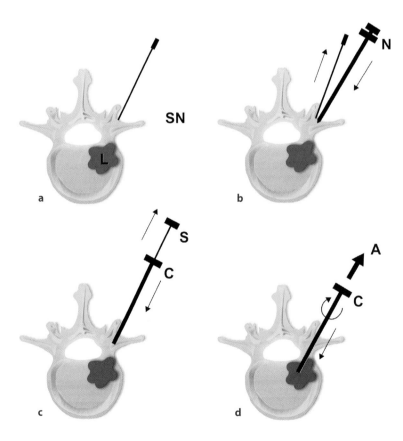

Fig. 3.2a–d. Tandem needle technique. Example of a tandem needle technique. **a** A first 22-gauge spinal needle (*SN*) is introduced next to the lesion (*L*) and its correct position is controlled. **b** The biopsy needle (*N*) is then advanced parallel to the spinal needle until the lesion is reached. **c** Once the needle is inserted into the lesion, the inner stylet (*S*) of the biopsy needle is removed from the cannula (*C*). **d** The cannula (*C*) progresses into the lesion propelled by sufficient pressure and a rotating motion to obtain a larger bone sample. A syringe can be connected to the cannula to aspirate the sample (*A*, *bold arrow*)

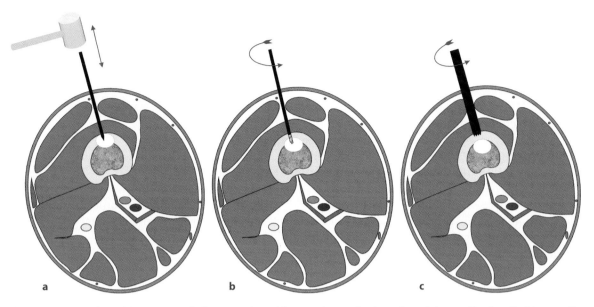

Fig. 3.3a–c. Long bone biopsy. **a** Cortical penetration with an orthogonal orientation of the needle, thus limiting needle slippage. A surgical hammer offers more precise control than manual pressure in thickened cortical bone. Cortical penetration performed by drilling (**b**) with a Bonopty penetration set or (**c**) with a trephine

disadvantages are poor soft-tissue contrast and radiation exposure for both patient and operator. CT is well-suited for precise needle guidance as its high resolution can differentiate bone from surrounding soft tissues, and vascular, neurological, and visceral structures. Its disadvantages are a slight delay in the timing and single (axial) plane of imaging.

To address these concerns, a combination of CT and fluoroscopy for interventional procedures has been recommended (GANGI et al. 1994). For fluoroscopy, a mobile C-arm is used, positioned in front of the CT-gantry. By using a rotating fluoroscope and CT, the structure of interest can be visualized three dimensionally and with exact differentiation of anatomic structures, which in many cases is not possible with fluoroscopy alone. Two mobile monitors are placed in front of the physician, displaying the last CT image and the fluoroscopic image. The operator can switch from CT to fluoroscopy and vice versa at any time (Fig. 3.4).

A percutaneous biopsy usually begins with CT and continues with fluoroscopy. Fluoroscopy is better than CT when real time control is necessary; thus fluoroscopy is preferred for drilling. With dual guidance the operator can switch to CT whenever precise control is required.

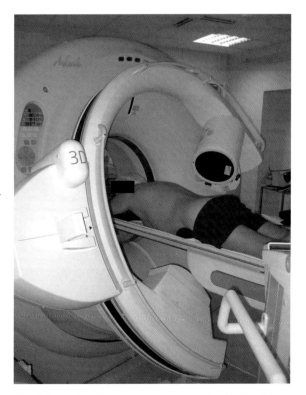

Fig. 3.4. Dual guidance procedure. Combined CT and fluoroscopic guidance. CT allows correct axial needle localization, while fluoroscopy permits real-time monitoring of the needle progression

3.4.5
Interest and Specificity of MR Guidance

The major indication for biopsy under MR guidance is pregnancy, when radiation must be avoided. However, MR imaging shows bone marrow abnormalities precisely (the latter are not visible on CT) thus optimizing target selection. One disadvantage of MR imaging is that the methods used in CT and fluoroscopy to identify the correct level and entry point are not available. Both longitudinal and axial coordinates of the entry point must be directly determined on the patient skin by a specific grid placed successively in the longitudinal and axial axis of the patient (Fig. 3.5a,b). A less specific but still useful method is to point directly at the entry point with a finger (Fig. 3.5c).

3.5
Procedure

3.5.1
Material

- Sterile drapes, tampons
- Hat, mask, sterile gloves
- Povidone-iodine (Betadine®)
- Alcohol scrub
- Syringe: 20 mL with 25-gauge, 1.5-inch needle with 10 mL of 1% lidocaine for local anesthesia
- Protective lead apron for personnel
- Spinal 22-gauge needle
- Selected biopsy system
- Surgical scalpel
- Surgical orthopedic hammer

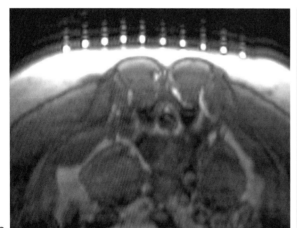

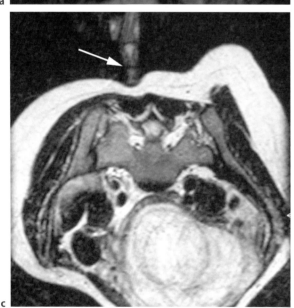

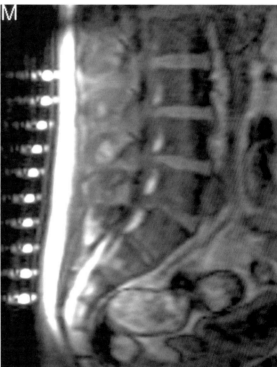

Fig. 3.5a–c. MR guided bone biopsy in a 56-year-old woman with discal hernia. **a** Axial TSE T1-weighted MR image of the lumbar spine shows a specific grid oriented axially allowing the axial axis determination of the cutaneous entry point. **b** Sagittal TSE T1-weighted MR image of the lumbar spine shows a specific grid oriented longitudinally allowing the longitudinal axis determination of the cutaneous entry point. **c** Axial TSE T2-weighted MR image of the pelvis demonstrates direct determination of the correct entry point by the operator pointing with a finger (*arrow*) on the patient's skin during MR acquisition

3.5.2
Medications

Most of these procedures can be performed under local anesthesia (subcutaneous and periosteal), with lidocaine hydrochloride 1%, (Xylocaine®, 1%) with a maximum dose of 300 mg. The skin's subcutaneous layers, muscles and the periosteum are infiltrated by local anesthesia (lidocaine hydrochloride 1%, with maximum dose of 300 mg) with a 22-gauge needle (Fig. 3.6).

Intravenous sedation may be necessary with larger needle sizes (greater than 14-gauge), with painful lesions such as osteoid osteoma or osteoblastoma, and with anxious patients. Midazolam hydrochloride, 50–100 µg/kg IM or IV, with maximal dose of 5 mg is suitable. Painful procedures may be completed with local injection of long acting anesthetics (Ropivacaine chlorhydrate [Naropeine®, 0.2%, 0.75%, 1%], 2.5–3 mg/kg with maximal dose of 200–225 mg).

Atropine should be readily available during spinal procedures to ameliorate possible vasovagal reaction risk (atropine sulfate, 0.25–1 mg IV).

Stronger anesthesia may be necessary with frail or elderly patients, who may find it difficult to collaborate during what can be a difficult and painful procedure. In such cases, an anesthesiologist should be consulted.

3.5.3
Needles

3.5.3.1
Ostycut Biopsy Needle

3.5.3.1.1
Characteristics

The Ostycut biopsy needle is a direct puncture needle (Angiomed-Bard, Karlsruhe, Germany) (Fig. 3.7a). It is minimally invasive and fine and therefore fragile, and it can be dangerously bent or broken inside bone, especially when the needle core is removed. Therefore it is best suited for lytic to mixed or mild condensing lesions. We do not use this needle for very dense bone lesions.

- Size: 13-, 14- and 15-gauge; 100 and 150 mm length
- Diamond-tip stylet, filleted cannula (Fig. 3.7b)

Fig. 3.6a,b. Percutaneous musculoskeletal biopsy. **a** Planning for the needle pathway. **b** Administration of local anesthesia in which the skin's subcutaneous layers, muscles and the periosteum are infiltrated by 1% lidocaine with a 22-gauge needle

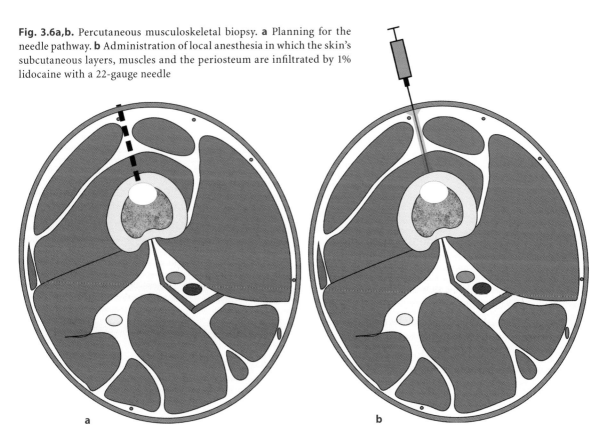

a   b

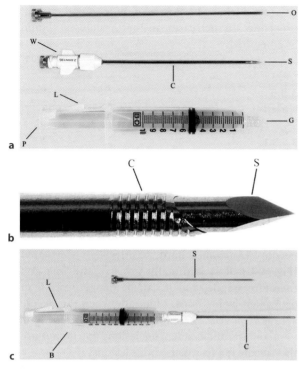

Fig. 3.7a–c. Ostycut Biopsy Needle Set. **a** Ostycut set composed of 13-gauge cannula (*C*) with diamond-tip stylet (*S*) and lateral wings (*W*), 20-mL syringe (*G*) with negative pressure locking device (*L*) connected to the plunger (*P*); blunt-tip obturator (*O*). **b** Magnified view of the diamond-tip of the stylet (*S*) and the filleted cannula tip (*C*). **c** Separation of the inner stylet (*S*) and connection of the syringe to the cannula (*C*); the plunger is withdrawn until the locking device (*L*) stops on the syringe barrel (*B*), ensuring negative pressure inside the syringe

- 20 mL syringe with negative pressure locking device
- Blunt-tip obturator

3.5.3.1.2
Procedure

Following subcutaneous administration of local anesthesia, the needle is inserted through an appropriate skin incision. It is propelled forward with continuous rotation. Bone penetration is achieved manually or by careful percussion using a surgical hammer. The top of the stylet may be hammered to allow cortical penetration or in case of difficult progression in condensed bone. Once in contact with the lesion or the pathologic region to be sampled, the stylet is removed and the 20-mL syringe is connected to the cannula (Fig. 3.7c). Samples are acquired by advancing the needle into the lesion: the syringe is kept in negative pressure by withdrawing the plunger (which may be locked in place) and the cannula advanced within the lesion with continuous rotation. The cannula should not be hammered without the stylet in place.

The system is also rotated during withdrawal, thus keeping the sample inside the cannula. The specimen is expelled from the needle by a dedicated obturator. The aspirated material is sent for cytological examination.

3.5.3.2
Bonopty Penetration Set

3.5.3.2.1
Characteristics

The Bonopty penetration set is a direct puncture needle (RADI Medical Systems, Uppsala, Sweden) (Fig. 3.8a). It is minimally invasive and fine. The cannula should not be hammered without the stylet in place. Bone penetration is achieved manually or by careful percussion using a surgical hammer or especially in dense lesions by using the manual drill. The Bonopty is well suited for lytic or mixed lesions but it is best suited for very condensed lesions, which is how we use it.

- Size: 14-gauge cannula with 15-gauge stylet; 95 mm length
- Diamond-tip stylet (Fig. 3.8b)
- Drill of 15-gauge, 122 mm length (Fig. 3.8b), an additional extended drill is available in 160 mm length

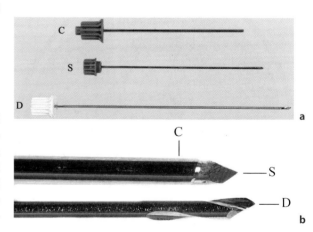

Fig. 3.8a,b. Bonopty biopsy system. **a** Bonopty biopsy system kit composed of 14-gauge cannula (*C*) with 15-gauge diamond-tipped stylet (*S*), 15-gauge drill (*D*). **b** Magnified view of the diamond shaped tip of the inner stylet (*S*) inside the cannula (*C*), and of the 15-gauge drill tip (*D*)

- Depth gauge: adjustable length 0–45 mm, break indicators every 5 mm

3.5.3.2.2
Procedure

The needle is introduced through an appropriate skin incision. The top of the stylet may be hammered to allow cortical penetration. Drilling devices, especially when they are eccentric like the Bonopty drill, often slip at the cortical entry point. Therefore we usually do a short cortical perforation (1–2 mm) using a hammer before drilling; this can be done coaxially by using the diamond shaped inner stylet. The cannula should not be hammered without the stylet in place. The bone is penetrated with the manual drill, especially in dense lesions. The manual drill is a precise tool and can penetrate even very dense bone safely. The drill will produce bone fragments which will obturate the device, so the drill must often be cleaned manually with a scalpel. If these bone fragments are part of the lesion they can be used as samples. The needle is advanced to the margin of the lesion. Once in contact, the stylet or drill is removed and a syringe connected to the cannula. The cannula is advanced within the lesion with continuous rotation.

3.5.3.3
Laredo Needle Set

3.5.3.3.1
Characteristics

There are three different sets (Fig. 3.9a–c):
- Laredo 1000: 11-gauge graduated cannula and diamond-tip 12-gauge stylet, 100 mm length; 12-gauge trephine, 12-gauge obturator
- Laredo 2000: 11-gauge graduated cannula and tapered-tip 12-gauge stylet, 100 mm length; 12-gauge trephine, 12-gauge obturator, 2 mm metallic wire, 18-gauge needle
- Laredo 3000: 11-gauge graduated cannula and cutting tip 12-gauge stylet, 100 mm length, 12 mm metallic wire

These needles are larger and less fragile, but more invasive, than the Bonopty or Ostycut needles. Bone penetration is achieved manually or by percussion using a surgical hammer or especially in dense lesions by using the manual trephine. These needles can be used for lytic or mixed or condensed lesions.

3.5.3.3.2
Procedure

The choice of the type of the tip (tapered or diamond) depends on the nature of the tissue to traverse; the diamond tip is better for lesions with difficult cortical penetration. The coaxial needle is advanced to the proximal margin of the lesion. The blue handle is unlocked and the inner stylet is removed. If drilling is necessary, the trephine may be introduced into the cannula (Fig. 3.9d). A 20-mL syringe is connected to the cannula and a slight continuous negative pressure is maintained which allows for cytologic aspiration with the specimen remaining inside the cannula. The needle progresses by continuous rotation and mild forward advancement; the combination of motions offers efficient retrieval of the sample. The rotating motion is sustained during removal to maintain the specimen inside the cannula. Once retrieved, the obturator is inserted into the cannula to extract the sample.

The Laredo 2000 set may be introduced by direct puncture, or by use of the metal wire (Fig. 3.9e). In the latter case, a Seldinger-like technique is used: installation of the wire next to the lesion through an 18-gauge spinal needle, retrieval of the 18-gauge, introduction of the biopsy device over the wire, retrieval of the wire. The progression of the needle is as previously described.

In case of thick cortices or intense condensation, the Laredo 3000 set should be used. The metal wire is firmly inserted into the cortex and serves as a guide for introducing the outer cannula. Once in contact with the bone, the metallic wire is removed and the inner cutting stylet introduced, and the needle progresses as already described.

3.5.3.4
Surgical Biopsy Set

3.5.3.4.1
Characteristics

The Surgical Biopsy Set (Aesculap, Center Valley, PA, USA) is made of surgical stainless steel (Fig. 3.10):
- Metal handle with locking device
- 10-Gauge cannula
- 11-Gauge trephine
- 11-Gauge spike
- 12-Gauge extracting device
- Obturators of 11- and 12-gauge

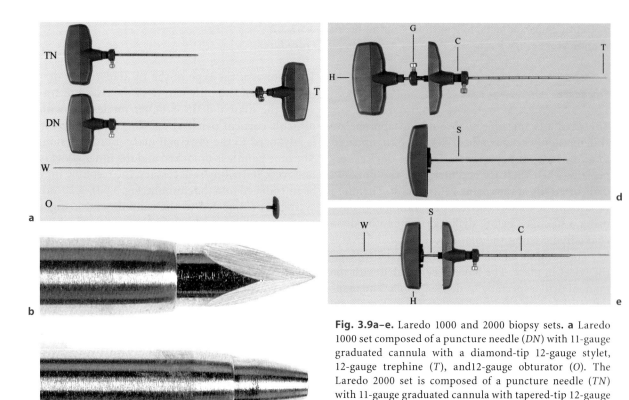

Fig. 3.9a–e. Laredo 1000 and 2000 biopsy sets. **a** Laredo 1000 set composed of a puncture needle (*DN*) with 11-gauge graduated cannula with a diamond-tip 12-gauge stylet, 12-gauge trephine (*T*), and12-gauge obturator (*O*). The Laredo 2000 set is composed of a puncture needle (*TN*) with 11-gauge graduated cannula with tapered-tip 12-gauge stylet, 1-mmmetallic wire (*W*), 12-gauge trephine (*T*), and 12-gauge obturator (*O*). **b** Magnified view of the Laredo 1000 needle with diamond-tip stylet. **c** Magnified view of the Laredo 2000 needle with tapered-tip stylet. **d** Laredo 1000 needle with the handle (*H*) unlocked by a counter-clockwise rotation and the stylet (*S*) is retrieved from the cannula (*C*). When the needle contacts the lesion, a syringe is connected to the cannula which may then be further inserted by continuous rotation and mild pressure. If drilling is necessary, the trephine (*T*) is introduced into the cannula; depth of drilling may be controlled by a depth gauge (*G*). **e** Laredo 2000 biopsy set composed of the metallic wire (*W*) which is first introduced by the Seldinger method through an 18-gauge needle until contact with the bone. The biopsy needle is passed over the wire which can be removed. The needle progression is assured by rotation and forward pressure. If drilling is necessary, the two parts of the handle (*H*) are unlocked and the stylet (*S*) removed from the cannula (*C*) to insert the trephine

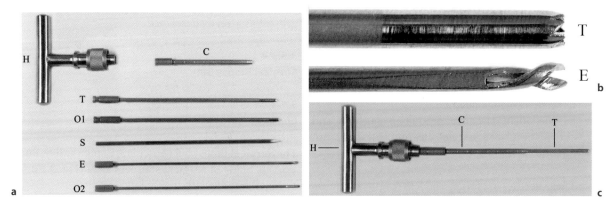

Fig. 3.10a–c. Surgical biopsy set. **a** Surgical biopsy set composed of handle (*H*) with locking device which can support an 11-gauge trephine (*T*); 10-gauge outer cannula (*C*); 11-gauge spike (*S*); 12-gauge special extracting-tipped device (*E*); two obturators of 11 and 12-gauge (*O1*, *O2*). **b** Magnified view of the 11-gauge trephine (*T*) and of the extracting-tipped device (*E*) which allows efficient removal of bone samples. **c** The spike is first firmly inserted into the concerned bone. Then, the 10-gauge outer cannula (*C*) is passed along the spike until it contacts bone. The spike is removed and the selected tool (here the trephine [*T*] mounted on the handle [*H*]) is introduced inside the cannula; several bone biopsies may be obtained using the coaxial principle

3.5.3.4.2
Procedure

The surgical biopsy set is used with a particularly thick cortex or when significant drilling is expected. A well-planned incision is necessary, more so than for the other biopsy devices. The first step of the procedure is the introduction of the 11-gauge spike into the involved bone; a surgical hammer may aid in cortical penetration. The 10-gauge cannula is passed over the spike and advanced into the cortex, then the spike is retrieved. Through the cannula, the trephine mounted on the handle may be passed several times into the lesion with a coaxial technique. The design of the trephine tip permits retention of the sample inside while the trephine is removed. An extracting device with a special tip shape assures that the sample stays in the device while it is removed. Once inside the trephine, bone samples can be extracted with a dedicated blunt tip obturator.

3.5.3.5
Temno Biopsy Device

3.5.3.5.1
Characteristics

The Temno biopsy set (Allegiance Healthcare Corporation, Dublin, OH, USA) contains:
- Spring-loaded mechanism, semiautomatic or automatic (Fig. 3.11a)
- Simple needle or coaxial use (Fig. 3.11b)
- Non-removable notched inner stylet
- Size: 18-, 20- and 22-gauge biopsy device with corresponding 17-, 19- and 21-gauge coaxial needle; 6, 9, 15 and 20 cm length
- These needles are used only for soft tissue samples; they cannot be used alone for bone penetration

3.5.3.5.2
Procedure

Temno biopsy devices are intended for soft tissue tumor and paravertebral soft tissue mass biopsies. When the needle is used directly, it is advanced until it approaches the lesion. The needle is loaded by withdrawing the plunger, which results in a slight retraction of the cannula and the inner stylet (Fig. 3.11c). The plunger is then pushed until resistance is felt; this causes the inner stylet to move forward about 15 mm (Fig. 3.11d). The operator must

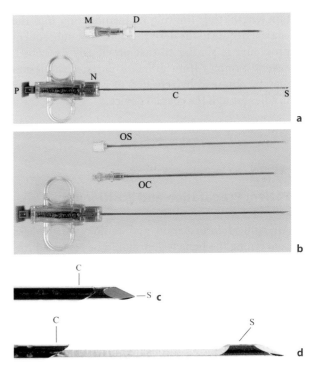

Fig. 3.11a–d. Temno semiautomatic coaxial biopsy system. **a** System is composed of spring-loaded biopsy needle (*N*) with plunger (*P*), with notched inner stylet (*S*) and outer 16-gauge cannula (*C*); and 15-gauge outer coaxial needle (*M*) with depth gauge (*D*). **b** Separation of the outer needle stylet (*OS*) allows insertion of the biopsy needle into the 15-gauge cannula (*OC*). **c** Magnified view of the cannula (*C*) and the stylet (*S*). After pulling back the plunger, both stylet and cannula are retracted, the stylet still covered by the cannula. **d** Slight pressure on the plunger makes the inner stylet (*S*) project beyond the cannula (*C*); further pressure fires the mechanism, with the cannula sliding over the stylet

keep in mind that the inner stylet extends beyond the needle tip and a sufficient margin must be maintained between the needle and normal structures (vessels, nerves, viscera). Once the stylet is in the correct position inside the lesion, supplementary pressure on the plunger unlocks the outer cannula which slides swiftly over the stylet. A sample of material is cut and remains in the notched part of the stylet. Before triggering the needle, the operator must check that the stylet is not bent and that the needle is correctly held with two fingers in the loop and the thumb on the plunger.

When using the coaxial system, one has to first deploy the coaxial needle at the appropriate site. The inner stylet of this outer needle is then removed and replaced with the biopsy needle (Fig. 3.11b). A ring placed on this needle can be blocked at a certain length, thus limiting its introduction into the coaxial needle to the desired depth. The subsequent procedure is similar to that previously described. Several samples from different parts of the lesion may be obtained by repeated passes of the biopsy needle through the coaxial device.

3.6
Patient Preparation and Positioning

All clinical information and radiological images concerning the bone lesion should be reviewed immediately before the procedure. Lesions suspected to be primary malignancies often require different entry points and trajectories than metabolic or infectious lesions. Some primary malignant lesions can be treated by surgical resection after PMSB. In such cases a path for the biopsy should be chosen that allows surgical resection via the same route. Collaboration with clinicians and pathologists before the biopsy is important to define the proper pathway and the amount of tissue to be acquired. The hemostatic profile must be evaluated with laboratory tests before PMSB (blood cell count, platelet count, prothrombin time, INR).

General positioning of the patient is similar to axial and appendicular biopsy. The patient is appropriately positioned on the CT or fluoroscopic table (prone, supine or decubitus; head or feet first). A large area around the entry point is cleansed three times with povidone-iodine and alcohol; the skin surrounding the entry point is covered with sterile drapes (Fig. 3.12). Most biopsies can be performed without general anesthesia. Local anesthesia allows the patient to cooperate, especially in reporting neurological pain if there is nerve impingement, which can facilitate correction of needle position. Local anesthesia of subcutaneous tissue is obtained with lidocaine with a 25-gauge, 1.5-inch needle. Then, local anesthetic is injected all along the needle pathway and in the periosteum. A small skin incision facilitates introduction of the biopsy needle through soft tissues. After the procedure, the skin is cleaned and any residual povidone is removed. The skin incision is covered with an adhesive bandage and the patient advised to keep it dry for at least 48 h. PMSB is normally an outpatient procedure and the patient can be sent home after a short recovery period.

3.7
Needle Biopsy Technique

Needles are selected based on several criteria: whether the lesion is lytic or sclerotic, the type of tissue involved (bone or soft tissue mass), the site of the lesion, and the preference and experience of the operator.

The following indications for needle selection are based on our institutional experience:

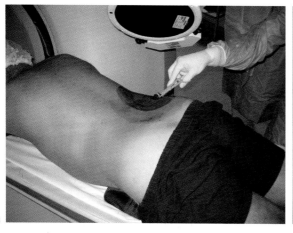
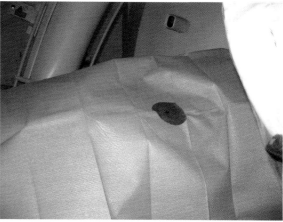

a   b

Fig. 3.12a,b. Installation and preparation of the patient. **a** The patient is comfortably installed on the CT or fluoroscopy table and a large area around the entry point is scrubbed three times. **b** The entry point area is delimited by sterile adhesive drapes. The drapes must be large enough to allow sufficiently sterile conditions and operator comfort

- Lytic lesions, soft tissue tumor: coaxial automatic or semi-automatic spring loaded needles, 14- to 16-gauge (Temno) (SCHWEITZER and DEELY 1993)
- Mild ossification or normal thin cortex surrounding the lesion: 14-gauge Ostycut bone biopsy needle and penetration by surgical hammer (Ostycut, Angiomed-Bard, Karlsruhe, Germany)
- Dense ossification, thick cortex surrounding the lesion, drilling necessary: 14-gauge Bonopty penetration set with drilling device or Laredo needle with 18-gauge trephine

3.8
Examination of Tissue Samples

Solid or semi-solid samples are sent for pathologic examination, completely immersed in formaldehyde solution. Solid and aspiration products may be sent in a sterile tube or directly in the syringe used for aspiration, sealed with a sterile cap. If there is a Pathology Department nearby, immediate pathologic analysis can be obtained from frozen section or by rapid cytologic interpretation, especially if the tumor appears heterogeneous or if treatment is to begin immediately. The blood clots obtained in the sample should not be discarded as they can be embedded in paraffin for histologic study and may provide significant information (AYALA and ZORNOSA 1983). Sampling of sclerotic lesions can retrieve dense sticks of bone. The dense bony material is usually of good value but has to be specially prepared by pathologists using decalcification before coloration.

3.9
Spine Biopsy

For spinal lesions, the preferential order for biopsy is: subcutaneous soft tissue mass, paraspinal soft tissue mass, vertebral bone, epidural mass. The latter should be subject to biopsy only if all other methods have failed to yield a diagnosis.

3.9.1
Lumbar Spine Biopsy

3.9.1.1
Bone Biopsy

3.9.1.1.1
Transpedicular Approach

Fluoroscopic guidance. The transpedicular approach is indicated for the majority of vertebral lesions and is mandatory for lesions that may be cancerous and require surgery (Fig. 3.13a,b). An initial lateral view

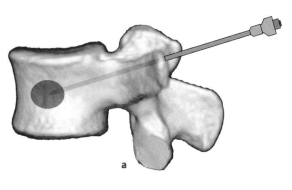

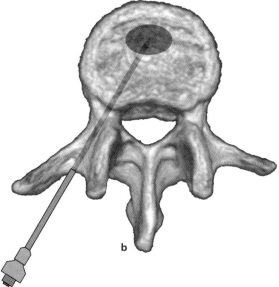

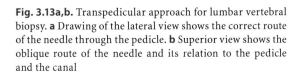

Fig. 3.13a,b. Transpedicular approach for lumbar vertebral biopsy. **a** Drawing of the lateral view shows the correct route of the needle through the pedicle. **b** Superior view shows the oblique route of the needle and its relation to the pedicle and the canal

is obtained to correctly identify the concerned vertebra. Once localized, the vertebra is kept in the center of the field of view while the C-arm is rotated to a direct anteroposterior (AP) view; the pedicle is then seen as a ring. The skin is marked about 4–5 cm laterally to the outer border of the pedicle; this lateral position provides an oblique trajectory through the vertebra. After cutaneous disinfection and administration of local anesthesia (c.f. Sect. 3.5), the needle is introduced into the pedicle through the skin mark. The safe pathway is delineated by the ring defined by the pedicle in the AP projection. By keeping the tip of the needle in this ring, which indicates a pathway between the lateral and medial cortical margins, the operator may be assured of avoiding the spinal canal. Once the needle tip is centered in the pedicle, axial loading via rotation ensures cortical penetration. Care is taken to keep the needle straight during loading, and its progress is closely monitored by alternating AP and lateral views. When the posterior cortical margin is breached, it is felt as a sudden cessation of resistance. Attention is drawn to the conscious and careful avoidance of traversing the lateral and medial cortical margins; easily achieved by keeping the needle tip "in the ring" of the pedicle on AP view (Fig. 3.14a). After the pedicle is completely crossed, the progression of the needle can be monitored solely in the lateral view (Fig. 3.14b).

The needle direction can be very slightly altered by lateral pressure on the needle associated with axial loading, bearing in mind the potential risk of needle breakage. The coaxial technique is the best for lytic vertebral lesions as it allows several biopsies without removing the needle. A major alternative to this procedure consists of rotating the C-arm from 10° to 40° to obtain the classical "Scotty dog" image where the pedicle is represented by the eye of the dog (Fig. 3.15). A mark is made on the skin at the eye level and defines the cutaneous entry point. This procedure allows a more oblique penetration of the needle inside the vertebral body, but presents a significant risk of cortical or canalar penetration.

CT guidance. This is preferred with small lesions that are difficult to identify with fluoroscopy, or when precise needle insertion is required. Axial images obtained at the level of the concerned vertebra help to localize the pedicles. The field of view must be large enough to see both the target and the skin surface. A pertinent slice is selected, where the target and the correct needle route are clearly visible. In most cases no gantry tilt is necessary, but when it is necessary, care must be taken to correctly identify the z-axis of the entry point. The pathway can then be drawn on the CT screen: the route leads to the target by passing into the groove delineated by

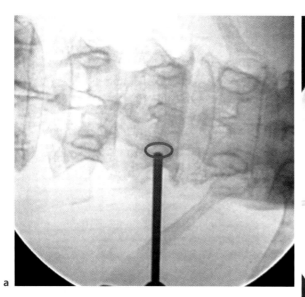
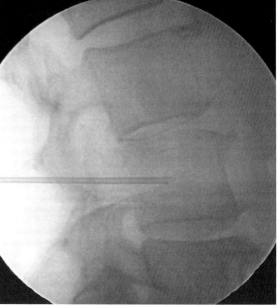

Fig. 3.14a,b. Fluoroscopic-guided transpedicular approach for bone biopsy in a 55-year-old woman with myeloma. **a** Anteroposterior radiograph of the lumbar spine shows "stay in the ring" technique. The pedicle is seen as a closed ring (*red circle*). The needle has to be kept inside this ring, avoiding any trespass of cortical margins and canalar penetration. **b** Lateral radiograph demonstrates the anteroposterior progression is monitored in lateral view. This view can be used alone once the pedicle is completely traversed

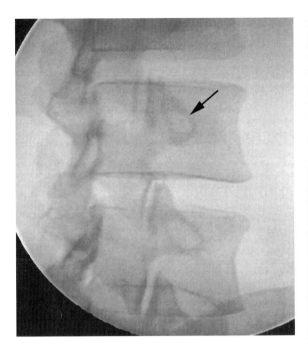

Fig. 3.15. "Scotty dog" view. Oblique radiography shows the pedicle is seen as the eye (*arrow*) of the "Scotty dog". The needle has to be kept in this eye until the pedicle is completely crossed

the transverse process and the articular processes (Fig. 3.16a). The intersection of the pathway and the skin is the entry point. Its vertical position corresponds to the CT z-axis defined on the screen and is shown on the patient's skin by the CT laser light beam. The lateral position may be localized on the patient by two methods: with a radio-opaque graduated grid placed on the skin, or by measuring the distance to the spinous processes line and placing a radio-opaque marker. Once this entry point is defined, the needle may be introduced under CT guidance. The pedicle is penetrated at the level of the transverso-articular groove (Fig. 3.16b). Real-time fluoroscopy is not necessary and sequential, regular CT slices are, in most cases, sufficient to achieve correct needle placement. The procedure is similar to that described in the preceding paragraph.

3.9.1.1.2
Posterolateral Extrapedicular Approach

This approach is specially suited for localized lesions of the lateral portions of the vertebra. CT guidance is used to ensure precision. The pathway is more oblique and the entry point more lateral than in the transpedicular approach and care must be taken

not to puncture a spinal nerve root (Fig. 3.17). The progression must be carried out with continuous communication with the patient so that the needle may be quickly retrieved if inadvertent contact occurs. The cortex is approached tangentially and is often difficult to penetrate. Extra pressure is needed when the needle meets the bone, and there is an increased risk of shearing.

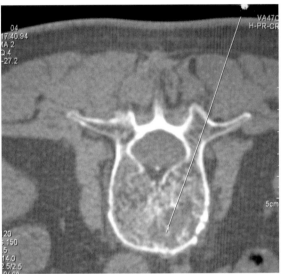

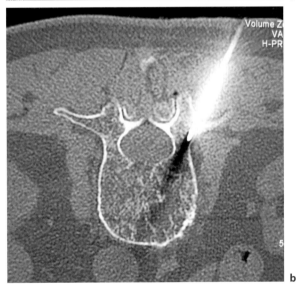

Fig. 3.16a,b. CT-guided transpedicular approach for bone biopsy in a 48-year-old woman with breast cancer. **a** Axial CT scan of the lumbar spine shows determination of the entry point and pathway on the CT screen. The pathway is drawn from the lesion to the skin through the pedicle with an oblique route. The entry point is located on the skin by a radioopaque marker. **b** Axial CT scan shows the introduction of the needle into the transverso-articular groove. Histologic examination revealed bone metastasis

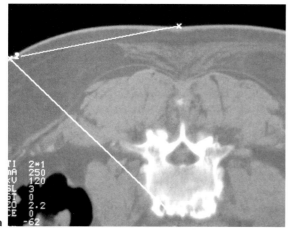

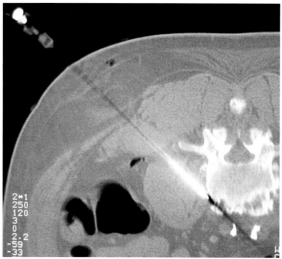

Fig. 3.17a,b. CT-guided extrapedicular approach for bone biopsy in a 68-year-old man with prostate cancer. **a** Axial CT scan of the lumbar spine shows entry point through right paravertebral and iliopsoas muscles. A longer needle is necessary compared to transpedicular biopsy. **b** Axial CT scan shows the introduction of the needle which has to pass through the paravertebral and iliopsoas muscles with a risk of spinal root puncture. Histologic examination revealed bone metastasis

3.9.1.2
Paraspinal Mass Biopsy

The procedures are in general performed under CT guidance which allows better visualization of the soft tissue masses. The majority of paraspinal masses are located in the anterolateral paravertebral area and the preferred pathway runs along the

vertebral body, at the lower part of the foramen so to avoid spinal nerve root puncture (Fig. 3.18a). Posterior masses are often easily reached with a direct puncture (Fig. 3.18b). Almost all needle devices can be used for paraspinal masses biopsies, but 16- to 18-gauge coaxial needles seem most appropriate as multiple samples can be obtained without crossing bony structures.

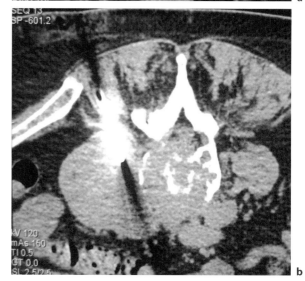

Fig. 3.18a,b. CT-guided paraspinal mass biopsy in a 54-year-old man with suspected septic discitis. **a** Axial CT scan of the lumbar spine shows determination of the entry point and pathway. A posterolateral approach is determined on the CT screen. **b** Axial CT scan shows the L4 paravertebral mass biopsied by a direct route from the skin entry point. Histologic examination revealed septic discitis

3.9.1.3
Posterior Structures Biopsy

Posterior structure biopsies are performed under CT control, because of its singular ability to visualize spinal cord, nerve roots and epidural spaces. These structures must be clearly identified to avoid inadvertent injury and to prevent the formation of an epidural hematoma. Posterior arch biopsies include bone biopsies and synovial articulations or synovial cyst aspirations.

The pathway for posterior bone biopsies must be as tangential as possible, in such a way that the needle does not enter the canal space (Fig. 3.19). This angulation reduces the risk of penetrating the canal if there is a sudden bony rupture or the needle slides. The procedure is similar to the procedure in Section 3.9.1.1.

Diagnostic aspiration of the posterior articular compartment can be performed to exclude articular infection, as well as for therapeutic synovial cyst decompression. MR guidance is an elegant alternative to CT, providing additional information about the surrounding soft tissues. Articular aspiration is performed with 20- to 22-gauge needle introduced by a direct posterior approach (Fig. 3.20). The fluid aspirated is sent for bacteriological examination. Repeat aspirations may be necessary for complete synovial cyst drainage.

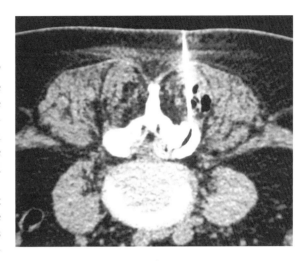

Fig. 3.20. CT-guided synovial cyst aspiration in a 61-year-old man. CT scan of the lumbar spine shows aspiration by needle in the posterior part of the joint

The indication for epidural mass biopsy must be counterbalanced with the significant risk of an epidural hematoma formation, and it is important to warn the orthopedic spinal surgeon of this possible occurrence. An epidural mass should only be biopsied if no other more accessible lesions are present. A smaller caliber needle is preferred; automatic or semi-automatic spring loaded needles must be avoided. Simple syringe aspiration is sufficient in most cases, providing small amounts of material for cytologic examination. The number of samples must be limited to reduce the risk of bleeding.

3.9.1.4
Disc Biopsy

Disc biopsies are indicated to evaluate clinical suspicion of discitis or spondylodiscitis. Fluoroscopic guidance is ideal as it allows real time needle observation and multiplanar visualization.

3.9.1.4.1
Fluoroscopic Guidance

A lateral view is obtained to precisely localize the concerned level. During this fluoroscopic evaluation, the adjacent endplates must be as parallel as possible utilizing the craniocaudal angulation and lateral translation of the C-arm. The C-arm is rotated until the "Scotty dog" appears, and then rotated further until the inferior articular process of the more cranial vertebra (ear of the "Scotty dog") is located

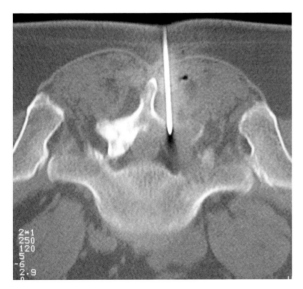

Fig. 3.19. CT-guided posterior arch biopsy in a 72-year-old woman with breast cancer. Axial CT scan of L5 shows the lesion is reached by a direct posterior oblique route. CT guidance allows precise localization of neural structures. Histologic examination revealed bone metastasis

at the center of the disc to puncture (Fig. 3.21). This position will lead to a central puncture of the disc. For a more anterior or posterior puncture, the inferior process has to be placed at the junction between the anterior third and posterior two-thirds or the anterior two-thirds and posterior-third respectively. It is important to remember that for diagnosing spondylodiscitis the sample has to be procured in the anterior part of the disc, as it is more frequently involved than the posterior part. Moreover, the central part of the infected disc is often necrotic with negative yield on bacteriological evaluation.

The needle is introduced through the skin entry point, and oriented to the inferior articular process (ear of the "Scotty dog"). The needle must stay as close as possible to the articular process to avoid puncturing the spinal root which crosses the disc space more anteriorly. Once the articular process is reached, one can induce a slightly craniocaudal orientation to contact the endplate and obtain both disc and bony samples. Contact with the disc is felt as a sudden increase of resistance to further progress, associated with moderate to acute pain expressed by the patient; but, in major infections, the contact can be soft and painless.

The L5–S1 level may be difficult to access, as the iliac crest interposes the trajectory. Craniocaudal angulation of the C-arm is necessary to create a pathway over the superior edge of the iliac crest. The entry point into the disc appears as a triangle delimited by the superior endplate, the superior articular process of the underlying vertebra and the iliac crest (Fig. 3.22). The needle must be kept as close as possible to the articular process to avoid puncturing the spinal root.

In general, large needles (i.e. Ostycut, 14-gauge) are recommended for disc biopsies, as they allow the acquisition of both disc and bony samples. Moreover, disc decompression with large needles appears to be useful for pain and disc infection management (ARYA et al. 1996). In patients with a low pain threshold or excruciating pain, smaller needles, (i.e. 18- to 20-gauge) used coaxially are sufficient for disc samples; bone samples may be deferred. Material is sent for bacteriological examination including culture and Gram stain, and for pathologic examination.

3.9.1.4.2
CT Guidance

Fluoroscopic localization of the correct disc level is followed by selection of CT gantry angle to facilitate an axial image parallel to the disc. The pathway is determined as the direct route from the center of the disc to the skin, tangential to the articular process (Fig. 3.23). As with fluoroscopic guidance, the close

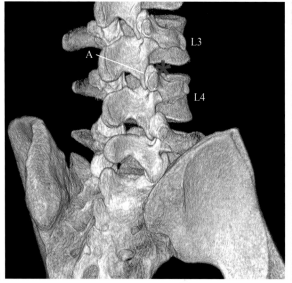
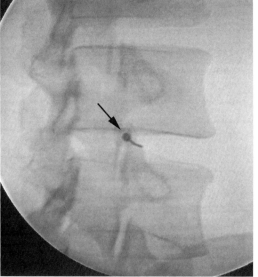

Fig. 3.21a,b. Determination of the target for disc biopsy in a 31-year-old woman with discitis. **a** Three-dimensional view of the lumbar spine shows the spine rotated until the superior articular process of the underlying vertebra (*A*) projects in the middle of the involved disc (here L3–L4). The needle is introduced just next to the articular process (***). **b** The C arm is rotated until the corresponding fluoroscopic view is obtained. The needle (*arrow*) appears as a spot superimposed on the target

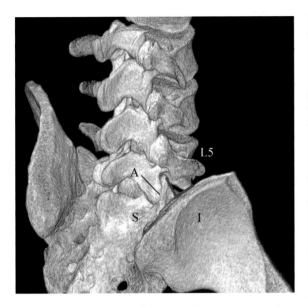

Fig. 3.22. Determination of the target for lumbar L5–S1 disc biopsy. A craniocaudal orientation is given to the C-arm to make the classical "triangle" appear on the three-dimensional view of the lumbar spine. This triangle delimited by the iliac crest (*I*) ahead, the superior articular process (*A*) of S1 (*S*) behind, and the inferior endplate of L5 above, is the target for an L5–S1 disc biopsy

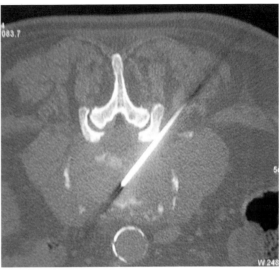

Fig. 3.23. Lumbar disc biopsy under CT guidance in a 75-year-old woman. Axial CT scan of the lumbar spine shows an adequate slice parallel to the disc is selected. The entry point is determined by drawing a line from the disc region to biopsy tangentially to the articular process. The needle is slowly inserted into the disc after contacting the articular process, thus avoiding a spinal root puncture. Histologic examination revealed septic discitis

proximity of the needle pathway to the articular processes greatly reduces the risk of puncturing the spinal nerve root. The z-axis of the entry is determined on the patient with the laser light beam, and the lateral position by use of a radio-opaque grid or marker (c.f. Sect. 3.8). Major gantry angulation is sometimes necessary, especially for L5–S1 level biopsy. Dual guidance can be very helpful in such circumstances (c.f. Sect. 3.7.1). Needle selection and insertion are similar to those described in the preceding fluoroscopic guidance section.

3.9.2
Thoracic Spine Biopsy

3.9.2.1
Bone Biopsy

3.9.2.1.1
Transpedicular Approach

The transpedicular approach is almost exclusively performed under CT guidance (Fig. 3.24). CT provides better visualization of pleural structures, reducing the risk of complications. Thoracic vertebra

pedicles are often small and susceptible to fracture risk and there is little opportunity to correct the trajectory of the needle. This approach is indicated for massive lesions involving a great part of the vertebra or for lesions located next to the pedicle. The transpedicular approach is mandatory for lesions that may be cancerous and require surgery.

The needle size must correspond to the pedicle; in general 13- to 16-gauge needles are the largest practical size. Both fluoroscopic and CT guidance are similar to those described for lumbar spine biopsy.

3.9.2.1.2
Extrapedicular Approach

The extrapedicular approach is the preferred technique for thoracic spine biopsy. CT and fluoroscopic guidance are both suitable. The use of larger needles than in the transpedicular approach is possible and the trajectory can be modified, but the pathway through paraspinal tissues is longer than in the transpedicular approach.

Costovertebral approach. This must be preferred for thoracic spine biopsy whenever possible. It is indicated in almost all vertebral lesions, especially an-

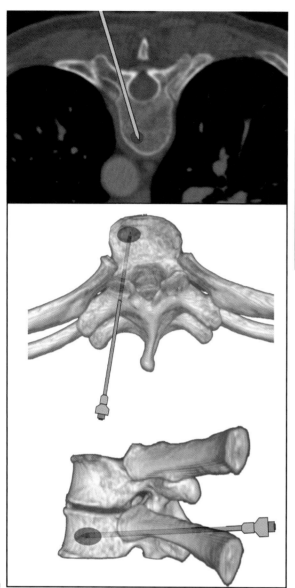

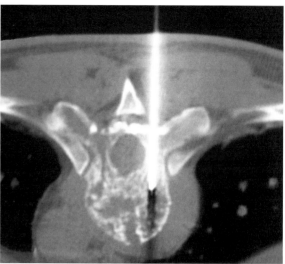

Fig. 3.24a,b. Transpedicular approach for thoracic spine biopsy in a 44-year-old man with lung cancer. **a** Axial CT scan and drawings show the needle transverses the pedicle; a slightly oblique trajectory is often necessary to access central lesions. This approach can be difficult in the thoracic level because of the relative tightness of the thoracic pedicles. **b** Axial CT scan shows the transpedicular approach of the needle, parallel to the pedicle axis. Histologic examination revealed bone metastasis

terior and anterolateral. The needle is introduced between the pedicle and the head of the adjacent rib through an oblique route (Fig. 3.25a). The patient is prone and with fluoroscopy a lateral view is obtained to localize the involved level. The C-arm is then rotated until the pedicle appears as a ring and the articular processes are located at the middle of the disc space. The posterior pleura can be identified as the "pleural line", external to the projection of the head of the rib. The correct pathway is between the pedicle and the rib, at the superior part of the endplate (Fig. 3.25b,c). Great care must be exercised not to cross the pleural line; as long as the needle stays

medial to this pleural line, no pleural transgression will occur. Needle progression is monitored with this fluoroscopic angulation until the vertebra is reached following which repeated AP and lateral views are utilized. Dual guidance (c.f. Sect. 3.8) is useful in this instance; regular CT image acquisition confirms the correct needle position. Under CT guidance, the pathway to the target is determined between the head of the rib and the pedicle after selection of the correct level (Fig. 3.26). The entry point is defined with a radio-opaque grid or marker (c.f. Sect. 3.7.1.1). Needle progression is monitored by successive CT slices. Fluoroscopic CT is rarely necessary.

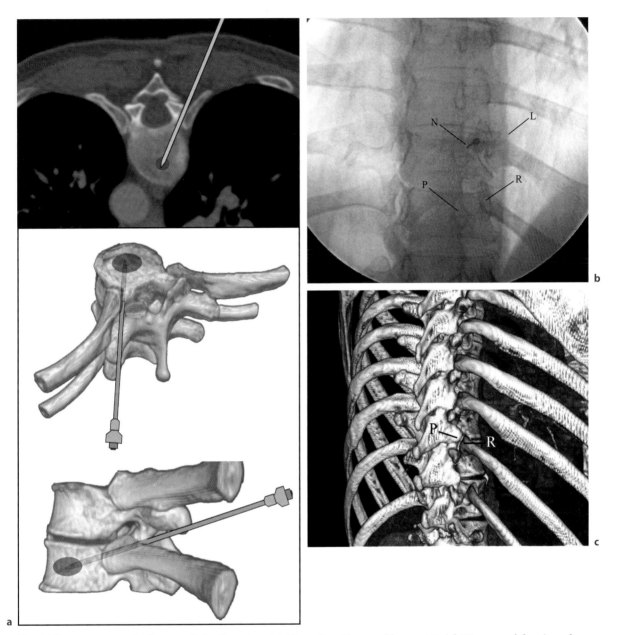

Fig. 3.25a–c. Costovertebral approach for thoracic spine biopsy in a 58-year-old man. **a** Axial CT scan and drawings show the needle passes between the head of the rib and the pedicle, under the transverse process, at the level of the posterior joint. **b** Fluoroscopic view of the thoracic spine demonstrates the route of the needle (*N*) is circumscribed by the pedicle (*P*) and the head of the rib (*R*); the pleural line (*L*) should never be trespassed. **c** Three-dimensional CT view of the thoracic spine better shows the correct pathway between the pedicle (*P*) and the rib (*R*)

Costotransversal approach. This is performed exclusively under CT guidance, as it presents a major risk of pleural injury. The indications for this approach are similar to those for the costovertebral approach. The pathway corresponds to an oblique trajectory between the transverse process and the posterior part of the corresponding rib (Fig. 3.27). Frequent CT images are mandatory as the needle passes very close to the pleural line; anterior needle slippage through the pleural space is relatively limited anteriorly by the tubercle of the rib, while posterior slippage through the spinal canal is limited by the transverse process. The determination of the entry point is as previously described.

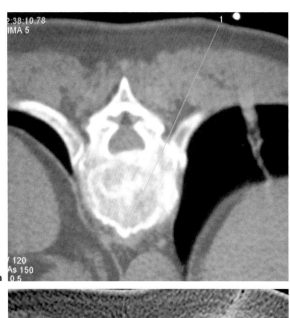
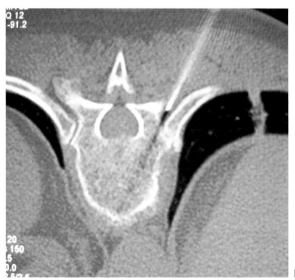
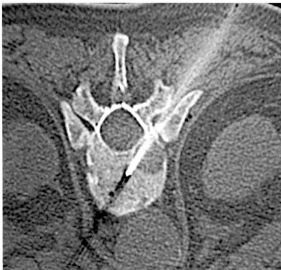

Fig. 3.26a–c. CT-guided costovertebral approach for thoracic vertebral biopsy in a 57-year-old woman with breast cancer. **a** Axial CT scan of the thoracic spine shows the route passes between the pedicle and the head of the rib, at the level of the posterior joint, with an oblique angulation. **b** Axial CT scan shows the introduction of the spinal needle and anesthesia of the periosteum and of the paraspinal muscles. **c** Axial CT scan demonstrates that a pathway between the head of the rib and the pedicle will avoid pleural and canalar injuries. An oblique angulation of the needle during the introduction allows biopsy of central lesions. Histologic examination revealed bone metastasis

3.9.2.2
Paraspinal and Posterior Structures Biopsy

Biopsies of posterior structures at the thoracic level are similar to those in the lumbar level. Thoracic paraspinal masses are reached by an intercostal approach and a pleural separation from parietal structures may be performed (as previously described) to allow for safer introduction of the needle.

3.9.2.3
Disc Biopsy

For fluoroscopic guidance, the positioning is similar to the thoracic vertebral biopsy; the C-arm is ro-tated to obtain the same configuration as previously described. The entry point is located at the level of the disc, between the superior articular process of the underlying vertebra and the posterior part of the corresponding rib. Again, care must be taken not to cross the pleural line, thus avoiding pleural penetration (Fig. 3.25b,c). Needle progression is monitored by alternating lateral and AP views (Fig. 3.28).

Under CT guidance, the route is a costovertebral approach between the rib and the pedicle at the level of the disc concerned (Fig. 3.29). The progression of the needle must be watched carefully to avoid neural puncture.

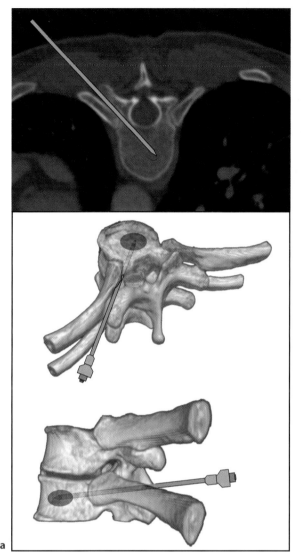

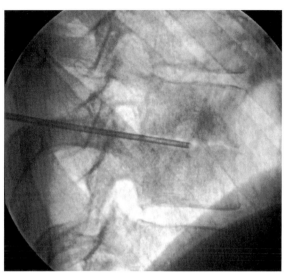

Fig. 3.28. Thoracic disc biopsy in a 78-year-old woman. Lateral fluoroscopic view shows a costovertebral approach of T10–11 disc biopsy. The slightly oblique trajectory of the needle permits both disc and vertebral endplate bone sampling. Histologic examination revealed septic discitis

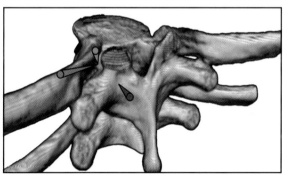

Fig. 3.27a,b. Costotransversal approach for thoracic biopsy in a 48-year-old man. **a** Axial CT scan and drawings show the needle transverses the costotransverse joint between the transverse process and the rib at the level of the rib tubercle. **b** Three-dimensional view of thoracic spine shows the different approaches for biopsy with a *blue arrow* for the costotransversal approach, *green arrow* for the costovertebral approach, and *red arrow* for the transpedicular approach

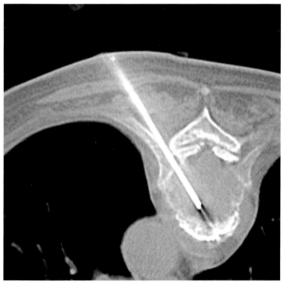

Fig. 3.29. CT-guided thoracic disc biopsy in a 43-year-old woman with discitis. Axial CT scan of the thoracic spine shows the pathway runs between the head of the rib and the articular processes, at the level of the posterior joints. An adequate slice parallel to the disc must be selected for the lumbar spine

3.9.3
Cervical Spine Biopsy

All radiological, clinical and biological complementary information must be thoroughly discussed with clinicians before performing any cervical biopsy. Cervical biopsies should be performed only if no other investigation can provide a definitive diagnosis. Complications are more likely to occur at the cervical level than in the thoracic and lumbar levels as there is a higher density of vascular, neurological and visceral structures.

3.9.3.1
Vertebral and Disc Biopsy

The anterolateral approach is the preferred route for biopsies of the anterior structures. CT is the guidance modality of choice, although fluoroscopic guidance is possible and widely used. The major drawback of this approach is the interposition of the carotid artery which lies under the sternocleidomastoid muscle. The artery has to be posteriorly displaced, manually by the operator, and kept in this position until the tip of the needle has overcome it. The needle is introduced at the anterior part of the sternocleidomastoid muscle, just in front of the operator's hand displacing the carotid artery (Fig. 3.30). The longitudinal level of the target (vertebra or disc) has been previously determined by CT examination and marked on the patient skin. Injection of contrast medium during screening allows visualization of the vascular structures and is recommended.

Anterolateral access to the upper vertebras (C1, C2 and C3) is often difficult, and these levels may be reached by a transoral approach, through the pharynx, under general anesthesia (Fig. 3.31).

Vertebral bodies and discs are generally biopsied with a 16- to 20-gauge coaxial needle allowing multiple samples and a relatively reduced bleeding risk. Smaller caliber needles (20- or 22-gauge) may be sufficient for paraspinal masses.

3.9.3.2
Posterior Arch

Posterior elements (articular processes, laminae, spinous processes, paraspinal posterior masses)

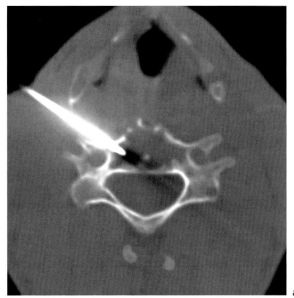

a

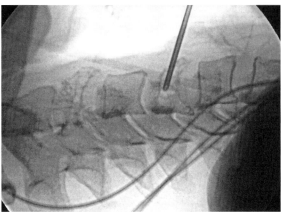

b

Fig. 3.30a,b. Cervical spine biopsy in a 28-year-old man. **a** Axial CT scan shows the classic anterolateral route for cervical spine biopsy, here of C5. The internal carotid artery is moved manually during needle introduction. Once the ICA level is passed, regular controls can assure the absence of vertebral artery puncture. **b** Lateral fluoroscopic view shows the needle within the C5 body. Histologic examination revealed vertebral hemangioma

are easily accessible by a posterior or posterolateral approach. CT guidance is recommended only to ensure the absence of canalar penetration, as no major vascular or peripheral neurological structures are threatened with this approach.

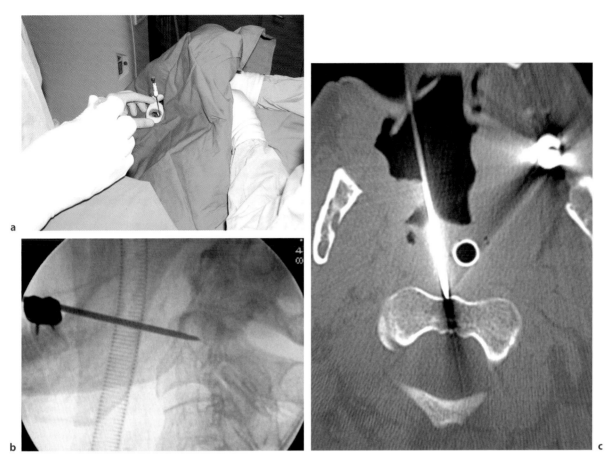

Fig. 3.31a–c. Transoral upper cervical spine biopsy in a 57-year-old woman with breast cancer. **a** Installation of the patient for transoral upper cervical spine biopsy. A Guedel cannula is placed in the patient's mouth through a perforated drape. The hypopharynx is sprayed with lidocaine, and scrubbed with povidone. **b** Lateral fluoroscopic view shows the odontoid lesion reached by transoral approach. **c** Axial CT scan shows the needle reaches the odontoid after passing through the pharynx muscles. Histologic examination revealed bone metastasis

3.10
Appendicular Skeleton Biopsy

PMSB of appendicular bone lesions are mostly performed under CT guidance, which allows identification of surrounding soft tissue involvement and of adjacent vascular, neurological and musculo-ligamentous structures. Lesions of superficial bones such as ribs, clavicles or sacroiliac joints can be reached under fluoroscopic guidance, as no major vascular or neurological elements lie between them and the skin entry point.

To obtain representative samples, the less mineralized portion of the lesion with the more aggressive aspect should be the target of the biopsy (BICKELS et al. 2001). Moreover, the more calcified areas are the more differentiated sites.

3.10.1
Flat Bones

For flat bones, the preferred approach is oblique with 30° to 60° angulation (Fig. 3.32). This tangential route reduces the risk of damage to underlying structures by limiting the possibility of direct penetration if the bone ruptures suddenly or the needle slips (Fig. 3.33). The needle is more likely to slip with such an oblique approach than with a strictly orthogonal approach and hence the needle must be introduced very cautiously.

CT guidance is mandatory for skull biopsy, as direct and precise visualization of the needle position and its relations with epidural spaces and parenchymal surface is necessary during the whole procedure (Fig. 3.34).

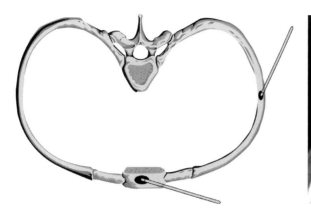

Fig. 3.32. Flat bones biopsy approach. Correct oblique approaches for sternum and rib biopsy. This oblique route is more secure than a direct route because pleural penetration is limited in case of needle shearing

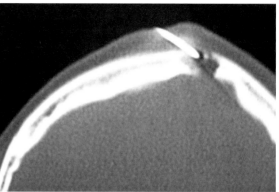

Fig. 3.34. Skull biopsy in a 21-year-old man. Axial CT scan shows the oblique trajectory during the skull biopsy which is mandatory to avoid meningal or parenchymal lesions. Histologic examination revealed eosinophilic granuloma

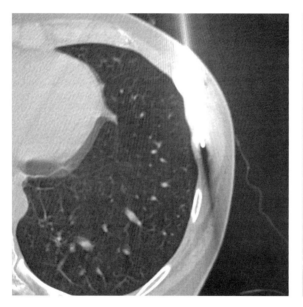

Fig. 3.33. Rib biopsy in a 71-year-old man with lung cancer. Axial CT scan of the thorax shows the tangential trajectory of the left 6th rib biopsy. A parenchymal window allows direct visualization of any pleural penetration. Histologic examination revealed bone metastasis

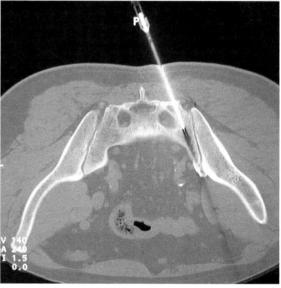

Fig. 3.35. CT-guided sacral biopsy in a 69-year-old man with lung cancer. Axial CT scan shows the needle within the lytic lesion of the sacrum. The posterior oblique approach is recommended, with a safe distance maintained from the sacral foramen. Histologic examination revealed bone metastasis

3.10.2
Pelvis

Needle biopsy is particularly useful at this site since tumors can be reached without complex surgery and the biopsy can be easily repeated.

The majority of pelvic lesions have specific, safe approaches: sacral lesions via a posterior route avoiding the sacral canal and nerves (Fig. 3.35); acetabular lesions by a direct anterior or posterior path, depending on the site of the lesions (Figs. 3.36 and 3.37). Iliac wings lesions are, whenever possible, reached by a trans-osseous approach which avoids any muscular involvement (Figs. 3.38 and 3.39). However, for unreachable lesions (distal lesions), the shorter trans-muscular route is preferred.

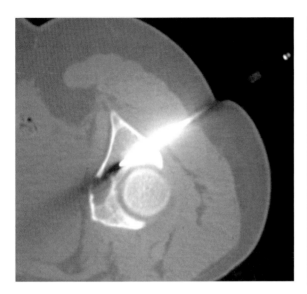

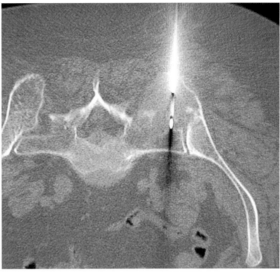

Fig. 3.36. CT-guided acetabular biopsy in a 17-year-old man. Axial CT scan shows the needle within the lytic lesion of the posterior wall of the left acetabulum. A posterior approach was chosen due to the presence of the femoral neurovascular structures located anteriorly. The sciatic nerve must be identified and avoided. Histologic examination revealed eosinophilic granuloma

Fig. 3.38. CT-guided iliac wing biopsy in a 75-year-old woman with breast cancer. Axial CT scan shows the 16-gauge semi-automatic spring-loaded needle within the lytic lesion of the posterior aspect of the left iliac bone. The needle is armed and the stylet is visible inside the lesion. Histologic examination revealed bone metastasis

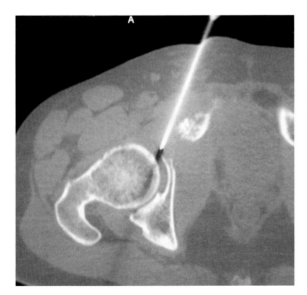

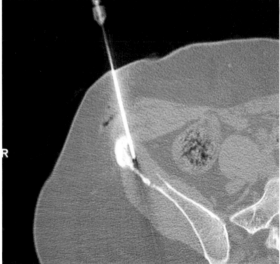

Fig. 3.39. CT-guided iliac wing biopsy in a 58-year-old man with colon cancer. Axial CT scan shows the needle within the lytic lesion of the distal third of the right iliac wing. The trajectory to the bone must be as short as possible, and ideally passes through the wing longitudinally to reach the lesion. In this case, the entry point was chosen at the level of the anterior superior iliac spine. Histologic examination revealed bone metastasis

Fig. 3.37. CT-guided acetabular biopsy in a 47-year-old man with colon cancer. Axial CT scan shows the needle within the lytic lesion of the anterior column of the right acetabulum. The anterior location allows an oblique anterior approach far from the femoral vessels. Histologic examination revealed bone metastasis

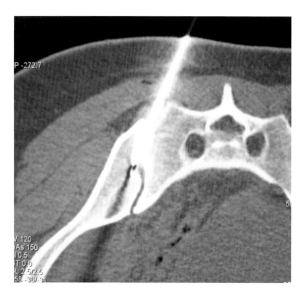

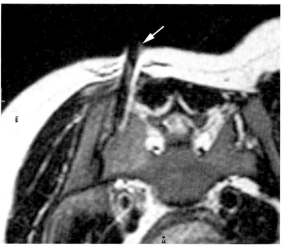

Fig. 3.40. CT-guided sacroiliac joint biopsy in a 38-year-old woman with sacroiliitis. Axial CT scan shows the needle within the right sacroiliac joint. The classical approach is posterior and oblique in the axis of the joint. Histologic examination revealed infectious sacroiliitis

Fig. 3.41. MR imaging-guided sacroiliac joint biopsy in a 26-year-old pregnant woman with suspected streptococcus sacroiliitis. Axial FSE T2-weighted MR image shows the non-magnetic needle (*arrow*) within the left sacroiliac joint following a similar oblique trajectory. Histologic examination revealed infectious sacroiliitis

Biopsies of the sacroiliac joints should take a direct oblique posterior approach (Figs. 3.40 and 3.41).

3.10.3
Upper and Lower Limbs

3.10.3.1
Compartmental Anatomy and Consequences

Two rules determine the needle pathway: avoid neurological and vascular structures and stay in the anatomical compartment with the lesion. The extremities present different compartments separated by fasciae and aponeurosis (Figs. 3.42 and 3.43) (ANDERSON et al. 1999; BICKELS et al. 2001). The route of the biopsy needle must cross only compartments involved with the lesion and avoid contaminating uninvolved compartments. This is particularly important with primary bone tumors: a lesion which extends beyond the limit of its original compartment, called an extracompartmental lesion, would be treated by a wider resection than a strictly intracompartmental lesion (TOOMAYAN et al. 2005). By staying in the involved compartment when performing the biopsy, one avoids the possibility of transforming an intracompartmental lesion into an extracompartmental lesion by disseminating cells along the tract (Figs. 3.42 and 3.43) (ANDERSON et al. 1999; TOOMAYAN et al. 2005). If a single-compartment procedure is not possible, the shorter route to the lesion must be preferred, minimizing tissue injury during needle passage. The entry point of the biopsy can be tattooed on the skin with permanent ink in case surgery is later performed.

3.10.3.2
Classical Approaches

The cutaneous penetration point must be chosen so as not to compromise an eventual surgical procedure, especially a limb-salvage procedure, and it is mandatory that the needle pathway and entry point be completely resectable with the lesion (BICKELS et al. 2001). While strictly avoiding the uninvolved compartments, the needle entry point and route must be similar to the classical oncologic surgical incisions (BICKELS et al. 2001). The following approaches are recommended, but it is evident that the biopsy route must be adapted to the site of the lesion. For example, a lateral lesion should be biopsied by the shortest lateral approach; even if the corresponding classical surgical approach is medial. In such cases, the biopsy route should be discussed with the orthopedic surgeon prior to the biopsy, and

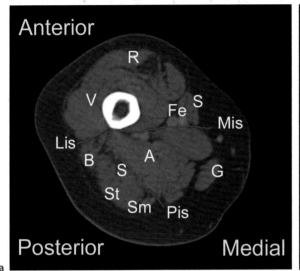

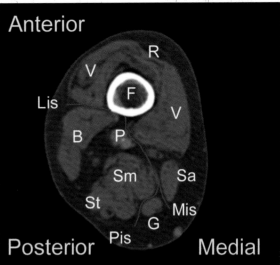

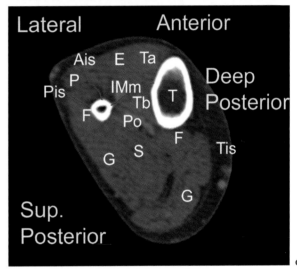

Fig. 3.42a–c. Compartmental anatomy of the lower extremity. **a** Drawing shows the compartmental anatomy of the upper thigh composed of three compartments. Anterior compartment limited by the lateral (*Lis*) and medial (*Mis*) intermuscular septa, containing the rectus femoris (*R*), the vastus muscles (*V*), the sartorius (*Sa*) and the femoral pedicle (*Fe*). Posterior compartment limited by the lateral (*Lis*) and posterior (*Pis*) intermuscular septa, containing the biceps femoris (*B*), the semi-tendinous muscle (*St*), the semi-membranous muscle (*Sm*), and the sciatic nerve (*S*). Medial compartment limited by the medial (*Mis*) and posterior (*Pis*) intermuscular septa, containing the adductor muscles (*A*) and the gracilis (*G*). **b** Compartmental anatomy of the lower thigh, also composed of three compartments. The medial compartment contains only the gracilis muscle at this level; in the posterior compartment, the femoral pedicle becomes the popliteal pedicle (*P*), behind the femur (*F*), and the sciatic nerve divides into tibial and peroneal nerves. **c** Compartmental anatomy of the mid-lower leg composed of four compartments. Anterior compartment limited by the anterior intermuscular septum (*Ais*) and the interosseous membrane (*IMm*), containing the tibialis anterior (*TA*), extensor hallucis longus and extensor digitorum longus (*E*). Lateral compartment limited by the anterior intermuscular septum (*Ais*) and lateral intermuscular septum (*Lis*), containing the peroneus longus and brevis (*P*). Deep posterior compartment limited by the fibula (*F*), the tibia (*T*), and interosseous membrane (*IMm*) containing the tibialis posterior (*TP*), flexor hallucis longus and flexor digitorum longus (*F*). The peroneal artery and vein (*Po*) are located laterally in this compartment. Superficial posterior compartment, separated from the deep posterior compartment by the transverse intermuscular septum (*Tis*), containing the gastrocnemius (*G*) and soleus (*S*) muscles

the entry point clearly described. Joint penetration should be avoided as much as possible, as capsular involvement may lead to a total joint excision.

3.10.3.2.1
Shoulder

The approach is anterior through the anterior third of the deltoid muscle. It is absolutely necessary to avoid penetrating the pectoralis major muscle, as it is necessary for optimal joint reconstruction (Fig. 3.44).

3.10.3.2.2
Femur

Proximal femur. The classical oncologic route is posterolateral (Figs. 3.45 and 3.46) through the vastus

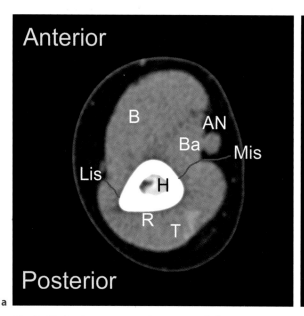 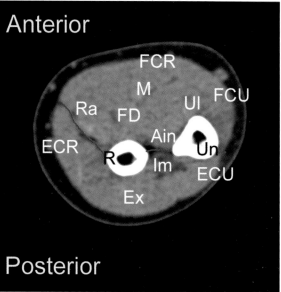

a   b

Fig. 3.43a,b. Compartmental anatomy of the upper extremity. **a** Compartmental anatomy of the arm composed of two compartments delimited by the lateral (*Lis*) and medial intermuscular septa (*Mis*) connected to the humerus (*H*). Anterior compartment: biceps brachii (*B*), brachialis (*Ba*), brachial artery and vein (*A*), ulnar and median nerve (*N*). Posterior compartment: triceps brachii (*T*), radial nerve (*R*). **b** Compartmental anatomy of the forearm composed of two compartments separated by the interosseous membrane (*Im*) joining the ulna (*Un*) and the radius (*R*). Anterior compartment: flexor digitorum profundus and superficialis (*FD*), flexor carpi ulnaris (*FCU*), flexor carpi radialis (*FCR*), median nerve (*M*), ulnar nerve (*Ul*), radial artery and superficial radial nerve (*Ra*), anterior interosseous neurovascular pedicle (*Ain*); posterior compartment: extensor digitorum, and extensors pollicis brevis and longus (*Ex*), extensors carpi radialis (*ECR*), extensor carpi ulnaris (*ECU*)

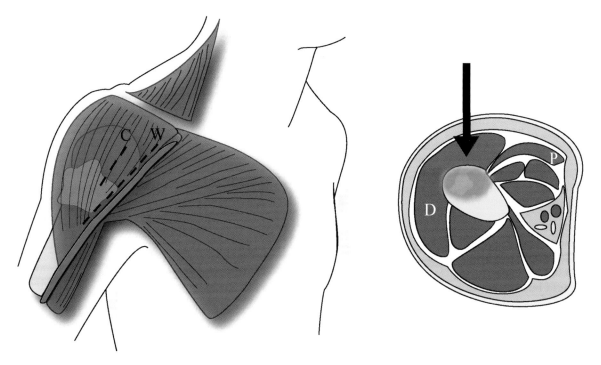

Fig. 3.44. Classical surgical approach for proximal humeral lesions. Drawings show the incision (*C*) is made through the deltoid (*D*) which is resected in almost all primary tumors. An incision through the deltopectoral groove is prohibited (*W*) as this would require pectoralis major (*P*) resection

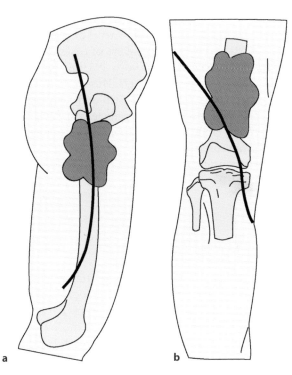

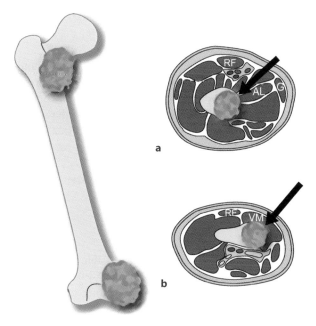

Fig. 3.47a,b. Medial femoral lesions. Drawings show medial approaches for (**a**) proximal and (**b**) distal medial femoral lesions. Rectus femoris (*RF*), gracilis (*G*), adductor longus (*AL*), vastus medialis (*VM*)

Fig. 3.45a,b. Classical surgical approach for proximal femoral lesions. Drawings show the approach is (**a**) posterior or postero-lateral and could be (**b**) extended anteriorly or medially in case of complete femur resection or medial involvement. The recommended biopsy approach is thus lateral through the vastus lateralis

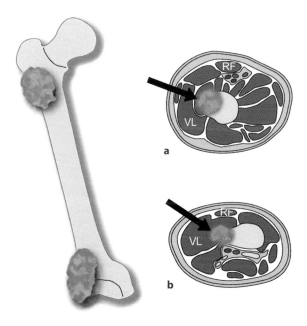

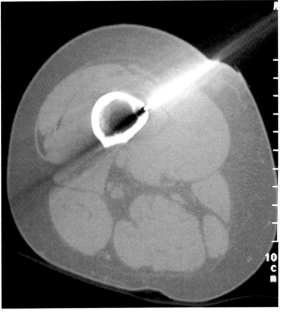

Fig. 3.46a,b. Lateral femoral lesions. Drawings show lateral approaches for (**a**) proximal and (**b**) distal lateral femoral lesions. Rectus femoris (*RF*), vastus lateralis (*VL*)

Fig. 3.48. CT-guided proximal femoral biopsy in a 25-year-old woman. Axial CT scan shows a medial approach of the medial femoral cortical lesion, avoiding penetration of the rectus femoris. Histologic examination revealed osteoid osteoma

lateralis. If that is not possible, a medial approach is possible through the adductor longus (Figs. 3.47 and 3.48).

Distal femur. The classical oncologic route is medial (Figs. 3.47, 3.49 and 3.50) through the vastus medialis for femoral lesions. If the medial route is contraindicated, a lateral approach through the vastus lateralis is an alternative (Fig. 3.46). An anterior approach through the rectus femoris is prohibited because the muscle is needed for optimal joint reconstruction if joint excision is necessary.

3.10.3.2.3
Tibia

The route has to be as medial as possible to follow the surgical oncologic approach (Fig. 3.49): anteromedial directly for medial lesions or anterior through the tibialis anterior for lateral lesions (Figs. 3.51 and 3.52).

Results

It has been widely proven that PMSB is an available and cost-effective procedure to obtain pathological or bacteriological diagnosis of musculoskeletal lesions. The literature reports accuracy similar and even superior to the classical surgical biopsy techniques: needle core biopsy (NCB) is described as accurate in 66%–100% of cases (DeSantos et al. 1978; Murphy 1983; Fraser-Hill and Renfrew 1992;

Ayala et al. 1995; Logan et al. 1996; Skrzynski et al. 1996; Dupuy et al. 1998; Yao et al. 1999; Hau et al. 2002) and FNA in 61%–90% of cases (Moore et al. 1979; Ayala and Zornosa 1983; El-Khoury et al. 1983; Layfield et al. 1993; Dupuy et al. 1998; Hau et al. 2002). Combining NCB and FNA seems to increase the specificity and reduce false negatives (White LM et al. 1996). Negative biopsies must always be interpreted carefully and repeated if there is reason to consider them unrepresentative (Berning et al. 1996).

3.11.1
General Results

It appears that PMSB is particularly effective for the diagnosis of metastatic lesions, with reported results from 82%–100% (Mink 1986; Fraser-Hill and Renfrew 1992; Kattapuram et al. 1992; Skrzynski et al. 1996; Dupuy et al. 1998). Best candidates are patients with one known lesion and another that is thought to be a metastasis (Fraser-Hill and Renfrew 1992), because a significant proportion of the second lesions may not to be metastatic (Mink 1986; Berning et al. 1996). PMSB is of lesser effectiveness with primary malignant tumors, with results reported from 74% to 93% (Fraser-Hill and Renfrew 1992; Logan et al. 1996; Skrzynski et al. 1996; Yao et al. 1999), but still similar or only slightly inferior to surgical biopsy results. For diagnosis of malignant tumors, PMSB is efficient for adults and children (Hussain et al. 2001). It should be kept in mind that the heterogeneous constitution of primitive bone tumors can lead to false negative results

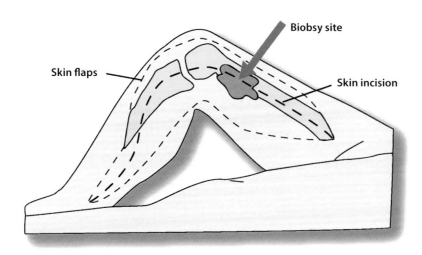

Fig. 3.49. Surgical oncologic approach for distal femoral and proximal tibial lesions at the knee. The approach is medial, offering optimal visualization of the neurovascular bundle. Percutaneous biopsies of regional lesions must be made through this medial approach as often as possible, reducing the necessity of extensive resection. Careful attention is required not to injure the neurovascular structures

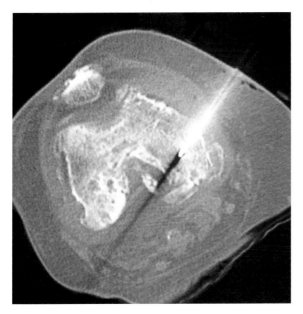

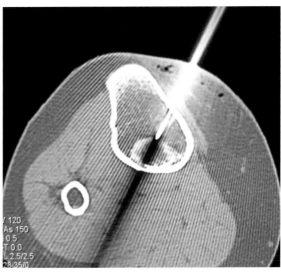

Fig. 3.52. CT-guided biopsy of a posteromedial tibial lesion in a 33-year-old man. Axial CT scan shows the anteromedial approach allows minimal muscular trespassing and avoids transgression of the uninvolved compartments. Histologic examination revealed chondroma

Fig. 3.50. CT-guided distal femoral biopsy in a 71-year-old woman with breast cancer. Axial CT scan shows a medial approach of the medial femoral condyle lytic lesion through the final part of the vastus medialis. Histologic examination revealed bone metastasis

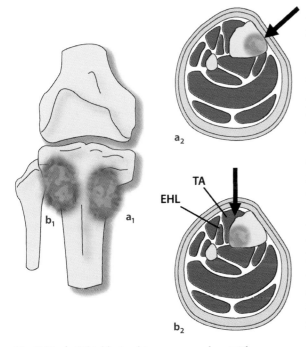

Fig. 3.51a,b. Tibial lesion biopsy approaches. **a** The recommended anteromedial approach, which avoids muscular penetration. **b** The anterior approach through the tibialis anterior (*TA*) and the extensor hallux longus (*EHL*) is possible for lateral lesions, but the interosseous membrane has to be preserved

and operators should be careful to obtain samples from different regions of the lesion (BERNING et al. 1996).

Poor results are reported with hematological diseases, probably because of the frequent lack of medullar biopsy, of the high frequency of necrotic lesions, and of the decalcification procedure which induces membrane antigen destruction (VIEILLARD et al. 2005). Good results have been reported for the diagnosis of lymphoma (AGID et al. 2003). The main reason for failed biopsies is a too-small sample for optimal pathologic analysis (JELINEK et al. 2002).

Some consideration should be given to the sole use of FNA in the diagnosis of tumoral disease; as the treatment of sarcomas is not dependent on the histological type of the lesion but on its malignancies and its grading, some authors argue that FNA should not be the only procedure for sarcoma diagnosis (WHITE VA et al. 1988; JONES et al. 2002). FNA is recognized as efficient for diagnosis of metastases (ZORNOZA 1982).

PMSB is particularly effective with infectious lesions; confirmation of infectious origin of bone and joint lesions ranges from 70% to 100% (FRASER-HILL and RENFREW 1992; LOGAN et al. 1996). Disc infections are recognized and the responsible agent identified in more than 70% of cases (FOUQUET et al. 1996; BRENAC and HUET 2001).

3.11.2
Specific Results

Any discussion of the accuracy of PMSB must take into account the type of tissue, the location of the lesion, and the radiological appearance of the lesion.

Results of soft tissue biopsies are discordant. Some authors reported the highest diagnostic rate (100%) (VIEILLARD et al. 2005), while others found a similar (YAO et al. 1999) or lower (SKRZYNSKI et al. 1996) rate compared to bone lesion biopsies. However, it may be that for bone lesions with adjacent soft tissue involvement (i.e. paravertebral mass or periosteal mass), the latter should be the target of the biopsy, mostly because of the relative ease of approach and execution. Furthermore, in patients with suspected metastases, biopsy of an eventual soft tissue mass avoids cortical penetration (DUPUY et al. 1998).

Location has little effect on the diagnostic utility of the biopsy (FRASER-HILL and RENFREW 1992), even if spinal biopsies seem to be more often positive (KATTAPURAM et al. 1992). Previous studies showed that the radiological aspect of the lesion has more influence on the results than the location; diagnostic rates were classically reported as lower for sclerotic lesions and vertebral compression fracture (FRASER-HILL and RENFREW 1992), while lytic lesions were associated with a higher diagnostic rate (VIEILLARD et al. 2005). A more recent publication (JELINEK et al. 2002) showed that, with improved needle technology, sclerotic lesion biopsy results are similar to those of lytic lesions. Cystic lesions with fluid and necrosis are more likely to yield false negative results, as necrotic areas offer little diagnostic information (JELINEK et al. 2002). In any case, prior to the procedure the lesion should be carefully analyzed to determine which areas are lytic; one of these will be the biopsy target because lytic areas are easier to biopsy. With a massive lytic lesion, the biopsy sample must be obtained from the periphery of the lytic region, as the central area will likely be necrotic and contain little useful material. Enhanced MR imaging and CT are useful tools for detecting active areas as optimal biopsy targets.

Aggressive lesions such as Ewing sarcoma or tumors with an osseous matrix like osteosarcomas are in general easily identified with PMSB. The histological interpretation of cartilaginous lesions may be very difficult and even impossible. As much as possible, the diagnosis should be made from radiologic evaluation and the histological proof brought by surgery (which consists of curettage, amputation, or local resection), as treatment of this kind of lesion is based mainly on surgery, independent of the malignancy grade. PMSB is probably of less interest for cartilaginous tumors.

3.11.3
Complications

Several complications can occur, but remain rare, about 0.2%–1% (MURPHY 1983; JELINEK et al. 2002). Surgical complications rates are reported as 2%–20% (MANKIN et al. 1982; SIMON 1982; BARTH et al. 1992).

3.11.3.1
General Complications

- Patient collapse from active bleeding
- Anaphylactic reactions to anesthetics
- Vasovagal reaction

3.11.3.2
Local Complications

- Local hematomas: more frequent with hypervascular tumors like thyroid, breast or renal carcinomas metastases, or osteosarcomas. In such lesions, the biopsy should be performed with a coaxial device and the biopsy site filled with a hemostatic device (i.e. Curaspon®).
- Infections: cellulitis, osteitis, osteomyelitis, arthritis, epidural abscess (but the incidence is lower with PMSB than surgical biopsies with delayed healing).
- Neurological complications, by puncture or compression by a hematoma: paresis, paraplegia, paresthesias.
- Vascular injuries.
- Visceral injuries: ureteral or digestive puncture.
- Arachnoiditis in case of thecal penetration, but most dural punctures remain asymptomatic.
- Pneumothorax and hemothorax in thoracic biopsies.
- Dissemination of tumoral cells is a rare but possible complication. The likelihood is reduced if

the correct pathway is chosen, in close collaboration with the surgeon (DeSantos et al. 1978). Dissemination of tumoral cells is assumed to be less likely with needle biopsy, as there is markedly reduced biopsy width and limited peri-tumoral bleeding (Bickels et al. 2001).

- Compromised surgery: incorrectly planned biopsies compromise surgical procedures in about 10% (Mankin et al. 1982; Simon 1982) with unnecessary amputations after surgical biopsies reported at about 5% (Mankin et al. 1982). Moreover, surgical biopsy with a large incision could be contraindicated when limb salvage surgery is planned, because of the significant risk of spreading contamination in the vessels after the tourniquet is released, and the theoretically possible contamination of the joint when the incision extends into the adjacent joint capsule (Ayala and Zornosa 1983). A well-planned needle biopsy should eliminate most of these problems as it causes little damage to surrounding normal tissue.
- Increased fracture risk of the sampled bone; PMSB is safer than surgical biopsy because less bone is removed, especially in vertebrae and load-bearing bones.
- Transitory recurrent laryngeal nerve palsy.

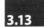

3.13
Conclusion

Histopathological and bacteriological studies are often needed in musculoskeletal lesions to establish a definitive diagnosis. In such cases, PMSB has become routine. Bone biopsies that once required open surgery have been successfully replaced by a minimally invasive procedure. PMSB has many advantages compared to surgical biopsy. Constant strict adherence to the asepsis rules for every interventional procedure is very important. Septic complications must absolutely be avoided. Proper needle, guidance and bone penetration techniques are also required to safely perform these procedures. Each PMSB should be performed after correct determination of the lesion type, as pathways may be different for primary malignant tumors. The whole medical team in charge of the patient must be aware of the limits of the diagnostic technique, in case of aspiration of insufficient material or sclerotic lesions. Every member of the team should be able to discuss the biopsy results, especially in difficult cases in which a definitive diagnosis may require combined and concordant histologic, clinical and multimodality imaging results.

3.12
Post-Procedure Management

The patient is kept under observation for at least 1 h, in a dependent position, on the side of the puncture site to limit hematoma formation. General parameters are monitored (blood pressure, pulse, heart rate, respiration) at 30-min intervals. Analgesics may be given, if necessary. If no problems are encountered, the patient can be discharged into the care of an accompanying responsible person. The patient should not drive or perform any tasks for the rest of the day. Written instructions should be provided that list possible significant problems: fever, swelling of the puncture site, abnormal pain, stiff neck, neurological deficit. Should any of these symptoms occur, the physician must be informed immediately. The instruction sheet should state clearly how to reach the physician.

References

Agid R, Sklair-Levy M, Bloom AI, Lieberman S, Polliack A, Ben-Yehuda D, Sherman Y, Libson E (2003) CT-guided biopsy with cutting-edge needle for the diagnosis of malignant lymphoma: experience of 267 biopsies. Clin Radiol 58:143–147

Anderson MW, Temple HT, Dussault RG, Kaplan PA (1999) Compartmental anatomy: relevance to staging and biopsy of musculoskeletal tumors. AJR Am J Roentgenol 173:1663–1671

Arya S, Crow WN, Hadjipaviou AG, Nauta HJ, Borowski AM, Vierra LA, Walser E (1996) Percutaneous transpedicular management of discitis. J Vasc Interv Radiol 7:921–927

Ayala AG, Zornosa J (1983) Primary bone tumors: percutaneous needle biopsy. Radiologic-pathologic study of 222 biopsies. Radiology 149:675–679

Ayala AG, Ro JY, Fanning CV, Flores JP, Yasko AW (1995) Core needle biopsy and fine-needle aspiration in the diagnosis of bone and soft-tissue lesions. Hematol Oncol Clin North Am 9:633–651

Barth RJ Jr, Merino MJ, Solomon D, Yang JC, Baker AR (1992) A prospective study of the value of core needle biopsy and fine needle aspiration in the diagnosis of soft tissue masses. Surgery 112:536–543

Berning W, Freyschmidt J, Ostertag H (1996) Percutaneous bone biopsy, techniques and indications. Eur Radiol 6:875–881

Bickels J, Jelinek J, Shmookler B, Malawer M (2001) Biopsy of musculoskeletal tumors. In: Malawer M, Sugarbaker PH (eds) Musculoskeletal cancer surgery. Kluwer Academic Publishers, Dordrecht Boston London, pp 38–45

Brenac F, Huet H (2001) Diagnostic accuracy of the percutaneous spinal biopsy. Optimization of the technique. J Neuroradiol 28:7–16

Coley BL, Sharp GS, Ellis EB (1931) Diagnosis of bone tumors by aspiration. Am J Surg 13:215–224

deSantos LA, Lukeman JM, Wallace S, Murray JA, Ayala AG (1978) Percutaneous needle biopsy of bone in the cancer patient. AJR Am J Roentgenol 130:641–649

Dupuy DE, Rosenberg AE, Punyaratabandhu T, Tan MH, Mankin HJ (1998) Accuracy of CT-guided needle biopsy of musculoskeletal neoplasms. AJR Am J Roentgenol 171:759–762

El-Khoury GY, Terepka RH, Mickelson MR, Rainville KL, Zaleski MS (1983) Fine-needle aspiration biopsy of bone. J Bone Joint Surg Am 65:522–525

Faugere MC, Malluche HH (1983) Comparison of different bone-biopsy techniques for qualitative and quantitative diagnosis of metabolic bone diseases. J Bone Joint Surg Am 65:1314–1318

Fouquet B, Goupille P, Gobert F, Cotty P, Roulot B, Valat JP (1996) Infectious discitis diagnostic contribution of laboratory tests and percutaneous discovertebral biopsy. Rev Rhum Engl Ed 63:24–29

Fraser-Hill MA, Renfrew DL (1992) Percutaneous needle biopsy of musculoskeletal lesions. 1. Effective accuracy and diagnostic utility. AJR Am J Roentgenol 158:809–812

Fraser-Hill MA, Renfrew DL, Hilsenrath PE (1992) Percutaneous needle biopsy of musculoskeletal lesions. 2. Cost-effectiveness. AJR Am J Roentgenol 158:813–818

Gangi A, Kastler BA, Dietemann JL (1994) Percutaneous vertebroplasty guided by a combination of CT and fluoroscopy. AJNR Am J Neuroradiol 15:83–86

Hau A, Kim I, Kattapuram S, Hornicek FJ, Rosenberg AE, Gebhardt MC, Mankin HJ (2002) Accuracy of CT-guided biopsies in 359 patients with musculoskeletal lesions. Skeletal Radiol 31:349–353

Hussain HK, Kingston JE, Domizio P, Norton AJ, Reznek RH (2001) Imaging-guided core biopsy for the diagnosis of malignant tumors in pediatric patients. AJR Am J Roentgenol 176:43–47

Jelinek JS, Murphey MD, Welker JA, Henshaw RM, Kransdorf MJ, Shmookler BM, Malawer MM (2002) Diagnosis of primary bone tumors with image-guided percutaneous biopsy: experience with 110 tumors. Radiology 223:731–737

Jones C, Liu K, Hirschowitz S, Klipfel N, Layfield LJ (2002) Concordance of histopathologic and cytologic grading in musculoskeletal sarcomas: can grades obtained from analysis of the fine-needle aspirates serve as the basis for therapeutic decisions? Cancer 96:83–91

Kattapuram SV, Khurana JS, Rosenthal DI (1992) Percutaneous needle biopsy of the spine. Spine 17:561–564

Layfield LJ, Armstrong K, Zaleski S, Eckardt J (1993) Diagnostic accuracy and clinical utility of fine-needle aspiration cytology in the diagnosis of clinically primary bone lesions. Diagn Cytopathol 9:168–173

Logan PM, Connell DG, O'Connell JX, Munk PL, Janzen DL (1996) Image-guided percutaneous biopsy of musculoskeletal tumors: an algorithm for selection of specific biopsy techniques. AJR Am J Roentgenol 166:137–141

Mankin HJ, Lange TA, Spanier SS (1982) The hazards of biopsy in patients with malignant primary bone and soft-tissue tumors. J Bone Joint Surg Am 64:1121–1127

Martin HE, Ellis EB (1930) Biopsy by needle puncture and aspiration. Ann Surg 92:169–181

Mink J (1986) Percutaneous bone biopsy in the patient with known or suspected osseous metastases. Radiology 161:191–194

Moore TM, Meyers MH, Patzakis MJ, Terry R, Harvey JP Jr (1979) Closed biopsy of musculoskeletal lesions. J Bone Joint Surg Am 61:375–380

Murphy WA (1983) Radiologically guided percutaneous musculoskeletal biopsy. Orthop Clin North Am 14:233–241

Ruhs SA, el-Khoury GY, Chrischilles EA (1996) A cost minimization approach to the diagnosis of skeletal neoplasms. Skeletal Radiol 25:449–454

Schweitzer ME, Deely DM (1993) Percutaneous biopsy of osteolytic lesions: use of a biopsy gun. Radiology 189:615–616

Simon MA (1982) Biopsy of musculoskeletal tumors. J Bone Joint Surg Am 64:1253–1257

Skrzynski MC, Biermann JS, Montag A, Simon MA (1996) Diagnostic accuracy and charge-savings of outpatient core needle biopsy compared with open biopsy of musculoskeletal tumors. J Bone Joint Surg Am 78:644–649

Toomayan GA, Robertson F, Major NM (2005) Lower extremity compartmental anatomy: clinical relevance to radiologists. Skeletal Radiol 34:307–313

Vieillard MH, Boutry N, Chastanet P, Duquesnoy B, Cotten A, Cortet B (2005) Contribution of percutaneous biopsy to the definite diagnosis in patients with suspected bone tumor. Joint Bone Spine 72:53–60

White LM, Schweitzer ME, Deely DM (1996) Coaxial percutaneous needle biopsy of osteolytic lesions with intact cortical bone. AJR Am J Roentgenol 166:143–144

White VA, Fanning CV, Ayala AG, Raymond AK, Carrasco CH, Murray JA (1988) Osteosarcoma and the role of fine-needle aspiration. A study of 51 cases. Cancer 62:1238–1246

Yao L, Nelson SD, Seeger LL, Eckardt JJ, Eilber FR (1999) Primary musculoskeletal neoplasms: effectiveness of core-needle biopsy. Radiology 212:682–686

Zornoza J (1982) Needle biopsy of metastases. Radiol Clin North Am 20:569–590

Percutaneous Spinal Facet and Sacroiliac Joint Injection

4

Galina Levin, Jonathan S. Luchs, and A. Orlando Ortiz

CONTENTS

4.1   Introduction   73

4.2   **Facet-Related Back Pain**   73
4.2.1   Clinical Features of Facet-Related Back
        Pain   74
4.2.2   Facet Joint Anatomy   74

4.3   **Lumbar Facet Block**   76

4.4   **Lumbar Synovial Cysts**   77

4.5   **Cervical Facet Block**   79

4.6   **Sacroiliac Joint**   80
4.6.1   Sacroiliac Joint Anatomy   80
4.6.2   Sacroiliac Joint Injection Technique   80

4.7   **Post-Procedure Follow-Up**   81

4.8   **Complications Related to Facet and
        Sacroiliac Joint Injections**   81

4.9   **Conclusion**   82

        References   82

G. Levin, MD, Fellow
A. O. Ortiz, MD, MBA, FACR, Professor and Chairman
Department of Radiology, Winthrop University Hospital,
259 First Street, Mineola, NY 11501, USA
J. S. Luchs, MD, Assistant Professor,
Director of Musculoskeletal Imaging and Intervention
Department of Radiology, Winthrop University Hospital,
259 First Street, Mineola, NY 11501, USA

4.1 Introduction

Back pain is a major cause of patient-related primary care visits in the United States. Facet and sacroiliac joint disease have been recognized as an important cause of back pain for nearly a century. The development of percutaneous spine procedures has enabled not only the diagnostic evaluation of this patient population but also, in specific instances, therapeutic intervention.

In recent years these procedures have become more and more popular with physicians and patients due to their efficacy, short procedure time, and low rate of complications. This chapter describes some of the most common percutaneous interventions, as well as relevant anatomy and research data.

4.2 Facet-Related Back Pain

Facet joint disease was first recognized and described as a cause of back pain by Goldthwait in 1911. Then in the 1960s Hirsch et al. confirmed the theory by injecting hypertonic saline solution into facet joints of patients and reproducing symptoms of facet joint disease. Further studies demonstrated that pain caused by injection of zygapophyseal joints is not only reproducible but occurs in a certain distribution depending on the level injected (April et al. 1990; Dwyer et al. 1990).

The cause of facet-related back pain is believed to be a result of osteoarthritic changes, as these joints are constantly subjected to movement and shear forces. Other derangements in the spine can influence or accelerate facet joint disease. For instance, one study demonstrated that in the context of disc space narrowing, most of the compressive forces usually applied to the disc space are actually transferred to the facet joints (Adams et al. 1983). Osteoarthritis-related facet joint pain is mediated by special neuropeptides, in particular substance P, by mechanoreceptors in the facet joint capsule, as well as by nerve fibers in the facet joint and adjacent soft tissues (Cavanaugh et al. 1997).

4.2.1
Clinical Features of Facet-Related Back Pain

Clinical presentation in patients with spinal facet syndrome can be quite variable. The pain may be localized to the region of the facet joint or it may be referred distally. For example, pain in the upper cervical regions may refer to the occipital region and even cause headaches. Similar referred pain patterns can be seen with lumbar facet syndrome. One retrospective study showed that sacroiliac and spinal facet diseases are the most common causes of referred pain. A frequently overlooked presentation of spinal facet disease is Maigne syndrome. This entity involves disease of the thoracolumbar facet joints that creates significant referred pain or hypersensitivity of the skin overlying the iliac crests (Bernard and Kirkaldy-Willis 1987).

Clinical diagnosis of facet joint disease is frequently complicated by other etiologies of back pain such as trauma, muscular pain or disc disease. The following symptoms are suggestive of, although not entirely specific to, facet syndromes: unilateral/bilateral paravertebral pain that is worst at rest and is aggravated by twisting or rotation and extension, tenderness on palpation of the affected joint, and morning stiffness (Fenton and Czervionke 2003). Although MR imaging at times can demonstrate inflammatory changes within the facet joints, clinical evaluation and physical examination remain the most important factors in diagnosing patients with facet syndromes.

Patients in whom the clinical evaluation is suggestive of facet joint syndrome and who fail to respond to conservative medical treatment are candidates for diagnostic facet blocks. This procedure involves injection of small amounts of anesthetic agents and steroids either directly into the facet joint (intra-articular block) or in the region of the capsule (extra-articular block). Diagnostic facet joint injections can be performed by utilizing controlled and comparative techniques. In the controlled method placebo and anesthetic agents are injected sequentially on different occasions. In comparative facet

blocks, the effects of a short-acting anesthetic are compared to the effects of a long-acting anesthetic. In both of these methods the patient remains blinded to the agent being injected, and thorough records of the patient's pain levels are crucial to establishing the efficacy of these procedures.

The major contraindications to facet injections include infection and uncorrected coagulopathy (Table 4.1). Patients with ongoing serious infections should not undergo these procedures due to potential immunosuppression from steroids. Congestive heart failure, poorly controlled diabetes and bleeding gastric and duodenal ulcers can also be exacerbated by steroid injections. Although most of the facet joint injections are performed with small amounts of iodinated contrast agents, in patients with a history of serious allergic reactions to iodinated dyes, these procedures can be performed without contrast agents by confirming the needle position with additional radiographic projections.

Table 4.1. Contraindications to facet injections

1. Major hypersensitivity to anesthetic solutions or glucocorticoids
2. Systemic infection
3. Local infection in the region of planned injection
4. Medical conditions that could be exacerbated by glucocorticoids
5. Uncorrected coagulopathy
   (a) Bleeding disorders
   (b) Thrombocytopenia ($<50,000/mm^3$)
   (c) Anticoagulant therapy
   (d) Other medications that affect bleeding time (e.g., anti-platelet agents)
6. Pregnancy

4.2.2
Facet Joint Anatomy

Each facet joint is covered by a two layer capsule. The outer layer is comprised of parallel collagen fibers. The inner layer consists of irregularly arranged elastic fibers (Yamashita et al. 1996). Superiorly and inferiorly, the capsule contains small openings that allow movement of fat between intracapsular and extracapsular spaces (Fig. 4.1). Superior and inferior reflections of the fibrous capsule are also slightly looser than in other parts of the joint, forming sub-

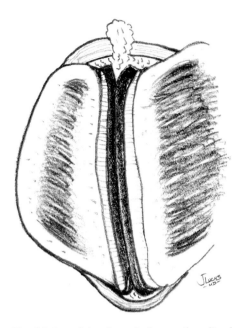

Fig. 4.1. Facet joint. An articular cartilage-lined synovial joint with fat at either end, contained by a joint capsule, is depicted. Notice the fat extending through a tear in the capsule on the upper portion of the joint

capsular pockets. Anteriorly, the capsule is replaced by the ligamentum flavum (LEWIN et al. 1962).

The articular surface is composed of a facet cortex that, in a healthy joint, is uniformly covered by articular cartilage. Facet joints affected by osteoarthritis usually demonstrate erosions of articular cartilage to a variable extent. Facet joints are synovial joints. They contain a synovial lining nearly identical to the synovium in extraspinal joints.

Intra-articular structures can be subdivided into fat and meniscoid components. The fat occupies any free space under the capsule. Within the joint the fat is covered by the synovium. As mentioned previously, intra-articular and extra-articular fat communicate via tiny holes in the superior and inferior parts of the capsule. The meniscoid structures in the facet joints do not have any histological resemblance to the menisci found in the large extraspinal joints. There is significant variation in the number and types of meniscoid structures between different individuals. One of the meniscoid structures is a connective tissue rim, which is a focal thickening of the internal aspect of the capsule involving the dorsal and ventral margins of the joints. It is present in about 20% of joints. An adipose tissue pad is the second meniscoid structure and is seen in approximately 88% of joints. It is normally found in

the superoventral and inferodorsal aspects of the joint. It is comprised of blood vessels and fat surrounded by synovial folds. The fat within the adipose tissue pads is continuous with the rest of the fat within the joint. Fibroadipose meniscoid is the third major type of meniscoid intra-articular structure, and consists of vessels and fat surrounded by the synovial membrane. Adipose tissue pads are usually larger than other meniscoids, and may project into the joint cavity. They are seen in approximately 54% of joints. Meniscal structures are thought to serve a protective function during joint movement (BOGDUK 1997b; BOGDUK and ENGEL 1984).

Knowledge of the facet joint innervation is crucial to understanding and treating facet joint disease. Each facet joint is innervated by branches from two adjacent segmental levels: the same level medial branch and a branch arising one level above (Fig. 4.2). For example, the L2-3 facet joint receives innervation from the L2-3 level and the L1-2 level.

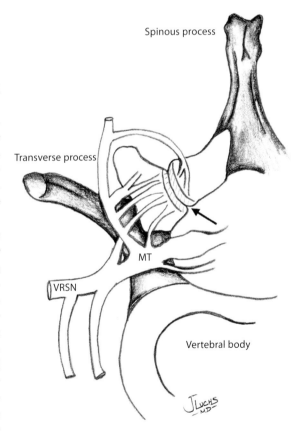

Fig. 4.2. Facet joint and its innervation. Multiple neural fibers originating from both the main trunk (*MT*) of the exiting spinal nerve and a branch from the exited ventral ramus spinal nerve (*VRSN*) are depicted. The complexity of the facet innervation originating from the same level and a level above the facet joint is also shown (*arrow*)

4.3

Lumbar Facet Block

The lumbar facet joints have an arcuate configuration formed by concave surfaces of the superior and inferior articular processes. The lumbar facet joints are best seen in an oblique view resembling the "Scotty dog," which requires an approximately 30–45° angulation of the X-ray tube. A shallower angle (10–20°) is usually required for actual access to the joint. There is a gradual change in facet joint orientation from the upper to the lower lumbar spine. In the upper lumbar spine the facet joints are oriented in a more vertical position, and in the lower lumbar spine a more coronal orientation of the joints is observed. The lumbar facet joint has an arcuate (concave) configuration, and the plane of orientation is usually oblique with respect to the true sagittal plane. The joint can be injected anywhere in the posterior recess that is accessible from a posterior approach. The inferior aspect of the posterior recess is larger than the superior, making it an ideal site for puncture. The posterior recess is covered by a fibrous capsule that creates resistance during the needle puncture. Ideally, the needle tip will be just superior to the neck of the "Scotty dog" when the needle is in the inferior recess. The needle does not have to be deep in the joint space for successful injection. In fact, advancing the needle too deep may result in damage to the synovial membrane or articular cartilage.

The procedure can be performed under fluoroscopic guidance with the patient in the prone position. The back is prepped and draped in a sterile fashion. After the skin and the soft tissues in the region of interest are anesthetized with a short-acting anesthetic such as 1% lidocaine, a 22- or 25-gauge spinal needle is directed toward the posterior and inferior aspect of the facet joint (Fig. 4.3). After the needle passes through the fibrous capsule, 0.1–0.5 ml of nonionic contrast is injected to verify the intraarticular position of the needle tip (Fig. 4.3c). Alternatively, needle position can be confirmed by rotating the fluoroscope and demonstrating a constant relationship between the needle tip and the inferior joint space. Then a mixture of bupivacaine (2 ml, 0.5%) and methylprednisolone (40 mg) or betamethasone (3 mg) is prepared (STALLMEYER and ORTIZ 2002). The volume of the facet joint rarely exceeds 1 ml. Injection of larger amounts of fluid can lead to extravasation and even rupture of the joint bursa (DESTOUET et al. 1982). At times, extensive hypertrophic changes in the joint can prevent needle access despite adequate fluoroscopic visualization. The operator may have to settle for a peri-articular

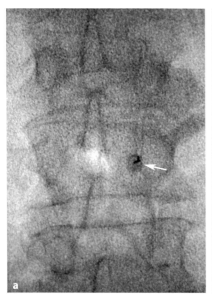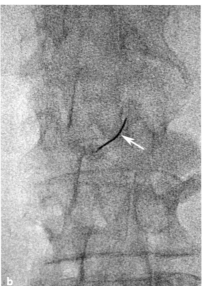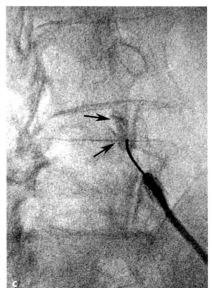

Fig. 4.3a–c. Lumbar facet block in a 67-year-old woman with left side nonradiating low back pain at L4-5 level. **a** Oblique radiograph of the lumbar spine demonstrates a "down the barrel" approach (*arrow*) to the oblique lumbar facet joint. **b** Oblique radiograph of the lumbar spine demonstrates a slight bend in the distal needle (*arrow*) confirming facet joint access and proper placement. **c** Left L4-5 facet arthrogram view confirms plane of injection (*arrows*) for subsequent steroid and anesthetic injection

injection. Alternatively, facet joint injection can be performed with computed tomographic (CT) guidance. With the patient in the prone position, the facet joint(s) of interest can be localized. Skin markers are used to plan an appropriate needle trajectory that will allow access to the joint. The spinal needle is then advanced under CT guidance. The position of the needle tip within the joint can be confirmed by CT. An arthrogram can be performed using 0.1 to 0.5 ml of low osmolar non-ionic contrast media. Once the joint is accessed, the appropriate injectate can be administered. It is important to note that regardless of the type of imaging, an arthrogram should always be performed when a synovial cyst is suspected.

4.4
Lumbar Synovial Cysts

Lumbar synovial cysts are juxta-articular cysts that comprise the majority of peri-facet cysts (WILLIAMS and MURTAGH 2002). These cysts arise from hypertrophied, redundant synovium in an osteoarthritic joint. Occasionally they may arise from small periarticular ganglia and are actually ganglion cysts.

Juxta-articular cysts are often located within the lumbar spine at the L4-5 level or, less commonly, at the L5-S1 level. Rarely, juxta-articular cysts may be found in the cervical or thoracic spine segments. When present in the lumbar spine they arise more frequently from the ventral aspect of the facet joint surface (Figs. 4.4a, 4.5a,b). These cysts can sometimes be considered an incidental finding when they arise from the dorsal surface of the facet joint. Ventrally located synovial cysts can exert a mass effect upon adjacent neural structures, such as exiting nerve roots, and therefore may cause radiculopathy.

Symptomatic lumbar synovial cysts are often amenable to image-guided therapy (WILLIAMS and MURTAGH 2002; PARLIER-CUAU et al. 1999) Those cysts that maintain their communication with the facet joint can be accessed indirectly through the facet joint via posterior facet joint injection (Fig. 4.5c,d). A facet joint arthrogram is particularly helpful in this case as it helps to identify whether or not the cyst communicates with the facet joint. If contrast extends from the joint into the cyst then a direct communication is established. The cyst can be treated in one of three ways: aspiration, injection with steroid and anesthetic, or cyst rupture. An attempt can be made to aspirate the cyst, but this may not be feasible (Fig. 4.4).

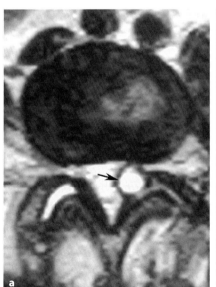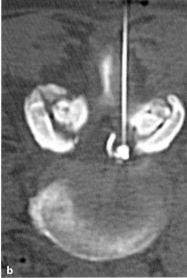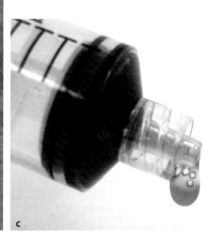

Fig. 4.4a–c. Lumbar synovial cyst in a 50-year-old woman with left side L4 radiculopathy. **a** Axial T2-weighted MR image demonstrates a left lumbar facet cyst (*arrow*) originating from the ventral surface of the joint and displacing the adjacent thecal sac. **b** Axial CT scan in prone patient demonstrates needle placement into a left synovial cyst through an interlaminar approach. The needle directly penetrates the cyst wall. **c** Tenacious synovial fluid aspirated from lumbar facet cyst

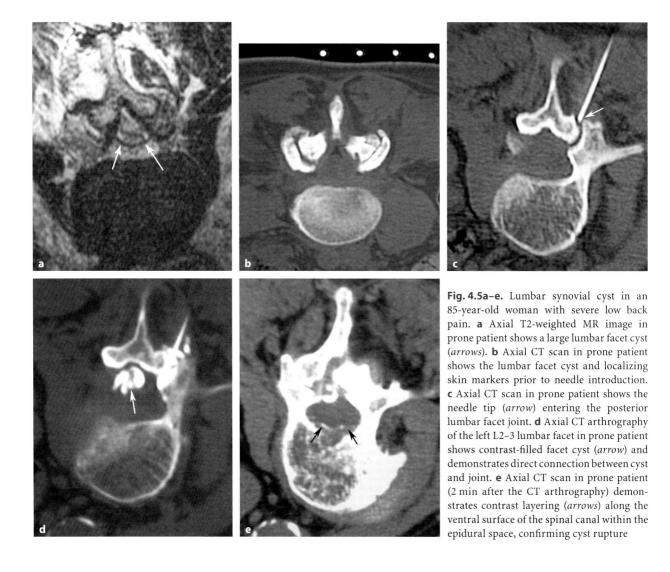

Fig. 4.5a–e. Lumbar synovial cyst in an 85-year-old woman with severe low back pain. **a** Axial T2-weighted MR image in prone patient shows a large lumbar facet cyst (*arrows*). **b** Axial CT scan in prone patient shows the lumbar facet cyst and localizing skin markers prior to needle introduction. **c** Axial CT scan in prone patient shows the needle tip (*arrow*) entering the posterior lumbar facet joint. **d** Axial CT arthrography of the left L2–3 lumbar facet in prone patient shows contrast-filled facet cyst (*arrow*) and demonstrates direct connection between cyst and joint. **e** Axial CT scan in prone patient (2 min after the CT arthrography) demonstrates contrast layering (*arrows*) along the ventral surface of the spinal canal within the epidural space, confirming cyst rupture

Cyst rupture can be attempted by injecting at least 3 to 5 ml of a steroid and anesthetic mixture [2 ml of DepoMedrol (80 mg) mixed with 3 ml of 0.5% bupivacaine] with a 5- or 10-ml Luer-Lok syringe (Fig. 4.5d). Cyst rupture can be very painful, and the use of patient sedation and analgesia are therefore strongly recommended (Fig. 4.5e). Some cysts may be resistant to rupture and can be aspirated and injected with 1 to 2 ml of a steroid and anesthetic mixture. If the initial facet arthrogram does not conclusively show communication between the facet joint and cyst, or the facet joint cannot be accessed due to advanced degenerative change, then an interlaminar approach to the cyst should be considered. An interlaminar approach can be attempted when the cyst lies in close proximity to the dorsolateral epidural space, a not uncommon location for these lesions, as they often arise from the facet joint (Fig. 4.4b). Interlaminar access can be obtained with CT guidance using a contralateral oblique posterior approach with a 22-, 20- or 18-gauge spinal needle. The needle tip is carefully advanced into the cyst. Localization of the needle tip within the cyst is confirmed by injecting 1 ml of a low osmolar non-ionic contrast agent and obtaining axial images through the cyst. Cyst rupture can be attempted. Axial CT images through the level of a ruptured cyst will show residual contrast agent within the epidural space. Regardless of whether the cyst is aspirated, injected or ruptured, the patient should be made aware that the cyst can recur. A recurrent cyst can be re-treated. Failure of these cyst injection techniques should indicate open surgical decompression or resection of the cyst.

Cervical Facet Block

This procedure can be performed with the patient placed in either the prone position, with the neck flexed and turned away from the side of the injection, or in the lateral decubitus position. Again, either fluoroscopic- or CT-guided techniques may be utilized.

The cervical facet joint is oriented in the oblique coronal plane and is most easily accessed via a posterior oblique or lateral trajectory (Fig. 4.6). As with the lumbar facet joints, the cervical facet joints are also covered by a fibrous capsule. The protocol regarding the injection of anesthetic agents is essentially similar to the one used for lumbar facet blocks (Fig. 4.7).

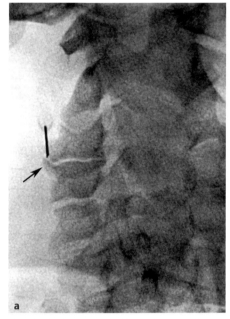
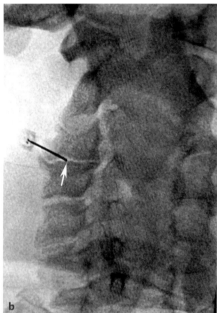

Fig. 4.6a,b. Cervical facet block in a 59-year-old man with left side C3–4 level neck pain. **a** Oblique fluoroscopic image demonstrates lateral needle placement, with the needle unable to advance due to facet osteophyte (*arrow*). **b** Oblique fluoroscopic image demonstrates repositioning of the needle, which now enters the center of the facet joint (*arrow*)

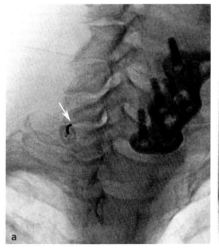
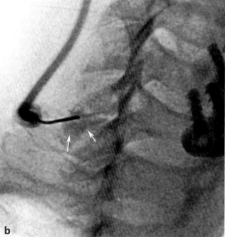

Fig. 4.7a,b. Cervical facet block in a 49-year-old woman, status post anterior cervical fusion with left side lower neck pain. **a** Oblique fluoroscopic image demonstrates posterior oblique needle approach and placement (*arrow*). **b** Oblique fluoroscopic image of facet arthrogram confirms injection plane (*arrows*) for subsequent therapeutic injection

4.6
Sacroiliac Joint

Treatment of sacroiliac conditions dates back to the 1930s, when this technique was first described by HALDEMAN and SOTO-HALL (1938). In the early 1990s studies conducted in healthy volunteers demonstrated that injection of saline into the sacroiliac joint produces localized pain over the joint. These results suggested that sacroiliac joints can also be a source of back pain, similar to spinal facet joints (FORTIN et al. 1994). Further studies have shown that pathologic sacroiliac joints may account for between 13% and 30% of low back pain symptoms (BERNARD and KIRKALDY-WILLIS 1987; MAIGNE et al. 1996; SCHWARZER et al. 1995).

There are numerous causes of sacroiliac-related low back pain. These include spondyloarthropathies, infections, metabolic diseases, trauma, osteitis condensans ilii, and idiopathic sacroiliitis. One study showed that approximately 35% of patients have idiopathic onset of pain (CHOU et al. 2004). Patients with sacroiliac joint pain may complain of focal asymmetric low back pain with or without a radiating component that extends to the hip. Clinically, sacroiliac joint syndrome may present as pain on palpation of the affected sacroiliac joint or anterior superior iliac spine, and decreased sacroiliac joint motion. The patient's symptoms can sometimes be provoked with Patrick or Gaenslen maneuvers. Patients with sacroiliac joint pain do not demonstrate sensory, motor or reflex deficits in contrast to nerve root compression syndromes (BERNARD and KIRKALDY-WILLIS 1987). Sacroiliac joint syndrome cannot be definitively diagnosed by physical examination alone (SCHWARZER et al. 1995). In addition, most radiologic findings correlate poorly with clinical symptoms. For example, in sacroiliitis, skeletal scintigraphy has a sensitivity of 12.9%–65%, single photon emission CT 9%, and MR imaging 54% (CHOU et al. 2004). Sacroiliac joint blocks, on the other hand, are currently accepted as the gold standard for diagnosis of sacroiliac joint syndrome. A review of the literature shows a wide spectrum of success rates ranging from mild or transient improvement of symptoms to significant decrease in pain (BOLLOW et al. 1996; MAIGNE et al. 1996; MAUGARS et al. 1992; PEREIRA et al. 2000; SLIPMAN 2001; SCHWARZER et al. 1995).

4.6.1
Sacroiliac Joint Anatomy

The sacrum consists of five fused vertebrae that gradually become smaller in posterior dimension and wider in anterior dimension when the sacrum is examined in craniocaudal direction. The sacrum tightly articulates with two ilia, forming two sacroiliac joints. Posteriorly, the sacroiliac joint is secured by the interosseus sacroiliac ligament. Ventrally, the sacrum is bound to the ilia by the anterior sacroiliac ligament. Sacrospinous and sacrotuberous ligaments attach the lower sacrum to the ischium, thus preventing upward tilting of the lower sacrum. The sacroiliac joint lacks a true well-defined capsule, as is seen in spinal facet joints. Isolating the capsule from the dense anterior and posterior sacroiliac ligaments is extremely difficult. The posterior capsule is absent or rudimentary, and the anterior capsule is thickened (BOGDUK 1997a).

At this time there is no consensus regarding innervation of the sacroiliac joints. Variable innervation from as high as L2 to as low as S3 has been reported (BOGDUK 1997a).

4.6.2
Sacroiliac Joint Injection Technique

This procedure may be performed with fluoroscopic or CT guidance. After the patient is placed in the prone position, a wide area over the sacrum and buttock is prepped using a sterile technique. Following injection of a local anesthetic such as 1% lidocaine, a 22-gauge spinal needle is directed into the inferior joint space. With fluoroscopy, the frontal projection may show two apparent joint spaces; the upper fibrous portion of the sacroiliac joint and the lower synovial portion of the true sacroiliac joint. The latter portion of the joint is located more medially on the frontal projection. Furthermore, rotation of the fluoroscope away from the site of injection in the transverse plane will demonstrate the inferior joint space such that a medial to lateral needle trajectory relative to the midline will allow access to the joint (Fig. 4.8). With CT guidance, the inferior joint space is directly visualized such that the needle can be directly advanced into the joint (Fig. 4.9a). Once the needle enters the sacroiliac joint, a small amount of low osmolar non-ionic contrast agent is injected to confirm intra-articular position (Fig. 4.9b). Then a mixture of 1–3 ml bupivacaine (0.5%) and 40 mg methylprednisolone is injected.

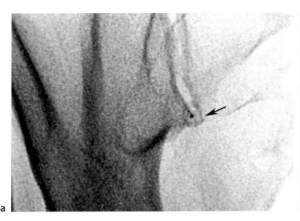
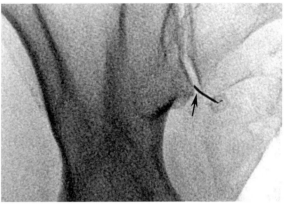

Fig. 4.8a,b. Sacroiliac injection in a 41-year-old woman with left side sacroiliac joint pain. **a** Anteroposterior fluoroscopic image shows a "down the barrel" approach into the sacral iliac joint (*arrow*). **b** Anteroposterior fluoroscopic image confirms needle tip placement in the sacroiliac joint demonstrated by a slight bend in the needle tip (*arrow*)

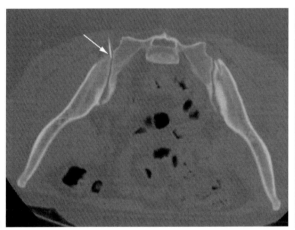
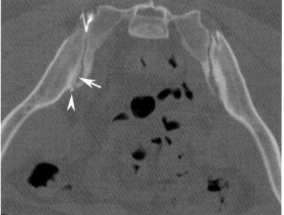

Fig. 4.9a,b. Sacroiliac injection in a 34-year-old woman with right side sacroiliac joint pain. **a** Axial CT scan through the sacrum demonstrates needle tip placement (*arrow*) in the posterior right sacroiliac joint. **b** Axial CT arthrography of the sacroiliac joint demonstrates that the contrast extends in an anterior superior direction, and confirms injection into the synovium-lined portion of the joint (*arrow*). Small amount of contrast decompresses out of the anterior-superior sacroiliac joint (*arrowhead*)

4.7
Post-Procedure Follow-Up

Spinal facet block and sacroiliac joint injections are usually performed on an outpatient basis. The patient is instructed to arrange for transportation home, as driving is not advisable immediately following the procedure. After the procedure the patient is given 30 to 60 minutes to recover. If there are no motor/sensory deficits or any other complications related to the procedure, the patient may be discharged. Some patients may experience localized pain that is usually relieved with oral analgesics.

4.8
Complications Related to Facet and Sacroiliac Joint Injections

Complications of facet and sacroiliac joint injections are very rare. Hypersensitivity reactions to either iodinated contrast agents or steroids are relatively rare. Patients with a history of prior hypersensitivity reactions to iodinated contrast agents should undergo procedures without contrast. Some other possible complications are epidural or soft tissue hematoma, epidural abscess and infectious arthritis. Other potential complications of facet injection procedures are listed in Table 4.2.

Table 4.2. Potential complications of facet joint procedures

1. Infectious
   - Soft tissue abscess
   - Epidural abscess
   - Septic arthritis
2. Traumatic
   - Soft tissue hematoma
   - Epidural hematoma
   - Arterial injury
3. Injectate-related
   - Anaphylactic reaction to contrast agent, anesthetic or steroids
   - Transient hypercorticism
   - Retinal hemorrhage
   - Epidural lipomatosis

4.9
Conclusion

This chapter demonstrates why joint arthropathies are important etiological factors in neck and low back pain. Although further studies regarding efficacy and long term effects of radiologically-guided procedures would be of benefit, the current medical literature shows that these interventions are not only safe and effective in treating medically refractory facet or sacroiliac related pain syndromes, but may also allow patients to avoid more invasive surgical procedures.

References

Adams MA, Hutton WC (1983) The mechanical function of the lumbar apophyseal joints. Spine 8:327–330

Aprill C, Dwyer A, Bogduk N (1990) Cervical zygapophyseal joint pain patterns. II: A clinical evaluation. Spine 15:458–461

Bernard TN Jr, Kirkaldy-Willis WH (1987) Recognizing specific characteristic of nonspecific back pain. Clin Orthop Relat Res 217:266–280

Bogduk N (1997a) The sacroiliac joint. In: Bogduk N (ed) Clinical anatomy of the lumbar spine and sacrum. Churchill Livingstone, Edinburgh, pp 177–185

Bogduk N (1997b) The zygapophyseal joints. In: Bogduk N (ed) Clinical anatomy of the lumbar spine and sacrum. Churchill Livingstone, Edinburgh, pp 33–41

Bogduk N, Engel R (1984) The menisci of the lumbar zygapophyseal joints. A review of their anatomy and clinical significance. Spine 9:454–460

Bollow M, Braun J, Taupitz M et al. (1996) CT-guided intraarticular corticosteroid injection into the sacroiliac joints in patients with spondyloarthropathy: indication and follow-up with contrast-enhanced MRI. J Comput Assist Tomogr 20:512–521

Cavanaugh JM, Ozaktay AC, Yamashita T et al. (1997) Mechanisms of low back pain: a neurophysiologic and neuroanatomic study. Clin Orthop Relat Res 335:166–180

Chou LH, Slipman CW, Bhagia SM et al. (2004) Inciting events initiating injection-proven sacroiliac joint syndrome. Pain Med 5:26–32

Destouet JM, Gilula LA, Murphy WA et al. (1982) Lumbar facet joint injection: indication, technique, clinical correlation, and preliminary results. Radiology 145:321–325

Dwyer A, Aprill C, Bogduk N (1990) Cervical zygapophyseal joint pain patterns. I: A study of normal volunteers. Spine 15:453–457

Fenton DS, Czervionke LF (2003) Facet joint injection and medial branch block. In: Fenton DS, Czervionke LF (eds) Image-guided spine interventions. Saunders, Philadelphia pp 9–21

Fortin JD, Dwyer AP, West S et al. (1994) Sacroiliac joint: pain referral maps upon applying a new injection/arthrography technique. Spine 19:1475–1482

Goldthwait JE (1911) The lumbo-sacral articulation: an explanation of many cases of "lumbago", "sciatica" and paraplegia. Boston Med Surg J 164:365–372

Haldeman KO, Soto-Hall R (1938) The diagnosis and treatment of sacroiliac condition by injection of procaine. J Bone Joint Surg Am 20:675–685

Hirsch D, Inglemark B, Miller M (1963) The anatomic basis for back pain. Acta Orthop Scand 33:1–17

Lewin T, Moffet B, Viidek A (1962) The morphology of the lumbar synovial intervertebral joints. Acta Morphol Neerlando-Scandinav 4:299–319

Maigne JY, Aivaliklis A, Pfefer F (1996) Results of sacroiliac joint double block and value of sacroiliac pain provocation tests in 54 patients with low back pain. Spine 21:1889–1892

Maugars Y, Mathis C, Vilon P et al. (1992) Corticosteroid injection of the sacroiliac joint in patients with seronegative spondyloarthropathy. Arthritis Rheum 35:564–568

Parlier-Cuau C, Wybier M, Nizard R et al. (1999) Symptomatic lumbar facet joint synovial cysts: clinical assessment of facet joint steroid injection after 1 and 6 months and long-term follow-up in 30 patients. Radiology 210:509–513

Pereira PL, Gunaydin I, Trubenbach F et al. (2000) Interventional MR imaging for injection of sacroiliac joints in patients with sacroiliitis. AJR Am J Roentgenol 175:265–266

Slipman CW, Lipetz JS, Plastaras CT et al. (2001) Fluoroscopically guided therapeutic sacroiliac joint injections for sacroiliac joint syndrome. Am J Phys Med Rehabil 80:425–432

Stallmeyer MJ, Ortiz AO (2002) Facet blocks and sacroiliac joint injections. Tech Vasc Interv Radiol 5:201–206

Schwarzer AC, Aprill CN, Bogduk N (1995) The sacroiliac joint in chronic low back pain. Spine 20:31–37

Wagner AL, Murtagh FR (2002) Intraspinal cyst aspiration. In: Williams AL Murtagh FR (eds) Handbook of Diagnostic and Therapeutic Spine procedures. Mosby, St.Louis, pp 92–106

Yomashita T, Minaki Y, Ozaktay AC, Cavanaugh JM, King AI (1996) A morphological study of the fibrous capsule of the human lumbar facet joint. Spine 21: 538–543

Percutaneous Infiltration of the Craniovertebral Region

ALAIN CHEVROT, JEAN-LUC DRAPÉ, DIDIER GODEFROY, and ANTOINE FEYDY

CONTENTS

5.1 Introduction 83

5.2 Anatomy 83

5.3 Technique 84
5.3.1 Practical Application 84
5.3.2 Results 86
5.3.2.1 Normal Arthrography 86
5.3.2.2 Pathology 86

5.4 Accidents 87

5.5 Indications 87

5.6 Conclusion 91

References 91

5.1
Introduction

C1-2 arthrography and steroid injection is a radiological approach to the treatment of cervical spine pathology of the first two vertebrae. Arthrography is the first step for treatment with a long acting steroid injection (CHEVROT et al. 1995; HOVE and GYLDENSTED 1990). For the moment, there is no other technique for pain management in the craniovertebral region.

The atlanto-axial junction is frequently affected by osteoarthritis and sometimes by inflammatory diseases, such as rheumatoid arthritis and ankylosing spondylitis. The described technique is fluoroscopy-guided, permitting opacification and steroid injection directly into the atlantoaxial joint cavity.

5.2
Anatomy

The first two vertebrae have a complex anatomy, which is different from the general structure of the other vertebrae (BLAND and BOUSHEY 1990; BOGDUK 1982; ELLIS et al. 1991; LAZORTHES et al. 1962; PFIRRMANN et al. 2001; SCHWEITZER et al. 1992). The first cervical vertebra has neither body nor spinous process; it consists of an anterior and a posterior arch extended between two lateral bone masses, forming a ring. Each lateral mass has a superior and an inferior articular facet. The superior facet articulates with the condyles of the occipital bone; the inferior facet is adapted to the facet of the transverse processes of the axis.

The second cervical vertebra has a vertical conical process called the odontoid process on the upper surface of the body, and on the lateral sides it has two transverse processes with laterally inclined upper articular surfaces. The odontoid process presents two articular facets: one anterior, corresponding to the anterior arch of the atlas, and one posterior, corresponding to the transverse atlantal ligament extended between the two lateral masses of the first vertebra. The articulating surfaces of the lateral atlanto-axial joints are both convex, but the poor congruence is corrected by a thick cartilage. The joint capsule is attached at a distance from the edges of the vertebral surfaces, allowing wide movement. There are synovial-lined joints in the lateral atlanto-axial, the anterior atlanto-axial and the syndesmo-odontoid joints, with possible interarticular communication.

A. CHEVROT, MD, Professor and Chairman
J.-L. DRAPÉ, MD, PhD, Professor
D. GODEFROY, MD, Professor
A. FEYDY, MD, PhD, Associate Professor
Department of Radiology B, Cochin University Hospital, Assistance Publique - Hôpitaux de Paris, Paris Descartes University, 27 rue Faubourg Saint Jacques, 75679 Paris Cedex 14, France

From a functional point of view, there is a unique trochoid articulation, which permits extensive rotational movements due to a loose capsule. The lateral flexion is principally facilitated by the atlanto-occipital joint. The atlanto-axial stability depends on the complex ligament apparatus of the transverse, alar and apical ligaments.

A detailed study of all anatomic structures on axial sections is necessary to find the safest approach to the atlanto-axial junction (CACCIOLA et al. 2004). The puncture of the joint should avoid the vessels and nerves situated anterolaterally (the carotid artery, the jugular vein, the vagus and phrenicus nerves) and postero-laterally (the vertebral artery and vein, plus the root of the second cervical nerve) (Fig. 5.1).

The second cervical dorsal nerve is located just below the lateral atlanto-axial joint; its branches supply the atlanto-occipital and the atlanto-axial synovial spaces. The main branch, called the greater occipital nerve, innervates the skin and muscles of the upper neck and skull. The C2 dorsal ramus, running a few millimeters behind the atlanto-axial joint, can be in contact with the posterior recess. Some authors describe a different anatomy, and contest the proximity of the C2 dorsal ramus to the atlanto-axial joint, questioning its relationship with occipital neuralgia (BOVIM et al. 1991; LAZORTHES et al. 1962).

There are postmortem arthrography experiments in the medical literature that provide a better knowledge of the synovial joint spaces than anatomic studies (DIRHEIMER et al. 1977; DUSSAULT and NICOLET 1985; MELLSTRÖM et al. 1980).

5.3
Technique

The posterolateral approach appears to be the safest technique (CHEVROT et al. 1995; CHEVROT et al. 1997). The needle is inserted directly behind the mastoid process, advanced behind the vertebral artery, then directed towards the posterior aspect of the atlanto-axial joint and inserted into the posterior recess. The point of puncture is chosen under lateral fluoroscopy: the posterior aspect of the atlanto-axial joint. A 20- or 22-gauge needle is introduced, following the central X-ray beam, which highlights the target area. The needle is inserted until it comes into contact with the C2 lamina.

5.3.1
Practical Application

The patient is seated in profile in front of the radiological plane, which is in an upright position (Fig. 5.2a). The procedure can also be performed with the patient in lateral decubitus and radiological plane horizontal. The patient lies on the side opposite the punctured side. Light premedication (perlingual diazepam®) is administered several minutes before the injection. The patient is informed that the procedure may elicit a sharp pain, which will soon disappear. Due to the lethal risk of a local anesthetic acting on the cervical nerve structures, it is imperative to avoid using any form of local anesthetic.

After skin asepsis, a sterile auto-adhesive windowed draping is placed to cover the head and the neck of the patient. A 20-gauge, 8-cm, spinal needle is used. For some doctors this needle is a little too wide, and they prefer a 22-gauge needle. A 20-gauge needle is easier to guide, due to its rigidity. In addition, the technique does not provoke spinal puncture, and it is not expected to create a post puncture headache. Thus it is not necessary to use a 22- or 25-gauge needle. Only nonionic, nonneurotoxic contrast media must be used.

Under fluoroscopic guidance, the entry point is chosen on the skin at the point of projection of the lamina of the axis, and of the posterior aspect

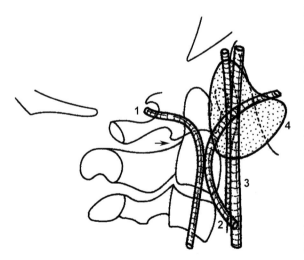

Fig. 5.1. C1-2 relationship with the vessels, illustrating the point of puncture of the C1-2 joint at the posterior aspect of the C1-2 joint (*arrow*). (*1*, vertebral artery; *2*, external carotid artery; *3*, internal carotid artery; *4*, parotid gland)

of the lateral mass of the atlas. The needle is then gently introduced until lamina bone contact is felt and slightly bent toward the inferior aspect of the posterior mass of the atlas.

Injection of a small amount of contrast media indicates the intra-articular position of the tip of the needle (Fig. 5.2b). If the opacification is stagnant, the position of the needle is not intra-articular and must be corrected. After opacification of the joint cavity, and with the needle placed in the articulation, 0.5–1 ml of a long-acting steroid is injected into the joint cavity, according to the articular cavity capacity. Finally, after removing the needle, lateral and anteroposterior radiographs are obtained (Fig. 5.3).

If the vertebral artery is accidentally punctured, injection of contrast media under fluoroscopic guidance will demonstrate rapid opacification of this artery. The needle should be withdrawn gently out of the vessel and repositioned in to the C1-2 joint. No drug should be injected unless radiologist is certain the needle tip is away from the vertebral artery.

The patient is questioned about the location of the pain provoked by the injection and whether it has appeared in the usual symptomatic area. If the usual pain is produced during the injection, it is a good sign that the procedure will be successful (ZAPLETAL et al. 1996). This is an out-patient procedure.

Another technique has been described using a true posterior approach under fluoroscopic needle guidance. Its aim is to use an anteroposterior view of the C1-2 joint as obtained in the "open mouth" position (Fig. 5.4a). In this position the C1-2 joint space

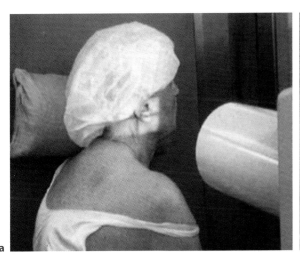
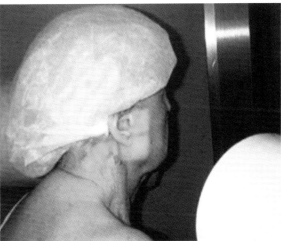

Fig. 5.2a,b. Puncture of the C1-2 joint in a man. **a** Position of the patient. **b** Correct site of needle introduction

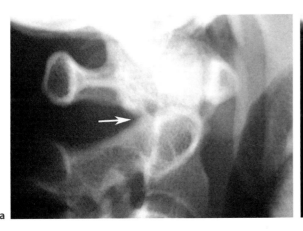
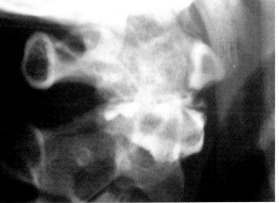

Fig. 5.3a,b. Fluoroscopic control in a 60-year-old woman who underwent C1-2 infiltration. **a** Lateral radiograph of the craniovertebral region shows the point of puncture is easily demonstrated at the posterior aspect of the C1-2 joint (*arrow*). **b** Lateral arthrographic view shows the normal pattern of the C1-2 joint cavity

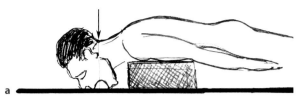

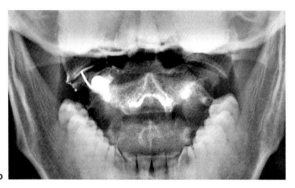

Fig. 5.4a,b. Posterior approach. **a** Position of the patient for posteroanterior view control of the C1-2 joint space. The *arrow* indicates the position of the needle. **b** Posteroanterior view control of the C1–2 joint space. The needle is seen in the target area and a small amount of contrast fills the joint cavity

is clearly visible. It is possible to insert a needle directly into the joint cavity from a direct posterior approach (Fig. 5.4b). This approach is further from the vertebral artery, which makes it potentially safer. However, the position of the patient is somewhat uncomfortable: lying face down on the horizontal radiological table with the mouth wide open. The joint itself is well seen if the anatomy is normal. The safety of the procedure is reduced due to the long path of the needle, which could deviate internally or externally. In the case of destructive modifications, the joint is often not clearly visible and the puncture is impossible.

There is no described C1-2 arthrography technique with CT as an approach control.

5.3.2
Results

5.3.2.1
Normal Arthrography

The lateral atlanto-axial joint cavity is triangular with an external basis. The capsule is attached in the postero-internal part near the edges of the articulating faces, and at a distance anteriorly and later-

ally, enclosing cartilage and vertebral bone. Opacification permits analysis of the articular surfaces and subchondral bone (Figs. 5.3, 5.5). The articular cavity presents an anterior and a particularly well-developed posterior recess.

When filling a normal cavity, the contrast media opacifies the joint space homogenously, and the borders are regular. In 15% of cases, during the injection we have observed opacification of the contralateral atlanto-axial articular cavity (Fig. 5.6). The joint spaces of the medial atlanto-axial and syndesmodental articulations are very small in healthy subjects.

5.3.2.2
Pathology

In the majority of cases, arthrography shows either minimal degenerative patterns, or diverticular capsule widening, or simply a large posterior extension, possibly in contact with the C2 posterior branch.

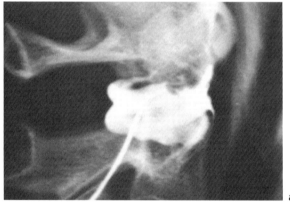

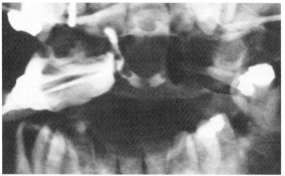

Fig. 5.5a,b. Steroid infiltration in a 55-year-old man with C1-2 osteoarthritis. **a** Lateral arthrographic view shows the reduction of the cavity size. **b** Open mouth arthrographic view demonstrates seepage of the contrast media into the central joint from a right articular injection

Fig. 5.6. Normal arthrographic view in a 62-year-old man. Open mouth arthrographic view shows normal C1–2 arthrography with simultaneous opacification of both sides

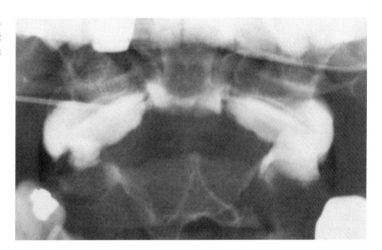

In osteoarthritis, which is commonly diagnosed on plain radiographs, arthrography sometimes shows a very small cavity (GENEZ et al. 1990; ZAPLETAL et al. 1996). Articular puncture is thus impossible. In this particular case, it is possible to inject the steroid locally, hoping that similar pain relief will be achieved.

In rheumatoid arthritis, arthrography shows a wider cavity due to the effects of synovitis on cartilage destruction, bone erosion and ligamentous disruption (HALLA et al. 1989; MORIO et al. 2003; SCHWEITZER et al. 1992). Arthrography usually reveals a large articular cavity with important diverticular extensions, especially on the superior aspects. The borders of the articular cavity are sometimes irregular, and contrast media leakage may be observed.

In ankylosing spondylarthritis, the pattern of the articular cavity varies from small atrophic to normal with very large posterior recesses.

It is not safe to inject the contrast medium into the vertebral artery, although, in the past, this was a way to perform vertebral arteriography. Doing so will cause blood to seep into the syringe. Under fluoroscopy, however, it is easy to control the problem by observing the opacification of the vertebral artery when contrast media injection is tested. If this occurs, withdraw the needle immediately. Replace it a little lower down. This also explains why it is strictly forbidden to inject gas (risk of gas-induced cerebral embolism) or crystal steroids (risk of crystal-induced cerebral embolism).

Infection is avoided by strict asepsis.

If the puncture is performed by a well-trained radiologist, and on a cooperative patient, it is a safe technique. The approach is very similar to the lateral method of puncture in suboccipital myelography already referred to in the medical literature.

5.4
Accidents

The anatomic particularities of the atlanto-axial joint, especially its proximity to major neck vessels and nerves, necessitate a very precise and meticulous procedure for the puncture. In the above-described method, puncture of the pharyngeal spaces is not a risk.

Accidental puncture of the vertebral artery may occur, but is usually devoid of any clinically significant problems. However, hemostasis should be achieved before arthrography.

5.5
Indications

When it is possible to identify the C1-2 radiological abnormalities as a source of pain, specific in situ treatment should be proposed. The efficacy of corticoid therapy in articular pathology has been described in a large number of studies (SCHELLHAS et al. 2000).

Arnold neuralgia could be caused by C2 root impingement due to a synovial cavity (Fig. 5.7).

Osteoarthritis is a good indication with or without neuralgia (Figs. 5.8, 5.9) (GENEZ et al. 1990; SCHWEITZER et al. 1992).

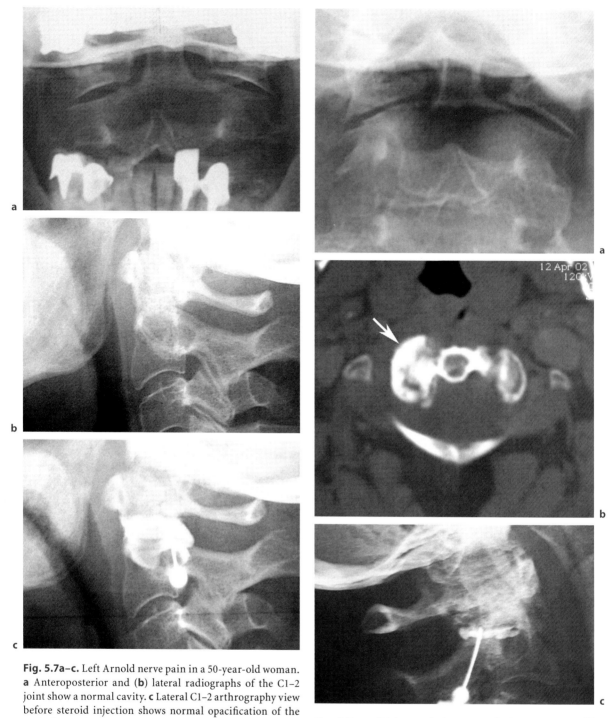

Fig. 5.7a–c. Left Arnold nerve pain in a 50-year-old woman. **a** Anteroposterior and (**b**) lateral radiographs of the C1–2 joint show a normal cavity. **c** Lateral C1–2 arthrography view before steroid injection shows normal opacification of the articular cavity

Fig. 5.8a–c. Right cervical upper pain in an 85-year-old woman. **a** Anteroposterior open mouth C1-2 view shows narrowing of the right C1–2 joint space. **b** Axial CT scan shows destructive right C1–2 area (*arrow*). **c** Lateral view of right C1–2 arthrography before steroid injection shows atrophic joint cavity

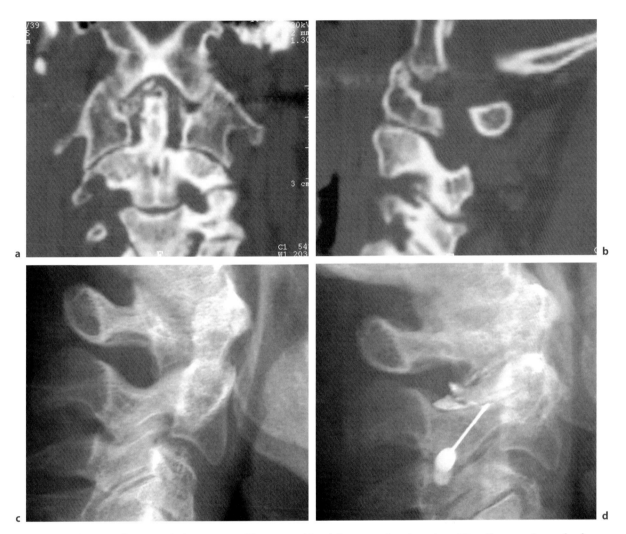

Fig. 5.9a–d. Cervical upper pain in a 67-year-old woman with calcium pyrophosphate deposition disease. **a** Coronal reformatted CT scan shows the narrowing of the joint spaces, and calcifications surrounding the odontoid process. **b** Sagittal reformatted CT scan crossing the right C1–2 joint shows the narrowing of the joint space. Lateral C1–2 (**c**) radiograph and (**d**) arthrography view before steroid injection show the small volume of the joint cavity

In rheumatoid arthritis, due to the cervical spine involvement, C1-2 arthrography permits destruction of the pannus (HALLA et al. 1989; MORIO et al. 2003) and reduction of synovial inflammation in the anterior atlanto-axial and the posterior syndesmodental joint. This procedure may be indicated in the early stages of rheumatoid arthritis (Fig. 5.10).

This technique may also be applied to treatment of synovial cysts (MORIO et al. 2003; OKAMOTO et al. 2004; VERGNE et al. 1996). Patient follow up should demonstrate clinical improvement over several weeks or months, with some patients totally relieved of pain after the first corticoid injection.

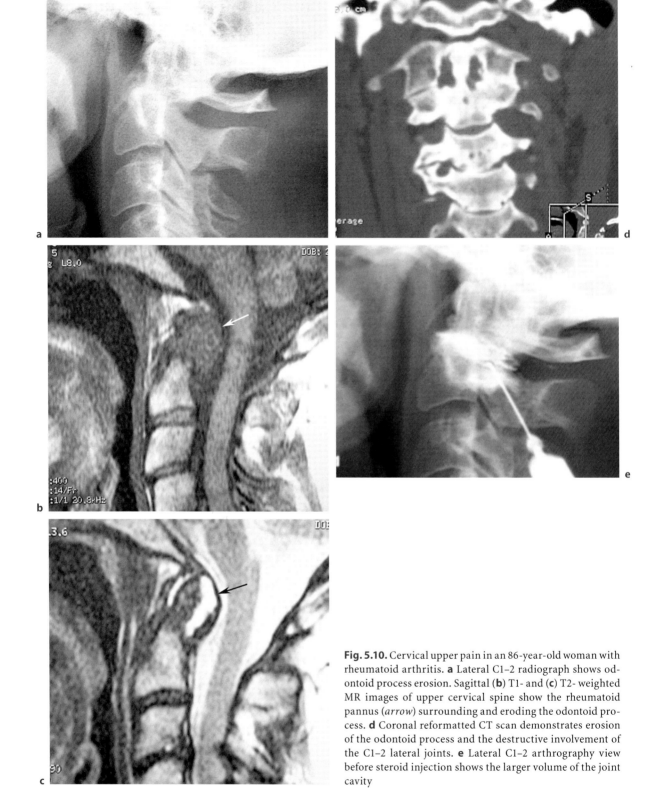

Fig. 5.10. Cervical upper pain in an 86-year-old woman with rheumatoid arthritis. **a** Lateral C1–2 radiograph shows odontoid process erosion. Sagittal (**b**) T1- and (**c**) T2- weighted MR images of upper cervical spine show the rheumatoid pannus (*arrow*) surrounding and eroding the odontoid process. **d** Coronal reformatted CT scan demonstrates erosion of the odontoid process and the destructive involvement of the C1–2 lateral joints. **e** Lateral C1–2 arthrography view before steroid injection shows the larger volume of the joint cavity

5.6
Conclusion

C1-2 arthrography and steroid injection is a safe means for intra-articular steroid injection. The lateral approach under fluoroscopy is safe and fast. It is indicated in case of pain due to osteoarthritis or inflammatory disease. It is an out-patient procedure, and demonstrates good efficacy.

References

Bland JH, Boushey DR (1990) Anatomy and physiology of the cervical spine. Sem Arthr Rheum 20:1–20

Bogduk N (1982) The clinical anatomy of the cervical dorsal rami. Spine 7:319–330

Bovim G, Bonamico L, Fredriksen TA (1991) Topographic variations in the peripheral course of the greater occipital nerve. Autopsy study with clinical correlations. Spine 16:475–478

Cacciola F, Phalke U, Goel A (2004) Vertebral artery in relation to C1-C2 vertebrae: an anatomical study. Neurol India 52:178–184

Chevrot A, Cermakova E, Vallee C, Chancelier MD, Chemla N, Rousselin B, Langer-Cherbit A (1995) C1-2 arthrography. Skeletal Radiol 24:425–429

Chevrot A, Drape JL, Godefroy D, Dupont AM, Gires F, Chemla N, Pessis E, Sarazin L, Minoui A (1997) Image-guided spinal steroid injections. Semin Musculoskelet Radiol 1:221–230

Dirheimer Y, Ramsheyi A, Reolon M (1977) Positive arthrography of the craniocervical joints. Neuroradiology 12:257–260

Dussault RG, Nicolet VM (1985) Cervical facet joint arthrography. J Can Assoc Radiol 36:79–80

Edwards RJ, David KM, Crockard HA (2000) Management of tuberculomas of the craniovertebral junction. Br J Neurosurg 14:19–22

Einig M, Heiger HP, Meairs S, Faust-Tinnefeldt G, Kapp H (1990) Magnetic resonance imaging of the craniocervical junction in rheumatoid arthritis: value, limitations, indications. Skeletal Radiol 19:341–346

Ellis JH, Martel W, Lillie JH, Aisen AM (1991) Magnetic resonance imaging of the normal craniovertebral junction. Spine 16:105–111

Genez BM, Willis JJ, Lowrey CE, Lauerman WC, Woodruff W, Diaz MJ, Higgs JB (1990) CT findings of degenerative arthritis of the atlantoodontoid joint. AJR Am J Roentgenol 154:315–318

Halla JT, Hardin JG, Vitek J, Alarcon GS (1989) Involvement of the cervical spine in rheumatoid arthritis. Arthritis Rheum 5:652–659

Hove B, Gyldensted C (1990) Cervical analgesic facet joint arthrography. Neuroradiology 32:456–459

Lazorthes G, Gaubert J, Chancholle AR, Lazorthes Y (1962) Les rapports de la branche postérieure des nerfs cervicaux avec les articulations interapophysaires vertébrales. Bull Assoc Anat 48:887–895

Mellström A, Grepe A, Levander B (1980) Atlantoaxial arthrography. A postmortem study. Neuroradiology 20:135–144

Morio Y, Yoshioka T, Nagashima H, Hagino H, Teshima R (2003) Intraspinal synovial cyst communicating with the C1-C2 facet joints and subarachnoid space associated with rheumatoid atlantoaxial instability. Spine 28:E492–495

Okamoto K, Doita M, Yoshikawa M, Manabe M, Sha N, Yoshiya S (2004) Synovial cyst at the C1-C2 junction in a patient with atlantoaxial subluxation. J Spinal Disord Tech 17:535–538

Pfirrmann CW, Binkert CA, Zanetti M, Boos N, Hodler J (2001) MR morphology of alar ligaments and occipitoatlantoaxial joints: study in 50 asymptomatic subjects. Radiology 218:133–137

Saway PA, Blackburn WD, Halla JT, Allarcon GS (1988) Life table analysis of survival in patients with rheumatoid arthritis and cervical spine involvement. Arthritis Rheum 31[suppl 1]:R47

Schellhas KP, Garvey TA, Johnson BA, Rothbart PJ, Pollei SR (2000) Cervical diskography: analysis of provoked responses at C2-C3, C3-C4, and C4-C5. AJNR Am J Neuroradiol 21:269–275

Schweitzer ME, Hodler J, Cervilla V, Resnick D (1992) Craniovertebral junction: normal anatomy with MR correlation. AJR Am J Roentgenol 158:1087–1090

Vergne P, Bonnet C, Zabraniecki L, Bertin P, Moreau JJ, Treves R (1996) Synovial cyst at the C1-C2 junction and spondyloarthropathy. J Rheumatol 23:1438–1440

Zapletal J, Hekster RE, Straver JS, Wilmink JT, Hermans J (1996) Relationship between atlanto-odontoid osteoarthritis and idiopathic suboccipital neck pain. Neuroradiology 38:62–65

Percutaneous Treatment of Intervertebral Disc Herniation

Xavier Buy, Afshin Gangi, Stéphane Guth, and Ali Guermazi

CONTENTS

6.1   Introduction   93

6.2   Periradicular Steroid Injection   94
6.2.1   Principle   94
6.2.2   Patient Selection   94
6.2.2.1 Indications   94
6.2.2.2 Contraindications   94
6.2.3   Technique   94
6.2.3.1 Lumbar Level   95
6.2.3.2 Cervical Level   96
6.2.3.3 Thoracic Level   96
6.2.4   Post-Procedural Instructions   98
6.2.5   Complications   98
6.2.5.1 Technical Complications   98
6.2.5.2 Drug Related Complications   98
6.2.6   Results   98

6.3   Percutaneous Disc Decompression   99
6.3.1   General Principles   99
6.3.2   Disc Puncture   100
6.3.2.1 Lumbar Disc Puncture   100
6.3.2.2 Thoracic Disc Puncture   101
6.3.2.3 Cervical Disc Puncture   102
6.3.3   Percutaneous Laser Disc
        Decompression   103
6.3.3.1 Principle of PLDD   103
6.3.3.2 Patient Selection for PLDD   104
6.3.3.3 Materials for PLDD   104
6.3.3.4 Technique of PLDD   104
6.3.3.5 Post-Operative Instructions   106
6.3.3.6 Complications of PLDD   106
6.3.3.7 Results   106
6.3.4   Bipolar Radiofrequency Nucleoplasty   107
6.3.4.1 Principle of Nucleoplasty   107
6.3.4.2 Patient Selection for Nucleoplasty   108
6.3.4.3 Materials   108
6.3.4.4 Technique of Nucleoplasty   109
6.3.4.5 Post-Operative Instructions   112
6.3.4.6 Complications of RF Nucleoplasty   113
6.3.4.7 Results of RF Nucleoplasty   113
6.3.5   Targeted Disc Decompression   114
6.3.6   Comparison of PLDD vs
        RF Nucleoplasty   114

6.4   Conclusion   116

        References   116

6.1 Introduction

Disc herniation is defined as rupture of the fibro-cartilagenous annulus fibrosus that surrounds the intervertebral disc, associated with the release of the central gelatinous nucleus pulposus. Most herniations take place in the lumbar area of the spine. They occur more frequently in middle aged and older men, especially those involved in strenuous physical activity. They cause physical disability with significant social and economic effects.

Although first described by Virshow in 1857, the physiopathology and therapeutics of disc herniation remain controversial (CASTRO et al. 2005). There is no single, clear explanation as to why disc rupture causes axial spinal pain and/or radicular pain. When disc herniation contacts a nerve root, radicular symptoms (leg, arm or intercostal pain) appear. However, physical pressure on a peripheral nerve alone produces paraesthesia but no pain. It is postulated that biochemical factors somehow cause pain.

Pain management in disc herniation relies mainly on conservative care combining rest, physiotherapy and oral medication (analgesics and anti-inflammatory drugs). If 6 weeks of conservative therapy and a minimum of one selective image-guided periradicular steroid injection fail, treatment turns to percutaneous techniques directed at the disc (GANGI et al. 1998a).

X. BUY, MD, Senior Radiologist
A. GANGI, MD, PhD, Professor of Radiology
S. GUTH, MD, Senior Radiologist
Department of Radiology B, University Hospital of Strasbourg, Pavillon Clovis Vincent BP 426, 67091 Strasbourg, France
A. GUERMAZI, MD, Associate Professor of Radiology Department of Radiology, Section Chief, Musculoskeletal, Boston University School of Medicine, 88 East Newton Street, Boston, MA 02118, USA

Despite its acceptance, open discectomy is a major surgical procedure. In a prospective study of 412 primary and 69 reoperations for lumbar disc herniations, Stolke et al. (1989) reported an intraoperative complication rate of 7.8% for microdiskectomies, 13.7% for macrodiskectomies and 27.5% for reoperations. Postoperative complications ranged from 1.4% for reoperation, 3.9% for microdiskectomies up to 4.2% for macrodiskectomies. The risk of complications correlates with the age of the patient and the operating time. In their review of 28,000 discectomy procedures, Ramirez and Thisted (1989) reported 1 in 64 patients having a major complication, 1 in 335 having a neurological complication, nearly 1 in 500 having a cardiovascular complication and 1 in 1,700 dying from the procedure. The long term outcome, complications and suboptimal results associated with open disc surgery have led to the development of minimally invasive techniques that avoid opening the spinal canal and extensive disc ablation.

The minimally invasive percutaneous techniques in use today aim at removing a small amount of central nucleus pulposus to reduce intradiscal pressure and thus obviate disco-radicular compression. Chemonucleolysis with papaine was introduced by Smith et al. (1963) in an early attempt to treat herniation without surgery. It was used for treating sciatica due to disc herniation and proved the effectiveness of disc decompression for treating disc herniation. Although the technique showed good results with a 70%–80% success rate, it had unacceptable adverse reactions and is no longer used in the USA or Europe. Since then, several alternative percutaneous nucleotomy techniques have been developed: purely mechanical decompression (automated percutaneous lumbar discectomy), chemical decompression (alcohol, oxygen-ozone) or thermal decompression (laser, radiofrequency) (Andreula et al. 2004).

6.2
Periradicular Steroid Injection

6.2.1
Principle

As proven by Ian Macnab (MB, CHB, FRCS, FRCS(C), 1921–1992), radicular pain due to disc herniation cannot be explained by a purely mechanical approach. The manifestation of pain has a close relationship with the release of mediators from macrophages. Inflammatory cytokines, prostaglandins, nitrous oxide (NO), phospholipase A2 (PLA2) and cyclooxygenase-2 (COX-2) may be involved in radiculitis caused by mechanical compression (Kawakami et al. 1999; Kobayashi et al. 2005). Periradicular steroid injection (PSI) is the first minimally invasive technique to be considered early in the treatment regime. PSI is effective, probably because of its anti-inflammatory effects. It should be performed under image guidance to ensure proper deposition of steroid.

6.2.2
Patient Selection

6.2.2.1
Indications

The main indication for PSI is radicular symptoms due to discal compression, resistant to conventional medical treatment. Patient selection is based on a precise clinical examination supported by discal abnormalities on CT or MR imaging at the corresponding level. This is mandatory to avoid misdiagnosing extra-discal causes of radiculitis.

Pure axial back or neck pain due to disc herniation and post-discectomy syndromes may sometimes benefit from epidural infiltration.

6.2.2.2
Contraindications

Steroids are contraindicated in patients with diabetes or gastric ulcers or who are pregnant. In patients with bleeding diathesis, epidural puncture is contraindicated and a foraminal approach should be performed carefully. In severe spinal stenosis, long-acting synthetic steroids should be avoided, due to their hyperosmotic effect. Adjuvants in long acting steroids can also produce allergic reactions in patients with atopic tendencies. This should be checked by prior interview.

6.2.3
Technique

The procedure is performed on an outpatient basis. Image guidance is provided by CT, MR imaging or C-arm fluoroscopy. CT guidance is preferred as it allows for exact planning and positioning of the needle extradurally, preventing intrathecal or intravascular injection. The needle tip should be positioned as close as possible to the disco-radicular interface.

6.2.3.1
Lumbar Level

The patient is prone. The entry point and the pathway are determined by axial CT, with scan thickness not exceeding 3 mm. The CT gantry does not need to be tilted to perform an interlaminar puncture. The approach is epidural-lateral for posteromedial or posterolateral herniation, foraminal for foraminal or extra-foraminal herniation.

6.2.3.1.1
Epidural Lateral Infiltration

After painting and draping, the skin of the entry point is infiltrated with local anesthetic. A 22-gauge spinal needle is positioned via a posterior approach near the painful nerve root under CT-control (Figs. 6.1 and 6.2). Fluoro-CT is not necessary. When the nerve root is inadvertently touched, the patient will immediately report an electric pain in the radic-

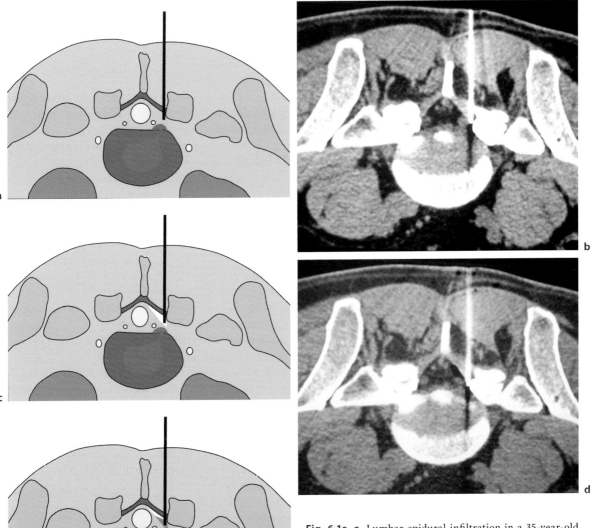

Fig. 6.1a–e. Lumbar epidural infiltration in a 35-year-old man with sciatic pain due to posterolateral hernia. Drawings and their corresponding axial CT scans show (**a,b**) needle tip in the epidural space, followed by (**c,d**) gaseous epidurography to confirm the proper position before (**e**) steroid injection

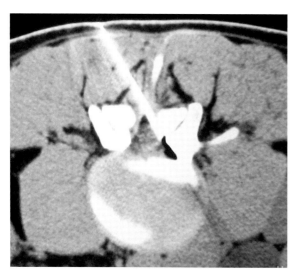

Fig. 6.2. Lumbar epidural infiltration in a 26-year-old man with crural pain due to posterolateral hernia. Axial CT scan shows posteromedial diagonal as an alternative approach when direct access is impossible

ular area and the needle should be withdrawn a few millimeters. A flexible sterile connecting tube is fixed to the needle to avoid displacement of the tip during injection. The extradural position of the needle is confirmed by negative aspiration of cerebrospinal fluid and blood followed by injection of 1 mL of iodine contrast. For CT-guided low epidural lumbar infiltration (from L3 to S1) only, gaseous epidurography using 1 mL of sterile air from the connecting tube can be used to check the position of the needle tip. Under fluoroscopic control, iodine contrast injection is used systematically; using flash or positive blood aspirate to predict intravascular injections is 97% specific, but only 45.9% sensitive (Furman et al. 2000). Then 1.5 mL of long acting steroid (cortivazol 3.75 mg, Aventis Pharma, Strasbourg, France) solution, mixed with 1 mL of lidocaine 1% is injected.

If the dura has been perforated because the dural sac has adhered to the ligamentum flavum or because of an incorrect maneuver, the needle must be pulled back slightly and its position checked by aspirating for cerebrospinal fluid and injecting iodine for contrast. In such cases, lidocaine should be avoided and hydrocortisone preferred; long acting steroids should never be used in intrathecal injection as they may precipitate in the cerebrospinal fluid and induce chemical arachnoiditis. Hydrocortisone is also preferred for severe spinal stenosis, as long acting synthetic steroids worsen symptoms due to their hyperosmotic effect.

6.2.3.1.2
Foraminal Infiltration

Foraminal infiltration is quite similar to epidural infiltration but with a more lateral entry point. The needle slips along the facet joint and is pushed 1 cm further so that its tip remains just behind the nerve root as it exits the foramen (Fig. 6.3). Too anterior positioning of the needle tip is dangerous and should be avoided, as rare cases of paraplegia have been reported. The mechanism of this very serious complication remains unclear, and for this reason, we prefer epidural infiltrations. If injections are performed under fluoroscopic guidance, iodine contrast is injected to check the correct periradicular position of the needle.

6.2.3.2
Cervical Level

The patient is placed in supine position head turned slightly to the opposite side and hyperextended with a cushion under the shoulders. The entry point and the pathway are determined by axial CT scan not exceeding 2 mm thickness. After painting, draping and superficial infiltration of local anesthesia, a 22-gauge spinal needle is placed by a lateral approach near the painful nerve root under CT control. The tip of the needle is positioned in contact with the anterior side of the facet joint, behind the nerve root, avoiding the anteriorly situated vertebral artery. A flush connecting tube is fixed to the needle to avoid unintentional displacement of its tip during injection. The needle position is checked by aspirating for blood, and by injecting 1–2 mL iodine for contrast. After excluding intravascular injection, 1.5 mL of long acting steroid (cortivazol 3.75 mg) solution is injected (Fig. 6.4).

Air must never be used as a contrast medium at the cervical level. Lidocaine should not be injected in the foramen as it may diffuse around the spinal cord and induce transient phrenic nerve palsy. A posterior approach with the patient lying prone has been described but because the dura and the ligamentum flavum are in contact the risk of intrathecal injection is high. The lateral approach is preferred.

6.2.3.3
Thoracic Level

Thoracic periradicular steroid injections have few indications as intercostal radicular pain due to disc herniation is rare. However, a foraminal injection

Percutaneous Treatment of Intervertebral Disc Herniation 97

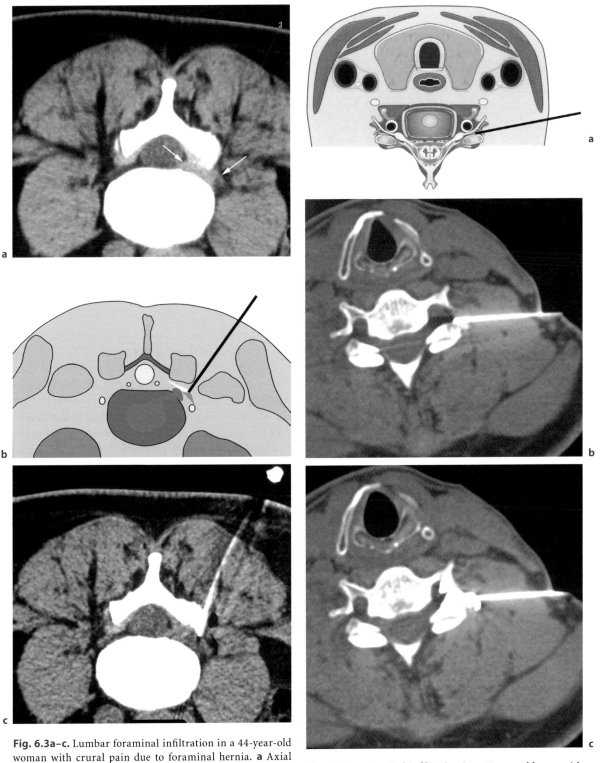

Fig. 6.3a–c. Lumbar foraminal infiltration in a 44-year-old woman with crural pain due to foraminal hernia. a Axial CT scan shows a right foraminal hernia of L3–L4 (arrows). b Drawing and its corresponding (c) axial CT scan show needle tip in the right foraminal space. The needle tip should remain behind the nerve root

Fig. 6.4a–c. Cervical infiltration in a 32-year-old man with cervico-brachial neuralgia due to disc herniation. a Drawing and its corresponding (b) axial CT scan show needle tip in the left cervical foramen in contact with the articular process. c Axial CT scan shows the needle position is checked by iodine contrast before steroid injection

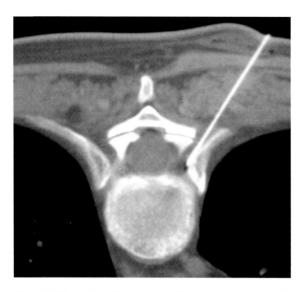

Fig. 6.5. Thoracic infiltration in a 32-year-old woman with intercostal pain. Axial CT scan demonstrates the right posterolateral approach at the level of T8

of long acting steroids mixed with 1 mL of lidocaine can be done safely by CT-guided posterolateral approach (Fig. 6.5). The needle tip should remain behind the nerve root; its precise position must be checked by injection of 1 mL of iodine contrast.

6.2.4
Post-Procedural Instructions

Patients can stand up immediately and return to their activities. The sterile dressing can be removed after 36 h. Although steroids are locally deposed, restricted sodium intake is recommended for a week.

6.2.5
Complications

Severe adverse events following periradicular steroid injections are rare (<0.05%), occurring more often with cervical injection (Ma et al. 2005).

6.2.5.1
Technical Complications

Major complications are extremely rare. Infectious complications such as meningitis with neurological damage (quadriplegia, multiple cranial nerve palsies, nystagmus, etc.), epidural abscesses (Huang et al. 2004) and spondylodiscitis have been reported

after epidural or intrathecal injection of steroids (Hooten et al. 2004; Yue and Tan 2003). Of course, strict sterility during the intervention is essential. Vascular complications are mainly due to vertebral artery injury or intra-arterial injection at the cervical level (Rosenkranz et al. 2004). Medullary infarction following lumbar infiltrations has been reported, possibly from damage to a low arising artery of Adamkiewicz (Houten and Errico 2002; Huntoon and Martin 2004). Hence, strict and careful observation of iodine contrast distribution is mandatory before injecting steroids, particularly with foraminal infiltrations. Epidural hematomas at cervical or lumbar levels have also been reported but these rarely require surgical decompression (Reitman and Watters 2002).

6.2.5.2
Drug Related Complications

Mild reactions like flushing (allergic reaction to the adjuvant in the steroid) or transient increase in pain at the injection site have been reported in less than 5% of cases. There is a high risk of thecal calcifications with triamcinolone hexacetonide and we do not recommend its use. Intrathecal injection of cortivazol causes chemical arachnoiditis and calcifications. Long acting synthetic steroids should be injected only if the needle is in the correct epidural position, otherwise natural steroids (hydrocortisone) should be used. Hydrocortisone should also be preferred for lumbar canal stenosis as the osmotic effect of long acting steroids may be responsible for transient increases in pain. Symptomatic epidural lipomatosis following local steroid infiltration has been reported but remains unusual (Sandberg and Lavyne 1999). However, there should be no more than four infiltrations in a year at the same level to avoid secondary lipodystrophy.

In lidocaine sensitive patients, immediate transient anesthesia in the distribution of the injected nerve root is possible. Complete neurological recovery is noted within 1 h and the patient can be discharged.

6.2.6
Results

Although periradicular steroid injection has been used for decades, its efficacy is still controversial. The literature is not at all clear, but the following points need to be kept in mind when considering the results of various studies. Puncture technique, approach, the diameter of the needle, the use of image guidance and contrast opacification prior to steroid injection all vary widely. Studies assessing the efficacy of epidural steroid injections should use an epidurogram to verify the injection site, as simple loss of air pressure resistance leads to 25.7%–30% of inaccurate needle tip placements (BARTYNSKI et al. 2005; JOHNSON et al. 1999; STOJANOVIC et al. 2002). Patient selection also varies. Radicular pains of varying causes (disc herniation, spinal stenosis, degenerative disorders, etc.) treated with PSI have variable outcomes. Non-controlled studies report success in 33%–72% of patients. Short-term benefit of percutaneous nerve root block is quite high with good pain relief especially in irritative radiculopathy. Irritative radiculopathy is described as sciatica alone, while compressive radiculopathy is described as sciatica with sensory, motor, or reflex disturbances. The irritative group responds significantly better than the compressive group. Periradicular steroid infiltrations seem to be less beneficial for more chronic radicular pain (CYTEVAL et al. 2006). Epidural steroid injection provides mild to moderate improvement in leg pain and sensory deficits and reduces the need for analgesics for up to 6 weeks. It also prevents surgery for contained disc herniations (KARPPINEN et al. 2001; KOLSTAD et al. 2005). Steroids speed the rate of recovery and return to function, allowing a reduction of medication, while awaiting the natural improvement expected in most spinal disorders (MCLAIN et al. 2005).

When the results of several controlled studies are combined, there is no difference between the steroid-treated groups and the control groups at long-term follow-up. This can be explained by the generally favorable long-term prognosis for these non-surgically treated patients. However, a beneficial effect is seen in patients with radicular pain syndromes at intermediate-term follow-up.

RIEW et al. (2000) performed a prospective randomized controlled double blinded study with 55 patients. A combined solution of bupivacaine and betamethasone obviated the need for surgical decompression in 20/28 (71%) patients. He suggested that patients suffering from lumbar radicular pain due to disc herniation should be considered for selective infiltrations before turning to surgery.

In our experience with over 5,000 periradicular steroid infiltrations performed under CT guidance, short-term benefit was high with good pain relief in 78% of extraforaminal herniations and 65% for other locations. The long-term result (persistence of relief for at least 6 months) was satisfactory only in extraforaminal herniations. We had no major complications. The use of image guidance for periradicular infiltrations significantly increases accuracy and decreases complication rates (WATANABE et al. 2002).

6.3
Percutaneous Disc Decompression

6.3.1
General Principles

When conservative therapies (oral analgesics, physiotherapy) associated with selective image-guided periradicular steroid injections fail to control radicular pain due to disc herniation, treatment is directed at the disc with the aim of decompressing or removing the herniation.

Conventional open surgery for disc herniation has limitations. It offers suboptimal results and its morbidity is not negligible, particularly with the risk of epidural fibrosis. Several less invasive percutaneous techniques have been developed, relying on the fundamental principle that the intervertebral disc is a closed hydraulic space; minor ablation of the nucleus pulposus induces significant decompression. Nucleolysis with injection of chemopapain was described in 1963 with good results (SMITH et al. 1963), but there is a small but definitive risk of serious adverse events and it is no longer being manufactured.

Oxygen-ozone and alcohol are also employed for chemical nucleolysis (ANDREULA et al. 2003; BURIC and MOLINO LOVA 2005), but are still under evaluation. The mechanism of action of oxygen-ozone remains unknown. Chemical techniques may suffer the disadvantage of uncontrolled ablation. Moreover, alcohol is contraindicated in a perforated annulus, as it can diffuse into the surrounding soft tissues with disastrous results.

Several mechanical and thermal nucleotomy techniques have been developed recently. Percutaneous techniques have many advantages over conventional open surgery: surrounding tissues are protected, there is no scar, only local anesthesia is needed and the patient can go home, and much reduced cost (25%–30% of conventional surgical treatment cost).

These techniques are limited, however, to contained disc herniations.

Automated percutaneous lumbar discectomy is rarely used today due to poor clinical design, high cost and patient discomfort.

Thermal techniques with high temperature (laser, targeted disc decompression) or low temperature (radiofrequency nucleoplasty) combine purely mechanical decompression with thermally induced modifications of intradiscal cytokines involved in disc degeneration. They may also destroy nociceptors in the periphery of the annulus. Moreover, fusion of collagen fibers in the annulus occurs at temperatures over 70 °C, with visible shrinkage at the periphery of the disc (WANG et al. 2005).These techniques are detailed in the following paragraphs.

6.3.2
Disc Puncture

6.3.2.1
Lumbar Disc Puncture

The procedure can be performed in the prone or lateral decubitus position. We prefer prone as the patient is more stable. A standard extra-pedicular posterior-lateral approach is used. To open up the posterior aspect of the disc space, pillows are positioned under the abdomen to place the lumbar spine in a semi flexed position (particularly helpful for L5-S1 level). Fluoroscopic guidance is used; CT is not necessary in routine practice. Of course, strict asepsis is mandatory with sterile draping of the patient, the operator and the head of the C-arm.

Under fluoroscopy, the desired disc level is marked. A paramedian line 8–10 cm (a hand's width) lateral and parallel to the midline is drawn depending on patient corpulence. The site of insertion of the needle is the point of intersection of the paramedian line with the plane of the disc as seen on lateral fluoroscopy (Fig. 6.6). For the L5-S1 level, the site of insertion is slightly higher and curved needles are necessary when prominent iliac wings block the direct approach.

Constant and complete neurological monitoring of the patient is required during the procedure. Hence, it is strongly advised not to use sedation and to anesthetize the nerve root. Local anesthesia is administered with lidocaine using a 22-gauge needle, infiltrating from skin to articular process. Under lateral fluoroscopy, the needle slips along the ar-

ticular process into the disc. Close contact with the articular process is mandatory to avoid puncturing the nerve root. When penetrating the disc, the needle must remain parallel to and midway between the two vertebral endplates (Fig. 6.7). The position of the needle tip must be confirmed on anteroposterior and lateral projections.

The "Scotty dog" technique requires an oblique projection. The C-arm is rotated until the superior articular process (ear of the "Scotty dog") is centered midway between the anterior and posterior aspects of the vertebral body. The superior endplate of the same vertebral body should superimpose. Disc puncture is performed in the axis of the X-ray beam, just anterior to the "ear of the dog" (Fig. 6.8). For the L5-S1 level, significant caudal angulation is required for optimal visualization.

For CT-guidance, the CT gantry is tilted if necessary to be parallel to the intervertebral disc plane. The entry point and the pathway are determined accurately by CT, avoiding the nerve root and visceral structures. At the L5-S1 level, curved needles may

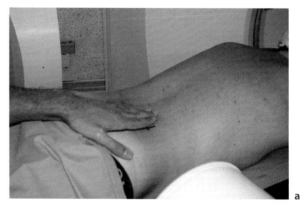

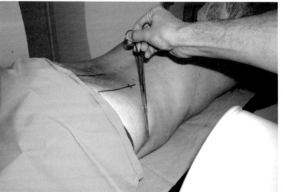

Fig. 6.6a,b. Technique of lumbar disc puncture. Skin entry point is at the intersection of (**a**) the paramedian line with (**b**) the plane of the disc, as marked by the sponge holder, using lateral fluoroscopy

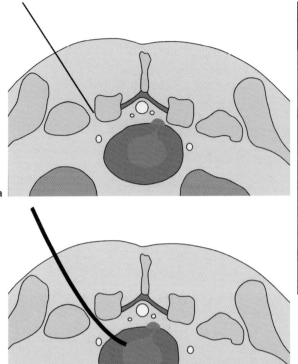

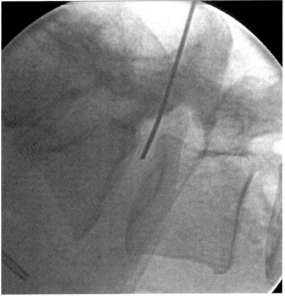

Fig. 6.7a–c. Lumbar disc puncture in a 29-year-old man with sciatica requiring L5-S1 percutaneous disc decompression. **a** Local anesthesia from the skin to the articular process. **b** Drawing and its corresponding (**c**) lateral radiograph of the lumbar spine show the needle inserted into the disc. Close contact with the articular process is mandatory to avoid the nerve root

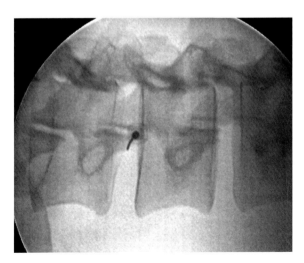

Fig. 6.8. Lumbar disc puncture using Scotty dog technique in a 33-year-old man with sciatica requiring percutaneous disc decompression. Scotty dog radiograph of the lumbar spine shows puncture performed at L4–L5 level, in the axis of the X-ray beam, just anterior to the articular process

be necessary. Once the entry point is determined, a lateral fluoroscopic view is obtained at the desired disc level. This way, the operator can visualize the pathway and correct angulation of the needle towards the intervertebral disc in real time. Discography can be performed just before the procedure to confirm that the disc herniation is contained if any doubt persists.

6.3.2.2
Thoracic Disc Puncture

The patient is prone and a posterolateral approach is used. The C-arm is rotated 35° laterally from the anteroposterior view. With this oblique projection, two rings are visible, the medial corresponding to the pedicle and the lateral corresponding to the head of the rib. Then, the C-arm is angulated craniocaudally so that the X-ray beam is parallel to the disc. The puncture is performed between the pedicle and the rib, in the axis of the beam (Fig. 6.9).

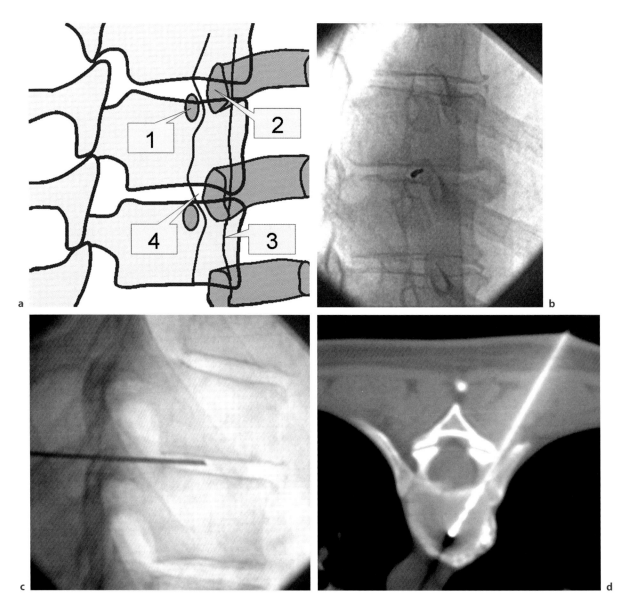

Fig. 6.9a–d. Thoracic disc puncture in a 42-year-old woman with right intercostal pain due to T7–T8 herniation, requiring percutaneous disc decompression. **a** Drawing and (**b**) oblique fluoroscopic view with 35° rotation from the sagittal plane show the approach for thoracic disc puncture (*1*= pedicle, *2*= head of the rib, *3*=pleural line, *4*=access point for disc). **c** Lateral fluoroscopy view and (**d**) axial CT scan show the access needle within the disc

6.3.2.3
Cervical Disc Puncture

Cervical puncture is performed by a standard anterolateral approach under fluoroscopic guidance. The patient is supine, with a cushion under the lower neck and upper thoracic spine to hyperextend the neck. A right side entry point is theoretically safer as the esophagus often deviates slightly to the left. The disc level is checked with fluoroscopy.

Asepsis must be strict as the proximity of oropharyngeal structures increases the risk of infection. After preparation of the skin and superficial local anesthesia, the carotid artery is detected by its pulsation. With two fingers, the operator presses against the spine, moving the carotid artery laterally. Then the disc is punctured directly between the two fingers, the needle passing between the carotid artery laterally and esophagus medially (Fig. 6.10).

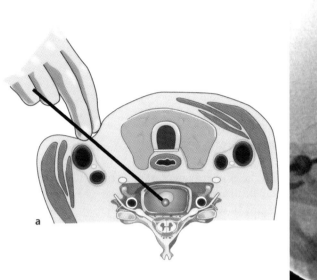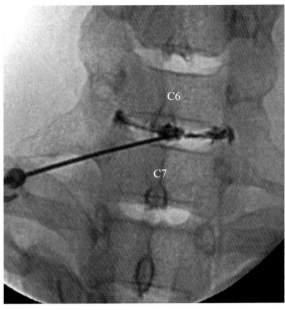

Fig. 6.10a,b. Cervical disc puncture in a 30-year-old man with right C7 neuralgia but no evidence of herniation on MR imaging. **a** Drawing shows antero-lateral approach with displacement of the carotido-jugular complex laterally by the operator's fingers. **b** Anteroposterior radiograph of the cervical spine shows the needle placement with discography of the C6–C7 disc

6.3.3
Percutaneous Laser Disc Decompression

Percutaneous laser disc decompression (PLDD) was pioneered by CHOY et al. (1987). The first case of laser decompression in a patient with symptomatic disc herniation was reported in the late 1980s (CHOY et al. 1987).

6.3.3.1
Principle of PLDD

The principle of percutaneous laser disc decompression is the transformation of light energy into thermal energy to vaporize a portion of the nucleus and achieve decompression (KNAPPE et al. 2004). Laser energy is transmitted into the disc through a thin optical fiber. Vaporization produces gas which is evacuated through the introducer needle. The ablation of a relatively small volume of nucleus (1.5–2 cm^3) results in an important reduction of intradiscal pressure which reduces disc herniation (CHOY et al. 1991), assuming that the herniation is still contained. Pressure reduction is not the only effect of laser. It also produces denervation of the pain receptors of the annulus fibrosus and spinal ligaments. Heating the disc with laser leads to the

destruction of nerve transmitter (L-glutamate, substance P, peptides and quinine) production sites. The levels of chemical factors (prostaglandin E2 and phospholipase E2) responsible for nerve root irritation are significantly reduced after PLDD, and nerve conduction velocities are increased (IWATSUKI et al. 2005). Experimental studies have shown that no temperature change is detected at the neural foramina or in the spinal canal during PLDD (CHOY et al. 1992; SCHLANGMANN et al. 1996). After laser irradiation, intradiscal pressure decreases and the nucleus pulposus is gradually replaced with fibrous tissue.

Whether to use laser or not depends on the tissue and the therapeutic objective. In laser nucleotomy, the aim is to vaporize the nucleus to achieve disc decompression (GANGI et al. 1998a, b). The laser wavelength has to be chosen to allow for good absorption to obtain the photothermal effect. Holmium:yttrium-aluminum-garnet (YAG) laser is effective in treating disc herniation. Its short penetration of 1–2 mm makes it safe, with low temperature and less risk of disc perforation. The drawbacks are slow vaporization with increased operating time, possible shock wave and high cost. Neodymium:YAG laser is actually the best compromise for discal procedures. Its penetration of 7 mm allows for fast vaporization of sufficient nuclear volume to achieve decompression. The major disadvantage is its high temperature (GANGI et al. 1996).

6.3.3.2
Patient Selection for PLDD

6.3.3.2.1
Indications

Patient selection is crucial for treatment effectiveness (OHNMEISS et al. 1994). For lumbar levels, the best indications for PLDD are sciatica or crural pain (leg pain of greater intensity than back pain, positive straight-leg-raising test, decreased sensation, normal motor response and tendon reflex) due to contained disk herniation determined by CT or MR imaging, and failure of 6 weeks of conservative therapy and selective steroid injections.

Less often, PLDD can be indicated for posteromedial contained disc herniation with pure axial low back pain resistant to 3 months of conservative care. Disc decompression is effective if the symptoms are produced by maneuvers which increase pressure on the posterior spinal ligament: positive cough sign and positive "memory pain" with provocative discography.

6.3.3.2.2
Contraindications

Contraindications of PLDD are nerve paralysis, hemorrhagic diathesis, spondylolisthesis, free fragments, spinal stenosis, significant psychological disorders, severe degenerative disc with collapse >50%, workplace injuries with monetary gain, and local infection of the skin, subcutaneous or muscular layers.

Previous surgery at the same level is considered a relative contraindication. An extruded disc is generally considered a contraindication to PLDD but, according to CHOY (2001), patients with extruded but nonsequestrated disc herniations may also benefit.

6.3.3.2.3
Limitations

PLDD produces high temperatures and the risk of thermal injury to the adjacent vertebral endplates increases when the height of the disc is reduced. Moreover, laser energy penetrates 5–8 mm from the tip of the optical fiber, depending on the wavelength used. This can be dangerous for the spinal cord and

foraminal nerve roots at the cervical level with an anterior approach (SCHMOLKE et al. 2004). For these reasons, low energy (300 J) and particular caution should be used to treat thoracic and cervical herniations (CHOY and FEJOS 2004). These levels are treated with radiofrequency (RF) nucleoplasty in our department.

6.3.3.3
Materials for PLDD

The laser energy necessary to treat disc herniations can be provided by many lasers in the near infra-red region or with visible green radiation (KNAPPE et al. 2004) with wavelength varying from 514 to 2150 nm, e.g. KTP, Ho:YAG and diode laser (CHOY 1993; GANGI et al. 1996; GEVARGEZ et al. 2000).We are currently using a diode laser with an 805 nm wavelength (Diomed Inc., Cambridge, UK).

The following materials are used:
- 18-Gauge spinal needle
- Side-arm fitting to remove by-products of vaporization and reduce pressure that would build up during the procedure
- Quartz optical fiber of 400 μm to transmit laser energy to the disc
- Laser protection eyewear

6.3.3.4
Technique of PLDD

For lumbar PLDD, a standard posterolateral approach is used. Local anesthesia is infiltrated from skin to articular process, using a 22-gauge spinal needle. Complete neurological monitoring is necessary during the whole procedure; sedation and anesthesia of the nerve root are avoided. An 18-gauge spinal needle is inserted into the disc using the tandem technique. Its tip is positioned at the posterior annulus/nucleus junction (Fig. 6.11) (CHOY et al. 1992).

Before insertion, the optical fiber must be connected to the laser and checked for integrity. The red spot must be circular and homogeneous. After removing the stylet of the 18-gauge needle the optical fiber is inserted into the disc. The distal part of the optical fiber should not extend more than 3–5 mm beyond the needle tip. The proper length of the fiber is marked with a sterile strip to avoid excessive advancement (Fig. 6.12).

When the fiber is in the right position, the laser procedure begins. Laser protection eyewear is man-

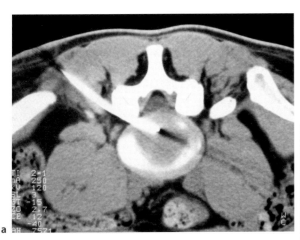
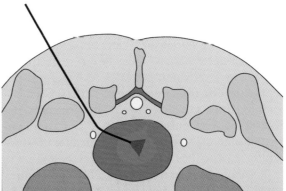
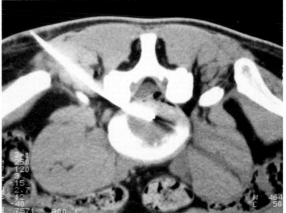

Fig. 6.11a–c. Percutaneous laser disc decompression in a 35-year-old man with right L5 sciatic pain. **a** Axial CT scan of the lumbar spine shows an 18-gauge spinal needle is positioned at the posterior annulus/nucleus junction. **b** Optical fiber inserted into the nucleus. **c** Axial CT scan at the same level as (**a**) shows that vaporization is visible with gas diffusion into the herniation after PLDD

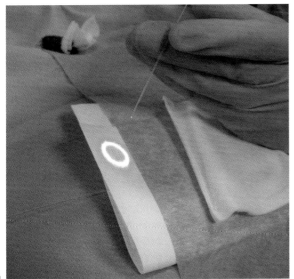
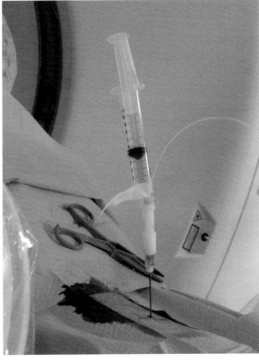

Fig. 6.12a,b. Technique of percutaneous laser disc decompression. **a** The integrity of the optical fiber is checked before insertion. **b** The proper length of the fiber is marked with a sterile strip. Aspiration on the side-arm fitting is applied to reduce pressure within the disc

datory. The laser is turned on to produce 15 W with 0.5- to 1-s pulses or "on" time, at 4- to 10-s intervals or "off" time, depending on patient comfort. During the laser procedure, small puffs of smoke can be seen exiting the needle. If any back pain occurs during the intervention, it may be due to heating of the adjacent vertebral endplates or hyperpressure within the disc from trapped gas. The last phenomenon is clearly visualized by CT. In such cases, the interval between pulses is increased and aspiration is applied to the side-arm fitting to reduce pressure within the disc (Fig. 6.12) (GANGI et al. 1996).

Recommended laser doses for PLDD procedures range from 1,200 to 1,500 J for L1–2, L3–4 and L5–S1 levels and 1,500 to 2,000 Joules for L4–L5. Vaporization depends on the color of the disc. When the disc is too transparent, it conducts light energy. If no vaporization is visible on CT after 400 Joules, the optical fiber is activated by dipping its tip into the patient's blood to produce the photothermal effect. At the end of the procedure, the needle and the fiber are withdrawn and the skin entry point is covered with sterile dressing.

6.3.3.5
Post-Operative Instructions

Patients are discharged after 3 h. A post-laser treatment instruction sheet stresses rest for a few days along with prescriptions for pain, muscle relaxation, and anti-inflammation. For 2 weeks after the intervention, sitting, bending and stooping are restricted. Athletic activities should be halted for a minimum of 6 weeks. Three weeks after PLDD, the patient should undergo physical therapy to stretch the trunk area. Some activities such as bathing are prohibited until the skin has fully healed, to prevent infection.

Follow-up relies mainly on clinical symptoms. CT or MR imaging of the lumbosacral spine is performed only if any complication is suspected. The shrinkage of the herniation is generally modest to moderate and only visible after several months.

6.3.3.6
Complications of PLDD

The overall rate of complication is 0.4%–0.5% for lumbar levels and 0.6%–1% for cervical levels (CHOY 2004; HELLINGER 2004).

The major complication of PLDD is septic spondylodiscitis. This can be avoided with strict sterility during the procedure. Thermal injury of adjacent vertebral endplates leading to aseptic spondylitis with severe backache has been reported (Fig. 6.13). If any back pain occurs during vaporization, laser energy delivery should be slowed. Thermal spondylitis is treated with NSAIDs but symptoms can last up to 6 months.

Recurrence of disc herniation or free fragment extrusion, with recurrence of leg pain has been reported in about 5% of patients. They often occur within the first month following the PLDD procedure and are usually due to reinjury. Strict adherence to post-operative instructions is mandatory to avoid excessive stress on the disc before healing is complete.

In our experience, we have had one septic discitis, two thermal spondylitis and one expulsion of free nucleus fragment into the canal (from gardening the day after the PLDD procedure) without need for surgery.

6.3.3.7
Results

Many studies with large series report a high success rate of PLDD with 70%–89% good results for radicular pain (BOSACCO et al. 1996; CASPER et al. 1996; CHOY 2004; GANGI et al. 2005; GEVARGEZ et al. 2000). These results are independent of the wavelength of the laser. Immediate pain relief on the intervention table is reported in 60% of patients. The decrease in pain is fast in the initial period and then stabilizes after 6 weeks. PLDD is also an effective and safe alternative to conventional open surgery for the treatment of contained disc herniation; its morbidity is low and it can be performed safely under local anesthesia on an outpatient basis. Considering the management of purely lower back pain with positive discogram treated by PLDD, BLACK et al. (2004) reported 88% good or fair results. Half of the patients treated with PLDD at the lumbar level return to work within four weeks (BOSACCO et al. 1996; GEVARGEZ et al. 2000). The success rate is similar at the cervical level (KNIGHT et al. 2001) but the optical fiber should be very precisely positioned to avoid thermal damage to the spinal cord or the nerve roots.

PLDD has been performed in our institution since 1991. From 1991 to 2000, 458 patients with herniated lumbar disk and radicular pain were treated by PLDD. The oldest was 71 years and the youngest was 12. Mean age was 42 years. The longest follow-up was 10 years, with average follow-up of 22 months. Macnab's criteria and the visual analog scale (VAS)

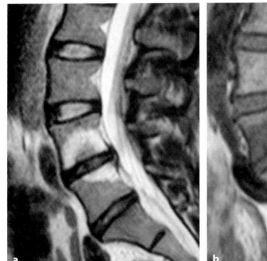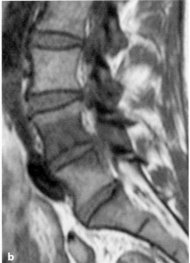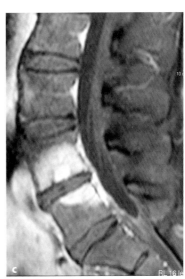

Fig. 6.13a–c. Thermal spondylitis in a 30-year-old woman treated with PLDD. **a** Sagittal T2, (**b**) unenhanced T1, and (**c**) contrast-enhanced T1-weighted MR imaging of the lumbar spine show mirror edema in the adjacent vertebral endplates, with normal signal of L4–5 disc

were used to grade the response to treatment. The overall success rate was 76% with 55.6% good and 20.2% fair results. In four cases, the PLDD was performed at two levels. Immediate relief of leg pain was achieved in 63% of patients. Thirty-six patients with poor results or recurrence were later treated surgically with a satisfying success rate (68%). After 6–12 months, disk herniation was reduced on CT or MR imaging. These cases were evaluated a second time with a mean follow-up of 53 months, with identical results. One patient suffered from spondylodiscitis. Another suffered for 6 weeks from severe backache due to aseptic discitis (at 3 years follow-up). One patient was readmitted 24 h after PLDD with severe recurrence of leg pain due to free fragment evacuation with upward migration. After 3 years, the results remained stable with 71% of patients free of radicular pain. This data is encouraging and substantiates the validity of percutaneous laser nucleotomy for contained lumbar disk herniation.

The three most critical elements for successful PLDD are: proper patient selection, correct needle placement and effective vaporization.

6.3.4
Bipolar Radiofrequency Nucleoplasty

Bipolar RF nucleoplasty relies on Coblation® technology to ablate soft tissue. This technique, initially used for arthroscopic surgery, was introduced for disc decompression in July 2000.

6.3.4.1
Principle of Nucleoplasty

This technique, developed by ArthroCare (Austin, TX, USA), uses a low-energy bipolar radiofrequency electrode (SpineWand®) that produces ionization of the sodium atoms in the nucleus. This creates a focused, high energy ionic plasma field which disintegrates the intra-molecular bonds in the nucleus. Unlike other radiofrequency systems that are temperature-driven, it does not rely on heat energy to ablate tissue, so thermal damage and tissue necrosis is avoided. Complex molecules are transformed into simple molecules, mainly gas, which evacuate through the introducer cannula. The temperature peak during the procedure is approximately 40–65 °C with a rapid decrease at the periphery of the disc (NAU and DIEDERICH 2004). Porcine intradiscal thermal mapping found an increase in temperature of less than 5 °C, 3 mm from the tip of the electrode. Nucleoplasty has a much lower temperature range than PLDD. This transmission of energy into a plasma field at low temperatures is called "Coblation®", a contraction of the words cold or controlled and ablation.

Several coblation channels are excavated as the electrode advances, removing a portion of the nu-

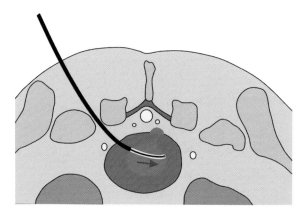

Fig. 6.14. Nucleoplasty principles. Drawing shows coblation with disintegration of tissue via an ionized plasma field as the electrode is advanced (low temperature). Coagulation with thermal treatment of tissue as the electrode is withdrawn (No longer recommended by the manufacturer in the new protocol)

cleus to achieve disc decompression (Fig. 6.14). These channels have sharp margins, with no signs of thermal injury (CHEN YC et al. 2003b; LEE et al. 2003). The low temperature plasma field activated with the coblation mode does not modify the fibrocartilage cells or the collagen matrix arrangement in the area immediately around the probe channels. When the electrode is withdrawn, each channel is thermally treated (coagulated) using a lower range of energy below the threshold that activates the plasma field. Coagulation induces higher temperatures, potentially shrinking the disc (through fusion of collagen fibers in the annulus). In its new protocol, Arthro-Care advises use of the coblation mode alone, without coagulation of the channels, to avoid the risk of thermal diffusion to the vertebral endplates.

As with laser nucleotomy, coblation technology relies on decompression but the low temperature ionized plasma field also induces biochemical modifications in the disc which may play an additional therapeutic role (ALEXANDRE et al. 2005). After nucleoplasty, O'NEILL et al. (2004) found a significant reduction of interleukin 1 (associated with tissue degeneration) and an increase of interleukin 8 (associated with tissue angiogenesis).

6.3.4.2
Patient Selection for Nucleoplasty

Indications of nucleoplasty are the same as for PLDD: contained focal disk herniation determined by CT or MR imaging with positive and consistent neurological findings of radicular pain greater than axial pain, decreased sensation, normal motor response and tendon reflex, refractory to a minimum of 6 weeks of conservative care and selective periradicular infiltrations. Less often, pure axial pain due to disc herniation can benefit from nucleoplasty (SINGH et al. 2002) when associated with positive provocative discography. Positive cough sign is also clinically important to evoke pain symptoms due to increased pressure on the posterior spinal ligament.

The contraindications of nucleoplasty are exactly the same as for PLDD.

The much lower range of temperatures makes it possible to treat small discs (thoracic, cervical) with coblation technology with much less risk of thermal injury to adjacent structures than with laser. The special nucleoplasty electrode designed for cervical levels creates spherical voids instead of channels. It appears to be safer as no energy diffuses towards the spinal canal.

Coblation technology requires sodium to transmit energy via an activated plasma field. This process cannot work if the disc is dehydrated. Pressure reduction after nucleoplasty is highly dependent on the degree of spine degeneration as shown by CHEN YC et al. (2003a) on a cadaveric study. However, decompression is not indicated for degenerative discs.

6.3.4.3
Materials

The material for RF nucleoplasty consists of an introducer needle, a bipolar radiofrequency probe (SpineWand®), and a radiofrequency generator.

An energy protocol adapted to the procedure is selected. The generator is directly controlled by the operator via a pedal. Coblation is activated and the electrode is advanced to disintegrate the nucleus. Coagulation of the channels is performed as the electrode is withdrawn if shrinkage of the disc is necessary, but the process should be fast so as not to allow thermal diffusion to adjacent structures.

For lumbar and thoracic nucleoplasty, the introducer needle is a 17-gauge graduated needle whose length is specially adapted to the radiofrequency probe. Once in appropriate position, the Perc-DLR SpineWand® radiofrequency electrode is placed through it in a coaxial fashion. Its curved tip allows creation of several coblation channels when the axis of the electrode is rotated (Fig. 6.15).

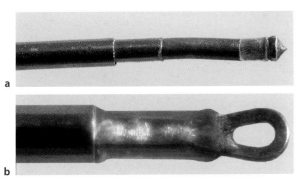

Fig. 6.15a,b. Nucleoplasty bipolar electrodes. **a** Bent tip for lumbar and thoracic levels. **b** Looped tip for cervical level

For cervical nucleoplasty, due to smaller discs, the introducer needle is 19-gauge with a luer lock. Once in the disc, the Perc-DC SpineWand® is fastened to the introducer needle hub. This specially designed cervical electrode has a looped tip that creates spherical voids in the nucleus (Fig. 6.15).

6.3.4.4
Technique of Nucleoplasty

6.3.4.4.1
Lumbar Level

Through a skin incision, the 17-gauge needle is inserted under lateral fluoroscopic control using the same standard extra-pedicular posterior-lateral approach as described for laser nucleotomy. The 17-gauge needle is quite stiff and difficult to bend into a curve. This can be problematic for the difficult L5-S1 approach. The tip of the 17-gauge needle is placed at the annulus/nucleus junction, so that when the radiofrequency electrode is introduced through the needle, the active tip may pass directly into the nucleus. The advancement of the electrode through the nucleus has a low resistance feel similar to cutting through butter. When the device touches the anterior part of the annulus, high resistance is encountered at the tip. The depth is marked with a wing-shaped stopper to prevent perforation and coblation beyond the nucleus. Prior to ablation, fluoroscopic control with anteroposterior and lateral views or CT control is necessary to confirm the proper placement and extent of the electrode (Fig. 6.16). Particular caution should be taken to keep the electrode parallel to the adjacent vertebral endplates to avoid touching them during the proce-

dure. Patients must be monitored for pain during the whole intervention; it is strongly advised not to use sedation. To confirm a contained disc herniation or if any doubt persists, discography can be performed just before nucleoplasty.

While monitoring the patient, the SpineWand® is advanced into the disc with the coblation plasma mode activated, so that tissue along the path of the device disintegrates (SINGH et al. 2002). The electrode is then withdrawn to the starting position in the coagulation mode, which thermally seals the ablation channel. Coagulation mode does not reach the threshold to activate the ionized plasma, but induces thermal diffusion into the disc. The manufacturer's new protocol does not recommend the use of coagulation, as thermal injury to the vertebral endplates could occur. However, coagulation of the coblation channels may induce shrinkage of the disc and also denervation of the annulus. These mechanisms may play an important role in pain management.

After the first channel is created, the SpineWand® is rotated clockwise. The SpineWand® device is curved and each rotation changes its direction and creates a new channel inside the nucleus. Six to ten channels are created in total, depending on the desired amount of tissue reduction. This procedure is very fast, lasting less than 2 min once the electrode is in proper position. CT control during nucleoplasty is not necessary in routine practice, but it does show the production of gas in the nucleus due to coblation (Fig. 6.17).

6.3.4.4.2
Thoracic Level

The technique is much like lumbar nucleoplasty. The 17-gauge introducer needle is inserted into the disc, using the standard posterolateral approach. Under fluoroscopic control, the C-arm is rotated 35° laterally from the posteroanterior view. The puncture is performed parallel to the disc, between the head of the rib and the transverse process. Combined CT and fluoroscopy can be helpful for a precise approach. The electrode is inserted coaxially in the 17-gauge needle and the wing-shaped stopper is positioned. A maximum of six coblation channels are created, three on the left side and three on the right. Due to the height of the thoracic discs, coblation with the tip of the electrode pointing cranially or caudally should not be performed to avoid harming the vertebral endplates (Fig. 6.18).

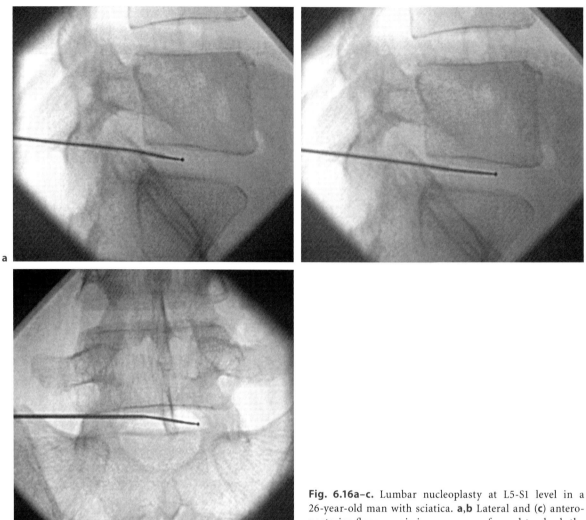

Fig. 6.16a–c. Lumbar nucleoplasty at L5-S1 level in a 26-year-old man with sciatica. **a,b** Lateral and (**c**) antero-posterior fluoroscopic images are performed to check the extent of the electrode and its proper position, parallel to the vertebral endplates, prior to coblation

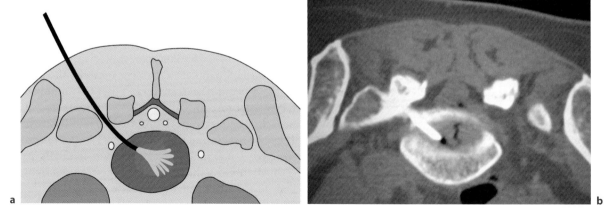

Fig. 6.17a,b. Lumbar nucleoplasty in a 40-year-old man with sciatica. **a** Drawing shows the creation of 6–10 channels in the nucleus by clockwise rotation of the electrode. **b** Axial CT scan shows the diffusion of gas into the herniation

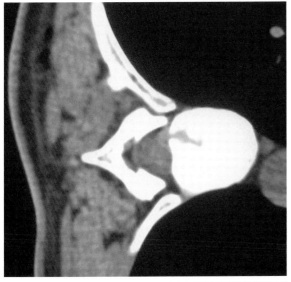

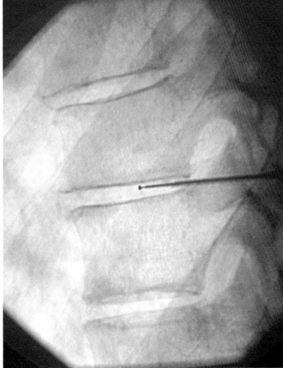

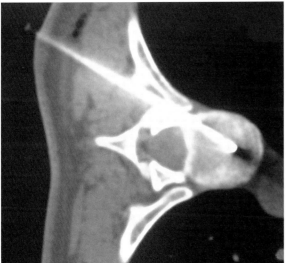

Fig. 6.18a–c. Thoracic nucleoplasty in a 32-year-old woman with right T7 intercostal pain. **a** Axial CT scan shows a right posterolateral thoracic herniation. **b** Lateral fluoroscopy image and (**c**) axial CT scan show the position of the electrode in the disc, parallel to the vertebral endplates, using an intercostopedicular approach. Due to the smaller disc, a maximum of six coblation channels are created, carefully avoiding contact with the vertebral endplate

6.3.4.4.3
Cervical Level

Cervical puncture is performed by a standard anterolateral approach under fluoroscopic guidance. The patient is placed in supine position, with a cushion under the lower neck and the upper thoracic spine to hyperextend the neck. A right side entry point is theoretically safer as the esophagus is often slightly deviated towards the left. Asepsis must be strict as the proximity of oropharyngeal structures increases the risk of infection. After preparation of the skin and superficial local anesthesia, the carotid artery is detected by its pulsation. With two fingers, the operator presses against the vertebral space, mov-

ing the carotid artery laterally, the trachea and the esophagus medially. The 19-gauge introducer needle is inserted between these two fingers into the disc.

The Perc-DC SpineWand®, specially designed for the cervical level, is introduced coaxially and fastened to the introducer needle hub. Fluoroscopic anteroposterior and lateral projections are mandatory to confirm the proper position of the device. The tip of the electrode should be advanced to the mid part of the disc, but never beyond the mid-third/posterior-third junction to avoid damage to the spinal cord or nerve roots. Sedation is prohibited to allow complete neurological monitoring of the patient during the whole procedure. Half a second of coagulation mode is performed to ensure absence of

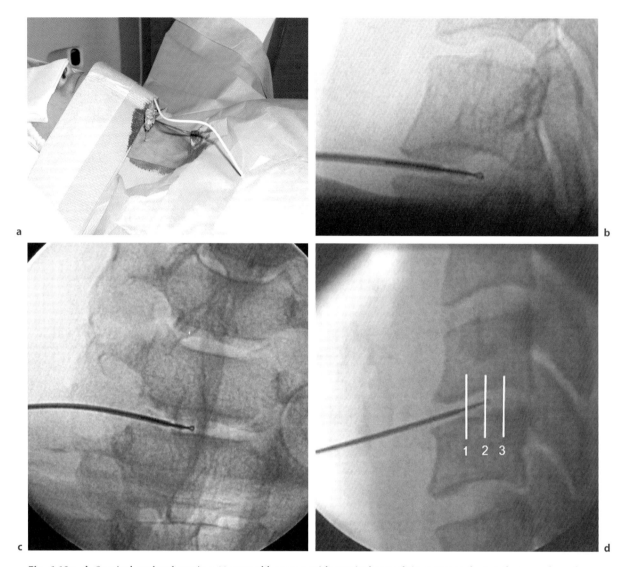

Fig. 6.19a–d. Cervical nucleoplasty in a 32-year-old woman with cervical neuralgia. **a** Image during the procedure shows cervical puncture with standard right anterolateral approach. **b** Lateral and (**c**) anteroposterior fluoroscopic images confirm the proper position of the electrode in the nucleus. **d** Lateral fluoroscopic image demonstrates the subsequent positions of the electrode within the nucleus represented by 1, 2, and 3. Three spherical voids are created in the mid part of the disc to achieve good decompression. The electrode should never be advanced beyond the mid-third/posterior-third junction (position 3) of the disc to avoid neurological damage

neurological stimulation. Then, coblation of the nucleus is performed, rotating the electrode on its axis through 180° over approximately 5 s. The device is withdrawn 1–2 mm without coagulation mode and coblation repeated to make a series of three spherical voids (Fig. 6.19). The SpineWand® is unlocked from the needle hub and withdrawn into the introducer needle before removing. This procedure is very fast, lasting less than 2 min once the electrode is in the proper position.

6.3.4.5
Post-Operative Instructions

Post-operative instructions following nucleoplasty are similar to laser nucleotomy (see above). For cervical decompression, a surgical collar is prescribed for the first week and neck rotation or bending is limited for two weeks. Follow-up relies mainly on clinical symptoms. CT or MR imaging of the spine is only performed if any complication is suspected.

The shrinkage of the herniation is visible only after several months.

6.3.4.6
Complications of RF Nucleoplasty

Literature reports transient minor side-effect with RF nucleoplasty (numbness, tingling or soreness at the puncture site) (BHAGIA et al. 2006). The only major complication following a nucleoplasty procedure is a fulminant and fatal mucormycosis spondylodiscitis (CHEN F et al. 2006). However, potential complications include discitis, hematoma, neural and vascular injuries, and pneumothorax for low-cervical or thoracic levels. Most complications can be avoided with strict respect for technique and adherence to all sterility measures.

The low temperature range during coblation makes the risk of thermal injury to the vertebral endplates much less than with laser nucleotomy. However, coagulation mode during withdrawal of the electrode (with possible shrinkage and denervation of the disc) causes thermal diffusion to adjacent structures. Coagulation is no longer recommended by the manufacturer, but in our opinion, with constant neurological monitoring, its prudent use is still possible.

In our practice, we have had two complications. Early on, following nucleoplasty a young patient had complete relief of leg pain but developed intense backache for several months requiring NSAIDS and analgesics. Clinical symptoms and MR imaging appeared similar to PLDD thermal spondylitis. This complication may have been caused by excessive use of coagulation mode. The second complication was a large nuclear free fragment that extruded 4 days post-nucleoplasty after heavy weight lifting by the patient. The resulting cauda equina compression required surgical treatment (Fig. 6.20). The importance of following post-operative instructions should be emphasized to the patient, especially during the early phase of disc healing.

6.3.4.7
Results of RF Nucleoplasty

Only a few studies of nucleoplasty are available. The selection criteria of those studies varies widely, with patients suffering from pure back pain and/or radicular pain included.

SHARPS and ISAAC (2002) studied 49 patients with a follow up of 12 months and reported a success rate of 79%. Since then, several authors have reported 75%–80% of patients showing significant improvement in

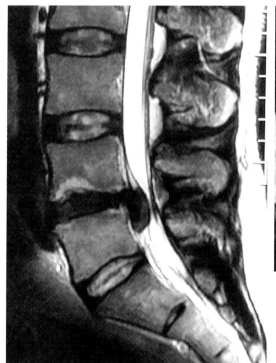
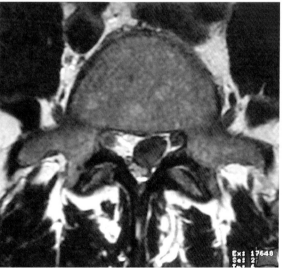

Fig. 6.20a,b. Nuclear fragment extrusion four days post nucleoplasty, after bending and lifting heavy weight, in a 48-year-old man. **a** Sagittal and (**b**) axial T2-weighted MR imaging show large nuclear free fragment extrusion within the left lumbar spinal canal with important mass effect on the dural sac

quality of life (ALEXANDRE et al. 2005; GERSZTEN et al. 2006; SINGH and DERBY 2006). These early success rates are comparable to, or slightly better than, those of previous percutaneous approaches. At the cervical level, BONALDI et al. (2006) and NARDI et al. (2005) obtained 80% complete resolution of pain with nucleoplasty, with a faster return to work, compared to conservative care. REDDY et al. (2005) also reported reduction of medication and functional improvement after nucleoplasty, with significant reduction in work and leisure impairment. RF nucleoplasty provides a safe and efficient alternative to microdiscectomy in selected cases (WELCH and GERSZTEN 2002).

In our department, from 2002 to 2006, 193 patients with sciatica due to herniated lumbar disk were treated by nucleoplasty on an out-patient basis. The shortest follow-up was 6 months and the longest 42 months. Post-procedural absolute radicular VAS equal to or less than 20 mm was considered a good result. The overall success rate was 81% according to Macnab's criteria with 50% good and 31% fair outcomes. The mean VAS decreased from 76 to 16 mm. The clinical outcome was fixed after 4–6 weeks and generally remained stable during the following months. This data provides encouraging information substantiating the validity of nucleoplasty for contained lumbar disc herniation. Nucleoplasty allows fast, safe and effective disc decompression when conservative therapies fail. Moreover, due to its low temperatures, the risk of thermal damage to the vertebral endplates is reduced. The specially designed cervical electrode allows for a safer treatment of cervical disc herniation compared to mechanical or laser decompression systems as the device avoids neural structures and no heat is transmitted to the spinal canal.

6.3.5
Targeted Disc Decompression

Targeted disc decompression (TDD) uses a flexible, heated, bipolar radiofrequency catheter (Acutherm®, Smith & Nephew Inc., Andover, MA, USA) to treat symptomatic disc herniation. The device is inserted through a 17-gauge needle into the disc, via a standard posterolateral approach. It winds around the nucleus so that its 1.5-cm active tip directly faces the herniation. The skin entry point side has to be contralateral to the herniation (Fig. 6.21). The deployment of the electrode may sometimes be difficult; the device kinks in 10% of cases.

The temperature is increased over 6 min to a plateau of 90 °C which is maintained for 6 min. This achieves focal thermal treatment of the contained herniated disc with shrinkage. TDD stems from intradiscal electrothermal therapy (IDET) but the range of temperatures are higher and the energy more focused. IDET is indicated for treatment of pure discogenic pain due to annular tears, while TDD is to decompress disc herniations.

TDD has the same indications and contraindications as other percutaneous decompression devices (PLDD, RF nucleoplasty). An interesting use of TDD is in the treatment of foraminal herniations. As the annulus is thicker in these herniations, treatment is difficult with standard nucleus removal. Use of TDD allows targeted thermal treatment of the herniation, with potential annulus shrinkage. One drawback is the proximity of the nerve root to the electrode. For this reason, the procedure should only be performed under local anesthesia with a fully conscious patient. Multiple annular tears make it difficult to position the electrode in about 10% of patients.

This recent and original technique seems to be promising, but no studies have been published yet.

6.3.6
Comparison of PLDD vs RF Nucleoplasty

Percutaneous techniques like nucleoplasty and PLDD have advantages over conventional open surgery:
- Performed under local anesthesia
- Outpatient basis, no extensive hospitalization
- Minimal recovery time (6 weeks or less)
- No risk of periradicular fibrosis, no scars
- Lower cost

However, only contained disc herniations can be treated.

Nucleoplasty is much like PLDD; the techniques are quite similar with the same patient criteria, the same approach to puncturing the disc and the same post-procedural instructions. Results are comparable with global efficacy ranging from 70%–80%.

However, there are differences:
- The 17-gauge introducer needle used for nucleoplasty is stiffer but not as sharp as the 18-gauge spinal needle used for PLDD. This makes it more difficult to bend and orientate which can be problematic in difficult L5-S1 access.
- Once the introducer needle is positioned into the disc, nucleoplasty decompression is achieved

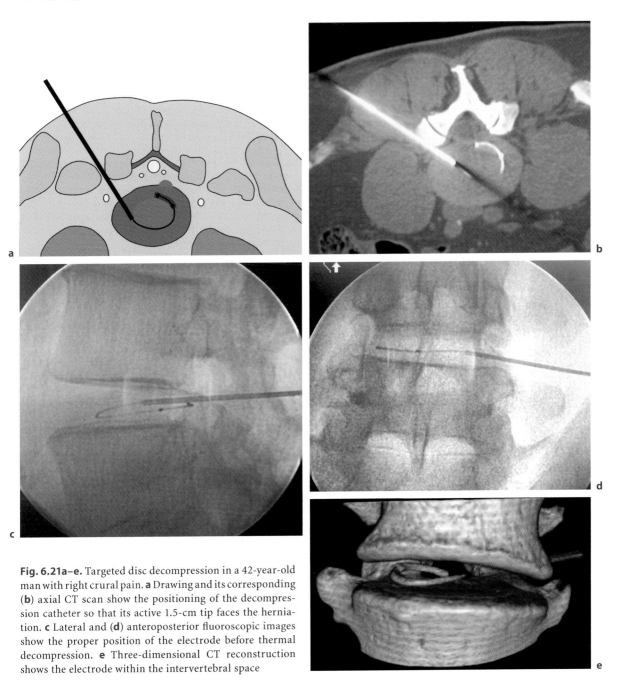

Fig. 6.21a–e. Targeted disc decompression in a 42-year-old man with right crural pain. **a** Drawing and its corresponding (**b**) axial CT scan show the positioning of the decompression catheter so that its active 1.5-cm tip faces the herniation. **c** Lateral and (**d**) anteroposterior fluoroscopic images show the proper position of the electrode before thermal decompression. **e** Three-dimensional CT reconstruction shows the electrode within the intervertebral space

within 2 min. In comparison, laser energy is delivered slowly to avoid thermal damage to surrounding structures and the vaporization requires 15 min once the optical fiber is positioned.

- The risk of thermal diffusion to the vertebral endplates (thermal spondylitis) is lower with nucleoplasty as coblation technology acts via a low temperature plasma field.
- The coblation effect is obtained systematically if the nucleus is hydrated, while the photother-

mal effect of laser depends on the color of the disc.

- The specially designed nucleoplasty Perc DC electrode is safer for treating cervical disc herniations as the energy source is kept away from neural structures.
- The nucleoplasty generator costs less than the laser generator, but the nucleoplasty electrode is roughly seven times more expensive than the optical fiber.

Conclusion

Disc herniation causing axial and/or radicular pain is a very common pathology with huge social and economic consequences. Initial conservative treatment relies on rest and oral medication with analgesics and NSAIDS.

If conservative treatment fails to control pain, selective periradicular steroid injection should be considered. Image-guided infiltrations are safer, particularly for the cervical level. They allow contrast opacification to control the proper positioning of the needle before steroid deposition. Short term results are satisfying, but the benefit often decreases after several weeks. Although periradicular steroid injections have been used for decades, their results remain controversial in the literature, probably due to significant variations in patient selection, technique, positioning of the needle and guidance modalities.

If 6 weeks of conservative therapy including steroid infiltrations has failed, then percutaneous disc decompression should be considered. Several techniques are available, all based on removing part of the nucleus pulposus to achieve decompression of the herniation. Among them, percutaneous laser disc decompression and radiofrequency nucleoplasty seem to be more efficient as they act not only by mechanical effect but also induce modifications in the disc biochemistry and innervations. These decompression techniques are much less invasive than conventional open surgery but can only be performed if the disc herniation is contained. Excellent pain relief is achieved in 75%–80% of patients with stable long term effects.

Interventional radiology plays an important role in pain management due to disc herniation. However, careful selection of patients after precise clinical examination remains essential to achieve successful treatment.

References

Alexandre A, Coro L, Azuelos A, Pellone M (2005) Percutaneous nucleoplasty for discoradicular conflict. Acta Neurochir Suppl 92:83–86

Andreula CF, Simonetti L, De Santis F, Agati R, Ricci R, Leonardi M (2003) Minimally invasive oxygen-ozone therapy for lumbar disk herniation. AJNR Am J Neuroradiol 24:996–1000

Andreula C, Muto M, Leonardi M (2004) Interventional spinal procedures. Eur J Radiol 50:112–119

Bartynski WS, Grahovac SZ, Rothfus WE (2005) Incorrect needle position during lumbar epidural steroid administration: inaccuracy of loss of air pressure resistance and requirement of fluoroscopy and epidurography during needle insertion. AJNR Am J Neuroradiol 26:502–505

Bhagia SM, Slipman CW, Nirschl M, Isaac Z, El-Abd O, Sharps LS, Garvin C (2006) Side effects and complications after percutaneous disc decompression using coblation technology. Am J Phys Med Rehabil 85:6–13

Black W, Fejos AS, Choy DS (2004) Percutaneous laser disc decompression in the treatment of discogenic back pain. Photomed Laser Surg 22:431–433

Bonaldi G, Baruzzi F, Facchinetti A, Fachinetti P, Lunghi S (2006) Plasma radio-frequency-based diskectomy for treatment of cervical herniated nucleus pulposus: feasibility, safety, and preliminary clinical results. AJNR Am J Neuroradiol 27:2104–2111

Bosacco SJ, Bosacco DN, Berman AT, Cordover A, Levenberg RJ, Stellabotte J (1996) Functional results of percutaneous laser discectomy. Am J Orthop 25:825–828

Buric J, Molino Lova R (2005) Ozone chemonucleolysis in non-contained lumbar disc herniations: a pilot study with 12 months follow-up. Acta Neurochir Suppl 92:93–97

Casper GD, Hartman VL, Mullins LL (1996) Results of a clinical trial of the holmium:YAG laser in disc decompression utilizing a side-firing fiber: a two-year follow-up. Lasers Surg Med 19:90–96

Castro I, Santos D, Christoph D, Landeiro J (2005) The history of spinal surgery for disc disease: an illustrated timeline. Arq Neuropsiquiatr 63:701–706

Chen F, Lu G, Kang Y, Ma Z, Lu C, Wang B, Li J, Liu J, Li H (2006) Mucormycosis spondylodiscitis after lumbar disc puncture. Eur Spine J 15:370–376

Chen YC, Lee SH, Chen D (2003a) Intradiscal pressure study of percutaneous disc decompression with nucleoplasty in human cadavers. Spine 28:661–665

Chen YC, Lee SH, Saenz Y, Lehman NL (2003b) Histologic findings of disc, end plate and neural elements after coblation of nucleus pulposus: an experimental nucleoplasty study. Spine J 3:466–470

Choy DS (1993) Percutaneous laser disc decompression (PLDD) update: focus on device and procedure advances. J Clin Laser Med Surg 11:181–183

Choy DS (2001) Response of extruded intervertebral herniated discs to percutaneous laser disc decompression. J Clin Laser Med Surg 19:15–20

Choy DS (2004) Percutaneous laser disc decompression: a 17-year experience. Photomed Laser Surg 22:407–410

Choy DS, Fejos AS (2004) Cervical disc herniations and percutaneous laser disc decompression: a case report. Photomed Laser Surg 22:423–425

Choy DS, Case RB, Fielding W, Hughes J, Liebler W, Ascher P (1987) Percutaneous laser nucleolysis of lumbar disks. N Engl J Med 317:771–772

Choy DS, Altman PA, Case RB, Trokel SL (1991) Laser radiation at various wavelengths for decompression of intervertebral disk. Experimental observations on human autopsy specimens. Clin Orthop Relat Res:245–250

Choy DS, Ascher PW, Ranu HS, Saddekni S, Alkaitis D, Liebler W, Hughes J, Diwan S, Altman P (1992) Percutaneous laser disc decompression. A new therapeutic modality. Spine 17:949–956

Cyteval C, Fescquet N, Thomas E, Decoux E, Blotman F, Taourel P (2006) Predictive factors of efficacy of periradicular corticosteroid injections for lumbar radiculopathy. AJNR Am J Neuroradiol 27:978–982

Furman MB, O'Brien EM, Zgleszewski TM (2000) Incidence of intravascular penetration in transforaminal lumbosacral epidural steroid injections. Spine 25:2628–2632

Gangi A, Dietemann JL, Ide C, Brunner P, Klinkert A, Warter JM (1996) Percutaneous laser disk decompression under CT and fluoroscopic guidance: indications, technique, and clinical experience. Radiographics 16:89–96

Gangi A, Dietemann JL, Mortazavi R, Pfleger D, Kauff C, Roy C (1998a) CT-guided interventional procedures for pain management in the lumbosacral spine. Radiographics 18:621–633

Gangi A, Dietemann JL, Gasser B, Guth S, de Unamuno S, Fogarrassi E, Fuchs C, Siffert P, Roy C (1998b) Interventional radiology with laser in bone and joint. Radiol Clin North Am 36:547–557

Gangi A, Basile A, Buy X, Alizadeh H, Sauer B, Bierry G (2005) Radiofrequency and laser ablation of spinal lesions. Semin Ultrasound CT MR 26:89–97

Gerszten PC, Welch WC, King JT Jr (2006) Quality of life assessment in patients undergoing nucleoplasty-based percutaneous discectomy. J Neurosurg Spine 4:36–42

Gevargez A, Groenemeyer DW, Czerwinski F (2000) CT-guided percutaneous laser disc decompression with Ceralas D, a diode laser with 980-nm wavelength and 200-microm fiber optics. Eur Radiol 10:1239–1241

Hellinger J (2004) Complications of non-endoscopic percutaneous laser disc decompression and nucleotomy with the neodymium: YAG laser 1064 nm. Photomed Laser Surg 22:418–422

Hooten WM, Kinney MO, Huntoon MA (2004) Epidural abscess and meningitis after epidural corticosteroid injection. Mayo Clin Proc 79:682–686

Houten JK, Errico TJ (2002) Paraplegia after lumbosacral nerve root block: report of three cases. Spine J 2:70–75

Huang RC, Shapiro GS, Lim M, Sandhu HS, Lutz GE, Herzog RJ (2004) Cervical epidural abscess after epidural steroid injection. Spine 29:E7–9

Huntoon MA, Martin DP (2004) Paralysis after transforaminal epidural injection and previous spinal surgery. Reg Anesth Pain Med 29:494–495

Iwatsuki K, Yoshimine T, Sasaki M, Yasuda K, Akiyama C, Nakahira R (2005) The effect of laser irradiation for nucleus pulposus: an experimental study. Neurol Res 27:319–323

Johnson BA, Schellhas KP, Pollei SR (1999) Epidurography and therapeutic epidural injections: technical considerations and experience with 5334 cases. AJNR Am J Neuroradiol 20:697–705

Karppinen J, Ohinmaa A, Malmivaara A, Kurunlahti M, Kyllonen E, Pienimaki T, Nieminen P, Tervonen O, Vanharanta H (2001) Cost effectiveness of periradicular infiltration for sciatica: subgroup analysis of a randomized controlled trial. Spine 26:2587–2595

Kawakami M, Matsumoto T, Kuribayashi K, Tamaki T (1999) mRNA expression of interleukins, phospholipase A2, and

nitric oxide synthase in the nerve root and dorsal root ganglion induced by autologous nucleus pulposus in the rat. J Orthop Res 17:941–946

Knappe V, Frank F, Rohde E (2004) Principles of lasers and biophotonic effects. Photomed Laser Surg 22:411–417

Knight MT, Goswami A, Patko JT (2001) Cervical percutaneous laser disc decompression: preliminary results of an ongoing prospective outcome study. J Clin Laser Med Surg 19:3–8

Kobayashi S, Baba H, Uchida K, Kokubo Y, Kubota C, Yamada S, Suzuki Y, Yoshizawa H (2005) Effect of mechanical compression on the lumbar nerve root: localization and changes of intraradicular inflammatory cytokines, nitric oxide, and cyclooxygenase. Spine 30:1699–1705

Kolstad F, Leivseth G, Nygaard OP (2005) Transforaminal steroid injections in the treatment of cervical radiculopathy. A prospective outcome study. Acta Neurochir (Wien) 147:1065–1070

Lee M, Cooper G, Lutz G, Doty S (2003) Histologic characterization of coblation nucleoplasty performed on sheep intervertebral disc. Pain Physician 6:439–442

Ma DJ, Gilula LA, Riew KD (2005) Complications of fluoroscopically guided extraforaminal cervical nerve blocks. An analysis of 1036 injections. J Bone Joint Surg Am 87:1025–1030

McLain RF, Kapural L, Mekhail NA (2005) Epidural steroid therapy for back and leg pain: mechanisms of action and efficacy. Spine J 5:191–201

Nardi PV, Cabezas D, Cesaroni A (2005) Percutaneous cervical nucleoplasty using coblation technology. Clinical results in fifty consecutive cases. Acta Neurochir Suppl 92:73–78

Nau WH, Diederich CJ (2004) Evaluation of temperature distributions in cadaveric lumbar spine during nucleoplasty. Phys Med Biol 49:1583–1594

O'Neill CW, Liu JJ, Leibenberg E, Hu SS, Deviren V, Tay BK, Chin CT, Lotz JC (2004) Percutaneous plasma decompression alters cytokine expression in injured porcine intervertebral discs. Spine J 4:88–98

Ohnmeiss DD, Guyer RD, Hochschuler SH (1994) Laser disc decompression. The importance of proper patient selection. Spine 19:2054–2058; discussion 2059

Ramirez L, Thisted R (1989) Complications and demographic characteristics of patients undergoing lumbar discectomy in community hospitals. Neurosurgery 25:226–230

Reddy A, Loh S, Cutts J, Rachlin J, Hirsch J (2005) New approach to the management of acute disc herniation. Pain Physician 8:385–389

Reitman CA, Watters W III (2002) Subdural hematoma after cervical epidural steroid injection. Spine 27:E174–176

Riew KD, Yin Y, Gilula L, Bridwell KH, Lenke LG, Lauryssen C, Goette K (2000) The effect of nerve-root injections on the need for operative treatment of lumbar radicular pain. A prospective, randomized, controlled, double-blind study. J Bone Joint Surg Am 82-A:1589–1593

Rosenkranz M, Grzyska U, Niesen W, Fuchs K, Schummer W, Weiller C, Rother J (2004) Anterior spinal artery syndrome following periradicular cervical nerve root therapy. J Neurol 251:229–231

Sandberg DI, Lavyne MH (1999) Symptomatic spinal epidural lipomatosis after local epidural corticosteroid injections: case report. Neurosurgery 45:162–165

Schlangmann BA, Schmolke S, Siebert WE (1996) [Temperature and ablation measurements in laser therapy of intervertebral disk tissue]. Orthopade 25:3–9

Schmolke S, Kirsch L, Gosse F, Flamme C, Bohnsack M, Ruhmann O (2004) Risk evaluation of thermal injury to the cervical spine during intradiscal laser application in vitro. Photomed Laser Surg 22:426–430

Sharps LS, Isaac Z (2002) Percutaneous disc decompression using nucleoplasty. Pain Physician 5:121–126

Singh V, Derby R (2006) Percutaneous lumbar disc decompression. Pain Physician 9:139–146

Singh V, Piryani C, Liao K, Nieschulz S (2002) Percutaneous disc decompression using coblation (nucleoplasty) in the treatment of chronic discogenic pain. Pain Physician 5:250–259

Smith L, Garvin P, Gesler R, Jennings R (1963) Enzyme dissolution of the nucleus pulposus. Nature 198:1311–1312

Stojanovic MP, Vu TN, Caneris O, Slezak J, Cohen SP, Sang CN (2002) The role of fluoroscopy in cervical epidural steroid injections: an analysis of contrast dispersal patterns. Spine 27:509–514

Stolke D, Sollmann WP, Seifert V (1989) Intra- and postoperative complications in lumbar disc surgery. Spine 14:56–59

Wang JC, Kabo JM, Tsou PM, Halevi L, Shamie AN (2005) The effect of uniform heating on the biomechanical properties of the intervertebral disc in a porcine model. Spine J 5:64–70

Watanabe AT, Nishimura E, Garris J (2002) Image-guided epidural steroid injections. Tech Vasc Interv Radiol 5:186–193

Welch WC, Gerszten PC (2002) Alternative strategies for lumbar discectomy: intradiscal electrothermy and nucleoplasty. Neurosurg Focus 13:E7

Yue WM, Tan SB (2003) Distant skip level discitis and vertebral osteomyelitis after caudal epidural injection: a case report of a rare complication of epidural injections. Spine 28:E209–211

Provocative Discography

WILFRED C. G. PEH

CONTENTS

7.1 Introduction 119

7.2 Disc Anatomy 120

7.3 Pathophysiology of Discogenic Pain 120

7.4 Imaging of Disc Disease:
An Overview 121

7.5 Discography 123
7.5.1 Indications 123
7.5.2 Contraindications 123
7.5.3 Technique 123
7.5.3.1 Pre-procedural Preparation 123
7.5.3.2 Equipment 124
7.5.3.3 Cervical Discography 125
7.5.3.4 Thoracic Discography 126
7.5.3.5 Lumbar Discography 126
7.5.3.6 Post-Discography Procedure 129
7.5.4 Interpretation 131
7.5.4.1 Disc Morphology 131
7.5.4.2 Dallas Discogram Description 132
7.5.4.3 Pain Provocation 133
7.5.5 Complications 137

7.6 Conclusion 137

References 139

7.1
Introduction

Provocative discography is an imaging-guided procedure in which a contrast agent is injected into the nucleus pulposus of the intervertebral disc. Discography provides both anatomical and functional information about the disc. Following intradiscal contrast injection, disc morphology is usually as-

W. C. G. PEH, MD, MBBS, FRCPG, FRCPE, FRCR
Clinical Professor, National University of Singapore, Senior
Consultant Radiologist, Alexandra Hospital, 378 Alexandra
Road, Singapore 159964, Republic of Singapore

sessed on anteroposterior and lateral radiographs, or axial thin section computed tomography (CT). The functional evaluation of discography consists of operator-induced pain provocation and assessment of the patient's response. The results of discography influence not only the surgical decision-making process but also the number of levels to be operated upon.

This procedure was first described by LINDBLOM in 1948 when he injected red lead contrast into a cadaveric disc. HIRSCH (1948) reported the first clinical series of 16 patients on whom discography was performed. Over subsequent years, provocative discography has been a subject of controversy, with both proponents and opponents. To date, however, provocative discography remains the only imaging technique that directly relates the patient's pain response to the morphological appearance of the disc (BOGDUK 1983; GUYER and OHNMEISS 1995; TEHRANZADEH 1998; ANDERSON and FLANAGAN 2000; BINI et al. 2002; ANDERSON 2004).

Low back pain is a common clinical problem. It may result from a variety of causes, including intervertebral disc disease. Magnetic resonance (MR) imaging is well-established for use in patients with suspected disc lesions. However, it is well known that many discs that appear abnormal on MR imaging are not symptomatic (COLHOUN et al 1988; LINSON and CROWE 1990; APRILL and BOGDUK 1992; SCHELLHAS et al 1996; LAM et al 2000; CARRAGEE et al 2000c; WEISHAUPT et al. 2001). Discs that appear normal on MR imaging have also been shown to be abnormal on discography (OSTI and FRASER 1992; BRIGHTBILL et al 1994).

Despite the lack of complete understanding of the pathophysiology of discogenic pain and the variable individual pain response (BOGDUK and MODIC 1996), many studies have supported provocative discography as a valuable diagnostic test in the investigation of discogenic pain (SIMMONS and SEGIL 1975; BRODSKY and BINDER 1979; SACHS et al. 1987; COLHOUN et al. 1988; SIMMONS et al. 1991; GRUBB and KELLY 2000; GUYER et al. 2003). However, being an invasive procedure, discography should not be used to screen patients with back pain. The procedure is useful provided that it is performed meticulously and interpreted precisely in carefully selected patients.

7.2
Disc Anatomy

The intervertebral disc is located between adjacent superior and inferior vertebral bodies. It is comprised of a central nucleus pulposus, surrounding annulus fibrosis and cartilaginous endplates (Fig. 7.1). The nucleus pulposus is composed of gelatinous material consisting of a collagen-proteoglycan complex that has a water content of approximately 70%–90% (BOGDUK 1997). The intranuclear cleft, located in the center of the nucleus pulposus, is mainly collagen and reticular fibers. The nucleus pulposus is avascular, and derives its nourishment through diffusion from blood vessels at the annulus fibrosis periphery and adjacent vertebral bodies.

The annulus fibrosis consists of concentric lamellae of collagen bundles that are attached to the rim of adjacent vertebrae by Sharpey fibers. The annulus fibrosis provides a strong link between adjacent vertebral bodies, while allowing some movement. The lamellae are thinner and less dense posteriorly than anteriorly or laterally, leading to a greater incidence of annular tears posteriorly (TEHRANZADEH 1998).

The cartilaginous endplates are located along the central osseous endplates of adjacent vertebral bodies, and overlie the superior and inferior margins of the nucleus pulposus. The posterior longitudinal ligament runs along, and is attached to, the posterior aspects of the vertebral bodies and intervertebral discs, from the level of the C2 vertebra to the sacrum. This ligament helps prevent hyperflexion of the vertebral column and posterior protrusion of the nucleus pulposus (TEHRANZADEH 1998).

The outer third of each lumbar intervertebral disc is innervated by penetrating branches of the sinovertebral nerves, gray rami communicantes and lumbar ventral rami (BOGDUK 1997). These nerve fibers are concentrated particularly at the posterolateral corners of the annulus fibrosis (GUARINO 1999). The nucleus pulposus acts as a shock absorber for axial forces, becoming broader when compressed.

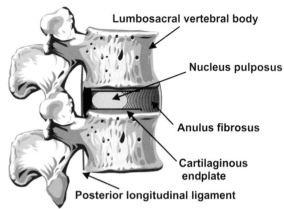

Lumbosacral disk anatomy   a

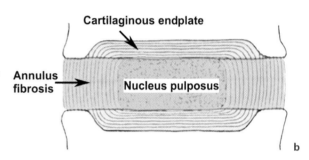

b

Fig. 7.1a,b. Disc anatomy. The intervertebral disc consists of a central nucleus pulposus surrounded by the annulus fibrosis and cartilaginous vertebral endplates

When the intervertebral disc is axially loaded, the nucleus pulposus absorbs approximately 70% of the force, with the rest being absorbed by the surrounding annulus fibrosis (GUARINO 1999).

7.3
Pathophysiology of Discogenic Pain

The pathophysiology of discogenic pain is still not completely understood, and a variety of mechanisms have been suggested. Internal disc degeneration is postulated to result from a series of events triggered by some type of initial stimulus (BOGDUK 1997). Early changes that occur in the nucleus pulposus include a progressive loss of hydration, pH decrease, and an increase in the level of substances such as enzyme phospholipase A2 (KITANO et al. 1993; SAAL 1989). With progression, there is a loss of nucleus viscoelasticity and resultant stress upon the surrounding annulus fibrosis, leading to development of an annular tear.

With further progression, part of the nucleus pulposus may herniate through the annular tear into the spinal canal or neural foramen. When the herniated disc material impinges upon an adjacent nerve root, typical radicular symptoms are produced. However, nerve root compression is responsible for pain in only approximately 5% or fewer patients with disc degeneration. Compression may lead to demyelination of nerve roots that are highly sensitive to hypoxia, chemical mediators, inflammation and pressure, leading to painful symptoms (TEHRANZADEH 1998). Radiating pain to the buttocks, hip, groin or lower limbs may however arise from the posterior annulus of the intervertebral disc, without direct involvement of the nerve root (SAIFUDDIN et al. 1998a).

Low back pain may occur in the absence of disc protrusion, as annular tears may be quite painful. A number of theories implicate various biochemical and biomechanical factors in the etiology of discogenic pain without focal disc protrusion. Discogenic pain may be due to leakage of chemical irritants, such as glycosaminoglycans and lactic acid, which come into contact with the pain fibers in the outer annulus fibrosis.

Discogenic pain may also be due to growth of granulation tissue in radial tears of the annulus fibrosis and nerve endings in the degenerated disc. Another theory is that when one portion of the annulus fibrosis fails because of a tear, the increased stresses are transferred to other parts of the annulus, leading to increased pressure and irritation of the nerve fibers. In a discographic study of porcine cadaveric discs, LEE et al. (2004) found that volumetric injection of discs with a torn annulus fibrosis can increase intra-annular pressure, but not in discs with an intact annulus fibrosis. Tears may also produce instability by decreasing the shock-absorbing qualities of the disc. It is likely that discogenic pain is due to a combination of different mechanisms, all causing stimulation of nerve fibers in the outer annulus fibrosis.

7.4
Imaging of Disc Disease: An Overview

Only a minority of patients presenting with low back pain require diagnostic imaging studies. Imaging is reserved for patients who have persistent painful symptoms, despite an adequate course of conservative treatment. Conventional radiographs are obtained initially and are useful for showing possible causes of back pain such as congenital anomalies, osteophytes, sacroiliitis, facet joint changes, bone destruction, pars interarticularis defects and soft tissue lesions such as renal calculi or aortic aneurysm calcification. CT supplements radiography by better showing bone lesions such as facet degeneration, fracture fragments, spinal canal stenosis and post-operative changes.

MR imaging is currently the most widely used imaging technique for the detection and characterization of disc disease. The normal nucleus pulposus is hyperintense on T2-weighted images, with the central nuclear cleft being seen as a hypointense area. The annulus fibrosis is normally hypointense on all pulse sequences. With disc degeneration, there is declining hydration of the nuclear pulposus, which is reflected as lower signal intensity on T2-weighted MR images (Fig. 7.2). MR imaging is also very useful for showing disc bulging, extrusion and sequestration. Loss of disc height or abnormal signal intensity is highly predictive of symptomatic tears extending into or beyond the outer annulus on discography (MILETTE et al. 1999). In a study correlating MR imaging with provocative discography, YOSHIDA et al. (2002) showed that T2-weighted MR imaging has high sensitivity and a high negative-predictive value in detecting symptomatic discs.

MR imaging may show a focal area of hyperintensity in the annulus fibrosis on T2-weighted images. This "high intensity zone" has been shown to correlate with an annular tear at that site (Fig. 7.3) (ITO et al. 1998). Some studies have reported a high correlation between the presence of the high intensity zone and discogenic pain (APRILL and BOGDUK 1992; SCHELLHAS et al. 1996; LAM et al. 2000), while others have argued that this sign is not specific enough for selection for surgery (HORTON and DAFTARI 1992; SMITH et al. 1998; RANKINE et al. 1999; CARRAGEE et al. 2000c).

Approximately 13% of patients with annular fissures that are visible on MR imaging are asymptomatic (SCHELLHAS et al. 1996). In another series, 30% of patients with normal MR imaging studies were found to have painful annular tears at discography (OSTI and FRASER 1992; BRIGHTBILL et al. 1994). Although MR imaging is generally useful for demonstrating various spine lesions, it is not as sensitive as discography for showing intrinsic annular tears or determining whether a particular disc is

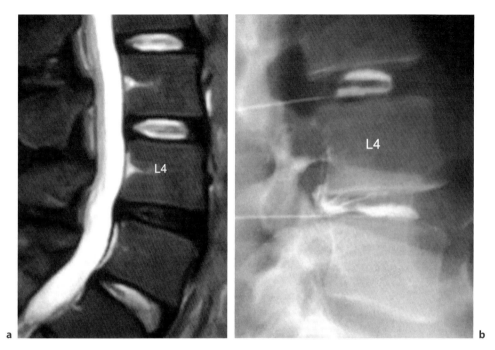

Fig. 7.2a,b. MR imaging-discographic correlation in a 39-year-old woman with low back pain and right sciatica. **a** Sagittal T2-weighted MR image shows a hypointense L4–5 disc, consistent with degeneration. The other lumbar discs are normal. **b** Lateral lumbar discogram shows a normal bilocular L3–4 disc and a degenerate L4–5 disc with a posterior annular tear and extradural extravasation

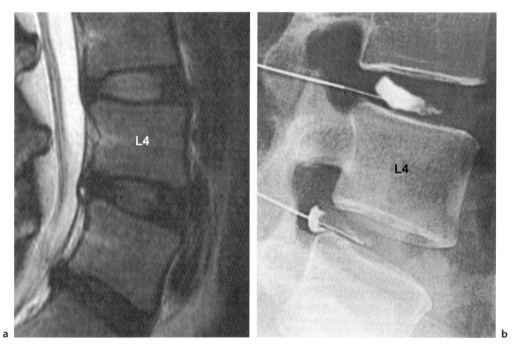

Fig. 7.3a,b. MR imaging-discographic correlation in a 29-year-old woman with low back pain and occasional right thigh radiation. **a** Sagittal T2-weighted MR image shows a hypointense L4–5 disc with a small focal "high intensity zone" consistent with a posterior annular tear in a degenerate disc. Posterior protrusions are present at L4–5 and L5–S1 disc levels. **b** Lateral lumbar discogram shows early contrast filling of a L4–5 disc annular tear with protrusion and a normal L3–4 disc

the cause of a patient's painful symptoms (Horton and Daftari 1992; Buirski and Silberstein 1993; Carragee et al. 2000c). Braithwaite et al. (1998) and Weishaupt et al. (2001) found a correlation between vertebral endplate signal changes and a painful lumbar disc, while Sandhu et al. (2000) found no significant relationship between provocative discography findings and vertebral endplate signal changes on MR imaging.

7.5.1
Indications

In general, discography should be performed only if the patient has failed adequate attempts at conservative management of persistent severe back or neck pain, and if noninvasive tests, such as MR imaging, have not provided sufficient diagnostic information. Nonresponding and persisting back pain should be of at least 4 months' duration (Kinard 1996; Guarino 1999). Discography should only be performed on patients being considered for surgery, as it assists in identifying the appropriate level for surgery. Pain due to facetogenic, neoplastic, inflammatory and traumatic causes should be excluded first (Fenton and Czervionke 2003).

Current indications for discography are (Guyer and Ohnmeiss 1995; Tehranzadeh 1998; Bini et al. 2002; Fenton and Czervionke 2003; Guyer et al. 2003; Anderson 2004):

- Further evaluation of demonstrably abnormal discs to assess the extent of abnormality or correlation of the abnormality with the clinical symptoms. These abnormalities include recurrent pain from a previously-operated disc and lateral disc herniation.
- Investigation of persistent, severe symptoms that do not correlate with discogenic-equivocal or inconsistent MR imaging or CT findings.
- To determine symptomatic disc level(s) where MR imaging or CT shows disc disease at multiple levels.
- Assessment of disc(s) before fusion to determine whether a disc within the proposed fusion segment is symptomatic, and whether the adjacent discs above and below are normal.

- Assessment of disc(s) prior to percutaneously-directed therapies such as intradiscal electrothermal therapy (IDET) (Saal and Saal 2000; Wetzel et al. 2002; Davis et al. 2004; Pauza et al. 2004).
- Assessment of candidates for minimally invasive surgery to confirm that the disc herniation is contained, or to investigate contrast distribution before chemonucleolysis or a percutaneous procedure.
- Assessment of postsurgical failed back syndrome in patients in whom MR imaging is nondiagnostic, particularly to determine if painful symptoms are related to lesions at the operated level or at an adjacent level. This includes differentiating recurrent disc herniation from a painful pseudoarthrosis or a symptomatic disc within a posteriorly-fused segment.

7.5.2
Contraindications

Current contraindications of discography are (Tehranzadeh 1998; Fenton and Czervionke 2003; Anderson 2004):

- Patients with a known bleeding disorder or who are undergoing anticoagulation therapy (International normalized ratio [INR] greater than 1.5, or platelets less than 50,000/mm^3).
- Pregnancy.
- Systemic infection or skin infection over the puncture site.
- Severe allergy to injectate, especially the contrast agent.
- Previously operated disc (which may yield a false-positive or false-negative result).
- Solid bone fusion that does not allow access to the disc.
- Severe spinal cord compromise at the disc level to be investigated.

7.5.3
Technique

7.5.3.1
Pre-procedural Preparation

Before the start of the procedure, the patient should be interviewed about the type, location and nature of the pain, as well as history of prior surgery. In some centers, the patient is asked to fill in a pain map or pain drawing to indicate the location of the pain and to grade the level of pain severity, preferably on a visual analog scale. Pain drawings may be helpful in identifying which specific discs are associated with pain complaints (OHNMEISS et al. 1999). The patient's medical and imaging records should be reviewed. It is important to compare MR images with radiographs to evaluate any ambiguity due to a transitional lumbosacral segment, the overall disc morphology and to identify a normal disc that can be used as a control.

Informed consent should be obtained. The patient needs to understand the purpose of the pain provocation test, particularly that the intradiscal injection aims to provoke the same pain that he or she experiences with movement or activity. The patient should fast for 6–8 h before the procedure. Giving prophylactic antibiotics is recommended. Intravenous cefazolin (Ancef, SmithKline Beecham, Philadelphia, PA/USA) 1g bolus is administered within 1 h prior to the procedure. In some centers, a mild sedative such as intravenous diazepam or midazolam is given prior to the procedure, with additional doses being given during the procedure if necessary. Others do not recommend sedation, as it may affect the patient's response to pain reproduction.

The patient ideally should be monitored by nursing staff during the procedure. Connection to an ECG monitor and pulse oximetry, and recording of pulse and blood pressure are suggested. Strict asepsis is mandatory. The patient should be cleaned and draped, and the radiologist should be fully scrubbed up and gowned.

7.5.3.2
Equipment

The discography tray should contain the following:
- 21-gauge 12.5-cm stainless steel spinal needle with stylet (Steriseal, Maersk Medical, Redditch, England) and 26-gauge 16.0-cm stainless steel spinal needle with stylet (Steriseal, Maersk Medical, Redditch, England) for thoracic and lumbar discography.
- 20-gauge 6.35-cm stainless steel spinal needle with stylet (Becton Dickenson, Rutherford, NJ/USA) and 26-gauge 8.9-cm stainless steel spinal needle with stylet (Becton Dickenson, Rutherford, NJ/USA) for cervical and thoracic discography.
- Curved needle set consisting of a 21-gauge 10.0-cm stainless steel straight needle with stylet, and a

26-gauge 15.0-cm nitinol curved needle (Pakter, Cook Inc, Bloomington, IN/USA) for the L5/S1 disc (Fig. 7.4).
- 25-gauge 3.8-cm needle for skin and subcutaneous local anesthesia.
- 1 ml tuberculin syringe for intradiscal injection.
- 5 ml syringe for local anesthesia.
- Alcohol and povidone-iodine scrubs.
- Sterile gauze and drapes.
- Lidocaine 1% (Xylocaine 1%, AstraZeneca LP, Wilmington, DE/USA).
- Nonionic contrast agent 300 mg I/ml (Omnipaque 300, Nycomed, Princeton, NJ/USA).

The size and type of needles varies with different centers and practitioners. For example, a 22-gauge inner needle may be placed within an 18-gauge outer needle. Some practitioners advocate the single needle approach using a 22-gauge styleted needle (FENTON and CZERVIONKE 2003). There are several reasons to adopt the double-needle approach: a lower rate of discitis (FRASER et al. 1987),a thinner 26-gauge inner needle can be used to decrease the size of the puncture in the annulus fibrosis, and there is the option of having a pre-shaped curve at the distal end of the inner needle to facilitate entry into the center of the L5-S1 nucleus. In the double-needle technique, the inner needle that enters the nucleus pulposus does not come into contact with the skin, theoretically reducing the infection rate.

Imaging is best performed in an interventional suite in the diagnostic radiology department. Biplane fluoroscopy is preferred (Fig. 7.5) but if it is not available, high-quality C-arm fluoroscopy is an acceptable alternative. In some centers, CT is used to guide needle placement. CT fluoroscopy allows near real-time evaluation of the procedure.

For patients who are allergic to iodinated contrast agents, MR discography using intradiscal gadolinium-chelate is a viable alternative and might be considered for patients who wish to limit their radiation exposure (HUANG et al. 2002; SLIPMAN et al. 2002; FALCO and MORAN 2003). Performing MR discography using an optical guidance tool attached to an MR compatible needle in a 0.23 T open magnet has been found to be accurate and relatively safe (SEQUEIROS et al. 2003). In a cadaveric study, KAKITSUBATA et al. (2003) found that MR discography was accurate in evaluating clinically significant radial tears of the annulus fibrosis, but was not as useful for identification of other types of annular tears.

Fig. 7.4. Needles used for discography. A curved needle set consisting of a 21-gauge 10.0-cm stainless steel straight needle with stylet, and a 26-gauge 15.0-cm long nitinol curved needle (Pakter, Cook Inc., Bloomington, IN, USA)

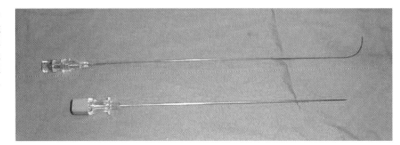

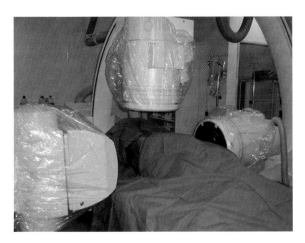

Fig. 7.5. Use of biplane fluoroscopy for discography. Patient positioned in a left lateral decubitus position in preparation for lumbar discography

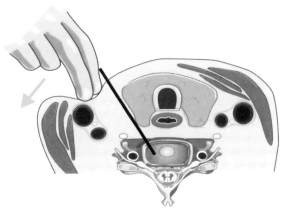

Fig. 7.6. Needle placement for cervical discography. The fingers are used to protect and laterally displace the carotid sheath contents. Other important structures to avoid are the trachea and esophagus

7.5.3.3
Cervical Discography

First described by SMITH and NICHOLS (1957), cervical discography remains a controversial procedure (PARFENCHUCK and JANSSEN 1994). Some investigators recommend that this procedure not be performed, as the information it provides does not outweigh the increased risk of complications, which have been reported in up to 13% of cases (CONNOR and DARDEN 1993). These complications include discitis, epidural abscess, hematoma, myelopathy and quadriplegia (ZEIDMAN et al. 1995). The risks versus benefits of performing cervical discography should be considered carefully prior to the procedure. Other practitioners have confirmed cervical discography to be a safe and useful procedure in selected patients with chronic intractable neck pain but negative or indeterminate imaging findings and who are being considered for surgery (GRUBB and KELLY 2000; MOTIMAYA et al. 2000; ZHENG et al. 2004).

The patient is placed supine on the fluoroscopy table, with the neck slightly hyperextended. The cervical disc to be punctured is identified and approached using an anterolateral approach. A right-side approach is normally used, as most operators are right handed, and it decreases the likelihood of inadvertently puncturing the esophagus, which runs slightly to the left of the midline. It is important to protect the carotid sheath contents; this is done by palpating the carotid pulse at the disc level and laterally displacing the carotid sheath structures using the middle and index fingers. Local anesthetic is administered, and the 20-gauge 6.35-cm outer needle is introduced just medial to the fingertips, displacing the carotid sheath structures (Fig. 7.6). The needle is directed parallel to the disc at an angle of approximately 40–45°, taking care to avoid the trachea and esophagus. The trachea can be easily identified by palpation.

Using intermittent anteroposterior and lateral fluoroscopy, the outer needle tip is positioned at the outer annulus fibrosis of the disc. The needle tip should be in line with the anterior cortex of the adjacent vertebral bodies on the lateral projection, and in line with the ipsilateral pedicles of the adjacent vertebral bodies on the anteroposterior projection. The stylet is then removed and replaced with the 26-gauge 8.9-cm inner needle, which is directed under fluoroscopic guidance until its tip is in the center of the disc space on both anteroposterior and lateral fluoroscopic images (Fig. 7.7).

7.5.3.4
Thoracic Discography

Thoracic discography is rarely performed, as it has few indications. Severe and disabling thoracic pain secondary to disc degeneration that warrants discography has not been well studied (TEHRANZADEH 1998; FENTON and CZERVIONKE 2003). This procedure has been used to evaluate symptomatic Scheuermann disease (WINTER and SCHELLHAS 1996). In a prospective discographic study of asymptomatic and symptomatic individuals, WOOD et al. (1999) found that thoracic discs with prominent Schmorl nodes may be intensely painful, even in life-long asymptomatic subjects. They showed that thoracic discography can demonstrate disc pathology that is not seen on MR imaging.

The patient is usually placed in a prone position. The needle is inserted under fluoroscopic or CT guidance. The technique is essentially similar to lumbar discography (see Sect. 7.5.3.5). Depending on the depth of the thoracic disc to be punctured, shorter (for cervical discography) or longer (for lumbar discography) needles may be used. Care should be taken to avoid puncturing structures such as the lung and spinal cord. During posteroanterior fluoroscopy, the needle tip should be kept along the lateral aspect of the superior articular process to avoid entering the spinal canal, and medial to the costotransverse junction to avoid a pleural puncture (FENTON and CZERVIONKE 2003).

7.5.3.5
Lumbar Discography

The vast majority of discograms performed in clinical practice are for the lumbar discs, particularly the lower three levels. For lumbar discography, the patient may be placed in a prone or left lateral decubitus position, depending on operator preference. Advocates of the prone position find that the patient is more stable and immobile. Having the patient's more symptomatic side raised slightly to make needle placement easier is recommended, as is placing a pillow under the abdomen to straighten the lum-

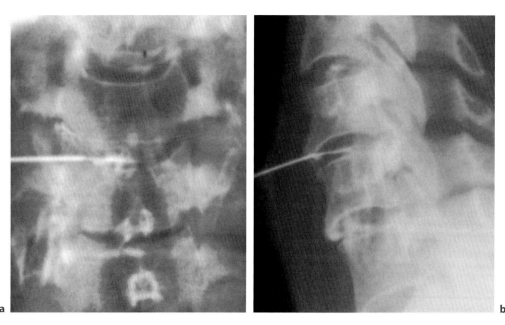

a   b

Fig. 7.7a,b. Cervical discography in a 36-year-old woman with neck pain and numbness of the left arm. **a** Anteroposterior and (**b**) lateral projections of the cervical spine show the needle positions for C4–5 discography. An anterolateral approach was adopted

bar curve (TEHRANZADEH 1998; FENTON and CZ-ERVIONKE 2003). This author prefers the left lateral decubitus position. The patient's knees are flexed to about 60–90°, with a pillow under the patient's waist to keep the spine straight. The left rather than right lateral decubitus position is preferred to decrease the chance of puncturing the artery of Adamkiewicz, which occurs four times more frequently on the left side. A patient in the decubitus position is also easier to manipulate physically, if necessary, to better visualize the disc during fluoroscopy (Fig. 7.5).

The skin puncture point is approximately 8–10 cm to the right of the midline (Fig. 7.8). For L4-5 and L5-S1 levels, the position of the iliac crest must be considered. Depending on operator preference, the tips of the spinous processes may be marked using indelible ink. After the patient is cleaned and draped, and local anesthesia is given, the outer needle is inserted (Fig. 7.9). The extradural approach, with the needle taking a posterolateral oblique path to the disc, is preferred to avoid puncturing the thecal sac (TEHRANZADEH 1998; FENTON and CZERVIONKE 2003; ANDERSON 2004). A 21-gauge 12.5-cm outer needle is inserted with an obliquity of about 45–60° to the sagittal plane. For the L5-S1 disc, due to the overlying iliac crest, an additional caudal angulation of up to 40° is usually necessary. When it is not possible to puncture the disc using a posterolateral oblique, extradural pathway, a para-midline transthecal pathway may be used (Fig. 7.10). This transthecal approach may be useful for post-operative patients with hardware or fusion masses along the desired path. Disadvantages include the risk of introducing infection into the subarachnoid space, subarachnoid hemorrhage with resultant arachnoiditis and post-procedural headache (ANDERSON 2004).

After repeated fluoroscopic imaging in the frontal and lateral directions, the 21-gauge outer needle is positioned with its tip at the right posterolateral corner of the annulus fibrosis of the target disc (Fig. 7.11). The needle tip should be located in line with the posterior cortex of the adjacent vertebral bodies on the lateral projection, and in line with the ipsilateral pedicles of the adjacent vertebral bodies on the posteroanterior projection. A mild degree of firm rubbery resistance is felt when the needle tip contacts the annulus fibrosis. The stylet of the outer needle is then removed, and a 26-gauge 16.0-cm inner needle is inserted inside the 21-gauge outer needle. Under fluoroscopic guidance in the two orthogonal directions, the tip of the inner needle is directed to

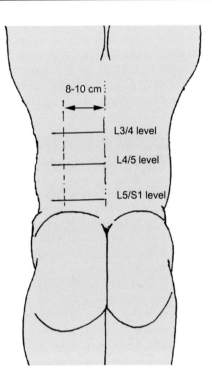

Fig. 7.8. Skin puncture points for lumbar discography. These are located approximately 8–10 cm from the midline. The spinous processes may be marked on the skin with ink

the center of the nucleus pulposus (Fig. 7.12). Sometimes, patients experience pain when the needle tip contacts the well-innervated outer annulus fibrosis. Some practitioners inject 1 ml of lidocaine prior to annular penetration to ease the pain.

The L5-S1 disc is often difficult to access, particularly for inexperienced discographers. A high-riding iliac crest, as well as disc space narrowing and a broad L5 transverse process, commonly produce bony obstructions and often lead to failure of the procedure (SMITH and BROWN 1967; TROSIER 1982). Failure rates of 15–30% have been reported (KUMAR and AGORASTIDES 2000). For the L5-S1 disc, it may be necessary to bend the tip of the inner needle prior to insertion (MCCULLOUGH and WADDELL 1978; TROSIER 1982; SACHS et al. 1990; ANDERSON 2004) or to use a dedicated curved needle set (Fig. 7.13). KUMAR and AGORASTIDES (2000) described the technique of manually pre-bending the outer needle, and found that the method has a better success rate than using a straight needle. The authors noted limitations of the technique, such as underestimating the needle curvature and maintaining correct orientation of the needle curve.

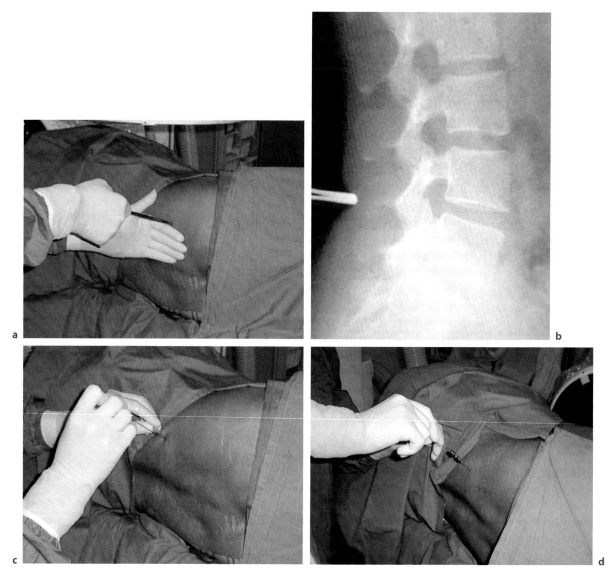

Fig. 7.9a–d. Lumbar discography skin puncture technique. **a** Surface marking of the skin puncture point, using four fingerbreadths as a rough measurement guide. **b** Lateral spine projection shows the puncture point for the L4–5 disc indicated by tip of the sponge forceps. **c** Insertion of the outer discogram needle during withdrawal of the small needle used for instillation of local anesthesia. The same skin puncture site is used. **d** Longer inner discogram needle placed within shorter outer needle

When the position of the inner needle is satisfactory, its stylet is removed and the needle is attached to a 1 ml tuberculin syringe with 0.1 ml markings. A nonionic contrast agent of 300 mg I/ml concentration is used. A test injection of 0.1 ml should confirm the needle's position. The injected contrast agent should form a rounded or curvilinear blob near the center of the disc space (Fig. 7.14). In a normal disc, there is moderate resistance during contrast injection; in a degenerate disc, there is mild or no resistance to injection. If there is marked resistance to contrast instillation at the beginning of the injection, with the contrast agent staying immediately at the needle tip, then the needle tip should be carefully viewed in two orthogonal planes to ensure it is not located within the annulus fibrosis. An annular injection may lead to a false-positive pain response. If the position of the needle tip is suboptimal, adjustment and fluoroscopic re-screening is required. Some practitioners use a manometer to measure opening and filling pressures during disc injection (MIN et al. 1996; DERBY et al. 1999; SOUTHERN et al. 2000).

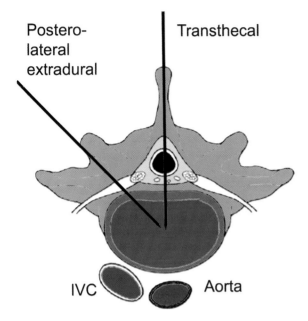

Fig. 7.10. Needle paths taken using the posterolateral extradural and transthecal approaches for lumbar discography

O'NEILL and KURGANSKY (2004) recommended that discography be performed under pressure control, to allow quantification of the pain threshold of discs and estimation of false-positive discs.

7.5.3.6
Post-Discography Procedure

After the needles are removed, the patient's back or neck is cleaned and small adhesive bandages are applied to the puncture sites. Following completion of post-discography imaging, the patient should be observed for 2 h in either a reclining or recumbent position. Pulse, blood pressure and respiratory rate should be monitored immediately and, if normal, should be taken again at discharge. If these parameters are abnormal, they should be monitored at 30-minute intervals until they return to baseline levels. The patient should be discharged to the care of a responsible person. Most practitioners will give their patients a prescription for a nonnarcotic painkiller,

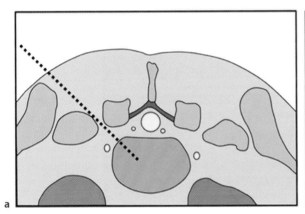

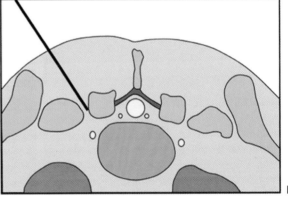

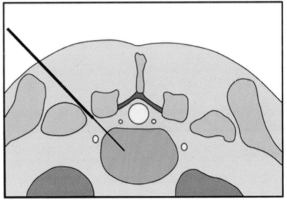

Fig. 7.11a–c. Positions of the outer and inner needles used in the posterolateral extradural approach for lumbar discography. **a** Anticipated needle path is shown by *dotted line*. **b** The outer needle is directed to the posterolateral corner of the annulus fibrosis. **c** The inner needle is placed within the outer needle and directed into the center of the nucleus pulposus

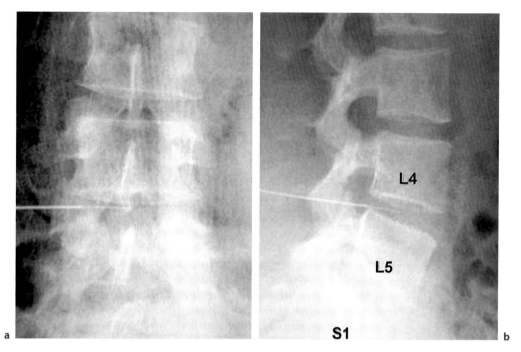

Fig. 7.12a,b. Needle positions for lumbar discography in a 35-year-old man with low back pain and right paraspinal pain. **a** Anteroposterior and (**b**) lateral lumbar spine projections show the positions of the outer needle at the posterolateral aspect of the annulus fibrosis (in line with the ipsilateral pedicles on the frontal view and the posterior vertebral body cortices on the lateral view) and the inner needle at the center of the nucleus pulposus of the L4–5 disc

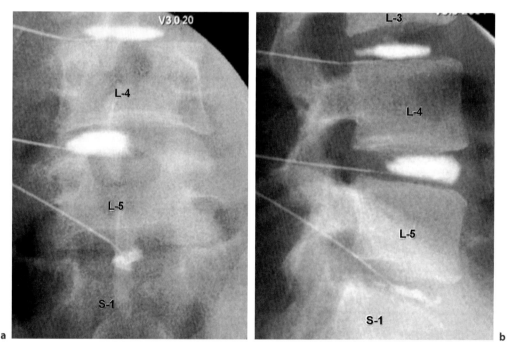

Fig. 7.13a,b. Curved needle set for L5–S1 discography in a 29-year-old man with chronic low back pain. **a** Anteroposterior and (**b**) lateral lumbar spine projections show the caudal angulation required to puncture the L5–S1 disc because of the high-riding iliac crests, compared with the relatively horizontal positions of the needles for the L3–4 and L4–5 discograms

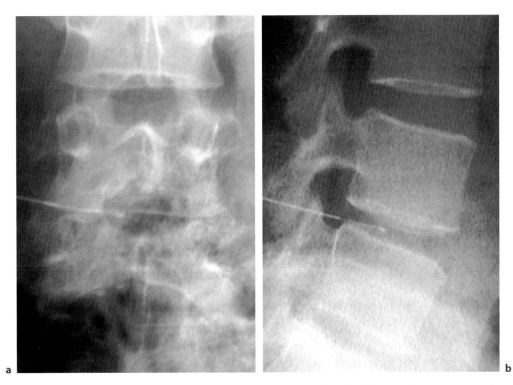

Fig. 7.14a,b. Initial test injection to confirm needle position in lumbar discography of a 41-year-old woman with low back pain and pain radiating down both legs. **a** Anteroposterior and (**b**) lateral lumbar spine projections show a tiny blob of contrast agent near the center of the L4–5 disc space

while others also add a short course of oral broad-spectrum antibiotics (FENTON and CZERVIONKE 2003).

7.5.4
Interpretation

The volume of contrast agent injected into the nucleus pulposus, and the amount of resistance during the injection, should be carefully recorded. The normal lumbar disc usually takes up to 1.5 ml of contrast agent, but a degenerated lumbar disc will typically have a volume of more than 2 ml. Most practitioners would not inject more than 3 ml of contrast agent into a single lumbar disc. For cervical discography, the volume of contrast agent should not exceed 0.5 ml per disc, while 0.5–1.0 ml is normally used for a thoracic discogram (TEHRANZADEH 1998). The injection is usually terminated when very firm resistance is met or if severe pain is elicited at low volumes (FENTON and CZERVIONKE 2003). Post-procedure imaging using CT (CT discography) and its classification is an option that supplements discographic interpretation. Patient position during discography should be standardized, as annular strains and bulges can be influenced by the position of the spine and the location of the disc and pressurization (REITMAN et al. 2001). The two major aspects to consider in the interpretation of discography are disc morphology and pain provocation.

7.5.4.1
Disc Morphology

Disc morphology is determined on evaluation of anteroposterior and lateral radiographs obtained after intradiscal contrast injection (Fig. 7.15). A normal disc retains its normal height on both AP and lateral radiographs. Injected contrast agent remains in the nucleus pulposus, and may be unilocular or bilocular ("hamburger bun" or "horseshoe") in shape. Unilocular discograms may be spherical ("cotton ball") or rectangular in shape (Fig. 7.16). Sometimes, a Schmorl node is seen as a focal protrusion of injected contrast agent into the adjacent vertebral endplate (BRIGHTBILL et al. 1994).

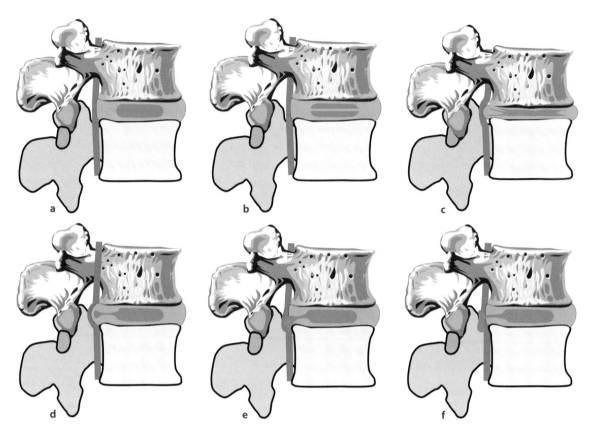

Fig. 7.15a–f. Various patterns of disc morphology on the lateral discographic projections. **a** Normal disc with unilocular shape. **b** Normal disc with bilocular shape. **c** Degenerate disc with annular disruption, disc height loss and posterior protrusion. **d** Protruded disc with radial tear. **e** Extruded disc with inferior migration (candle drip). **f** Extruded disc with posterior longitudinal ligament disruption. [Modified and reproduced with permission from Peh (2004)]

A degenerated disc loses water and height. Discography shows complex or multiple irregular fissures in the annulus fibrosis, with or without contrast leakage through annular tears. A bulging disc, often associated with degeneration, is characterized by circumferential, diffuse and symmetrical annular bulging. Discography may show annular fissures with an intact peripheral annulus. Disc protrusion refers to a focal protrusion of disc material that is often asymmetrical. The protrusion may be central or posterolateral, but with an intact posterior longitudinal ligament. A single annular fissure is often seen on discography. The nuclear material may migrate superiorly or inferiorly, producing a "candle drip" appearance in the latter case. A disc extrusion is a large protrusion that involves the posterior longitudinal ligament. An annular fissure with epidural space contrast extravasation is seen on discography (Fig. 7.17). A sequestrated disc is seen when extruded disc material is separated from the parent disc. The detached disc is usually located in the extradural space.

7.5.4.2
Dallas Discogram Description

CT discography refers to the CT images obtained following discography (Fig. 7.18). They provide excellent anatomical details in the axial plane. The Dallas discogram description (DDD) originally classified the appearance of the disc on CT into grades 0 to 3 (Sachs et al. 1987), but has been expanded to grades 0 to 4 (Aprill and Bogduk 1992).

- Grade 0: Contrast agent is confined entirely within the normal nucleus pulposus (Fig. 7.19a).
- Grade 1: Contrast agent extends radially along fissure involving the inner third of the annulus fibrosis.
- Grade 2: Contrast agent extends into the middle third of the annulus fibrosis.

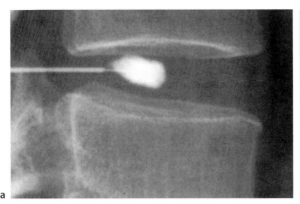
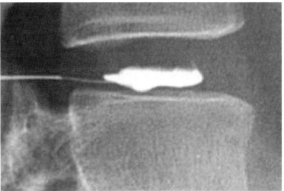
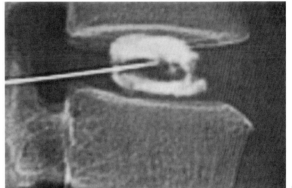

Fig. 7.16a–c. Discographic patterns of normal discs in different patients. Lateral radiographs show (**a**) unilocular (cotton ball) L3-4 disc, (**b**) unilocular (rectangular) L3–4 disc, and (**c**) bilocular (hamburger bun) L3–4 disc

- Grade 3: Contrast agent extends into the outer third of the annulus fibrosis, either focally or radially, to an extent not greater than 30° of the disc circumference.
- Grade 4: Contrast agent extends into the outer third of the annulus fibrosis, dissecting radially to involve more than 30° of the disc circumference (Fig. 7.19b).

Further modifications have been made: grade 5 indicates a full-thickness tear, either focal or circumferential, with extra-annular contrast leakage (SCHELLHAS et al. 1996); grade 6 indicates disc sequestration; and grade 7 indicates a diffuse annular tear in disc degeneration (Fig. 7.19c) (BERNARD 1990). With a spiral or multislice scanner to perform the CT discogram, good quality sagittal and coronal reconstructed images can provide additional information (Fig. 7.20) (VIVITMONGKONCHAI and PEH 2001).

CT discography has been found to be better than CT myelography and conventional discography (JACKSON et al. 1989). HODGE et al. (1994) recommended that CT discography be reserved for postoperative patients with recurrent symptoms who are unable to undergo MR imaging or in whom MR imaging is equivocal. BERNARD (1994) also found CT discography to be more accurate than contrast-enhanced MR imaging for distinguishing recurrent disc herniation from scar tissue.

7.5.4.3
Pain Provocation

Although the pathophysiology of discogenic pain is still not completely understood, it is likely due to a combination of several mechanisms, all causing stimulation of nerve fibers in the outer annulus fibrosis (WILEY et al. 1968; CROCK 1986). Suggested mechanisms of discogenic pain provocation are (WILEY et al. 1968; BRODSKY and BINDER 1979; MCNALLY et al. 1996):

- Stretching of fibers of the abnormal annulus fibrosis
- Extravasation of irritating chemical substances.
- Pressure on nerves
- Vascularized granulation tissue in the annulus fibrosis
- Posterior joint hyperflexion during injection
- Changes in loading patterns of the posterolateral annulus fibrosis or nucleus pulposus

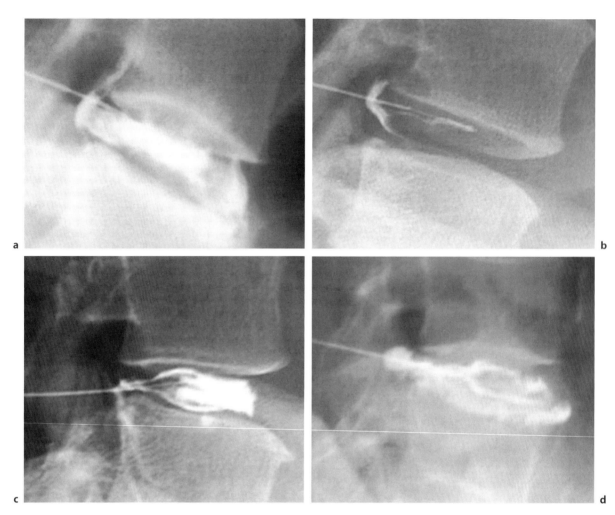

Fig. 7.17a–d. Discographic patterns of abnormal discs in different patients. Lateral radiographs show (**a**) degenerate L4–5 disc with multiple annular fissures and posterior protrusion with contrast extravasation, (**b**) early filling of L4–5 annular tear with posterior protrusion, (**c**) L4–5 posterior annular tear with inferior migration (candle drip), and (**d**) degenerate L4–5 disc with focal posterior protrusion

The degree of pain provocation from degenerative discs is variable. Abnormal discs may not be painful (WALSH et al. 1990). Pain provocation usually occurs in posterior annular tears of grade 3 or more, and less commonly in grade 1 or 2 disc lesions (VANHARANTA et al. 1987). Grade 3 annular disruption with a focal disc protrusion beyond the line of the vertebral body has a significantly higher frequency of symptomatic pain for all grades of degeneration compared to those without disc protrusion (MAEZAWA and MURO 1992). Delayed pain response following discography has been described. In patients with near-normal disc morphology, incomplete annular tears may not be filled at the time of injection and may instead fill with contrast agent up to 2.5 h later, causing pain (LEHMER et al. 1994).

Where possible, injecting an adjacent normal disc as a control is recommended (KINARD 1996; FENTON and CZERVIONKE 2003; ANDERSON 2004). The normal disc is identified from MR images prior to discography. This gives the practitioner an indication of the patient's level of pain tolerance, and also the reliability of the patient's responses at other levels. Pain from a normal disc is rare but patients may occasionally report feeling pressure or discomfort during injection. Up to 40% of asymptomatic patients with a previous lumbar discectomy have been found to have significant pain on injection of operated discs (CARRAGEE et al. 2000b).

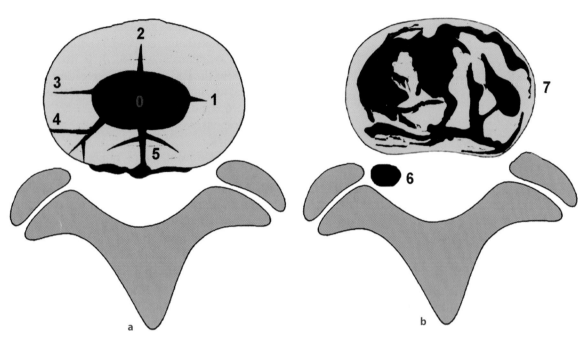

Fig. 7.18a,b. Modified Dallas discogram description for CT discography. The degrees of annular disruption are numbered from 0–7. **a** Grade 0, normal; grade 1, fissure inner third; grade 2, fissure middle third; grade 3, fissure outer third <30°; grade 4, fissure outer third >30°; grade 5, full-thickness tear with extra-annular contrast leakage. **b** Grade 6, sequestration; grade 7, diffuse tears in degenerate disc

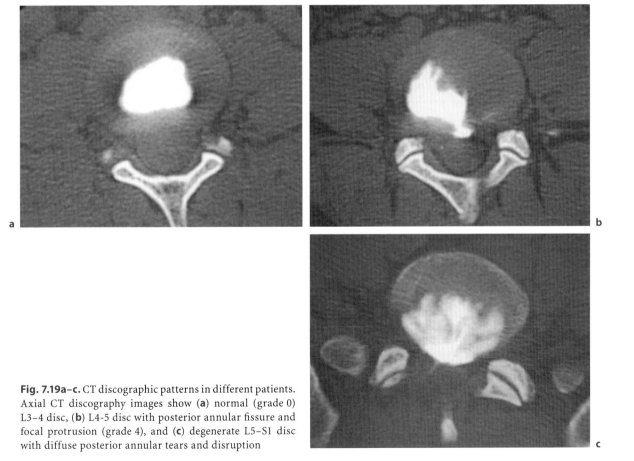

Fig. 7.19a–c. CT discographic patterns in different patients. Axial CT discography images show (**a**) normal (grade 0) L3–4 disc, (**b**) L4-5 disc with posterior annular fissure and focal protrusion (grade 4), and (**c**) degenerate L5–S1 disc with diffuse posterior annular tears and disruption

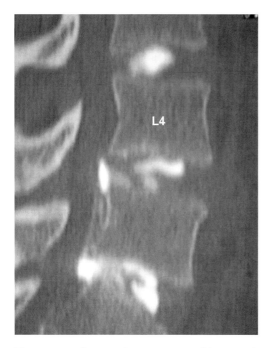

Fig. 7.20. CT discography in a 40-year-old man with severe low back pain. Sagittal reformatted CT image after discography shows a normal L3–4 disc, and posterior protrusions of degenerate L4–5 and L5–S1 discs

BLOCK et al. (1996) found that discographic pain reports are not only related to anatomic abnormalities but are also influenced by personality. Patients with abnormal scores on psychological tests may over-report pain during discography. The specificity of discography drops to 20% in patients with chronic pain and psychiatric risk factors, compared to specificity of up to 90% in healthy patients with no chronic pain and a normal psychiatric profile (CARRAGEE et al. 2000a). Use of pain drawings may be helpful in identifying patients who are likely to report pain on injection of a nondisrupted disc, as a correlation between pain drawings and discographic pain responses has been reported (OHNMEISS et al. 1994; OHNMEISS et al. 1999).

Pain provocation is the most useful and important aspect of discography. However, the individual patient's response is subjective and may be difficult to evaluate precisely. It is important to avoid bias during the procedure. The patient should not know when each injection begins or ends. Patients should instead be told before the start of the procedure, and intermittently reminded during the procedure, to immediately inform the practitioner when they experience any new or increasing pain. During injec-

tion, the location and character of the pain should be carefully noted and recorded. Leading questions should be assiduously avoided. It is useful to always observe the patient's facial expression or body movement for signs of pain response, particularly in patients who tend to be stoic.

Pain responses can be classified into the following categories:
- No, or insignificant, pain reproduction
- Pain different from the usual painful symptoms (discordant)
- Pain similar to some of the usual painful symptoms (partially concordant)
- Pain identical to the usual painful symptoms (concordant)

When taking the disc morphology and pain provocation aspects together, the categories of a discography study are:
- Normal study
- Abnormal but asymptomatic disc(s)
- Abnormal disc(s) with discordant symptoms
- Abnormal disc(s) with concordant (partially or fully) symptoms

The needles are left in place until completion of all the injections. Some practitioners inject a local anesthetic into discs that produce concordant pain. This additional test aims to help further determine whether a particular disc is a pain generator, particularly in cases where spinal fusion or intradiscal electrothermal therapy is being considered. In patients with a full-thickness annular tear, without the ability to increase intradiscal pressure, a false-negative discogram may be obtained. Hence, pain relief following intradiscal local anesthetic administration may be diagnostic of mechanoreceptor discogenic pain. This technique may also serve to diminish a false-positive pain response at a disc level that may be due to residual concordant pain at other levels. A 1:1 mixture of lidocaine 1% and bupivacaine 0.25%, giving both short- and longer-acting effects, has been recommended (FENTON and CZERVIONKE 2003).

KHOT et al. (2004) performed a prospective randomized study of the therapeutic effects of intradiscal steroid injection compared to a saline placebo in 120 patients with chronic low back pain of discogenic origin, and found that intradiscal steroid injections did not improve the clinical outcome. A pilot study of treatment of disc disease has shown promising results for the intradiscal injection of substances known to induce proteoglycan synthesis, such as glucosamine, chondroitin sulphate, hypertonic dextrose and dimethysulfoxide (KLEIN et al. 2003).

The finding of pain provocation during discography has a direct impact on the surgical outcome. COLHOUN et al. (1988) found, in their series of 137 patients with positive discograms, that 89% of cases obtained clinical benefit from surgery. GILL and BLUMENTHAL (1992) reported a 75% surgical success rate in patients with both positive discograms and MR imaging at the L5-S1 level, but a success rate of only 50% in patients with a combination of positive discograms and normal MR imaging. In a follow-up study of 96 patients who underwent pressure-controlled lumbar discography, DERBY et al. (1999) showed that highly chemically-sensitive discs appear to achieve better long-term outcomes with interbody/combined fusion than with intertransverse fusion, with patients without disc surgery having the least favorable outcome.

Others have questioned the predictive value of discography in surgical planning. MADAN et al. (2002) reported no significant difference in surgical outcome between a group of patients selected for surgery based on a positive discogram and another group that did not undergo preoperative discography. RHYNE et al. (1995) found that 68% of patients with a positive discogram showed significant symptomatic improvement with conservative treatment only. SMITH et al. (1995) retrospectively analyzed the nonoperative outcome of 25 patients with positive discograms who did not undergo surgery, and found that discogenic pain improved in patients without psychiatric disease.

7.5.5
Complications

The reported complication rate of discography is low, usually less than 1%. The most serious and frequently-encountered complication is discitis (Fig. 7.21). In an MR imaging study of patients undergoing lumbar discography, SAIFUDDIN et al. (1998b) suggested that any changes occurring in the vertebral endplate following discography should be considered due to infectious discitis. FRASER et al. (1987) reported a reduction of the discitis rate from 2.7% to 0.7%, using a double-needle instead of a single-needle technique. The incidence of infection can be decreased with use of prophylactic antibiotics and styleted needles (OSTI et al. 1990; GUYER and

OHNMEISS 1995). WILLEMS et al. (2004) analyzed ten discography studies in which prophylactic antibiotics were not given and found an infection rate of 0.25% in 4,891 patients and 0.094% in 12,770 discs. They concluded that the risk of post-discography discitis was minimal. Although there is no evidence to support the routine use of antibiotics in discography, many practitioners administer broad-spectrum antibiotics as prophylaxis against possible discitis (OSTI et al. 1990; TEHRANZADEH 1998; FENTON and CZERVIONKE 2003; ANDERSON 2004).

An experimental animal study has shown no evidence of discitis in sheep inoculated with *Staphylococcus epidermidis* and given prophylactic ceftriaxone (FRASER et al. 1989). LANG et al. (1994) confirmed good penetration of intravenous ceftriaxone into the disc 1–4 h following administration. In addition to an intravenous bolus 1 h prior to the procedure, some practitioners also use intradiscal antibiotics. In an in vitro study, KLESSIG et al. (2003) showed that intradiscal gentamycin, cefazolin and clindamycin remain efficacious in the presence of the contrast agent iohexol, and suggested that systemic antibiotic prophylaxis is not needed. For intradiscal injection, FENTON and CZERVIONKE (2003) combined 0.5 ml of cefazolin (10 mg/5 ml) with 2.3 ml of contrast agent, while ANDERSON (2004) mixed either cefazolin or vancomycin at a concentration of 1 mg per ml of contrast agent.

Nerve damage may also occur, although contact with the nerve usually causes only transient symptoms. A post-procedural headache may develop if the transthecal puncture route is used. Other possible complications are needle breakage, accidental intradural injection, intrathecal hemorrhage, meningitis, arachnoiditis, osteomyelitis and epidural abscess. As to whether discography causes injury to the disc itself, FLANAGAN and CHUNG (1986) and JOHNSON (1989) have shown that long term disc injury does not occur. Potential complications of discography should be preventable with strict asepsis and a meticulous technique.

7.6
Conclusion

Provocative discography has, since its initial description, been a subject of controversy, with both proponents and detractors. Some of the factors con-

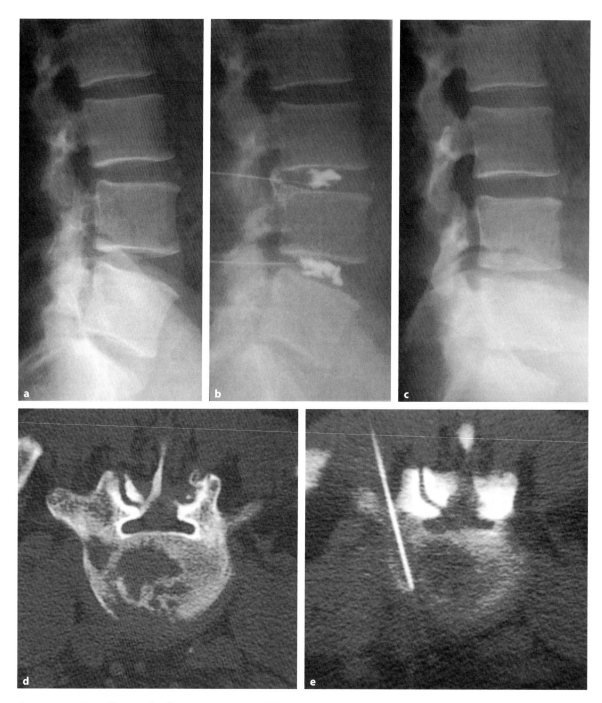

Fig. 7.21a–e. Post-discography discitis in a 46-year-old man with low back pain and right sciatica. **a** Initial lateral radiograph of lumbar spine shows normal disc spaces. **b** Lateral lumbar spine projection taken during discography shows a posterior annular tear and mild bulging of the L3–4 disc. Subsequent images showed a L4–5 posterior annular tear also. **c** Lateral radiograph of lumbar spine taken two months later shows loss of L4–5 disc height and upper L5 end-plate irregularity. The patient presented with persistent back pain, stiffness and fever, and raised inflammatory markers. **d** Axial CT scan (taken with patient prone) shows irregular destruction of the upper L5 vertebral body. **e** Axial CT scan shows position of the biopsy needle within the L4–5 disc. Disc and blood cultures were negative. The patient made a full recovery after antibiotic treatment

tributing to poor outcome – and hence to controversy – include: incorrect indications and patient selection, an inexperienced or inexpert practitioner, over-reporting of pain by hysterical patients, inaccurate assessment of pain response, needle misplacement and pain sources other than problematic discs (TEHRANZADEH 1998).

Provocative discography, however, remains the only diagnostic test that can provide both anatomical and functional information about a suspected disc lesion. It is a complementary test in patients whose painful symptoms are not explained by findings on noninvasive imaging modalities such as MR imaging or CT. Provided the patients are well selected, and the procedure precisely performed and carefully interpreted, provocative discography is a useful tool in the management of patients with low back pain, particularly for those who do not respond to conservative measures.

References

Anderson MW (2004) Lumbar discography: an update. Semin Roentgenol 39:52–67

Anderson SR, Flanagan B (2000) Discography. Curr Rev Pain 4:345–352

Aprill C, Bogduk N (1992) High intensity zone: a diagnostic sign of painful lumbar disc on magnetic resonance imaging. Br J Radiol 65:361–369

Bernard TN Jr (1990) Lumbar discography followed by computed tomography refining the diagnosis of low back pain. Spine 15:690–707

Bernard TN Jr (1994) Using computed tomography/ discography and enhanced magnetic resonance imaging to distinguish between scar tissue and recurrent lumbar disc herniation. Spine 19:2826–2832

Bini W, Yeung AT, Calatayud V et al. (2002) The role of provocative discography in minimally invasive selective endoscopic discectomy. Neurocirugia (Astur) 13:27–31

Block AR, Vanharanta H, Ohnmeiss DD et al. (1996) Discographic pain report: influence of psychological factors. Spine 21:334–338

Bogduk N (1983) The innervation of the lumbar spine. Spine 8:286-293

Bogduk N (1997) Clinical anatomy of the lumbar spine and sacrum, 3rd edn. Churchill Livingstone, New York

Bogduk N, Modic MT (1996) Controversy: lumbar discography. Spine 21:402–404

Braithwaite I, White J, Saifuddin A et al. (1998) Vertebral end-plate (Modic) changes on lumbar spine MRI: correlation with pain reproduction at lumbar discography. Eur Spine J 7:363–368

Brightbill TC, Pile N, Eichelberger RP et al. (1994) Normal magnetic resonance imaging and abnormal discography in lumbar disc disruption. Spine 19:1075–1077

Brodsky AE, Binder WF (1979) Lumbar discography: its value in diagnosis and treatment of lumbar disc lesions. Spine 4:110–120

Buirski G, Silberstein M (1993) The symptomatic lumbar disc in patients with low-back pain: magnetic resonance imaging appearances in both a symptomatic and control population. Spine 18:1808–1811

Carragee EJ, Chen Y, Tanner CM et al. (2000a) Can discography cause long-term back symptoms in previously asymptomatic subjects? Spine 25:1803–1808

Carragee EJ, Chen Y, Tanner CM et al. (2000b) Provocative discography in patients after limited lumbar discectomy: a controlled, randomized study of pain response in symptomatic and asymptomatic subjects. Spine 25:3065–3071

Carragee EJ, Paragioudakis SJ, Khurana S (2000c) 2000 Volvo Award winner in clinical studies: lumbar high-intensity zone and discography in subjects without low back problems. Spine 25:2987–2992

Colhoun E, McCall IW, Williams L et al. (1988) Provocation discography as a guide to planning operations on the spine. J Bone Joint Surg (Br) 70:267–271

Connor PM, Darden BV II (1993) Cervical discography complications and clinical efficacy. Spine 18:2035–2038

Crock HV (1986) Internal disc disruption. Spine 11:650–653

Davis TT, Delamarter RB, Sra P et al. (2004) The IDET procedure for chronic discogenic low back pain. Spine 29:752–756

Derby R, Howard MW, Grant JM et al. (1999) The ability of pressure-controlled discography to predict surgical and nonsurgical outcomes. Spine 24:364–372

Falco FJ, Moran JG (2003) Lumbar discography using gadolinium in patients with iodine contrast allergy followed by postdiscography computed tomography scan. Spine 28:E1–4

Fenton DS, Czervionke LF (2003) Discography. In: Fenton DS, Czervionke LF (eds) Image-guided spine intervention. Saunders, Philadelphia, pp 227–255

Flanagan MN, Chung BU (1986) Roentgenographic changes in 188 patients 10–20 years after discography and chemonucleolysis. Spine 11:444–448

Fraser RD, Osti OL, Vernon-Roberts B (1987) Discitis after discography. J Bone Joint Surg (Br) 69:26–35

Fraser RD, Osti OL, Vernon-Roberts B (1989) Iatrogenic discitis: the role of intravenous antibiotics in prevention and treatment. Spine 14:1025–1032

Gill K, Blumenthal SL (1992) Functional results after anterior lumbar fusion at L5-S1 in patients with normal and abnormal MRI scans. Spine 17:940–942

Grubb SA, Kelly CK (2000) Cervical discography: clinical implications from 12 years of experience. Spine 15:1382–1389

Guarino AH (1999) Discography: a review. Curr Rev Pain 3:473–480

Guyer RD, Ohnmeiss DD (1995) Lumbar discography. Position statement from the North American Spine Society Diagnostic and Therapeutic Committee. Spine 20:2048–2059

Guyer RD, Ohnmeiss DD, NASS (2003) Lumbar discography. Spine J 3:11S–27S

Hirsch C (1948) An attempt to diagnose the level of a disc lesion clinically by disc puncture. Acta Orthop Scand 18:132–140

Hodge JC, Ghelman B, Schneider R et al. (1994) Computed tomography (CT) discography and CT myelography. J Spinal Disord 7:470–477

Horton WC, Daftari TK (1992) Which disc as visualized by magnetic resonance imaging is actually a source of pain? A correlation between magnetic resonance imaging and discography. Spine 17:S164–S171

Huang TS, Zucherman JF, Hsu KY et al. (2002) Gadopentetate dimeglumine as an intradiscal contrast agent. Spine 27:839–843

Ito M, Incorvaia KM, Yu SF et al. (1998) Predictive signs of discogenic lumbar pain on magnetic resonance imaging with discography correlation. Spine 23:1252–1260

Jackson RP, Cain JE Jr, Jacobs RR et al. (1989) The neuroradiographic diagnosis of lumbar herniated nucleus pulposus. A comparison of computed tomography (CT), myelography, CT-myelography, discography, and CT-discography. Spine 14:1356–1361

Johnson RG (1989) Does discography injure normal discs? An analysis of repeat discograms. Spine 14:424–426

Kakitsubata Y, Theodorou DJ, Theodorou SJ et al. (2003) Magnetic resonance discography in cadavers: tears of the annulus fibrosus. Clin Orthop 407:228–240

Khot A, Bowditch M, Powell J et al. (2004) The use of intradiscal steroid therapy for lumbar spinal discogenic pain: a randomized controlled trial. Spine 29:833–837

Kinard RE (1996) Diagnostic spinal injection procedures. Neurosurg Clin North Am 7:151–165

Kitano T, Zerwekh JE, Usui Y et al. (1993) Biochemical changes associated with the symptomatic human intervertebral disk. Clin Orthop 293:372–377

Klein RG, Eek BC, O'Neill CW et al. (2003) Biochemical injection treatment for discogenic low back pain: a pilot study. Spine J 3:220–226

Klessig HT, Showsh SA, Sekorski A (2003) The use of intradiscal antibiotics for discography: an in vitro study of gentamicin, cefazolin, and clindamycin. Spine 28:1735–1738

Kumar N, Agorastides ID (2000) The curved needle technique for accessing the L5/S1 disc space. Br J Radiol 73:655–657

Lam KS, Carlin D, Mulholland RC (2000) Lumbar disc high-intensity zone: the value and significance of provocative discography in the determination of the discogenic pain source. Eur Spine J 9:36–41

Lang R, Saba K, Folman Y et al. (1994) Penetration of ceftriaxone into the intervertebral disc. J Bone Joint Surg (Am) 76:689–691

Lee SH, Derby R, Chen Y et al. (2004) In vitro measurement of pressure in intervertebral discs and annulus fibrosus with and without annular tears during discography. Spine J 4:614–618

Lehmer SM, Dawson MHO, O'Brien JP (1994) Delayed pain response after lumbar discography. Eur Spine J 3:28–31

Lindblom K (1948) Diagnostic puncture of intervertebral disks in sciatica. Acta Orthop Scand 17:213–239

Linson MA, Crowe CH (1990) Comparison of magnetic resonance imaging and lumbar discography in the diagnosis of disc disruption. Clin Orthop 250:160–163

Madan S, Gundanna M, Harley JM et al. (2002) Does provocative discography screening of discogenic back pain improve surgical outcome? J Spinal Discord Tech 15:245–251

Maezawa S, Muro T (1992) Pain provocation at lumbar discography as analyzed by computed tomography/ discography. Spine 17:1309–1315

McCullough JA, Waddell G (1978) Lateral lumbar discography. Br J Radiol 51:498–502

McNally DS, Shackleford IM, Orth E et al. (1996) In vivo stress measurement can predict pain on discography. Spine 21:2580–2587

Milette PC, Fontaine S, Lepanto L et al. (1999) Differentiating lumbar disc protrusions, disc bulges, and discs with normal contour but abnormal signal intensity. Magnetic resonance imaging with discographic correlations. Spine 24:44–53

Min K, Leu HJ, Perrenoud A (1996) Discography with manometry and discographic CT: their value in patient selection for percutaneous lumbar nucleotomy. Bull Hosp Jt Dis 54:153–157

Motimaya A, Arici M, George D et al. (2000) Diagnostic value of cervical discography in the management of cervical discogenic pain. Conn Med 64:395–398

Ohnmeiss DD, Guyer RD, Hochschuler SH (1994) Laser disc compression: the importance of proper patient selection. Spine 19:2054–2059

Ohnmeiss DD, Vanharanta H, Ekholm J (1999) Relation between pain location and disc pathology: a study of pain drawings and CT/discography. Clin J Pain 15:210–217

O'Neill C, Kurgansky M (2004) Subgroups of positive discs on discography. Spine 29:2134–2139

Osti OL, Fraser RD (1992) MRI and discography of annular tears and intervertebral disc degeneration. A prospective clinical comparison. J Bone Joint Surg (Br) 74:431–435

Osti OL, Fraser RD, Vernon-Roberts B (1990) Discitis after discography. The role of prophylactic antibiotics. J Bone Joint Surg (Br) 72:271–274

Parfenchuck TA, Janssen ME (1994) A correlation of cervical magnetic resonance imaging and discography/ computed tomographic discograms. Spine 19:2819–2825

Pauza KJ, Howell S, Dreyfuss P et al. (2004) A randomized, placebo-controlled trial of intradiscal electrothermal therapy for the treatment of discogenic low back pain. Spine J 4:27–35

Peh WCG (2004) Discography. Proceedings of the 23rd International Congress of Radiology. Medimond, Bologna, pp 343–350

Rankine JJ, Gill KP, Hutchinson CE et al. (1999) The clinical significance of the high-intensity zone on lumbar spine magnetic resonance imaging. Spine 24:1913–1920

Reitman CA, Hipp JA, Kirking BC et al. (2001) Posterior annular strains during discography. J Spinal Disord 14:347–352

Rhyne AL III, Smith SE, Wood KE et al. (1995) Outcome of unoperated discogram-positive low back pain. Spine 20:1997–2001

Saal JS (1989) High levels of phospholipase A2 activity in lumbar disc herniation. Spine 15:674–678

Saal JA, Saal JS (2000) Intradiscal electrothermal treatment for chronic discogenic low back pain: a prospective outcome study with minimum 1-year follow-up. Spine 25:2622–2627

Sachs BL, Vanharanta H, Spivey MA et al. (1987) Dallas discogram description: a new classification of CT discography in low-back disorders. Spine 12:287–294

Sachs BL, Spivey MA, Vanharanta H et al. (1990) Techniques for lumbar discography and computed tomography/ discography in clinical practice. Orthop Rev 19:775–778

Saifuddin A, Emanuel R, White J et al. (1998a) An analysis of radiating pain at lumbar discography. Eur Spine J 7:358–362

Saifuddin A, Renton P, Taylor BA (1998b) Effects on the vertebral end-plate of uncomplicated lumbar discography: an MRI study. Eur Spine J 7:36–39

Sandhu HS, Sanchez-Caso LP, Parvataneni HK et al. (2000) Association between findings of provocative discography and vertebral endplate signal changes on MRI. J Spinal Disord 13:438–443

Schellhas KP, Pollei SR, Gundry CR et al. (1996) Lumbar disc high-intensity zone: correlation of magnetic resonance imaging and discography. Spine 21:79–86

Sequeiros RB, Klemola R, Ojala R et al. (2003) Percutaneous MR-guided discography in a low-field system using optical instrument tracking: a feasibility study. J Magn Reson Imaging 17:214–219

Simmons EH, Segil CM (1975) An evaluation of discography in the localization of symptomatic levels in discogenic disease of the spine. Clin Orthop 108:57–69

Simmons JW, Emery SF, McMillin JN et al. (1991) Awake discography: a comparison study with magnetic resonance imaging. Spine 16:S216–221

Slipman CW, Rogers DP, Issac Z et al. (2002) MR lumbar discography with intradiscal gadolinium in patients with severe anaphylactoid reaction to iodinated contrast material. Pain Med 3:23–29

Smith GW, Nichols P (1957) The technique of cervical discography. Radiology 68:718–720

Smith L, Brown JE (1967) Treatment of lumbar disc lesions by direct injection of chymopapain. J Bone Joint Surg (Br) 49:502–519

Smith SE, Darden BV, Rhyne AL et al. (1995) Outcome of unoperated discogram-positive low back pain. Spine 20:1997–2000

Smith BM, Hurwitz EL, Solsberg D et al. (1998) Interobserver reliability of detecting lumbar intervertebral disc high-intensity zone on magnetic resonance imaging and association of high-intensity zone with pain and anular disruption. Spine 23:2074–2080

Southern EP, Fye MA, Panjabi MM et al. (2000) Disc degeneration: a human cadaveric study correlating magnetic resonance imaging and quantitative discomanometry. Spine 25:2171–2175

Tehranzadeh J (1998) Discography 2000. Radiol Clin North Am 36:463–495

Troisier O (1982) Technic of extradural diskography. J Radiol 63:571–578

Vanharanta H, Sachs BL, Spivey MA et al. (1987) The relationship of pain provocation to lumbar disc deterioration as seen by CT/discography. Spine 12:295–298

Vivitmongkonchai K, Peh WCG (2001) Provocative lumbar discography: current status. SGH Proc 10:302–309

Walsh TR, Weinstein JN, Spratt KF et al. (1990) Lumbar discography in normal subjects. A controlled prospective study. J Bone Joint Surg (Am) 72:1081–1088

Weishaupt D, Zanetti M, Hodler J et al. (2001) Painful lumbar disk derangement: Relevance of endplate abnormalities at MR imaging. Radiology 218:420–427

Wetzel FT, McNally TA, Phillips FM (2002) Intradiscal electrothermal therapy used to manage chronic discogenic low back pain: new directions and interventions. Spine 27:2621–2626

Wiley JJ, MacNab I, Wortzman G (1968) Lumbar discography and its clinical applications. Can J Surg 11:280–289

Willems PC, Jacobs W, Duinkerke ES et al. (2004) Lumbar discography: should we use prophylactic antibiotics? Study of 435 consecutive discograms and a systemic review of the literature. J Spinal Disord Tech 17:243–247

Winter RB, Schellhas KP (1996) Painful adult thoracic Scheuermann's disease: diagnosis by discography and treatment by combined arthrodesis. Am J Orthop 25:783–786

Wood KB, Schellhas KP, Garvey TA et al. (1999) Thoracic discography in healthy individuals. A controlled prospective study of magnetic resonance imaging and discography in asymptomatic and symptomatic individuals. Spine 24:1548–1555

Yoshida H, Fujiwara A, Tamai K et al. (2002) Diagnosis of symptomatic disc by magnetic resonance imaging: T2-weighted and gadolinium-DTPA-enhanced T1-weighted magnetic resonance imaging. J Spinal Disord Tech 15:193–198

Zeidman SM, Thompson L, Ducker TB (1995) Complications of cervical discography: analysis of 4400 diagnostic disc injections. Neurosurgery 37:414–417

Zheng Y, Liew SM, Simmons ED (2004) Value of magnetic resonance imaging and discography in determining the level of cervical discectomy and fusion. Spine 29:2140-2146

Percutaneous Joint Injections

Kathleen C. Finzel and Ronald S. Adler

CONTENTS

8.1   Introduction   143

8.2   Procedures Performed Under
        Fluoroscopic Guidance   143
8.2.1   Shoulder Injection   143
8.2.2   Hip Injection   145
8.2.3   Ankle/Foot Injection   146
8.2.4   Wrist Injection   148

8.3   Utility of Ultrasound   149
8.3.1   Technical Considerations   149
8.3.2   Injection of Joints   151

8.4   Therapeutic Joint Injections
        Performed Under CT Guidance   155

8.5   Conclusion   156

        References   156

8.1
Introduction

Image-guided diagnostic and/or therapeutic joint injections may be performed under fluoroscopic, CT or ultrasound guidance. In general, we find fluoroscopy or ultrasound to be more efficient than CT for the majority of joint procedures. The choice of imaging modality may depend on equipment availability or the expertise of the physician performing the procedure. Procedures performed on joints that have been significantly altered by previous trauma or prior surgery are more easily performed under fluoroscopy.

8.2
Procedures Performed Under Fluoroscopic Guidance

While contrast arthrography is less commonly performed now than in the past, it remains useful in the diagnosis of joint disorders. This is particularly true where MR imaging is not readily available. Fluoroscopically guided therapeutic injections of multiple joints are commonly performed at our institution. Evaluation for prosthetic loosening or the presence of joint infection remains a common reason for performing contrast arthrography in the hip. The popularity of MR arthrography of the shoulder and hip with many referring physicians is an additional reason one should know how to inject these joints.

8.2.1
Shoulder Injection

Shoulder arthrography is most often performed in preparation for an MR arthrogram in patients with suspected labral tears, and occasionally in patients with suspected rotator cuff tears who are unable to undergo MR imaging for some reason, usually due to the presence of a pacemaker. When performing shoulder arthrography, we most commonly use the anterior approach advocated by SCHNEIDER et al. (1975). The patient is supine on the radiography table, with the designated shoulder closest to the physician. The shoulder is placed in a neutral position, with the arm at the side and the thumb up. A slightly more tangential view of the joint may be obtained by

K. C. FINZEL, MD
Director, Diagnostic Imaging, ProHealth Care Associates, 2800 Marcus Avenue, Lake Success, NY 11042, USA
R. S. ADLER, MD, PhD
Professor of Radiology, Weill Medical College of Cornell University, Attending Radiologist, Chief, Division of Ultrasound and Body Imaging, Hospital for Special Surgery, 535 East 70th Street, New York, NY 10021, USA

placing a small amount of padding under the contralateral shoulder. However, if the glenohumeral joint is completely tangential, the fibrocartilaginous labrum may obstruct the needle path into the joint. A mark is placed on the skin at the level of the junction of the middle third of the glenoid with the inferior third overlying the space between the glenoid and the humeral head. After sterile preparation of the area and the use of local anesthesia, a 3.5-in. 22-gauge spinal needle is inserted vertically until it intercepts bone. At this point, the needle position may be checked fluoroscopically and the needle repositioned if it has strayed from the targeted site. When the needle tip is intra-articular, a test injection of contrast flows rapidly away from the needle, usually forming a thin crescentic line outlining the medial margin of the humeral head (Fig. 8.1). With an extra-articular position of the needle, contrast will pool around the needle tip.

If a conventional double contrast arthrogram is being performed, 4 ml of contrast can be injected into the joint, followed by 10 to 12 ml of room air. The patient is then imaged in an upright position usually before and after mild exercise of the joint. The presence of contrast and air immediately inferior to the acromion indicates a complete cuff tear, allowing the injected intra-articular contrast and air to enter the subacromial/subdeltoid bursa. The site of the tear cannot always be clearly visualized. In the presence of adhesive capsulitis, increased pressure is encountered when attempting to inject contrast, as well as diminished joint capacity. Sometimes, the injected contrast will bubble out of the hub of the needle due to the increased intra-articular pressure.

Therapeutic injection of the shoulder for adhesive capsulitis may be performed by injecting steroids to decrease inflammation and/or volume to lyse adhesions.

If the shoulder arthrogram is being performed for MR arthrography, 1 ml of iodinated contrast is injected to ensure the intra-articular position of the needle tip. Then, 10 to 14 ml of a 1:100 or 1:200 dilution of an MR contrast agent is injected into the joint. The patient is then escorted from the fluoroscopy suite to the MR suite. If a significant delay in MR scanning is anticipated, 1 ml of 1:1,000 epinephrine may be added to the contrast solution to delay joint resorption.

An alternative to this approach to the shoulder is the posterior approach (Farmer and Hughes 2002) or a modified anterior approach targeting the rotator interval as advocated by Depelteau et al. (2004). The rotator interval is a triangular space at the superomedial aspect of the humeral head created by the perforation of the anterosuperior part of the cuff by the coracoid process. This space is located between the supraspinatus and subscapularis tendons. The superior glenohumeral ligament and the long head of the biceps are located within the interval. Using this technique, patients are posi-

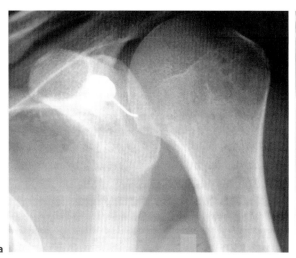 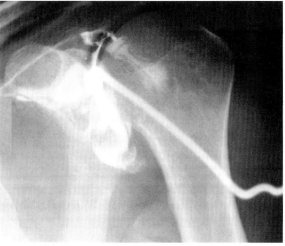

a   b

Fig. 8.1a,b. Anterior approach to shoulder arthrography in a 42-year-old man with limited range of motion of the left shoulder. With this approach, the shoulder is in a neutral position, with the arm at the side and the thumb directed up. **a** Anteroposterior radiograph shows the chosen site at the junction of the middle and inferior thirds of the glenoid. **b** Anteroposterior arthrogram shows how injected contrast initially forms a crescent along the humeral head. In this example, the axillary recess and subcoracoid recess of the joint are outlined by contrast

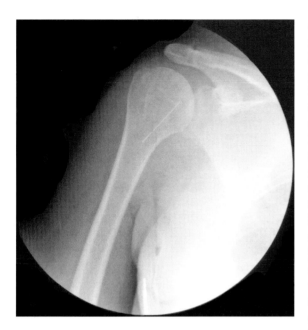

Fig. 8.2. Modified anterior approach to shoulder joint injection in a 38-year-old woman with shoulder pain after a sports injury. Anteroposterior radiograph shows the shoulder is externally rotated and the needle advanced vertically to intercept the superior medial aspect of the humeral head

tioned supine, with the arm externally rotated (palm up) to avoid the long head of the biceps tendon. The skin is marked over the upper medial quadrant of the humeral head just lateral to the joint line. After sterile preparation and administration of local anesthetic, a 1.5-in. 22-gauge needle can be used to enter the joint by advancing the tip to the humeral head. The shorter 1.5-in. needle can be used with this approach because the joint is more superficial than inferior at the level of the rotator interval (Fig. 8.2). Possible distortion of the inferior glenohumeral ligament and anteroinferior labrum with the anterior approach is avoided with the modified anterior approach targeting the rotator interval.

At our institution an anterior or modified anterior approach is used when accessing the shoulder joint via fluoroscopic guidance.

8.2.2
Hip Injection

For hip aspiration or arthrography the patient is positioned supine on the radiography table. A small cushion placed under the knee is useful for the patient's comfort, and relaxes the joint capsule. A sand bag may be placed along the outer border of the foot,

or the feet may be taped together to prevent external rotation of the femur. External rotation causes lateral displacement of the femoral vessels, which places them in jeopardy of accidental puncture during needle placement. The position of the femoral artery should be identified by palpating the pulse and the position marked to avoid needle puncture. If there is excessive abdominal pannus, the patient may be asked to manually lift it out of the way or it may be taped. Using fluoroscopy, the skin is marked at the level of the proximal femoral neck slightly to the medial side. After sterile preparation and draping, and infiltration of the area with local anesthetic, a 3.5-in. 22-gauge spinal needle is inserted into the joint. This may be done in a number of ways. In a native hip, the needle may be inserted vertically until it contacts the femoral neck (Fig. 8.3). However, a more inferior and lateral skin entry point with slanting of the needle superiorly and medially may be needed to avoid the femoral vessels and nerve. This approach may be required in patients with hip arthroplasty (Fig. 8.4). The needle is directed toward the proximal femoral neck and advanced until the tip intercepts bone. When the needle encounters the femoral neck, aspiration of synovial fluid can be attempted. If only a small amount of fluid is present, it

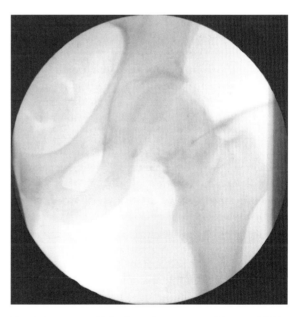

Fig. 8.3. Suspected labral tear in a 40-year-old man with hip pain. A vertical needle approach targeted the center of the femoral neck in this native hip. Anteroposterior radiograph of the left hip demonstrates how contrast outlines the joint with a smooth synovial lining. Therapeutic injection was performed with relief of hip pain

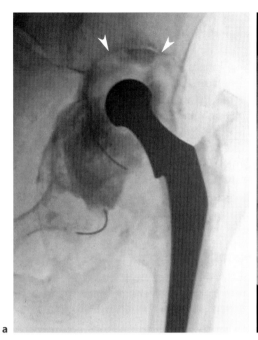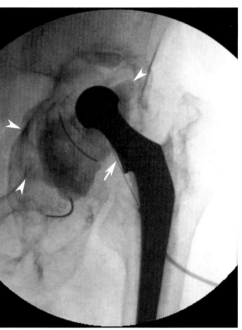

Fig. 8.4a,b. Left hip pain in a 76-year-old man many years postarthroplasty. **a** Anteroposterior radio-graph of the left hip joint shows both the radiolucent acetabular component (*arrowheads*) and the femoral stem have migrated proximally. **b** Arthrocentesis was performed to exclude infection prior to revision arthroplasty using an oblique approach. The needle was directed superomedially from the skin entrance site after palpating the femoral pulse. The needle (*arrow*) is lateral to the femoral vessels. Contrast is now visualized within the pseudocapsule (*arrowheads*)

may lie in a recess at the very medial margin of the femoral neck. The needle tip may be "walked" along the neck to the medial edge until successful aspiration of fluid for Gram stain, culture and sensitivity is accomplished. In the presence of a prosthesis, the needle tip may be more difficult to visualize fluoro-scopically, but it is directed to the medial aspect of the metallic femoral neck near its junction with the prosthetic head. If a test injection of contrast con-firms the intra-articular location of the needle tip by showing the injected contrast flowing across the femoral neck, but no synovial fluid can be aspirated, the joint can be lavaged. Lavage may be with either 10 ml of sterile saline or contrast, and the return aspirate sent for culture.

Injection of iodinated contrast, with a volume of up to 15 ml, may be performed through sterile tubing so it can be viewed fluoroscopically. When evaluat-ing for prosthetic loosening, very careful compari-son must be made between preliminary radiographs and those obtained after contrast administration. The entire prosthesis must be included in the postin-jection radiographs. The presence of a small amount of contrast at the bone-cement interface along the femoral stem or acetabular cup can be very subtle.

Digital subtraction fluoroscopy can make any subtle insinuation of contrast along the prosthesis or at the bone-cement interface more conspicuous.

To perform MR arthrography of the hip, a small amount of iodinated contrast is used to confirm the intra-articular position of the needle tip before injecting 15 ml of a 1:100 dilution of MR contrast agent.

Therapeutic injection of the hip is usually per-formed with 80 mg of Depo-Medrol (Pharmacia & Upjohn, Kalamazoo, MI, USA) and 5 ml 0.5% bupi-vacaine.

8.2.3
Ankle/Foot Injection

In our practice, requests for interventions involving the ankle joint are substantially less frequent than for the subtalar joint or the midfoot.

Inserting a needle into a nonarthritic ankle joint is straightforward. It is most easily accomplished by placing the patient on his or her side with the af-fected ankle on the tabletop. Overhead fluoroscopy produces a lateral view of the ankle. The joint is entered at its anterior margin. The dorsalis pedis pulse is palpated and its location marked on the skin to avoid injury. After sterile preparation of the field, and use of local anesthetic, a 22-gauge needle is inserted through the skin just below the joint. The needle is directed slightly cephalad and is advanced just underneath the anterior lip of the tibia into the joint (Fig. 8.5). When the needle tip is intra-articular, injection of contrast produces a thin band outlining the talar dome, or the contrast can be seen outlining the posterior recess of the joint (RUHOY et al. 1998).

Therapeutic injection of the posterior subtalar joint is more challenging than ankle joint injection. Pain originating in the posterior subtalar joint can be difficult to localize. Therefore, pain relief after therapeutic injection can be a valuable diagnostic tool implicating the joint as the pain source. The approach to the joint may be either posteromedial or anterolateral. When using the anterolateral approach, the patient lays on the opposite side, with the desired foot medial side down. The X-ray beam is angled cephalad until the anterior margin of the subtalar joint is parallel to the beam. A 22-gauge needle is then directed toward the anterior margin of the posterior subtalar joint space. If the anterior margin cannot be clearly seen, the needle tip may be directed toward the crucial angle of Gissane. This angle is formed at the intersection of the anterior

margin of the posterior subtalar joint and the body of the calcaneus. If needle placement is successful, injected contrast may outline both the joint and the posterior recess of the ankle joint, as this is a normal communication present in some patients.

In some patients, it is difficult to guide the needle tip past the fibula into the posterior subtalar joint. Therefore, it is also useful to know the posteromedial approach to the joint. For the posteromedial approach, the patient lies on the affected side with the lateral side of the foot down. The X-ray beam is tilted cephalad until the very posterior margin of the posterior subtalar joint is seen in profile. The location of the posterior tibial artery is identified by palpation. Its site is marked. After sterile preparation, a 22-gauge needle may be directed into the posterior margin of the posterior subtalar joint through a skin entry site 1 cm posteroinferior to the mark identifying the posterior tibial artery (Fig. 8.6). It is not uncommon when using the posteromedial approach to opacify one or more of the flexor tendon sheaths with a test injection of contrast. Since anesthetic or steroid injection into these structures may not be desirable, we more commonly use the anterolateral approach.

Midfoot injections are generally straightforward, with adjustments for any alterations in anatomy produced by trauma and/or arthrosis (Fig. 8.7).

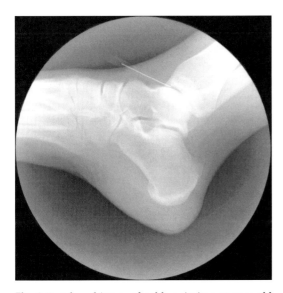

Fig. 8.5. A long history of ankle pain in a 52-year-old man who was referred for therapeutic injection. Lateral radiograph shows the ankle joint is entered through an anterior approach, with the needle passing just under the anterior lip of the tibia, usually just medial to midline to avoid the dorsalis pedis

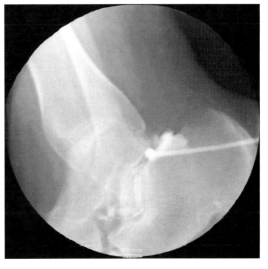

Fig. 8.6. Subtalar arthrosis following trauma in a 50-year-old man. Therapeutic injection was requested. Lateral radiograph demonstrates the use of the posteromedial approach to the subtalar joint. The X-ray tube is angled until the posterior facet of the joint is seen in profile and the needle tip is directed into the posterior margin

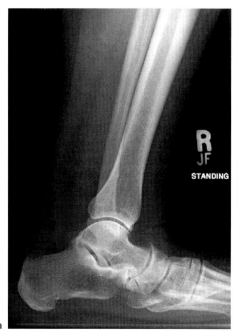

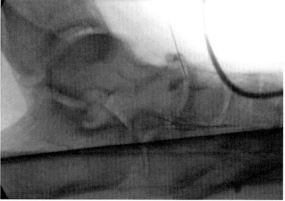

Fig. 8.7a,b. Severe talonavicular arthrosis in a 34-year-old woman. **a** Lateral radiograph of the right ankle shows a large dorsal osteophyte of the navicular bone. Therapeutic injection was performed with anteroposterior and (**b**) lateral fluoroscopy to guide the needle past the osteophyte. Depo-Medrol (40 mg) and bupivacaine 0.5% (2 ml) were injected into the joint after contrast injection confirmed the intra-articular position of the needle tip

8.2.4
Wrist Injection

Therapeutic wrist injections and wrist arthrography are rarely performed at our institution. To perform wrist arthrography, the patient is normally seated at the end of the fluoroscopy table, with the arm extended and the wrist flexed over a rolled towel. The chair on which the patient is seated must not be on rollers, as this circumvents the entire principle of providing a stable environment for the patient. If the patient raises any concern regarding a vasovagal reaction, it is important to take heed. In this case, it is better to position the patient prone on the fluoroscopy table with the arm extended overhead. A sterile field is created. Local anesthetic is provided with 1% lidocaine. The radial-carpal joint is entered at a point approximately 1 cm radial to the scapholunate interval. A 23- or 25-gauge needle is vertically directed into the space between the scaphoid and the distal radial articular surface, with the wrist held in flexion to maximize the size of this space. Contrast is injected under direct fluoroscopic visualization. It can be very helpful to use videofluoroscopy. If the contrast escapes from the radial-carpal joint into the midcarpal joint, the site of entry must be identified. This can occur very quickly, and it may be helpful to review the video to identify whether the contrast escaped through the torn scapholunate ligament or through the lunate-triquetral ligament. The radial-

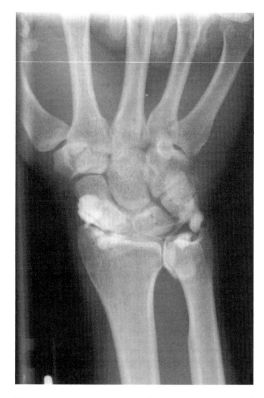

Fig. 8.8. Wrist arthrography in a 32-year-old woman. This waitress had severe ulnar sided wrist pain that impaired her ability to perform her job. Anteroposterior radial-carpal joint arthrography view demonstrates contrast extending into the distal radial-ulnar joint, indicating a tear of the triangulofibrocartilage

carpal joint is of small capacity, and only 2–4 ml of contrast are necessary to fill the joint. If the contrast remains in the radial-carpal joint during contrast injection, the needle is quickly removed. Again during direct fluoroscopic visualization, the wrist is put through a range of maneuvers, including radial and ulnar deviation to evaluate the integrity of the ligaments (Fig. 8. 8).

8.3
Utility of Ultrasound

The real-time nature of ultrasound makes it ideally suited to provide guidance for therapeutic delivery of corticosteroids and local anesthesia. A number of publications have illustrated the efficacy of this method for musculoskeletal interventional procedures (Adler and Allen 2004; Adler and Sofka 2003; Brophy et al. 1995; Cardinal et al. 1998; Grassi et al. 2001; Koski 2000; Sofka et al. 2001). Its real-time nature also allows continuous observation of needle position, thereby ensuring proper placement and providing continuous monitoring of the distribution of the therapeutic agent.

The current generation of high frequency small parts transducers further allows excellent depiction of the articular surfaces, particularly the small joints of the hand and foot. For this reason, needle placement in nonfluid distended structures, such as a nondistended joint, can be performed. Ultrasound guidance has broad appeal because it does not use ionizing radiation; this feature is particularly advantageous with the pediatric population and pregnant women.

Following a discussion of ultrasound technique, ultrasound-guided injections will be reviewed, with particular attention paid to the most commonly requested joint injections performed at our institution, which is an orthopedic and rheumatology specialty hospital. The most common clinical indication for ultrasound-guided injections is pain without response to other conservative measures, regardless of the anatomic site. This may occur as the result of a chronic repetitive injury from work, a sports-related injury, or from an underlying inflammatory disorder, such as rheumatoid arthritis. This chapter will concentrate on illustrative examples of several of the studies performed in the authors' practice, without dwelling on the specific clinical entities.

8.3.1
Technical Considerations

Diagnostic and subsequent interventional examinations are performed using either linear or curved phased array transducers, depending on depth and local geometry. Needle selection is based on specific anatomic conditions (i.e., depth and size of the region of interest). We employ a free hand technique in which the specular reflection of the needle is used to provide needle visualization (Fig. 8.9) (Sofka et al. 2001). The needle must be oriented so that it is perpendicular (or nearly so) to the insonating beam, and it then becomes a specular reflector, often having a strong ring-down artifact. While needle guides are available and may be of value, we have found that a free hand technique allows greater flexibility for adjusting the position of the needle during a procedure. Needle visualization can also be enhanced by injecting a small amount of anesthetic while observing in real-time.

Patient positioning to ensure comfort and optimal visualization of the anatomy should be assessed first. An offset may be required at the skin entry point of the needle relative to the transducer to allow for the appropriate needle orientation. Deep structures, such as the hip, are often better imaged using a curved linear or sector transducer, operating at center frequencies of approximately 3.5–7.5 MHz. Superficial, linearly oriented structures, such as in the wrist or ankle, are best approached using a linear array transducer with center frequencies from

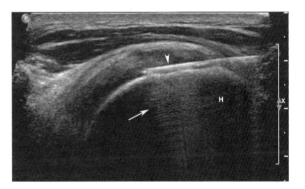

Fig. 8.9. Glenohumeral joint injection of the right shoulder in a 45-year-old woman with clinical symptoms of adhesive capsulitis. Ultrasound image shows a needle (*arrowhead*) placed into the posterior recess of the glenohumeral joint indicating the characteristic metallic ring-down artifact (*arrow*). This can often be made more conspicuous during injection with a small amount of local anesthetic vis à vis the introduction of microbubbles. Humerus (*H*)

7.5 to 17 MHz or higher. These factors should be assessed prior to skin preparation.

Once the transducer is properly positioned, the degree of joint distension can be assessed, as well as the needle position. When positioning the needle into a distended joint, the presence of an effusion and/or synovium often provides a contrasting background to better visualize the needle tip (Fig. 8.10). Alternatively, when injecting into a nonfluid distended structure, a test injection with local anesthetic often permits improved visualization of the needle tip by introducing microbubbles, as well as providing some fluid distension of the joint capsule (Fig. 8.11). The immiscible nature of the steroid anesthetic mixture may likewise produce a temporary contrast effect (Fig. 8.12).

The area in question is cleaned with iodine-based solution, and draped with a sterile drape. The transducer is immersed into an iodine-based solution and

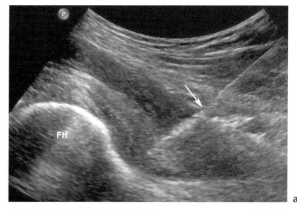

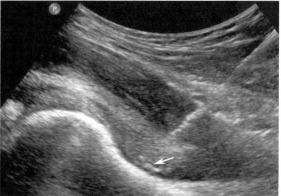

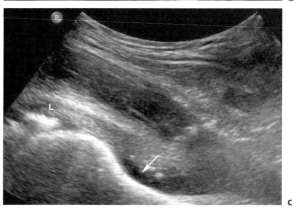

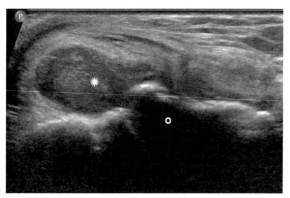

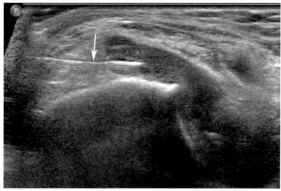

Fig. 8.10a,b. Left elbow joint injection in a 57-year-old woman with rheumatoid arthritis. **a** Transverse ultrasound image of the posterolateral recess shows portions of the olecranon (*O*) and the distended posterior capsule (*star*), which contains inflammatory pannus. The presence of a distended joint capsule significantly simplifies intra-articular injection of a steroid-anesthetic mixture. **b** A 25-gauge needle (*arrow*) is placed into the distended capsule under ultrasound guidance, and the therapeutic mixture is successfully injected

Fig. 8.11a–c. Hip pain and labral tear diagnosed on MR imaging in a 37-year-old woman. She was referred for therapeutic/diagnostic hip injection. **a** Hip injections may be performed using an intermediate frequency transducer operating with a curved linear or sector geometry. The needle (*arrow*) is directed toward the femoral neck, as shown. The femoral head (*FH*) is labeled. **b** The needle tip, which may not be conspicuous, can be enhanced following injection of a small amount of 1% lidocaine. The presence of microbubbles (*arrow*) below the joint capsule confirms appropriate needle placement. The injection is then performed, while observing in real-time. **c** Following needle removal, there is distension of the anterior capsule by hypoechoic fluid, with a few scattered bubbles along its nondependent surface (*arrow*). The acetabular labrum (*L*) has also become more conspicuous due to the presence of bubble redistribution

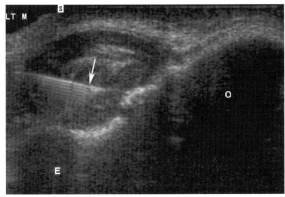

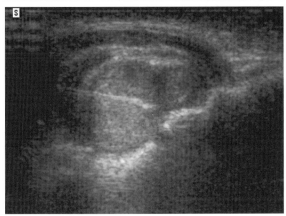

Fig. 8.12a,b. Long-standing rheumatoid arthritis and chronic elbow pain in a 40-year-old woman who was referred for therapeutic injection. **a** Ultrasound guided elbow injection in a patient with rheumatoid arthritis shows a distended posterior recess into which a needle (*arrow*) has been placed. This provides a simple method to ensure intra-articular injection without having to negotiate the joint proper. The olecranon (*O*) and epicondyle (*E*) are labeled. **b** During injection of the steroid-anesthetic mixture, the contrast effect of the suspension increases the overall echogenicity of the posterior recess. In real-time observation, material can usually be seen directly entering the joint proper. The contrast effect provides additional confirmation of the appropriate distribution of the injected material

surrounded by a sterile drape. A drape is also placed over portions of the ultrasound unit. A sonologist or radiologist positions the transducer, while a radiologist positions the needle and performs the procedure. We use 1% lidocaine (Abbot Laboratories, North Chicago, IL, USA) for local anesthesia. Once the needle is in position, the procedure is performed while imaging in real-time. Depending on anatomic location, either a 1.5-in. or spinal needle with a stylet is used to administer the anesthesia/corticosteroid mixture.

8.3.2
Injection of Joints

In general, either a high or medium frequency linear transducer is used for hand, wrist, elbow, foot and ankle injections. A longitudinal (across the joint) or a short axis (in the plane of the joint) approach can be used; however, a short axis approach is often technically easier for small joint injections (ADLER and SOFKA 2003). The needle should enter the skin parallel to the long axis of the transducer.

Superficial joints usually appear as separations between the normally continuous specular echoes produced by cortical surfaces (Fig. 8.13). As is true in other fluid-containing structures, the presence of an effusion is a helpful feature in visualizing the needle as it enters the joint, in as much as it provides a fluid stand-off. The short axis approach entails scanning across the joint and looking for the transition from one cortical surface to the next, marking the skin (with a surgical marker) and then placing a needle into the joint using ultrasound guidance (Figs. 8.10–8.15). It is helpful to rotate the transducer 90° degrees to a long axis view to confirm needle placement between the margins of the two bones.

Injection of a small amount of 1% lidocaine should display distension of the joint, as well as echoes filling the joint capsule. Small joint injections generally require 0.5 to 1 ml of the therapeutic mixture. In our experience, this approach works well in the great toe, midfoot, ankle and elbow. Occasionally, a long axis approach may be efficacious, as in the radiocarpal joint and lateral gutter of the ankle (Fig. 8.16). As is evident in some of the examples presented, ultrasound guidance allows one to negotiate osteophytes and joint bodies (Fig. 8.15). It allows identification of capsular out-pouching, thereby affording a more convenient indirect approach into a joint than slipping a needle into a small joint space.

We usually employ a long axis approach and a spinal needle when performing injections of larger, deeper joints such as the shoulder or hip (Figs. 8.9, 8.11, 8.17) (ADLER and ALLEN 2004; ADLER and SOFKA 2003). A larger volume is usually injected: between 2 and 4 ml of the steroid/anesthetic mixture. In the case of adhesive capsulitis, significantly larger volumes of local anesthetic (5–10 ml) may be added to provide additional joint distension.

We generally approach the glenohumeral joint using a posterior approach, with the patient in a decubitus position and the arm placed in cross adduc-

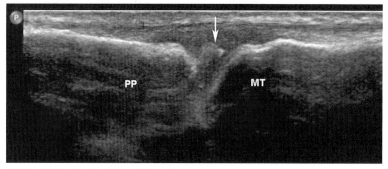

a

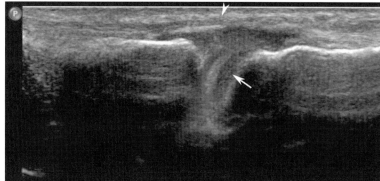

b

Fig. 8.13a,b. Left second MTP joint pain in a 42-year-old man referred for therapeutic injection. **a** Ultrasound image shows a needle (*arrow*) in cross-section as a punctate echogenic focus within this clinically inflamed joint. Distension of the dorsal recess is evident by abnormal soft tissue. In this image it is difficult to readily distinguish the joint capsule from the synovial proliferation. The proximal phalanx (*PP*) and metatarsal (*MT*) are labeled. **b** Following injection and needle removal, there is greater distension of the dorsal recess (*arrowhead*). The contrast effect of the injected material outlines the articular cartilage (*arrow*) of the second metatarsal head

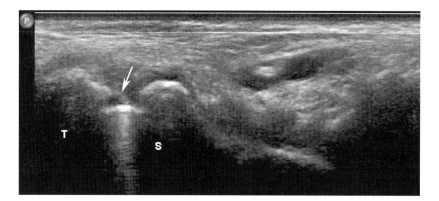

Fig. 8.14. Scaphotrapezial joint injection in a 50-year-old woman with left wrist pain. Longitudinal ultrasound image of the scaphoid (*S*) and trapezium (*T*) articulation obtained during joint injection. A bright central reflector within the joint (*arrow*) shows a 25-gauge needle in cross-section (short axis approach). The strong ring-down artifact confirms needle position. This can be further accentuated with a small test injection of 1% lidocaine. Fine adjustments in needle position are best made in this view when injecting small joints of the hand and feet. The scaphoid (*S*) and trapezium (*T*) are labeled

tion (ADLER and ALLEN 2004). An intermediate frequency linear transducer will suffice in the majority of cases, particularly if the transducer can display in a sector format. A linear transducer often results in better anatomic detail than curved arrays. The interface of the glenohumeral joint is usually seen with the patient in this position, as well as the hy-poechoic articular cartilage overlying the humeral head. We perform this injection using a long axis approach, with the needle directed toward the joint along the articular cartilage. A test injection with 1% lidocaine should show bright echoes filling the posterior recess, or distributed along the articular cartilage (Figs. 8.9, 8.17).

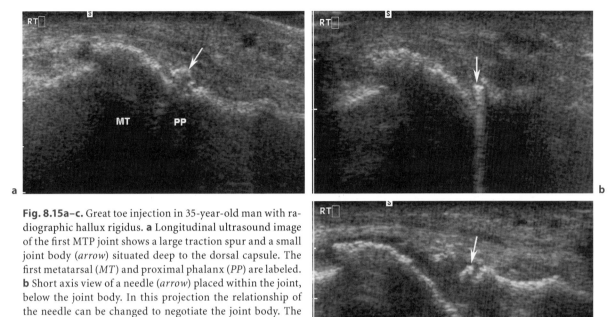

Fig. 8.15a–c. Great toe injection in 35-year-old man with radiographic hallux rigidus. **a** Longitudinal ultrasound image of the first MTP joint shows a large traction spur and a small joint body (*arrow*) situated deep to the dorsal capsule. The first metatarsal (*MT*) and proximal phalanx (*PP*) are labeled. **b** Short axis view of a needle (*arrow*) placed within the joint, below the joint body. In this projection the relationship of the needle can be changed to negotiate the joint body. The needle displays a characteristic ring-down artifact. **c** During the injection, the joint is distended by fluid containing low level echoes, and the joint body (*arrow*) floats to the nondependent surface. The ring-down from the needle becomes less conspicuous

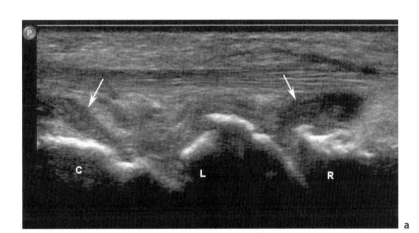

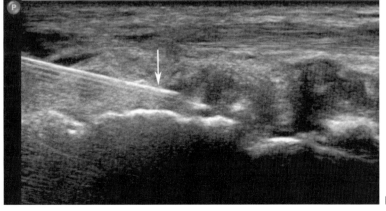

Fig. 8.16a,b. Wrist injection in a 75-year-old man with a painful swollen left wrist and suspected CPPD. **a** Longitudinal ultrasound image of the dorsal aspect of the radiolunocapitate joint (*CLR*) in a patient with pseudogout. Irregularity of the dorsal margins of the visualized radius and carpus are evident. There is distension of the proximal and midcarpal dorsal recesses by complex soft tissue (*arrows*). **b** With the wrist in mild palmar flexion, a 25-gauge needle (*arrow*) is positioned into the dorsal recess of the joint for therapeutic injection

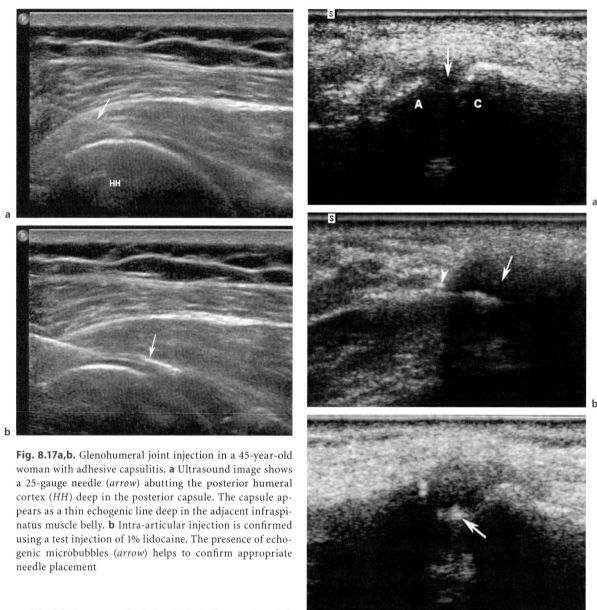

Fig. 8.17a,b. Glenohumeral joint injection in a 45-year-old woman with adhesive capsulitis. **a** Ultrasound image shows a 25-gauge needle (*arrow*) abutting the posterior humeral cortex (*HH*) deep in the posterior capsule. The capsule appears as a thin echogenic line deep in the adjacent infraspinatus muscle belly. **b** Intra-articular injection is confirmed using a test injection of 1% lidocaine. The presence of echogenic microbubbles (*arrow*) helps to confirm appropriate needle placement

Fig. 8.18a–c. Acromioclavicular joint injection in a 50-year-old man with shoulder pain localized to the acromioclavicular joint. **a** Longitudinal ultrasound image across the acromioclavicular joint (*AC*) in a patient for whom therapeutic injection was requested. A thin hypoechoic joint is apparent between the ends of the clavicle and acromion (*arrow*). **b** Turning the transducer 90° and observing in real-time, a needle (*arrowhead*) is positioned in the hypoechoic joint (*arrow*). **c** During the injection, the joint is best observed with the needle seen in cross-section (short axis approach). The needle (*arrow*) displays a characteristic ring-down artifact. The joint can be observed to expand in real-time with the appearance of a contrast effect from the injected material

The hip is approached similarly, in long axis, with the transducer placed anteriorly over the proximal thigh at the level of the joint (Fig. 8.11) (ADLER and SOFKA 2003). The approach is similar to that used in evaluating the joint for an effusion. Ideally, the anterior capsule is imaged at the head-neck junction of the femur. In this plane, the scan plane is lateral to the neurovascular bundle. The needle may be directed into the joint while maintaining its position in the scan plane of the transducer. A test injection of 1% lidocaine confirms the intra-articular needle position, and the therapeutic injection follows.

Finally, fibrous joints, such as the acromioclavicular joint, can likewise be injected using ultrasound guidance (Fig. 8.18) (ADLER and ALLEN 2004).

A short axis technique is employed similar to that used in the foot. The majority of these injections can be performed using a 1.5-in. needle with a small volume (0.5–1 ml) of therapeutic mixture. In addition to the acromioclavicular joint, this approach is useful in the sternoclavicular joint and pubic symphysis.

8.4
Therapeutic Joint Injections Performed Under CT Guidance

At our institution, we have only one CT scanner and it is in great demand. Therapeutic joint injections are almost always performed under fluoroscopic or ultrasound guidance. However, sacroiliac joint injections and facet injections in the spine are still sometimes performed under CT guidance. This is related to both the practitioner's choice and the rapidity with which these two procedures can usually be performed with CT guidance.

In each case, the patient is placed prone on the scanner table. After obtaining scout topograms,

5 mm contiguous axial images are obtained through the lower half of the sacroiliac joints in the case of sacroiliac joint injections. The route of needle placement is planned from these preliminary images. A 22-gauge 6-in. spinal needle is directed into the sacroiliac joint using a vertical approach. Local anesthetic is used very sparingly. Adjustments to needle placement are made as needed. Once proper needle position is confirmed, Depo-Medrol (40 mg) and bupivacaine 0.5% are injected (Fig. 8.19).

Facet joint injections in the lumbar spine are performed with the patient prone. After preliminary images are obtained through the level of interest,

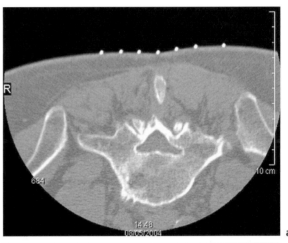
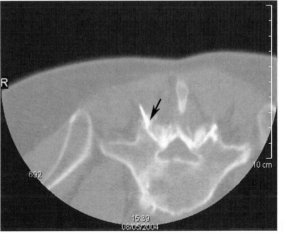

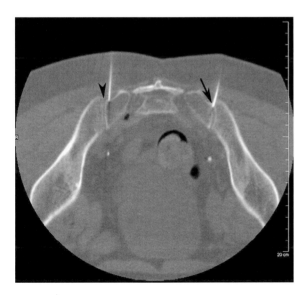

Fig. 8.19. Pain thought to be related to the sacroiliac joints in a 66-year-old man. Therapeutic sacroiliac joint injections were performed under CT guidance. Axial CT scan of the pelvis patient in prone position shows the needle tip is properly positioned in the left sacroiliac joint (*arrow*). The right needle needs to be repositioned 1 cm laterally (*arrowhead*). Depo-Medrol (40 mg) and bupivacaine 0.5% (3 ml) were injected into each joint

Fig. 8.20a,b. Facet joint arthrosis in a 70-year-old man referred for therapeutic injection. **a** Axial CT scan of the pelvis, with the patient in prone position and with skin markers showing the easiest access to the right L5–S1 facet joint. **b** The 22-gauge 3.5-in. spinal needle tip (*arrow*) was placed into the posterior margin of the right L5–S1 facet joint. Therapeutic injection consisted of Kenalog 0.5 ml (Kenalog-40 Injection, Bristol-Myers Squibb, Princeton, NJ, USA) and bupivacaine

and a sterile field is created, a 22-gauge needle is directed into the joint using a posterolateral oblique course. Since the osteophytes surrounding a very arthritic facet joint can be directly visualized under CT guidance, we find it is sometimes easier to accomplish the procedure with CT than fluoroscopy. If access to the joint is blocked by hypertrophic osteophytes, the posterior recess of the joint capsule can be accessed using a posteromedial approach (Fig. 8.20).

8.5
Conclusion

Diagnostic and therapeutic joint injections can be readily performed with imaging guidance. Ultrasound has several distinct advantages for guiding delivery of therapeutic injections. The most important of these is the ability to visualize the needle and make adjustments in real-time to ensure that medication is delivered to the appropriate location. As we have shown through a variety of clinical examples, the current generation of ultrasound scanners provides excellent depiction of the relevant anatomy. The needle has a unique sonographic appearance and can be monitored in real-time, as can the steroid-anesthetic mixture. No radiation exposure to the patient is an additional advantage of ultrasound guidance. Radiation exposure to the patient under fluoroscopy or CT guidance, however, is quite limited in the hands of a skilled, experienced radiologist. Knowledge of joint and para-articular anatomy is essential with either modality. Often the experience of the physician performing the procedure will dictate the choice of modality.

References

Adler RS, Allen A (2004) Percutaneous ultrasound guided injections in the shoulder. Techniques in Shoulder and Elbow Surg 5:122–133

Adler RS, Sofka CM (2003) Percutaneous ultrasound guided injections in the musculoskeletal system. Ultrasound Q 19:3–12

Brophy DP, Cunnane G, Fitzgerald O, Gibney RG (1995) Technical report: ultrasound guidance for injection of soft tissue lesions around the heel in chronic inflammatory arthritis. Clin Radiol 50:120–122

Cardinal E, Chhem RK, Beauregard CG (1998) Ultrasound-guided interventional procedures in the musculoskeletal system. Radiol Clin North Am 36:597–605

Depelteau H, Bureau N, Cardinal E, Aubin B, Brassard P (2004) Arthrography of the shoulder: a simple fluoroscopically guided approach for targeting the rotator interval. AJR Am J Roentgenol 182:329–332

Farmer KD, Hughes PM (2002) MR arthrography of the shoulder: fluoroscopically guided technique using a posterior approach. AJR Am J Roentgenol 178:433–434

Grassi W, Farina A, Filippucci E, Cervini C (2001) Sonographically guided procedures in rheumatology. Semin Arthritis Rheum 30:347–353

Koski JM (2000) Ultrasound guided injections in rheumatology. J Rheumatol 27:2131-2148

Ruhoy M, Newberg A, Yodlowski M, Mizel MS, Trepman E (1998) Subtalar joint arthrography. Semin Musculoskelet Radiol 2:433–437

Schneider R, Ghelman B, Kaye JJ (1975) A simplified injection technique for shoulder arthrography. Radiology 114:738–739

Sofka CM, Collins AJ, Adler RS (2001) Utilization of ultrasound guidance in interventional musculoskeletal procedures: a review from a single institution. J Ultrasound Med 20:21–26

Percutaneous Treatment of
Chronic Low Back Pain

Xavier Buy, Afshin Gangi, and Ali Guermazi

CONTENTS

9.1   Introduction   157

9.2   Discogenic Back Pain   157
9.2.1   Physiopathology, Clinical and
          Imaging Features   157
9.2.2   Provocative Discography   158
9.2.2.1   Indications   158
9.2.2.2   Technique   159
9.2.3   Minimally-Invasive Percutaneous Treatment
          of Discogenic Pain   161
9.2.3.1   Intradiscal Steroid Injection   162
9.2.3.2   Intradiscal Thermal Therapy   162

9.3   Facet Joint Syndrome   165
9.3.1   Physiopathology, Clinical and
          Imaging Features   165
9.3.2   Facet Block   166
9.3.3   Lumbar Cyst Infiltration   167
9.3.4   Facet Joint Denervation (Rhizolysis)   168
9.3.4.1   Indications   168
9.3.4.2   Technique   168
9.3.4.3   Results   169
9.3.4.4   Pulsed Radiofrequency   170

9.4   Sacroiliac Joint Syndrome   172
9.4.1   Physiopathology, Clinical and
          Imaging Features   172
9.4.2   Sacroiliac Block   173
9.4.2.1   Technique   173
9.4.2.2   Results   173
9.4.3   Sacroiliac Radiofrequency Denervation   174

9.5   Conclusion   175

          References   175

X. Buy, MD, Senior Radiologist
A. Gangi, MD, PhD, Professor of Radiology
Department of Radiology B, University Hospital of Strasbourg, Pavillon Clovis Vincent BP 426, 67091 Strasbourg, France
A. Guermazi, MD, Associate Professor of Radiology
Department of Radiology, Section Chief, Musculoskeletal, Boston University School of Medicine, 820 Harrison Avenue, FGH Building, 3rd Floor, Boston, MA 02118, USA

9.1
Introduction

Low back pain is a common problem with an important socio-economical impact. It is defined as chronic after 7–12 weeks of non-response to conservative therapies. Its estimated prevalence is 15% in adults, rising to 44% in the elderly (Jacobs et al. 2006). Unlike radicular pain where a cause of nerve root compression is often found, the precise etiology of back pain is difficult to establish as the clinical symptoms and the imaging features are often non-specific. Moreover, the fluctuation and subjectivity of pain and psychological factors make diagnosis and choice of therapy complex.

Three major causes of non-specific chronic low back pain will be discussed in this chapter: discogenic pain, facet joint syndrome and sacroiliac pain (Fig. 9.1). Other sources of back pain including vertebral body and disc herniation are described in specific chapters.

We will describe the physiopathology and clinical characteristics that must be understood to comprehend the pain mechanisms, and which are necessary for the interventional radiologist to establish a well-adapted therapeutic strategy. In doubtful cases, positive provocative tests or negative block tests may help to determine the source of pain. Proper patient selection is the key to successful treatment.

9.2
Discogenic Back Pain

9.2.1
Physiopathology, Clinical and Imaging Features

Degeneration of the intervertebral disc is a frequent source of back pain. Although the exact mechanisms

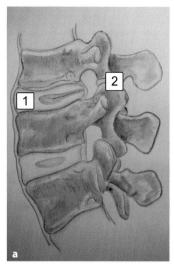 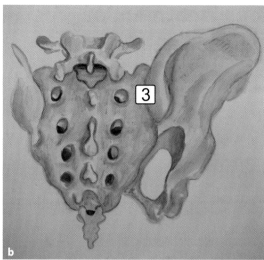

Fig. 9.1a,b. Three major causes of non-specific low back pain. **a** Drawing illustrates discogenic pain (*1*) and facet joint syndrome (*2*). **b** Drawing illustrates sacroiliac joint syndrome (*3*). (Drawings courtesy of C. Kauff)

of such pain remain unclear, mechanical and inflammatory factors are probably combined. Dehydration of the nucleus and fissures in the annulus fibrosus lead to a loss of weight-bearing properties and disc collapse. The biochemistry of the degenerative disc changes and high levels of pro-inflammatory mediators are found (interleukins, prostaglandins, tumor necrosis factor), with growth factors in the vascularized granulation tissues along torn fissures in the annulus (Burke et al. 2002; Peng et al. 2006b). Moreover, histological studies have shown extensive innervation in the severely degenerated human lumbar disc compared to normal discs, with an increase of substance P immuno-reactive nerve fibers known for their nociceptive properties (Coppes et al. 1997). This inflammatory reaction and nerve in-growth also involves the adjacent vertebral endplates (Ohtori et al. 2006).

Discogenic back pain is responsible for axial mechanical pain across the lumbar region, typically increasing after hyperflexion, but ceasing when prone and with rest. Paravertebral muscle contraction can be associated. Imaging provides only minor non-specific data: plain films and CT are often normal or show mild collapse of the disc. T2-weighted MR imaging sometimes shows a high intensity zone (HIZ) in the posterior part of the disc, which may represent an area of secondary inflammation as a consequence of an annular tear (Peng et al. 2006a; Schellhas et al. 1996). The HIZ of the lumbar disc on MR imaging in the patient with low back pain is considered by many authors to be a reliable marker of painful outer annular disruption (Lam et al. 2000). However, Carragee et al. (2000) in a prospective study

found HIZs in 25% of a non-symptomatic group. This prevalence is too high for meaningful clinical use (Fig. 9.2).

Buirski and Silberstein (1993) also found that no abnormal lumbar disc signal pattern could be identified on MR imaging that specifically indicated whether a disc would be painful. Subchondral edema can be found in the vertebral endplates adjacent to the painful disc. This edema is easily depicted on MR imaging with T1-weighted hyposignal and STIR/T2-weighted hypersignal (Modic et al. 1988). Axial MR sequences can also give information concerning paravertebral muscular atrophy which is a major factor of back pain and clinical outcome.

The non-specific information provided by clinical and imaging features makes discography a valuable test to determine the discal origin of a patient's symptoms.

9.2.2
Provocative Discography

9.2.2.1
Indications

Physical examination and non-invasive imaging are often non-specific (disc bulge, loss of T2-weighted MR imaging discal hypersignal, posterior high intensity zone on MR imaging, Modic I changes in the adjacent vertebral endplates), but can rule out potential underlying diseases. Provocative discography can overcome some of these limits and can be performed before planning treatment of any lumbar

Fig. 9.2a,b. A 34-year-old man with chronic low back pain. **a** Sagittal T2-weighted MR image of the lumbar spine shows hypointense discs from L3–4 to L5–S1. A high intensity zone (*arrow*) is visible in L5–S1, and confirmed on (**b**) axial balanced fast field-echo (BFFE) T2-weighted MR image. Discography in the three discs was only painful in L4–5

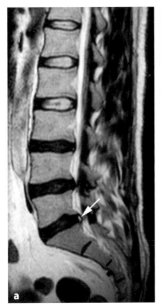
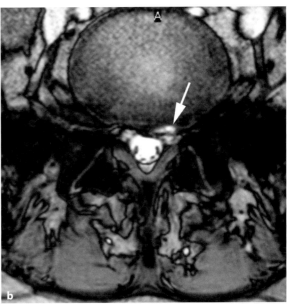

disc. CT can be added to discography to give the most precise information about the position and the extension of annular tears, but the additional information is often minimal. However, the major objective of this procedure is to revive the typical patient's usual back pain ("positive memory pain"), which confirms the discal origin of the symptoms.

Discography is considered the gold standard for diagnosing discogenic back pain. However, the ability of a patient to determine reliably the concordance of pain provoked during discography is poor. Specificity of discography is dramatically affected by the characteristics of the patient examined. It varies from 20% in patients with chronic pain and psychiatric risk factors, to 90% in healthy patients with no chronic pain states and a normal psychiatric profile (Carragee and Alamin 2001).

Because of this subjectivity, particular caution should be taken when interpreting the results of discography and determining the proper treatment for patients suffering from chronic low back pain.

9.2.2.2
Technique

Lumbar discography is performed in prone or lateral decubitus position, using a standard postero-lateral extrapedicular approach. The puncture technique is similar to percutaneous discal decompression (c.f. Chap. 6).

Under fluoroscopy, the desired disc level is marked. Local anesthesia with lidocaine is applied

and a 22-gauge needle is inserted into the nucleus. Close contact with the articular process is mandatory to avoid puncturing the nerve root (Fig. 9.3). The position of the needle tip must be confirmed on anteroposterior and lateral projections.

When prominent iliac wings block direct access to the disc (particularly for L5/S1 level), the needle needs to be bent (Fig. 9.4).

Then, 1–3 mL of iodine contrast is injected into the nucleus with low pressure. Some authors recommend the use of a manometer for precise monitoring of the intradiscal pressure, but we do not use one in routine practice. Discography gives morphologic information and can be supplemented if necessary by a disco-CT (Figs. 9.5 and 9.6). However, the major advantage of discography is that it provides enough physiological information to conclude that a degenerative disc is – or is not – responsible for the patient's symptoms. The discographic test is considered positive when the injection provokes the patient's usual pain ("memory pain"). To maximize the accuracy of the procedure, several points should be emphasized (Anderson 2004), as the assessment of the patient's pain remains subjective:

- Patients with psychological instability are poor candidates for this procedure
- A normal disc should also be injected as "control level"
- No information should be given to the patient concerning the disc level and the starting of injection, to avoid directed response

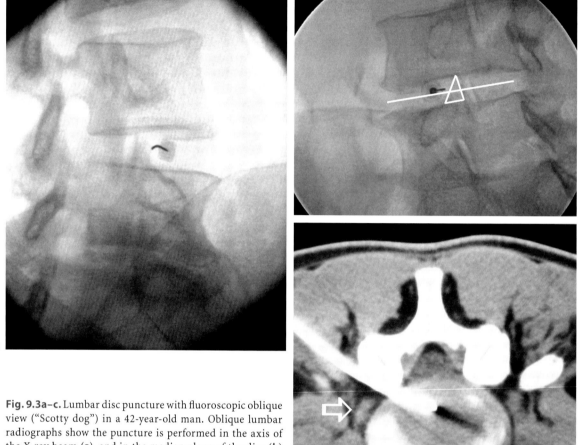

Fig. 9.3a–c. Lumbar disc puncture with fluoroscopic oblique view ("Scotty dog") in a 42-year-old man. Oblique lumbar radiographs show the puncture is performed in the axis of the X-ray beam (**a**), and in the median plane of the disc (**b**) (*white line*), just anterior to the facet (*white triangle*). Close contact with the articular process is mandatory to avoid the nerve root. **c** Axial CT scan shows the position of the nerve root (*arrow*)

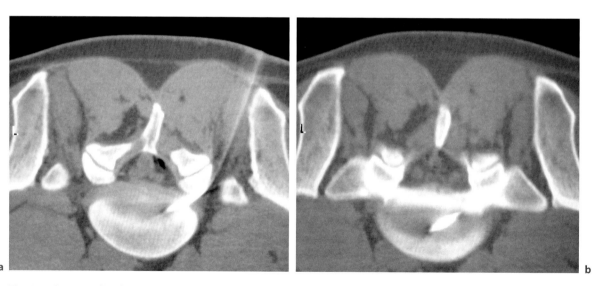

Fig. 9.4a,b. L5–S1 discal puncture in a 34-year-old man. **a,b** Axial CT scans at the level of L5–S1 confirm curved needle is necessary because of prominent iliac wings

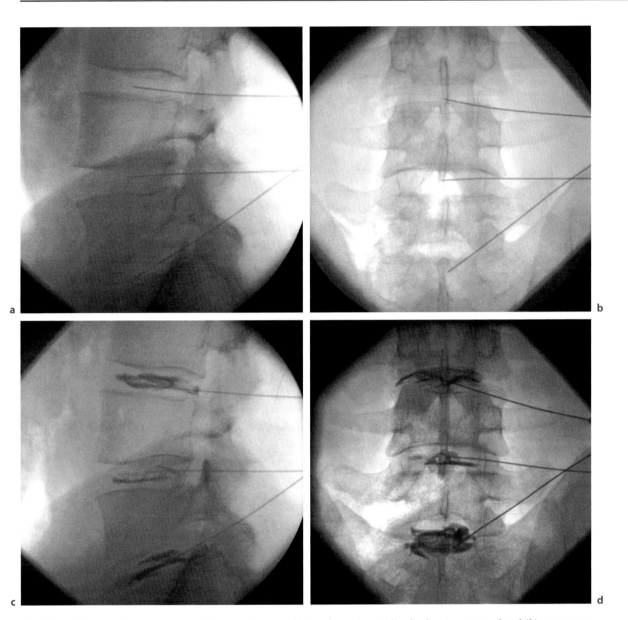

Fig. 9.5a–d. Lumbar discography in a 28-year-old man suffering from chronic low back pain. **a** Lateral and (**b**) anteroposterior radiographs of the lumbar spine show discal puncture at L3–4, L4–5 and L5–S1 levels. The proper positioning of the needles is confirmed by both lateral and anteroposterior fluoroscopic views before injection. **c** Lateral and (**d**) anteroposterior discography show degeneration in all three levels with epidural leak in L4–5. Only L4–5 injection was painful

Though it is considered the gold standard for assessing the discal origin of back pain, the procedure remains highly subjective; experience is necessary, including familiarity with the entire procedure and not just with discal puncture. According to CARRAGEE et al. (2006), the rate of low-pressure painful injections (false positive) in subjects without chronic low back pain is approximately 25%, and correlates with both anatomic and psychosocial factors.

9.2.3
Minimally-Invasive Percutaneous Treatment of Discogenic Pain

When the discal origin of back pain has been proven by provocative discography, several minimally-invasive percutaneous techniques are available. We describe below intradiscal steroid injections and intradiscal thermal therapy.

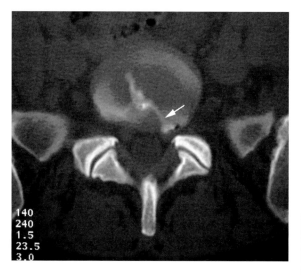

Fig. 9.6. Disco-CT in a 48-year-old woman. Axial disco-CT at L5–S1 level shows a left posterolateral annular tear (*arrow*). This additional information is important for treatment decisions

9.2.3.1
Intradiscal Steroid Injection

After a positive provocative discography, steroids can be injected directly into the nucleus, using the same approach (Fig. 9.7). Prednisolone can be safely used (Benyahya et al. 2004). Long acting synthetic steroids such as cortivazol or triamcinolone hexacetonide are contra-indicated as they may precipitate in the nucleus and induce extensive calcifications (Darmoul et al. 2005). The efficacy of intradiscal steroid injections remains controversial. Many authors report no improvement of clinical outcome compared with placebo (Khot et al. 2004). However, steroids may be more effective in patients with MR imaging findings of discogenic inflammation extending to the adjacent vertebral endplates (Modic I) (Buttermann 2004; Fayad et al. 2007). In patients with Modic I changes on MR imaging, intradiscal steroid injection may be an effective short-term treatment when conservative therapies have failed.

9.2.3.2
Intradiscal Thermal Therapy

9.2.3.2.1
Principles and Indications

Intradiscal electrothermal therapy (IDET) was introduced in the late 1990s. Its goal is to treat discogenic pain by progressively heating the posterior

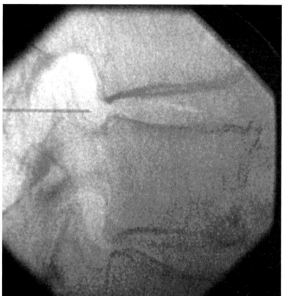

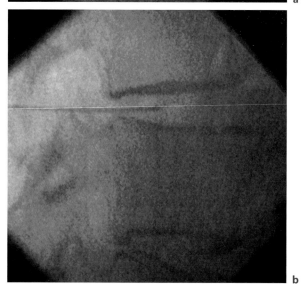

Fig. 9.7a,b. Intradiscal steroid injection in a 32-year-old man with chronic lumbar pain. **a** Lateral fluoroscopic view shows L3–4 degeneration with an intradiscal gaseous cleft. **b** Lateral fluoroscopic view after steroid injection demonstrates gas is no longer visible

annulus. Painful degenerative discs are often associated with annular tears and increased disc innervation. Moreover, the substance P immunoreactivity of these nerves tends to prove their nociceptive properties (Coppes et al. 1997). Heating the posterior part of the annulus may induce denervation of the painful disc but also shrinkage, as collagen type I fibers of the annulus fuse at 70 °C and above (Wang et al. 2005).

IDET is indicated for discogenic back pain without radicular compression, after failure of 4–6 months of conservative therapies. The socio-psychological context often associated with chronic low back pain requires a multidisciplinary approach and a high level of experience to get the most benefit from intradiscal thermal therapy. This minimally invasive percutaneous technique, an outpatient procedure, is a safe alternative to surgical fusion or disc prostheses which have similar outcomes but higher morbidity (ANDERSSON et al. 2006).

Contraindications include prior surgery at the same level, instability or spondylolisthesis, disc collapse >50%. Obesity is a relative contraindication of IDET as it is associated with therapy failure (COHEN et al. 2003). IDET is not indicated for facet syndrome and radicular pain due to disc herniation. In this last case, nucleotomy techniques are used to achieve nerve root decompression (c.f. Chap. 6).

9.2.3.2.2
Technique

IDET is an outpatient procedure. Lumbar disc puncture is achieved via a standard posterolateral extraforaminal approach, under fluoroscopic control. Strict sterility is mandatory. Local anesthesia is applied with a 22-gauge spinal needle up to the articular process, but not the foramen, to maintain complete neurological monitoring of the patient during the procedure. The 17-gauge introducer needle is positioned in tandem into the annulus. Then, a bipolar flexible loop radiofrequency electrode with a bent tip (Spinecath®, Smith & Nephew, London, UK) is inserted coaxially and deployed into the disc, so that its 5-cm active extremity faces the posterior annulus. This active tip is marked by two radio-opaque dots. The initial insertion is performed with lateral fluoroscopic control. Once the catheter curves along the posterior annulus, the anteroposterior view checks that it covers the interpedicular space (Fig. 9.8). Precise positioning must be controlled by both anteroposterior and lateral fluoroscopic views, to avoid extradiscal mispositioning through disc perforation.

The insertion is sometimes difficult when the tip of the electrode gets caught in annular tears. Incomplete deployment or kinking of the electrode occurs in about 20% of cases (Fig. 9.9). When the electrode is kinked, it should be removed simultaneously with the introducer needle to avoid inadvertent rupture of the electrode. To make the deployment easier, the 17-gauge introducer can be positioned slightly anterolaterally in the nucleus, so that the flexible loop electrode curves smoothly along the inner annulus without angulation. Also, the electrode should be wet before insertion, like hydrophilic guide wires in vascular interventions. In some cases where the deployment is incomplete, the procedure can be repeated or completed via a contralateral approach in the same setting.

Once the electrode is in proper position, increasing temperature is applied over several minutes to a plateau of 90 °C (corresponding to the temperature inside the catheter) and maintained for 4 min. The temperature in the tissues adjacent to the electrode is approximately 69 °C and rapidly decreases to 42 °C in the outer part of the annulus. The epidural temperature normally never exceeds 38 °C (SAAL and SAAL 2000b). If any leg pain occurs during the procedure, heating should stop immediately to avoid neural damage. Repositioning of the electrode should be reconsidered. For this reason, sedation and deep perineural anesthesia are strictly prohibited. If back pain occurs, the temperature can be decreased to 85 or 80 °C.

After the procedure, the electrode and the introducer are withdrawn and the wound is dressed. The patient is discharged after 2 h rest.

9.2.3.2.3
Post-Procedural Instructions

During the first 2 weeks, some activities are restricted to promote healing of the annulus. These activities include twisting and lifting. To reduce pressure on the posterior aspect of the lumbar discs, sitting time is limited. On the contrary, walking is encouraged. Normal activity can be resumed, slowly, over the next 4 weeks. Patients should not go back to intensive exercise such as sports or lifting before 8 weeks. A lumbar corset can be used in the early post-procedural phase.

9.2.3.2.4
Results

The therapeutic efficacy of IDET remains a controversial issue. Even the intradiscal physical effects of IDET are still unclear. Freeman et al. in animal studies found vascular granulation tissue consistent with healing response in the annular tears after IDET, but the temperature in the outer annulus was

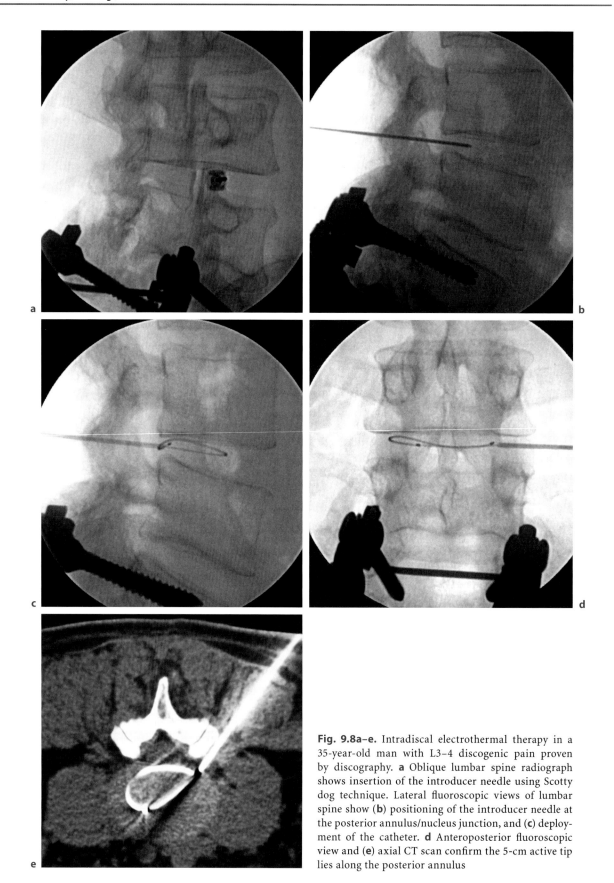

Fig. 9.8a–e. Intradiscal electrothermal therapy in a 35-year-old man with L3–4 discogenic pain proven by discography. **a** Oblique lumbar spine radiograph shows insertion of the introducer needle using Scotty dog technique. Lateral fluoroscopic views of lumbar spine show (**b**) positioning of the introducer needle at the posterior annulus/nucleus junction, and (**c**) deployment of the catheter. **d** Anteroposterior fluoroscopic view and (**e**) axial CT scan confirm the 5-cm active tip lies along the posterior annulus

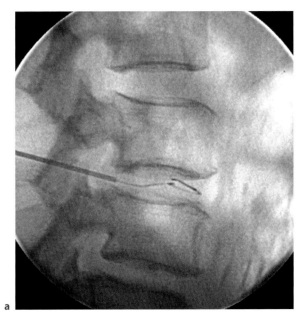

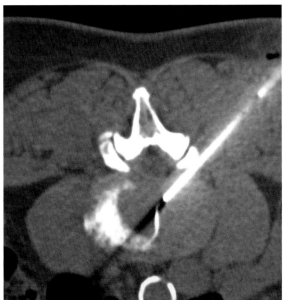

Fig. 9.9a,b. Kinking of the intradiscal electrothermal therapy catheter in a 38-year-old woman. **a** Lateral fluoroscopic view and (**b**) axial CT scan at the level of L4–5 show the introducer needle and catheter should be withdrawn simultaneously to avoid a rupture of the catheter inside the disc

insufficient to achieve denervation (Freeman et al. 2003).

Initial results of the procedure were promising with 71% of patients improved on both visual analogical and functional scores (Saal and Saal 2000a).

However, further prospective randomized studies found only about half of the patients reporting significant improvement of pain and functional scores after 1 or 2 years follow-up (Lee et al. 2003; Pauza et al. 2004). Several review studies deny the efficacy of IDET for treating discogenic pain, considering the benefit minimal compared to physiotherapy or even placebo (Davis et al. 2004; Freeman et al. 2005; Urrutia et al. 2007). Indeed, in our own experience, about half of the patients were satisfied with the procedure.

On the other hand, few complications have been reported for IDET. The major risk is thermal damage to the nerve roots when the electrode loops close to the dura. This is why continuous neurological monitoring during the heating phase is mandatory. Rare complications such as vertebral osteonecrosis (Djurasovic et al. 2002) or large disc herniation following the procedure (Cohen et al. 2002) have been reported.

9.3
Facet Joint Syndrome

9.3.1
Physiopathology, Clinical and Imaging Features

The term "facet syndrome" was introduced in the 1930s to describe back pain due to posterior articular facets (Ghormley 1933). The facet pain is attributed to segmental instability, synovitis, or degenerative arthritis. Facet joints have been implicated as the source of chronic pain in 15%–45% of patients with chronic low back pain (Manchikanti et al. 2002). Differentiation between disk disease and facet syndrome can sometimes be difficult, and the diagnosis is often made by exclusion. The clinical signs of facet syndrome are local paralumbar tenderness with mechanical pain on hyperextension; absence of neurological deficit, absence of radicular pain and negative straight leg rising also indicate facet syndrome (El-Khoury and Renfrew 1991; Helbig and Lee 1988; Lippitt 1984).

Imaging features are often minor or non-specific. Dynamic plain films can demonstrate posterior instability; CT or MR imaging can show gas or fluid in the joint with degenerative arthritis and hypertrophy of the facets (Fig. 9.10). T2-weighted MR sequences are very sensitive to degenerative-inflammatory changes of the posterior elements of the lumbar spine (D'APRILE et al. 2007). However, these imaging findings are often found in non-symptomatic patients.

In the absence of precise clinical features or criteria, the diagnosis of facet syndrome is confirmed by selective facet block tests. These tests can be performed by direct intra-articular injection of a mixture of steroids and local anesthetics, or by indirect neural block of the lumbar medial branch that innervates the facet joint. The choice of injection level is based on the presence of focal tenderness over a facet joint or the presence of osteoarthritis involving the joint. A block test must produce transient but complete pain relief to support the presumptive diagnosis of facet joint syndrome.

9.3.2
Facet Block

Facet joint injection is appropriate in two circumstances: as a diagnostic test when the facet origin of back pain remains unclear or when the painful levels have to be identified, and as a first minimally-invasive therapy when diagnostic blocks show that facet joints are the source of pain. Injection of a local anesthetic affects the nociceptive fibers within the synovium, whereas intracapsular injection of a corticosteroid may reduce inflammation of the synovium (DESTOUET et al. 1982). Facet block as diagnostic test is performed with local anesthetic only. A positive provocative test can also be performed with intra-articular injection of hypertonic saline.

Fig. 9.10a–c. Right paravertebral chronic lumbar tenderness in a 50-year-old man. **a** Axial CT scan shows right L4 laminar condensation. **b** Axial contrast-enhanced fat-suppressed T1-weighted and (**c**) sagittal T2 STIR MR images show right L4–5 facet inflammation with intra-articular effusion (*arrow*), synovitis and subchondral edema. Differential diagnosis should include infection

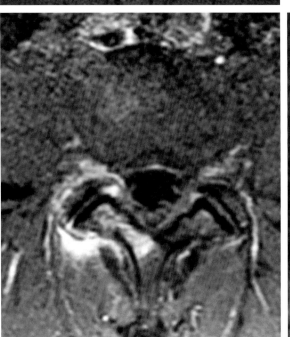

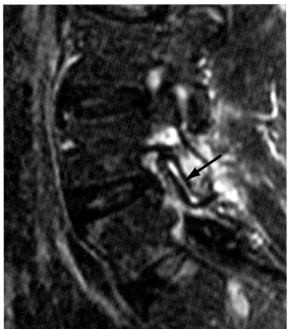

Injection of facet joints in the lumbar spine is simple and safe. CT or fluoroscopic control is best. Degenerative disease of facet joints usually affects multiple levels and both sides; thus, multilevel injection of facet joints on both sides is sometimes necessary. The patient is placed in the prone position on the operating table. The needle pathway and entry point are determined by CT or anteroposterior fluoroscopic view targeted on the affected level (Figs. 9.11 and 9.12). With fluoroscopic guidance, a slight lateral rotation of 5–10° from the strict anteroposterior view can help to get a better access to the joint. A 22-gauge spinal needle is then advanced vertically into each facet joint. The low recess of the facet joint is sometimes easier to puncture when osteophytes block the access to the articular space. Once the needle is in the joint, its proper position is checked by injection of 0.5 mL of iodine contrast, assuming fluoroscopic guidance.

The facet joint is small and the operator can feel elastic resistance during injection. Long acting steroids mixed with 1.5 mL of lidocaine are injected slowly. We use 1.5 mL of cortivazol solution (3.75 mg). This single dose of cortivazol per session should not be exceeded. If the injection is performed bilaterally, the total dose should be shared to avoid complications (flushing, tachycardia, sweating and increase of blood pressure).

The value of facet joint injection is controversial (LILIUS et al. 1989). In published studies, immediate relief was achieved in 59%–94% of cases and long-term relief was achieved in 27%–54% (DESTOUET et al. 1982; LIPPITT 1984; LYNCH and TAYLOR 1986; REVEL et al. 1998). In our experience over 15 years, immediate relief is achieved in about two thirds of cases and long-term relief is achieved in one third, with persistence of relief for at least 4 months. These results are in concordance with those of prospective studies (SCHULTE et al. 2006; SHIH et al. 2005). Complications of lumbar facet joint injection, with precise needle positioning, are highly unusual. Severe allergic reactions to local anesthetics are uncommon. Long acting steroid injection can produce local reactions, which most often occur immediately after the injection but stop after 24–48 h. The major complication is septic arthritis (ORPEN and BIRCH 2003), which can be avoided with strict sterility. Other complications are rare if the usual contraindications to steroid use are respected.

9.3.3
Lumbar Cyst Infiltration

Lumbar cysts are most frequent at L4/5 level and are associated with osteoarthritis of the adjacent facet joint or hypermobility. Synovial cysts have a lining of synovial cells and communicate with the facet joint. Ganglion cysts are due to myxomatous degeneration of fibrous tissue inside the ligamentum

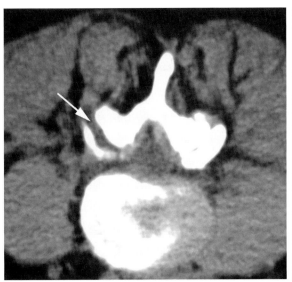
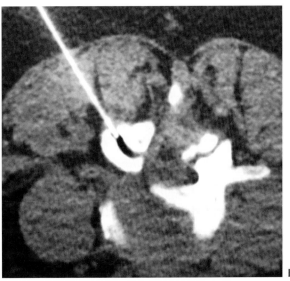

a   b

Fig. 9.11a,b. Right L4–5 facet infiltration in a 56-year-old woman. **a** Axial CT scan shows intra-articular effusion (*arrow*) of right L4–5 facet. **b** Axial CT scan shows aspiration via a 22-gauge spinal needle, followed by injection of cortivazol mixed with 1 mL of lidocaine

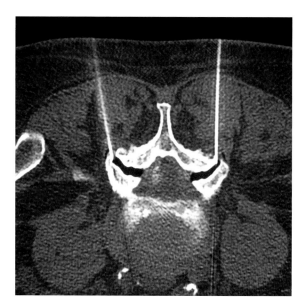

Fig. 9.12. Bilateral L4–5 CT-guided facet infiltration in a 57-year-old woman. Axial CT scan shows intra-articular void phenomenon due to degenerative disorders

flavum. Unlike synovial cysts, they do not have a lining of synovial cells and don't communicate with the facet joint (BUREAU et al. 2001). Synovial and ganglion cysts can extend into the spinal canal and cause radicular compression. When the symptoms are limited to back pain, the cyst is an epiphenomenon of facet osteoarthritis or posterior instability. These cysts are well depicted on CT and even better on MR imaging due to the higher contrast (SAUVAGE et al. 2000). As many as 32% of cysts show calcifications in the capsule (HEMMINGHYTT et al. 1982).

Surgical treatment with removal of symptomatic cysts is efficient (HSU et al. 1995; KHAN et al. 2005) but image-guided therapies with steroid infiltrations and percutaneous rupture are a minimally invasive alternative and should be considered first (BJORKENGREN et al. 1987). Steroid injections can achieve early pain relief in up to 75% of patients and also may result in complete regression of the cyst (BUREAU et al. 2001). After 6 months, 50% of patients still have good results (PARLIER-CUAU et al. 1999; SAUVAGE et al. 2000).

The puncture technique for synovial cysts is similar to facet joint injection. After injection of 1 mL of iodine contrast to show how the cyst communicates with the facet joint, 3 mL of prednisolone mixed with 1 mL of lidocaine are injected with hyperpressure to force out the contents of the cyst. After a sudden release of pressure, imaging control shows the dif-

fusion of contrast into the epidural space (Fig. 9.13). Cyst rupture is more difficult to achieve in cases of wall calcifications. In such cases, the cyst should be aspirated then injected with 1–2 mL of prednisolone. Prednisolone is preferred to cortivazol to reduce the risk of calcification.

For ganglion cysts (or for synovial cysts difficult to opacify by posterior facet puncture) the injection technique is similar but the puncture is directly into the cyst, as this myxomatous degeneration doesn't communicate with the facet joint (Fig. 9.14).

9.3.4
Facet Joint Denervation (Rhizolysis)

9.3.4.1
Indications

In some patients, facet joint injection with local anesthetics and steroids produces consistent but short-term pain relief. For these patients, facet joint denervation should be considered. This procedure, called rhizolysis, aims to destroy the sensitive branches innervating the facet joints to achieve a long lasting analgesic effect. Each facet joint is supplied by articular filaments arising from the medial branches of the dorsal rami above and below the joint (BOGDUK and LONG 1979). Therefore, rhizolysis must be performed on two levels to achieve denervation of one level (Fig. 9.15).

9.3.4.2
Technique

Rhizolysis is performed by injecting 1.5 mL of 95% ethanol at each point via a standard 22-gauge spinal needle, after having checked the precise position and distribution with injection of 1 mL of iodine contrast. However thermal rhizolysis using radiofrequency allows more selective treatment, without risk of inadvertent anterior diffusion towards the foramen. This procedure is performed under strict sterility, with fluoroscopic or CT control. The sensitive lumbar medial branches above and below the diseased joint have to be coagulated to achieve facet denervation. With the patient prone, entry points are determined so that the tip of the electrode touches the superior border of the medial part of the transverse processes (Figs. 9.16 and 9.17). Under fluoroscopic guidance, an anteroposterior view with a slight lateral rotation of 5–10° helps to avoid the facet

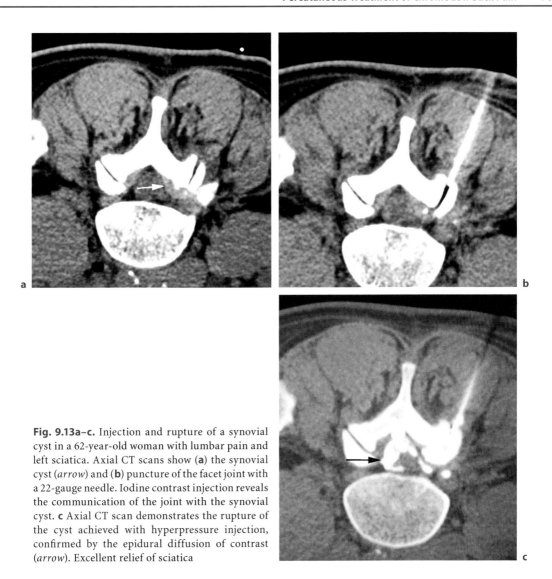

Fig. 9.13a–c. Injection and rupture of a synovial cyst in a 62-year-old woman with lumbar pain and left sciatica. Axial CT scans show (**a**) the synovial cyst (*arrow*) and (**b**) puncture of the facet joint with a 22-gauge needle. Iodine contrast injection reveals the communication of the joint with the synovial cyst. **c** Axial CT scan demonstrates the rupture of the cyst achieved with hyperpressure injection, confirmed by the epidural diffusion of contrast (*arrow*). Excellent relief of sciatica

joint. After bone contact with the superomedial part of the transverse process, a lateral view confirms the exact position before stimulation and coagulation. The electrodes used for rhizolysis should never be advanced beyond the transverse process, to avoid damaging the nerve root exiting the foramen. Continuous neurological monitoring is necessary and deep local anesthesia of the foramen is prohibited.

Once the electrode is in position, 90 s with a temperature over 60 °C are sufficient to achieve rhizolysis. Temperature-controlled radiofrequency can create reproducible lesion sizes and is preferred over voltage-controlled radiofrequency (Buijs et al. 2004). Many radiofrequency generators allow stimulation of the posterior lumbar medial branch before coagulation; contraction of the paravertebral muscles is visible during motor stimulation and the patient's usual back pain is provoked during sensory stimulation. If any pain or contraction occurs in the thigh, the radiofrequency electrode should be withdrawn slightly under fluoroscopy and the stimulation test repeated to avoid thermal damage of the foraminal nerve root. Active sensitivity and motor stimulation before rhizolysis highly increases the safety and the precision of the procedure.

9.3.4.3
Results

According to the literature, facet joint denervation provides good pain relief in 45%–69% of patients at long-term follow-up (Burton 1976; McCulloch 1976; Silvers 1990), but the procedure remains controversial (Leclaire et al. 2001). Pain relief is

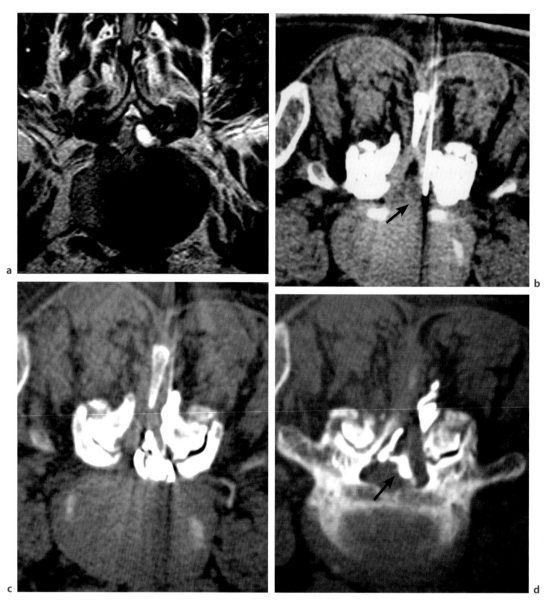

Fig. 9.14a–d. Injection and rupture of a ganglion cyst in a 62-year-old man with back pain and right sciatica. **a** Axial T2-weighted MR image shows the ganglion cyst and facet degeneration. Axial CT scans show (**b**) direct puncture of the cyst (*arrow*), with (**c**) no communication with the joint, and rupture of the cyst with (**d**) epidural leak (*arrow*) achieved by hyperpressure injection. Good relief of the sciatica

not reliably permanent because the nerve can regenerate, usually within 12–18 months. However, if pain recurs after several months, rhizolysis can be repeated effectively with more than 85% success (Schofferman and Kine 2004). Complications are uncommon, mainly minor transient pain at the puncture site (Kornick et al. 2004). Accidental damage to the foraminal nerve root can be avoided with careful attention to technique.

9.3.4.4
Pulsed Radiofrequency

Pulsed radiofrequency is newer in clinical practice and should not be confused with conventional continuous radiofrequency. Pulsed radiofrequency uses brief bursts of radiofrequency energy separated by relatively long pauses between bursts to allow heat to dissipate in the target tissue (Bogduk 2006). This low

Fig. 9.15a,b. Facet joint innervation. **a** Each facet joint is supplied by articular filaments arising from the medial branches of the dorsal rami above and below the joint. **b** Neurolysis is performed on the superomedial border of the transverse processes above and below the pathological facet. (Drawings courtesy of C. Kauff)

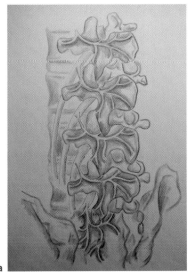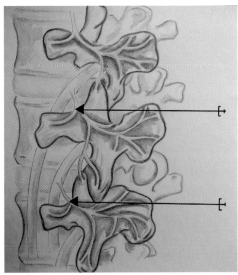

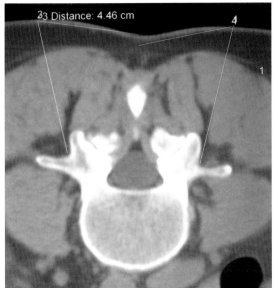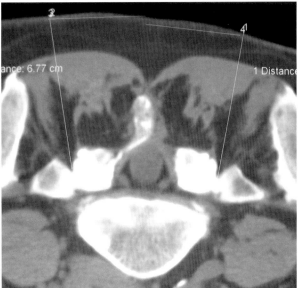

Fig. 9.16a,b. Examples of CT-guided determination of pathways for rhizolysis. Axial CT scans show the rhizolysis pathways through the superomedial borders of the transverse processes at (**a**) L4 and at (**b**) S1 levels

temperature therapy (about 42 °C) does not achieve neurotomy but acts like a neuromodulator, thereby minimizing the risk of adverse events compared to conventional continuous radiofrequency (AHADIAN 2004). Pulsed radiofrequency also avoids denervation of the deep paravertebral muscles. However, its mechanisms of action are not clearly elucidated and its clinical effect on back pain remain unproven. Only a little data is available in the literature but the efficacy seems less than continuous radiofrequency rhizolysis (MIKELADZE et al. 2003), particularly on long-term follow-up (TEKIN et al. 2007).

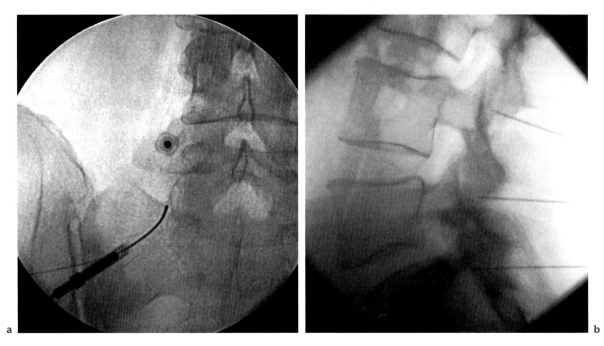

Fig. 9.17. Bilateral rhizolysis at L4–5 and L5–S1 levels. **a** Anteroposterior fluoroscopic view shows denervation has to be performed on the superomedial border of the transverse processes of L4, L5 and S1. **b** Needles should not go beyond the transverse processes on lateral fluoroscopic view

9.4
Sacroiliac Joint Syndrome

9.4.1
Physiopathology, Clinical and Imaging Features

The sacroiliac joint (SIJ) is a diarthrodial joint with hyaline cartilage on the sacral side in contact with fibrocartilage on the iliac side. The innervation of the SIJ is complex and still unclear (FORST et al. 2006; FORTIN et al. 1999; HANSEN et al. 2007). The anterior portion of the SIJ likely receives innervation from the posterior rami of the L2–S2 roots. Additional innervation to the anterior joint arises directly from the obturator nerve, superior gluteal nerve, and/or lumbosacral trunk. The posterior portion of the joint is innervated by the posterior rami of L4–S3 with a particular contribution from S1 and S2 (Fig. 9.18). The contribution from these roots differs among the joints of given individuals and could explain the high variability of pain referral patterns.

Pain from the SIJ appears mainly situated in the lumbar region and the buttocks, but can also be distributed more distally to the leg and even the foot (SLIPMAN et al. 2000). Elective pain is often provoked by finger pressure on the postero-superior iliac spine. Other provocation tests with different SIJ distraction maneuvers give inconsistent results.

With sacroiliitis, an inflammatory origin (spondylarthropathy) should be considered first, and should be excluded by appropriate lab exams before planning focal treatment. Chronic pain referred to SIJ may include traumas, lumbar fusion, and gait disorders, but is often idiopathic. The value of CT is limited in SIJ disease except to exclude differential diagnoses. MR imaging is not commonly used although it can occasionally show intra-articular effusion and subchondral edema.

Imaging techniques often make little contribution to the diagnosis of symptomatic SIJ, as their abnormal findings are generally minor and nonspecific. For this reason, intra-articular blocks with injection of steroids mixed with anesthetics represent the most reliable test to confirm the sacroiliac origin of pain (ELGAFY et al. 2001). Using SIJ blocks as gold standard, the prevalence of chronic low back pain due to SIJ is estimated at 10%–19% (MCKENZIE-BROWN et al. 2005).

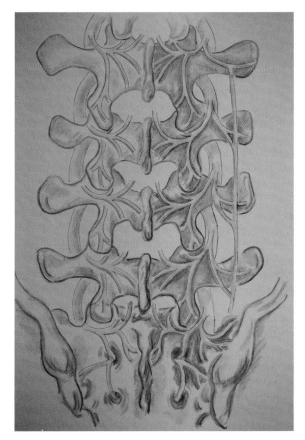

Fig. 9.18. Sacroiliac innervation. Posterior rami from L2 to S3 contribute to the anterior and the posterior innervation of the sacroiliac joint. Additional innervation directly arises from the obturator nerve, superior gluteal nerve, and/or lumbosacral trunk. (Drawing courtesy of C. Kauff)

9.4.2
Sacroiliac Block

Sacroiliac joint injections are a reliable test to establish the origin of back pain, but they are also the first step of minimally-invasive percutaneous treatment.

9.4.2.1
Technique

SIJ blocks are performed under strict sterility. Image guidance should be used systematically as the complex three-dimensional configuration and frequent osteophytes make a blind approach difficult. Blind injections reach the intra-articular space in only 22% cases, with a 24% chance of inadvertent epidural leak (ROSENBERG et al. 2000). With the patient in prone position, the low aspect of the SIJ

(over the distal 1–2 cm) is punctured under local anesthesia with a 22-gauge spinal needle, via a direct posterior approach, utilizing fluoroscopy, CT or MR imaging (DUSSAULT et al. 2000; PEREIRA et al. 2000; PULISETTI and EBRAHEIM 1999). If osteophytes block the low approach, an upper puncture can be performed through the fibrous part of the joint (Figs. 9.19–9.21). To check proper intra-articular positioning of the needle, 1 mL of contrast agent is injected if fluoroscopic control is used. Then, the block test is performed with injection of 2 mL of lidocaine into the joint. Relief of the usual pain, even transient, proves the sacroiliac origin of the symptoms. If long-term therapeutic effect is required, long acting steroids (3.75 mg of cortivazol) can be mixed with anesthetics. When bilateral SIJ injection is performed, the dose of steroids should be shared between the two articular compartments.

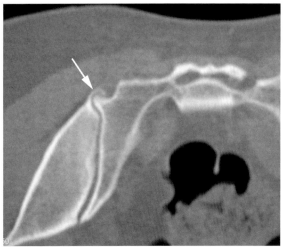

Fig. 9.19. Left sacroiliac pain in a 49-year-old woman. Axial CT scan precisely depicts how osteophytes (*arrow*) are blocking intra-articular access

9.4.2.2
Results

Percutaneous steroid injection of the SIJ often incriminates the joint as the cause of pain. Moreover, the procedure can provide significant but often temporary pain relief (STALLMEYER and ORTIZ 2002). Pain relief is fast and maximal with 80%–92.5% of patients improved for several months (BELLAICHE 1995; BOLLOW et al. 1996; BRAUN et al. 1996; KARABACAKOGLU et al. 2002; PULISETTI and EBRAHEIM 1999). After 6–12 months, pain often re-

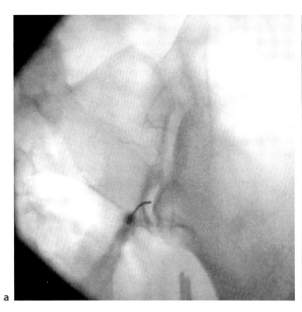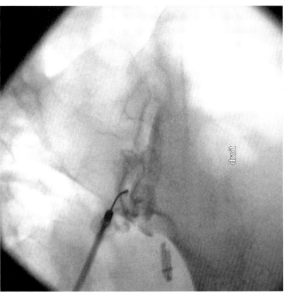

a   b

Fig. 9.20a,b. Sacroiliac joint injection under fluoroscopic guidance in a 43-year-old man. **a** Posteroanterior fluoroscopic views show direct posterior approach in the lower part of the right sacroiliac joint. **b** Proper position of the needle is confirmed by contrast injection

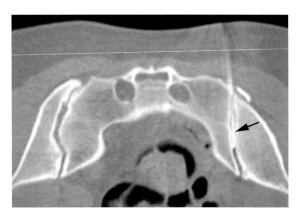

Fig. 9.21. Right sacroiliac joint injection in a 54-year-old woman. Axial CT scan shows the needle positioned in the left sacroiliac joint (*arrow*)

turns to the pre-injection level (HANLY et al. 2000). If the pain does return, SIJ injection can be repeated with good results (GUNAYDIN et al. 2006).

MR imaging can show a significant decrease of the subchondral edema and reduction of contrast enhancement in successful cases after steroid injection.

Review and guideline articles find moderate evidence for SIJ injections for short-term pain relief and limited evidence for long-term relief (BOSWELL et al. 2007; HANSEN et al. 2007).

9.4.3
Sacroiliac Radiofrequency Denervation

In patients with only short-term benefit after sacroiliac injection, radiofrequency therapy should be considered for prolonged pain relief. The theoretical principles are similar to facet joint denervation. However, due to the complex innervation of SIJ, its denervation remains controversial and there is no standard technique: most common are denervation of the sensitive roots supplying the SIJ (BURNHAM and YASUI 2007; VALLEJO et al. 2006; YIN et al. 2003), direct intra-articular thermal therapy (FERRANTE et al. 2001), or a combination of the two approaches (GEVARGEZ et al. 2002). The therapeutic effect of intra-articular SIJ radiofrequency is not clear but its success rate seems less than radiofrequency neurotomy of the sensitive nerve roots of the SIJ. However, only posterior denervation of the SIJ is achieved as the anterior nerves remain inaccessible to a percutaneous approach (Fig. 9.22).

The efficacy of radiofrequency denervation of the SIJ remains unclear. This procedure is efficient in about two thirds of patients during the first months, but only one third have consistent pain relief after 6 months.

According to several review articles, the evidence for radiofrequency neurotomy to treat chronic SIJ pain is limited (BOSWELL et al. 2007; HANSEN et al. 2007; MCKENZIE-BROWN et al. 2005).

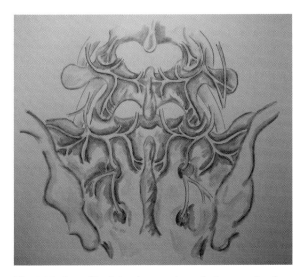

Fig. 9.22. Sacroiliac joint denervations. Only posterior denervations of the sacroiliac joint as the anterior nerves remain inaccessible to a percutaneous approach. (Drawing courtesy of C. Kauff)

9.5
Conclusion

Management of chronic low back pain is challenging. A strong understanding of the mechanisms that produce pain is essential to select precisely the patients and to offer them the optimal therapy. Disc, facet joint and sacroiliac joint should always be considered as the most likely causes of chronic back pain.

Several points must be clearly understood to maximize the results of any image guided percutaneous technique for treating chronic back pain:

- Precise clinical exam and imaging are necessary to orientate the diagnosis, even if their findings are often non-specific.
- Positive provocative tests such as discography, or block tests such as facet blocks and sacroiliac blocks, can help to clarify the origin of pain (diagnostic test). The same puncture technique can also be used for steroid injection (therapeutic test).
- Intradiscal thermal techniques should only be considered after a positive discography.
- Facet joint denervation (rhizolysis) should only be considered when the pain relapses after a positive facet block test.
- Sacroiliac radiofrequency remains a controversial technique as the denervation concerns only the posterior aspect of the joint.

References

Ahadian FM (2004) Pulsed radiofrequency neurotomy: advances in pain medicine. Curr Pain Headache Rep 8:34–40

Anderson MW (2004) Lumbar discography: an update. Semin Roentgenol 39:52–67

Andersson GB, Mekhail NA, Block JE (2006) Treatment of intractable discogenic low back pain. A systematic review of spinal fusion and intradiscal electrothermal therapy (IDET). Pain Physician 9:237–248

Bellaiche L (1995) Cortisone injection into the sacroiliac joint. Ann Radiol (Paris) 38:192–195

Benyahya R, Lefevre-Colau MM, Fayad F, Rannou F, Demaille-Wlodyka S, Mayoux-Benhamou MA, Poiraudeau S, Revel M (2004) Intradiscal injection of acetate of prednisolone in severe low back pain: complications and patients' assessment of effectiveness. Ann Readapt Med Phys 47:621–626

Bjorkengren AG, Kurz LT, Resnick D, Sartoris DJ, Garfin SR (1987) Symptomatic intraspinal synovial cysts: opacification and treatment by percutaneous injection. AJR Am J Roentgenol 149:105–107

Bogduk N (2006) Pulsed radiofrequency. Pain Med 7:396–407

Bogduk N, Long DM (1979) The anatomy of the so-called "articular nerves" and their relationship to facet denervation in the treatment of low-back pain. J Neurosurg 51:172–177

Bollow M, Braun J, Taupitz M, Haberle J, Reibhauer BH, Paris S, Mutze S, Seyrekbasan F, Wolf KJ, Hamm B (1996) CT-guided intraarticular corticosteroid injection into the sacroiliac joints in patients with spondyloarthropathy: indication and follow-up with contrast-enhanced MRI. J Comput Assist Tomogr 20:512–521

Boswell MV, Trescot AM, Datta S, Schultz DM, Hansen HC, Abdi S, Sehgal N, Shah RV, Singh V, Benyamin RM, Patel VB, Buenaventura RM, Colson JD, Cordner HJ, Epter RS, Jasper JF, Dunbar EE, Atluri SL, Bowman RC, Deer TR, Swicegood JR, Staats PS, Smith HS, Burton AW, Kloth DS, Giordano J, Manchikanti L (2007) Interventional techniques: evidence-based practice guidelines in the management of chronic spinal pain. Pain Physician 10:7–111

Braun J, Bollow M, Seyrekbasan F, Haberle HJ, Eggens U, Mertz A, Distler A, Sieper J (1996) Computed tomography guided corticosteroid injection of the sacroiliac joint in patients with spondyloarthropathy with sacroiliitis: clinical outcome and followup by dynamic magnetic resonance imaging. J Rheumatol 23:659–664

Buijs EJ, van Wijk RM, Geurts JW, Weeseman RR, Stolker RJ, Groen GG (2004) Radiofrequency lumbar facet denervation: a comparative study of the reproducibility of lesion size after 2 current radiofrequency techniques. Reg Anesth Pain Med 29:400–407

Buirski G, Silberstein M (1993) The symptomatic lumbar disc in patients with low-back pain. Magnetic resonance imaging appearances in both a symptomatic and control population. Spine 18:1808–1811

Bureau NJ, Kaplan PA, Dussault RG (2001) Lumbar facet joint synovial cyst: percutaneous treatment with steroid injections and distention-clinical and imaging follow-up in 12 patients. Radiology 221:179–185

Burke JG, Watson RW, McCormack D, Dowling FE, Walsh MG, Fitzpatrick JM (2002) Intervertebral discs which cause low back pain secrete high levels of proinflammatory mediators. J Bone Joint Surg Br 84:196–201

Burnham RS, Yasui Y (2007) An alternate method of radiofrequency neurotomy of the sacroiliac joint: a pilot study of the effect on pain, function, and satisfaction. Reg Anesth Pain Med 32:12–19

Burton CV (1976) Percutaneous radiofrequency facet denervation. Appl Neurophysiol 39:80–86

Buttermann GR (2004) The effect of spinal steroid injections for degenerative disc disease. Spine J 4:495–505

Carragee EJ, Alamin TF (2001) Discography. a review. Spine J 1:364–372

Carragee EJ, Paragioudakis SJ, Khurana S (2000) 2000 Volvo Award winner in clinical studies: lumbar high-intensity zone and discography in subjects without low back problems. Spine 25:2987–2992

Carragee EJ, Alamin TF, Carragee JM (2006) Low-pressure positive discography in subjects asymptomatic of significant low back pain illness. Spine 31:505–509

Cohen SP, Larkin T, Polly DW (2002) A giant herniated disc following intradiscal electrothermal therapy. J Spinal Disord Tech 15:537–541

Cohen SP, Larkin T, Abdi S, Chang A, Stojanovic M (2003) Risk factors for failure and complications of intradiscal electrothermal therapy: a pilot study. Spine 28:1142–1147

Coppes MH, Marani E, Thomeer RT, Groen GJ (1997) Innervation of "painful" lumbar discs. Spine 22:2342–2349; discussion 2349–2350

D'Aprile P, Tarantino A, Jinkins JR, Brindicci D (2007) The value of fat saturation sequences and contrast medium administration in MRI of degenerative disease of the posterior/perispinal elements of the lumbosacral spine. Eur Radiol 17:523–531

Darmoul M, Bouhaouala MH, Rezgui M (2005) Calcification following intradiscal injection, a continuing problem? Presse Med 34:859–860

Davis TT, Delamarter RB, Sra P, Goldstein TB (2004) The IDET procedure for chronic discogenic low back pain. Spine 29:752–756

Destouet JM, Gilula LA, Murphy WA, Monsees B (1982) Lumbar facet joint injection: indication, technique, clinical correlation, and preliminary results. Radiology 145:321–325

Djurasovic M, Glassman SD, Dimar JR, Johnson JR (2002) Vertebral osteonecrosis associated with the use of intradiscal electrothermal therapy: a case report. Spine 27:E325–328

Dussault RG, Kaplan PA, Anderson MW (2000) Fluoroscopy-guided sacroiliac joint injections. Radiology 214:273–277

El-Khoury GY, Renfrew DL (1991) Percutaneous procedures for the diagnosis and treatment of lower back pain: diskography, facet-joint injection, and epidural injection. AJR Am J Roentgenol 157:685–691

Elgafy H, Semaan HB, Ebraheim NA, Coombs RJ (2001) Computed tomography findings in patients with sacroiliac pain. Clin Orthop Relat Res 382:112–118

Fayad F, Lefevre-Colau MM, Rannou F, Quintero N, Nys A, Mace Y, Poiraudeau S, Drape JL, Revel M (2007) Relation of inflammatory modic changes to intradiscal steroid injection outcome in chronic low back pain. Eur Spine J 16:925–931

Ferrante FM, King LF, Roche EA, Kim PS, Aranda M, Delaney LR, Mardini IA, Mannes AJ (2001) Radiofrequency sacroiliac joint denervation for sacroiliac syndrome. Reg Anesth Pain Med 26:137–142

Forst SL, Wheeler MT, Fortin JD, Vilensky JA (2006) The sacroiliac joint: anatomy, physiology and clinical significance. Pain Physician 9:61–67

Fortin JD, Kissling RO, O'Connor BL, Vilensky JA (1999) Sacroiliac joint innervation and pain. Am J Orthop 28:687–690

Freeman BJ, Walters RM, Moore RJ, Fraser RD (2003) Does intradiscal electrothermal therapy denervate and repair experimentally induced posterolateral annular tears in an animal model? Spine 28:2602–2608

Freeman BJ, Fraser RD, Cain CM, Hall DJ, Chapple DC (2005) A randomized, double-blind, controlled trial: intradiscal electrothermal therapy versus placebo for the treatment of chronic discogenic low back pain. Spine 30:2369–2377; discussion 2378

Gevargez A, Groenemeyer D, Schirp S, Braun M (2002) CT-guided percutaneous radiofrequency denervation of the sacroiliac joint. Eur Radiol 12:1360–1365

Ghormley R (1933) Low back pain with special reference to the articular facets with presentation of an operative procedure. JAMA 101:1773–1777

Gunaydin I, Pereira PL, Fritz J, Konig C, Kotter I (2006) Magnetic resonance imaging guided corticosteroid injection of sacroiliac joints in patients with spondylarthropathy. Are multiple injections more beneficial? Rheumatol Int 26:396–400

Hanly JG, Mitchell M, MacMillan L, Mosher D, Sutton E (2000) Efficacy of sacroiliac corticosteroid injections in patients with inflammatory spondyloarthropathy: results of a 6 month controlled study. J Rheumatol 27:719–722

Hansen HC, McKenzie-Brown AM, Cohen SP, Swicegood JR, Colson JD, Manchikanti L (2007) Sacroiliac joint interventions: a systematic review. Pain Physician 10:165–184

Helbig T, Lee CK (1988) The lumbar facet syndrome. Spine 13:61–64

Hemminghytt S, Daniels DL, Williams AL, Haughton VM (1982) Intraspinal synovial cysts: natural history and diagnosis by CT. Radiology 145:375–376

Hsu KY, Zucherman JF, Shea WJ, Jeffrey RA (1995) Lumbar intraspinal synovial and ganglion cysts (facet cysts). Ten-year experience in evaluation and treatment. Spine 20:80–89

Jacobs JM, Hammerman-Rozenberg R, Cohen A, Stessman J (2006) Chronic back pain among the elderly: prevalence, associations, and predictors. Spine 31:E203–207

Karabacakoglu A, Karakose S, Ozerbil OM, Odev K (2002) Fluoroscopy-guided intraarticular corticosteroid injection into the sacroiliac joints in patients with ankylosing spondylitis. Acta Radiol 43:425–427

Khan AM, Synnot K, Cammisa FP, Girardi FP (2005) Lumbar synovial cysts of the spine: an evaluation of surgical outcome. J Spinal Disord Tech 18:127–131

Khot A, Bowditch M, Powell J, Sharp D (2004) The use of intradiscal steroid therapy for lumbar spinal discogenic pain: a randomized controlled trial. Spine 29:833–836; discussion 837

Kornick C, Kramarich SS, Lamer TJ, Todd Sitzman B (2004) Complications of lumbar facet radiofrequency denervation. Spine 29:1352–1354

Lam KS, Carlin D, Mulholland RC (2000) Lumbar disc high-intensity zone: the value and significance of provocative discography in the determination of the discogenic pain source. Eur Spine J 9:36–41

Leclaire R, Fortin L, Lambert R, Bergeron YM, Rossignol M (2001) Radiofrequency facet joint denervation in the treatment of low back pain: a placebo-controlled clinical trial to assess efficacy. Spine 26:1411–1416; discussion 1417

Lee MS, Cooper G, Lutz GE, Lutz C, Hong HM (2003) Intradiscal electrothermal therapy (IDET) for treatment of chronic lumbar discogenic pain: a minimum 2-year clinical outcome study. Pain Physician 6:443–448

Lilius G, Laasonen EM, Myllynen P, Harilainen A, Gronlund G (1989) Lumbar facet joint syndrome. A randomised clinical trial. J Bone Joint Surg Br 71:681–684

Lippitt AB (1984) The facet joint and its role in spine pain. Management with facet joint injections. Spine 9:746–750

Lynch MC, Taylor JF (1986) Facet joint injection for low back pain. A clinical study. J Bone Joint Surg Br 68:138–141

Manchikanti L, Singh V, Vilims BD, Hansen HC, Schultz DM, Kloth DS (2002) Medial branch neurotomy in management of chronic spinal pain: systematic review of the evidence. Pain Physician 5:405–418

McCulloch JA (1976) Percutaneous radiofrequency lumbar rhizolysis (rhizotomy). Appl Neurophysiol 39:87–96

McKenzie-Brown AM, Shah RV, Sehgal N, Everett CR (2005) A systematic review of sacroiliac joint interventions. Pain Physician 8:115–125

Mikeladze G, Espinal R, Finnegan R, Routon J, Martin D (2003) Pulsed radiofrequency application in treatment of chronic zygapophyseal joint pain. Spine J 3:360–362

Modic MT, Steinberg PM, Ross JS, Masaryk TJ, Carter JR (1988) Degenerative disk disease: assessment of changes in vertebral body marrow with MR imaging. Radiology 166:193–199

Ohtori S, Inoue G, Ito T, Koshi T, Ozawa T, Doya H, Saito T, Moriya H, Takahashi K (2006) Tumor necrosis factor-immunoreactive cells and PGP 9.5-immunoreactive nerve fibers in vertebral endplates of patients with discogenic low back pain and Modic type 1 or type 2 changes on MRI. Spine 31:1026–1031

Orpen NM, Birch NC (2003) Delayed presentation of septic arthritis of a lumbar facet joint after diagnostic facet joint injection. J Spinal Disord Tech 16:285–287

Parlier-Cuau C, Wybier M, Nizard R, Champsaur P, Le Hir P, Laredo JD (1999) Symptomatic lumbar facet joint synovial cysts: clinical assessment of facet joint steroid injection after 1 and 6 months and long-term follow-up in 30 patients. Radiology 210:509–513

Pauza KJ, Howell S, Dreyfuss P, Peloza JH, Dawson K, Bogduk N (2004) A randomized, placebo-controlled trial of intradiscal electrothermal therapy for the treatment of discogenic low back pain. Spine J 4:27–35

Peng B, Hou S, Wu W, Zhang C, Yang Y (2006a) The pathogenesis and clinical significance of a high-intensity zone (HIZ) of lumbar intervertebral disc on MR imaging in the patient with discogenic low back pain. Eur Spine J 15:583–587

Peng B, Hao J, Hou S, Wu W, Jiang D, Fu X, Yang Y (2006b) Possible pathogenesis of painful intervertebral disc degeneration. Spine 31:560–566

Pereira PL, Gunaydin I, Duda SH, Trubenbach J, Remy CT, Kotter I, Kastler B, Claussen CD (2000) Corticosteroid injections of the sacroiliac joint during magnetic resonance: preliminary results. J Radiol 81:223–226

Pulisetti D, Ebraheim NA (1999) CT-guided sacroiliac joint injections. J Spinal Disord 12:310–312

Revel M, Poiraudeau S, Auleley GR, Payan C, Denke A, Nguyen M, Chevrot A, Fermanian J (1998) Capacity of the clinical picture to characterize low back pain relieved by facet joint anesthesia. Proposed criteria to identify patients with painful facet joints. Spine 23:1972–1976; discussion 1977

Rosenberg JM, Quint TJ, de Rosayro AM (2000) Computerized tomographic localization of clinically-guided sacroiliac joint injections. Clin J Pain 16:18–21

Saal JA, Saal JS (2000a) Intradiscal electrothermal treatment for chronic discogenic low back pain: a prospective outcome study with minimum 1-year follow-up. Spine 25:2622–2627

Saal JS, Saal JA (2000b) Management of chronic discogenic low back pain with a thermal intradiscal catheter. A preliminary report. Spine 25:382–388

Sauvage P, Grimault L, Ben Salem D, Roussin I, Huguenin M, Falconnet M (2000) Lumbar intraspinal synovial cysts: imaging and treatment by percutaneous injection. Report of thirteen cases. J Radiol 81:33–38

Schellhas KP, Pollei SR, Gundry CR, Heithoff KB (1996) Lumbar disc high-intensity zone. Correlation of magnetic resonance imaging and discography. Spine 21:79–86

Schofferman J, Kine G (2004) Effectiveness of repeated radiofrequency neurotomy for lumbar facet pain. Spine 29:2471–2473

Schulte TL, Pietila TA, Heidenreich J, Brock M, Stendel R (2006) Injection therapy of lumbar facet syndrome: a prospective study. Acta Neurochir (Wien) 148:1165–1172

Shih C, Lin GY, Yueh KC, Lin JJ (2005) Lumbar zygapophyseal joint injections in patients with chronic lower back pain. J Chin Med Assoc 68:59–64

Silvers HR (1990) Lumbar percutaneous facet rhizotomy. Spine 15:36–40

Slipman CW, Jackson HB, Lipetz JS, Chan KT, Lenrow D, Vresilovic EJ (2000) Sacroiliac joint pain referral zones. Arch Phys Med Rehabil 81:334–338

Stallmeyer MJ, Ortiz AO (2002) Facet blocks and sacroiliac joint injections. Tech Vasc Interv Radiol 5:201–206

Tekin I, Mirzai H, Ok G, Erbuyun K, Vatansever D (2007) A comparison of conventional and pulsed radiofrequency denervation in the treatment of chronic facet joint pain. Clin J Pain 23:524–529

Urrutia G, Kovacs F, Nishishinya MB, Olabe J (2007) Percutaneous thermocoagulation intradiscal techniques for discogenic low back pain. Spine 32:1146–1154

Vallejo R, Benyamin RM, Kramer J, Stanton G, Joseph NJ (2006) Pulsed radiofrequency denervation for the treatment of sacroiliac joint syndrome. Pain Med 7:429–434

Wang JC, Kabo JM, Tsou PM, Halevi L, Shamie AN (2005) The effect of uniform heating on the biomechanical properties of the intervertebral disc in a porcine model. Spine J 5:64–70

Yin W, Willard F, Carreiro J, Dreyfuss P (2003) Sensory stimulation-guided sacroiliac joint radiofrequency neurotomy: technique based on neuroanatomy of the dorsal sacral plexus. Spine 28:2419–2425

Percutaneous Interventions

in the Management of Soft Tissue Conditions

10

DAVID MALFAIR and PETER L. MUNK

CONTENTS

10.1   **Introduction**   *179*

10.2   **General Principles**   *180*

10.3   **Cystic Masses in the Soft Tissues**   *180*
10.3.1   General   *180*
10.3.2   Abscess   *181*
10.3.2.1 Rationale and Patient Selection   *181*
10.3.2.2 Procedure   *181*
10.3.3   Subacromial-Subdeltoid Bursitis   *182*
10.3.3.1 Anatomic Considerations   *182*
10.3.3.2 Rationale and Patient Selection   *182*
10.3.3.3 Procedure   *183*
10.3.4   Olecranon Bursitis   *183*
10.3.4.1 Rationale and Patient Selection   *183*
10.3.4.2 Procedure   *183*
10.3.5   Greater Trochanteric Bursitis   *184*
10.3.5.1 Rationale and Patient Selection   *184*
10.3.5.2 Procedure   *184*
10.3.6   Retrocalcaneal and Achilles Bursitis   *184*
10.3.6.1 Rationale and Patient Selection   *184*
10.3.6.2 Procedure   *185*
10.3.7   Ganglion Cysts   *185*
10.3.7.1 Rationale and Patient Selection   *185*
10.3.7.2 Procedure   *185*

10.4   **Tendons**   *186*
10.4.1   Tendinosis   *186*
10.4.1.1 Rationale and Patient Selection   *186*
10.4.1.2 Procedure   *187*
10.4.2   Tenosynovitis and Tenography   *187*
10.4.2.1 Rationale and Patient Selection   *187*
10.4.2.2 Procedure   *187*

10.4.3   Calcific Tendinosis   *188*
10.4.3.1 Anatomic Considerations   *188*
10.4.3.2 Rationale and Patient Selection   *188*
10.4.3.3 Ultrasound Procedure   *191*
10.4.3.4 Fluoroscopic Procedure   *191*

10.5   **Snapping Hip**   *192*
10.5.1   Rationale and Patient Selection   *192*
10.5.2   Procedure   *193*

10.6   **Muscle**   *193*
10.6.1   Piriformis Syndrome   *193*
10.6.1.1 Anatomic Considerations   *193*
10.6.1.2 Rationale and Patient Selection   *194*
10.6.1.3 Procedure   *195*

10.7   **Conclusion**   *195*

      References   *196*

D. MALFAIR, MD, FRCPC, Assistant Professor
P. L. MUNK, MD, CM, FRCPC, Professor and Head,
Musculoskeletal Division
Department of Radiology, Vancouver General Hospital,
University of British Columbia, 899 West 12th Avenue,
Vancouver, BC V5Z 1M9, Canada

10.1
Introduction

Over the past several decades a wide variety of diagnostic and therapeutic imaging-guided interventions have been developed. Initially these were performed under fluoroscopy, and changed little until newer modalities emerged. The use of computed tomography (CT) and ultrasound, among others, has led to new and still evolving techniques for percutaneous treatment of soft tissue disorders. Ultrasound has proven particularly well-suited to these tasks, as it provides multiplanar imaging of the target with real-time visualization of the needle and its relationship to adjacent tendons and neurovascular structures. This chapter provides an overview of common diagnostic and therapeutic imaging-guided soft tissue musculoskeletal interventions.

10.2
General Principles

Most of the treatments described here share common features in terms of preparation and basic technique. Relevant imaging should be reviewed prior to the procedure to confirm the clinical diagnosis, rule out other causes of symptoms and to assist planning. General contraindications to percutaneous treatment include bleeding diathesis, allergies (i.e., contrast, local anesthetics) and the presence of skin infection. A brief interview with the patient should review the characteristics, duration and severity of the presenting clinical problem. Informed consent is procedure-specific but should always include the risk of bleeding, infection and allergy to local anesthetic.

Any time corticosteroids are injected, local and systemic complications should be discussed. The most important local complication is the risk of tendon rupture in the case of tendinous or peritendinous injection (Kleinman and Gross 1983). Other local soft tissue complications may include cosmetic changes such as local atrophy, alopecia, telangectasia and depigmentation. Diabetic patients may experience transient elevation of blood sugar levels.

Proper positioning permits both patient comfort and optimal anatomic access for the procedure. Initial imaging with CT, ultrasound or fluoroscopy is performed with careful attention to the entry site and the appropriate trajectory of the needle. The procedure is carried out under sterile conditions using local anesthetic. Occasionally some patients may also require mild sedation. Changes in symptoms should be documented (e.g., pain relief after injection of local anesthetic). Instructions on preventing and recognizing complications should be reiterated.

10.3
Cystic Masses in the Soft Tissues

10.3.1
General

Ultrasound is the modality of choice for diagnosing and guiding percutaneous therapy of superficial cystic masses, including abscesses, hematomas, ganglia and bursae. A high frequency linear probe is ideal for imaging such lesions. Cystic masses are characteristically anechoic or hypoechoic, with increased through-transmission (Fig. 10.1). Occasionally, a cyst may contain hyperechoic contents. In these cases, increased through-transmission, and fluctuance with compression, confirm its cystic nature. Power Doppler should always be used with ultrasound prior to aspirations to exclude vascular causes of a pseudocystic lesion, such as an aneurysm.

Many of these structures are amenable to clinical percutaneous treatment using surface anatomy and direct palpation. Advantages of ultrasound include increased accuracy in needle placement with real-time visualization of injection and aspiration. Superficial structures such as tendons and vessels are also more easily avoided.

A curvilinear ultrasound probe is useful for deep cystic lesions. CT guidance may be necessary in patients when a deep mass is poorly visualized by any sonographic technique (Fig. 10.2). Fluoroscopy may be a useful adjunct to ultrasound when placing a drain or dilating a tract over a wire. Injections of some deep bursae such as the subacromial and greater trochanteric bursae can be performed under fluoroscopy. While these are amenable to ultrasound treatment, fluoroscopic visualization of the entire bursa as it fills with contrast provides excellent confirmation of correct placement, as well as additional anatomic information.

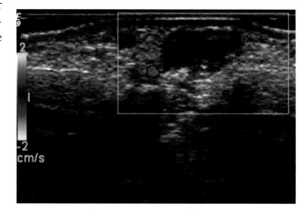

Fig. 10.1. Ganglion cyst dorsal to metacarpals in a 53-year-old woman. Sagittal ultrasound image demonstrates an anechoic uniform collection. Fluctuance with palpation and posterior acoustic enhancement confirms its cystic nature

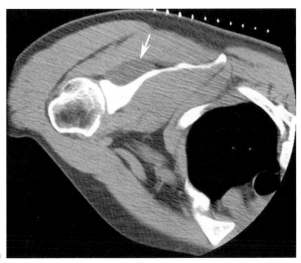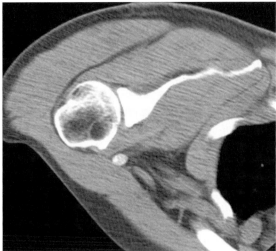

Fig. 10.2a,b. CT-guided paralabral cyst injection in a 41-year-old woman. Axial CT scans of the right shoulder show a para-labral cyst (*arrow*) (**a**) before and (**b**) after treatment. The cyst was aspirated and 40 mg of triamcinolone injected

10.3.2
Abscess

10.3.2.1
Rationale and Patient Selection

Soft tissue infections are a common problem often caused by trauma, a foreign body, osteomyelitis or immunosuppression. Most soft tissue infections are uncomplicated and are easily treated with antibiotics. When infections form abscesses, it is difficult to achieve a therapeutic concentration of antibiotic within these collections. Percutaneous drainage of an abscess provides microbial sensitivities and assists therapy by removing the collected fluid that is poorly treated by antibiotics alone.

Ultrasound is the modality of choice for diagnosing and guiding percutaneous therapy of soft tissue abscesses. It easily identifies a cystic collection within areas of subcutaneous edema. CT is also an effective imaging modality for these purposes (STRUK et al. 2001). Associated gas within an abscess causes "dirty" shadowing on ultrasound, which may be correlated with radiographs or CT. It should be noted that, in some circumstances such as pyomyositis, there may be more than one abscess.

10.3.2.2
Procedure

After routine preparation, an 18-gauge needle is used for aspiration of the frequently viscous material un-

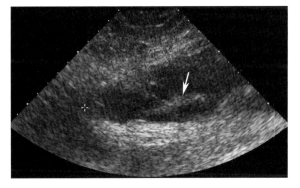

Fig. 10.3. Soft tissue abscess in a 26-year-old man. Sagittal ultrasound image shows an 18-gauge needle (*arrow*) placed within the abscess. Pus was aspirated and sent for culture and sensitivities

der imaging guidance. After pus has been aspirated for diagnostic confirmation and microbial sensitivities, there are several options. For small collections, the abscess may be nearly completely drained via the 18-gauge needle (Fig. 10.3). This process may be improved by lavage with sterile normal saline. For larger collections, often in the hip or buttock, placement of a drainage catheter is required. A guide wire is placed into the abscess through the 18-gauge needle. The wire is looped within the collection, and serial dilation of the tract is performed. A 10-French or larger drainage catheter is recommended because it is less likely to be obstructed by the viscous material (Fig. 10.4).

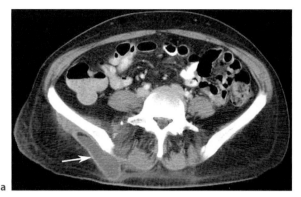
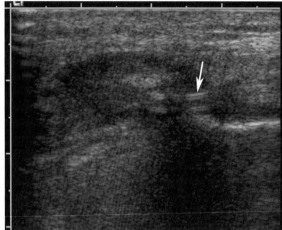

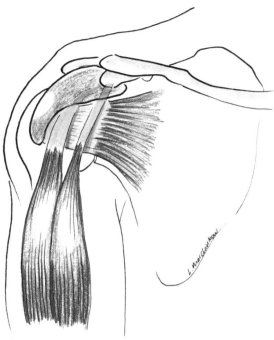

Fig. 10.5. Subacromial bursa. The subacromial bursa lies between the acromion and joint capsule. It extends laterally 2 cm distal to the greater tuberosity. In 95% of cases it is continuous with the subdeltoid bursa, and continues inferiorly to the level of the surgical neck of the humerus

Fig. 10.4a,b. Abscess in a 41-year-old woman. **a** Axial CT scan shows the abscess (*arrow*) posterior to right iliac crest. **b** The abscess was drained under ultrasound, and a 10-French drainage catheter was placed (*arrow*)

10.3.3
Subacromial-Subdeltoid Bursitis

10.3.3.1
Anatomic Considerations

The subacromial bursa lies just inferior to the acromioclavicular joint. Its chief function is to protect the rotator cuff from friction with the adjacent coracoacromial arch and deltoid muscle. It normally extends from the coracoid process medially to a variable distance laterally, as much as 3 cm below the greater tuberosity (Fig. 10.5) (PETERSILGE et al. 1993). The bursa often contains only minimal fluid. Pathologic causes of increased fluid within this potential space include bursitis secondary to impingement, glenohumeral instability, tendinopathy of the rotator cuff and full thickness cuff tears.

10.3.3.2
Rationale and Patient Selection

Patients with rotator impingement and tendinosis often have increased pain with activity worsening abduction. The pain is usually focal, just under the acromion. The usefulness of subacromial injections in the treatment of impingement syndrome is controversial. Some authors have found that injection with local anesthetic and steroids improves symptoms on an acute and subacute basis (AKGUN et al. 2004). Others have reported that injections did not help in blinded prospective trials (BLAIR et al. 1996; MCINERNEY et al. 2003). These studies did not use imaging guidance for subacromial injections. Ultrasound-guided injection has been shown to be more efficacious than blind injection (NAREDO et al. 2004). The injection of steroids is best performed in close consultation with the referring physician.

The subacromial bursa is also injected for purposes other than the treatment of impingement. Injection of local anesthetic into this bursa is an important adjunct to the percutaneous treatment of calcific tendinosis (section 10.4.3). Aspiration also may be required to rule out infection or crystal arthropathy.

10.3.3.3
Procedure

The subacromial bursa is amenable to injection using either ultrasound or fluoroscopic guidance. Ultrasound has many advantages, including real-time positioning with the needle under the acromion, and visualization of soft tissue structures. Fluoroscopy is preferred at some institutions, as it allows visualization of the contrast as it pools in the bursa.

The patient is placed in a supine position with the imaging intensifier over the shoulder. A lateral approach is often taken at a level just inferior to the lateral aspect of the acromion. As local anesthetic is injected, the 25-gauge needle is directed just under the surface of the acromion. At the level of the acromion, local anesthetic flows freely with little resistance. Next, 2 ml of contrast (Optiray) is injected under fluoroscopic guidance to confirm correct placement (Fig. 10.6), followed by injection with 40 mg of triamcinolone and 5 ml of 0.5% marcaine. Post-injection fluoroscopy confirms dilution of the initial contrast bolus within the bursa. The patient is reminded of possible complications, such as infection, and told to document changes in symptoms.

10.3.4
Olecranon Bursitis

10.3.4.1
Rationale and Patient Selection

The olecranon bursa lies just superficial to the proximal ulna, adjacent to the triceps attachment. This bursa is most commonly inflamed secondary to chronic mechanical irritation. Other causes include acute trauma, infection and systemic inflammatory processes such as gout. In cases where there is a history of trauma, plain radiographs should be obtained to rule out an associated fracture. Aspiration is often indicated to rule out infection or crystal arthropathy. In addition to standard complications, patients should be advised of possible recurrence of swelling and occasional fistulous connection with the skin.

10.3.4.2
Procedure

Ultrasound examination confirms a cystic mass just superficial to the olecranon. After routine preparation, an 18-gauge needle is inserted into the cystic mass under direct sonographic visualization. A posterolateral approach is recommended to avoid the ulnar nerve. A "zigzag" needle path may reduce the incidence of fistulous connection to the skin. Aspirated fluid can be tested for microbes or crystals. Removal of fluid often reduces symptoms caused by local pressure effects. If the collection recurs, repeat aspiration with steroid injection may be indicated.

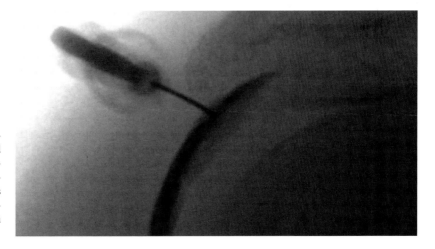

Fig. 10.6. Subacromial-subdeltoid bursitis in a 48-year-old man. Fluoroscopy-guided subacromial-subdeltoid bursa injection image shows the contrast is smoothly distributed in the expected curvilinear distribution of the bursa

10.3.5
Greater Trochanteric Bursitis

10.3.5.1
Rationale and Patient Selection

The greater trochanteric bursa lies just superficial to the greater trochanter of the femur. It is most commonly inflamed by repetitive trauma. Chronic friction with the adjacent iliotibial band or gluteus medius muscle may be seen in runners and in patients with leg length discrepancy. Other common causes include acute trauma, rheumatoid arthritis and previous lateral hip surgery. Patients complain of point tenderness at the greater trochanter that worsens during external rotation of the hip. Radiographs of the pelvis should be obtained prior to the procedure to rule out other causes of symptoms such as trauma, hip arthropathy or primary bone lesion. If rest, ice and NSAIDs are insufficient to treat the bursitis, percutaneous injection of steroids has been shown to relieve symptoms (SHBEEB et al. 1996). Injection accuracy improves with the use of fluoroscopy (COHEN et al. 2005). Standard informed consent is obtained, including complications of steroid administration and the possibility of continued or recurrent symptoms.

10.3.5.2
Procedure

After routine preparation, a 22-gauge spinal needle is placed with its tip against the greater trochanter from a lateral approach using fluoroscopic or ultrasound guidance. As the needle is removed from the bony surface, a free flow of anesthetic signifies entry into the bursa. This can be confirmed with the injection of contrast (Optiray) under fluoroscopic visualization. Next, 40 mg of triamcinolone and 5 ml of 0.5% marcaine are injected. Post-injection images demonstrate dispersion of contrast within the distended bursa (Fig. 10.7).

10.3.6
Retrocalcaneal and Achilles Bursitis

10.3.6.1
Rationale and Patient Selection

Two bursae are closely related to the Achilles tendon near its calcaneal insertion. The Achilles bursa is found just superficial to the tendon, while the retrocalcaneal bursa lies between the tendon and posterior calcaneus (Fig. 10.8). These bursae are most

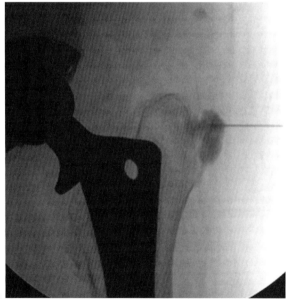 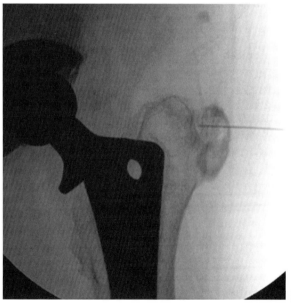

Fig. 10.7a,b. Trochanteric bursitis in a 68-year-old woman. **a** Anteroposterior radiograph shows a 22-gauge spinal needle opacifies the greater trochanteric bursa. **b** Correct placement can be distinguished from intratendinous injection by the ease of infiltration and the dispersion of contrast with steroids

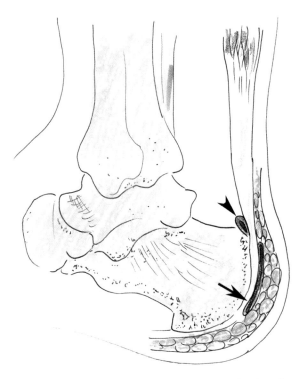

Fig. 10.8. The Achilles bursa (*arrow*) is superficial to the Achilles tendon and easily injected. The retrocalcaneal bursa is deep to the tendon (*arrowhead*) and is best injected via a lateral approach

commonly inflamed secondary to chronic mechanical irritation, including repetitive movements such as jogging. Tight shoes are another common cause of bursitis in this region. Other causes include systemic conditions such as gout and rheumatoid arthritis.

Most of these patients have symptomatic improvement with conservative therapy such as rest, NSAIDs and different shoes. In patients who do not improve with conservative measures, percutaneous steroids improve symptoms. Careful consultation with the referring specialist and the patient is recommended prior to steroid injection because of the reported risk of Achilles tendon rupture. In cases where the posterior heel pain is not directly attributable to the Achilles tendon, plain films are recommended to rule out a calcaneal stress fracture.

10.3.6.2
Procedure

Ultrasound may show an inflamed retrocalcaneal or Achilles bursa. More than 3 mm of fluid within the retrocalcaneal bursa is pathologic (FESSEL and VON HOLSBEECK 1998). Power Doppler may identify as-

sociated inflammation surrounding the cystic component of the bursa. In all cases, the Achilles tendon should be closely examined for any partial tear. The presence of a partial tear contraindicates steroid treatment. Associated tendinosis of the Achilles is a common finding.

A 22-gauge needle is placed within the cystic structure under direct ultrasound guidance. A lateral approach is preferred to avoid the neurovascular bundle. Aspiration is attempted to rule out gout or infection. A 1:1 combination of triamcinolone and 0.5% marcaine is then injected under direct visualization. This mixture is echogenic and is seen to disperse throughout the anechoic bursa. Patients should be advised to avoid strenuous activity until clearance from their referring physician.

10.3.7
Ganglion Cysts

10.3.7.1
Rationale and Patient Selection

Ganglia are the most common soft tissue masses of the wrist, and are most frequently found just dorsal to the scapholunate joint. The volar aspect of the wrist, the DIP joints and the ankle are also common locations. Ganglion cysts are often asymptomatic but may present with pain or sensation of fullness. The patient's main complaint is often cosmetic.

Numerous studies demonstrate successful percutaneous treatment of ganglia. In most studies, ganglion injection with local anesthetic and steroid gives a 60%–80% cure rate (HOLM and PANDEY 1973). Patients considering treatment should be advised of routine complications. Chances of local steroid effect, such as atrophy and depigmentation, should be emphasized. These complications are potentially less likely with injection under direct sonographic vision. Ultrasound is an ideal modality in patients with small, symptomatic ganglia that are difficult to palpate clinically. Surgery remains the definitive treatment.

10.3.7.2
Procedure

After routine preparation, a 20-gauge needle is placed with its tip within the ganglion using sonographic visualization. If the ganglion is greater than 6 mm, aspiration is attempted. The thick gelatinous material may be difficult to aspirate and an 18-gauge needle may be required. After aspiration, a 1–2 ml mixture of equal parts 0.5% marcaine and 40 mg/ml triamcinolone is injected. Ultrasound shows dispersion of the echogenic mixture throughout the ganglion. A larger volume of steroid is needed for larger ganglia involving the ankle or knee (Fig. 10.9).

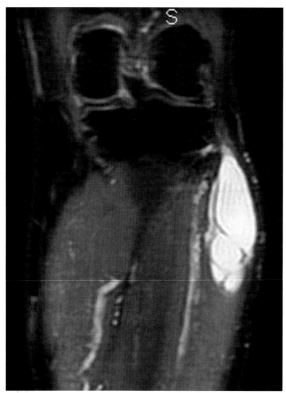

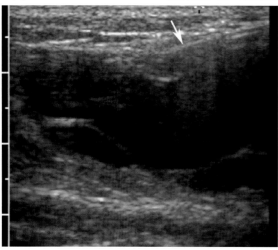

Fig. 10.9a,b. Tibiofibular ganglion cyst in a 37-year-old man. **a** Coronal T2-weighted MR image of the left knee demonstrates a multiseptated ganglion arising from the tibiofibular joint. **b** The patient was symptomatic, and needle (*arrow*) aspiration and injection with steroid yielded good results

10.4.1
Tendinosis

10.4.1.1
Rationale and Patient Selection

Repetitive movement of a joint often leads to chronically painful tendons. Poorly conditioned athletes just beginning an exercise program are especially at risk. The Achilles and patellar tendons are most often affected. Other common sites include the rotator cuff tendons, the flexor and extensor tendons of the forearm and the posterior tibial tendon. Tendinosis is likely caused by numerous microscopic mechanical disruptions. How these microtears lead to painful symptoms is a matter of debate. Many authors maintain that pain in tendinosis is secondary to inflammation (KOENIG et al. 2004). They believe that judicious treatment with intratendinous corticosteroids is warranted and has been shown to be effective. Other authors postulate that the pain is caused by the neurovascular ingrowth found in chronic tendinosis (ALFREDSON et al. 2003). Early data on percutaneous sclerosants that reduce this vascular ingrowth have shown promise in reducing pain (OHBERG and ALFREDSON 2003). Intratendinous injections of sclerosants or steroid require close consultation with the referring physician.

Initial management is conservative, and includes rest, physiotherapy and anti-inflammatories. If these treatments fail, percutaneous therapy may be necessary. Ultrasound is the modality of choice for injection of tendons. The tendon is usually enlarged, heterogeneously hypoechoic and hyperemic (Fig. 10.10). Focal tenderness is often observed while scanning. The tendon should be carefully inspected for partial or full thickness tears.

Procedure-specific complications include the risk of the injected fluid rupturing the tendon. These ruptures, reported anecdotally, are likely caused by injection of steroid into partially torn tendons. Corticosteroids are known to inhibit collagen synthesis and tendon repair. It is prudent to withhold steroids in a tendon with a visualized partial tear. Other complications of corticosteroids include transient hyperglycemia and local atrophy of skin and soft tissues. Long term complications of injections of sclerosants (polidocanol, dextrose, platelets) are unknown.

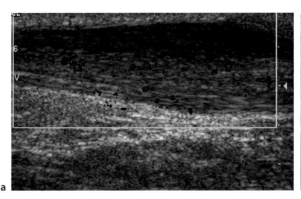 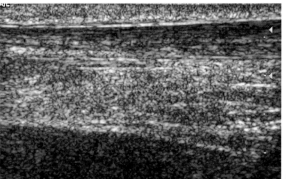

Fig. 10.10a,b. Achilles tendinosis in a 33-year-old man. Longitudinal ultrasound images of (**a**) Achilles tendinosis and (**b**) the normal contralateral Achilles tendon. The abnormal tendon is enlarged, heterogeneous and hyperemic

Other sites of tendinopathy have also responded favorably to percutaneous injection. Lateral epicondylitis has been shown to respond to an injection of autologous blood when traditional conservative therapy failed (EDWARDS and CALANDRUCCIO 2003).

10.4.1.2
Procedure

A diagnostic ultrasound including color Doppler is performed initially. After routine preparation, a 25-gauge needle is placed just ventral to the tendon under direct sonographic visualization using a free hand technique. A medial approach avoids the sural nerve. The needle is placed within the regions of increased vascularity just outside the tendon, and the sclerosant is injected under direct sonographic vision. The process is continued until the abnormal neovascularity is largely diminished or eliminated. After the injection, the patient is asked to report any relief of symptoms.

10.4.2
Tenosynovitis and Tenography

10.4.2.1
Rationale and Patient Selection

Tenosynovitis is inflammation of the tendon and adjacent tendon sheath. It is most commonly found in the tendons of the wrist and the ankle. Predisposing factors include trauma, repetitive motion and infection. Rheumatoid arthritis and psoriasis are also risk factors. Patients complain of local tender-

ness that worsens with activity. Decreased range or motion, chronic pain and loss of smooth movement may also occur.

MR imaging is highly accurate in diagnosing tenosynovitis in patients who are imaged for chronic ankle or wrist pain, and it can assess the integrity of the tendons. In experienced hands ultrasound can provide similar information. The presence of fluid surrounding the tendons can be documented, and image-guided aspiration can help rule out infection. Ultrasound-guided injection of steroids has been shown to be effective in de Quervain tenosynovitis (KAMEL et al. 2002). Tenography may also be used as an alternative to ultrasound to confirm and treat tenosynovitis, especially in the ankle tendons.

Initial treatments for noninfectious causes of tenosynovitis include rest and NSAIDs. If this is unsuccessful, an anesthetic/steroid injection should improve symptoms as well as confirm the diagnosis. Therapeutic effects likely result from anti-inflammatory properties of the steroids and the mechanical disruption of adhesions during distention of the tendon sheath. Published studies show a 50% remission rate after injecting the tendon sheath with steroids (JAFFE et al. 2001). When infection is a consideration, ultrasound-guided aspiration is often indicated to obtain culture and sensitivities.

10.4.2.2
Procedure

Ultrasound-guided aspiration is ideal for tenosynovitis when the main purpose of the procedure is to obtain fluid for culture and sensitivity (Fig. 10.11). A 22-gauge needle is adequate for this indication. This technique is useful for fluid sampling, espe-

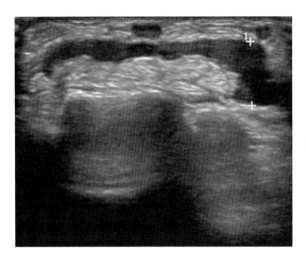

Fig. 10.11. Flexor tendonitis of the wrist in a 24-year-old woman. Transverse ultrasound image of the wrist demonstrates fluid around the flexor tendons. The patient had fluid aspirated with no evidence of infection

cially in the tendons of the wrist. However, if a diagnostic and therapeutic injection is required, fluoroscopy can better demonstrate an endpoint for contrast administration. Increased resistance to fluid administration may be due to adhesions rather than a completely distended tendon sheath. Fluoroscopy demonstrates peritendinous adhesions, which can at times be disrupted by increased syringe pressure under direct visualization. Complete tendon sheath distension is the end point for contrast administration.

A tenogram demonstrates inflammation by the presence and severity of sacculations, irregularities and stenoses (JAFFE et al. 2001). Extrinsic masses may also be observed impinging on the tendons. Normal narrowing of the tendon sheath is secondary to overlying retinaculae and should not be mistaken for a pathologic process (SCHREIBMAN 2004). Percutaneous treatment is often curative for chronic tenosynovitis. Recalcitrant cases may require surgical debridement.

Under sterile conditions, a 25-gauge needle filled with local anesthetic and contrast is placed directly into the tendon. As the needle is withdrawn, free flow of the mixture signifies that the needle tip was within the tendon sheath. Correct placement is confirmed with fluoroscopy.

Localization of the correct tendon can be performed using surface anatomy or ultrasound. The posterior tibial tendon can be palpated just superior to the medial malleolus. Contrast should extend to and terminate at the medial process of the navicular

to confirm correct placement. If contrast continues inferiorly below the navicular, the flexor digitorum longus tendon has been opacified. Repositioning of the needle anteriorly with re-injection of the contrast/anesthetic solution will opacify the posterior tibial tendon sheath.

The common peroneal tendon sheath is found just posterior to the lateral malleolus. The common tendon sheath divides into the peroneus brevis, which terminates on the base of the fifth metatarsal, and the peroneus longus, which continues to attach to the inferior surface of numerous tarsal bones (Fig. 10.12).

Usually, 6 ml of 0.5% marcaine and 3 ml of Optiray are sufficient. The flow of contrast may be impeded at the site of the adhesions. Increased pressure on the syringe results in adhesion disruption and further filling of the sheath. Injection is continued until the tendon sheath is completely opacified, followed by 1 ml of betamethesone (6 mg/ml) or other steroid. Exertion should be avoided for six weeks after injection to avoid the small but significant risk of tendon rupture.

10.4.3
Calcific Tendinosis

10.4.3.1
Anatomic Considerations

The rotator cuff muscles help stabilize the shoulder joint and assist in abduction and internal and external rotation of the shoulder. The supraspinatus muscle is a conical muscle that originates from the supraspinous fossa of the scapula and attaches to the superior aspect of the greater tuberosity. The infraspinatus and teres minor muscles arise from the infraspinous fossa and attaches to the posterior aspect of the greater tuberosity. The subscapularis arises from the costal margin of the scapula to insert into the lesser tuberosity. Knowledge of the relationship of these tendons and their position on radiographs in internal and external rotation is important in determining the location of periarticular calcifications (RE and KARZEL 1993).

10.4.3.2
Rationale and Patient Selection

Rotator cuff calcification is not uncommon, with an estimated prevalence of 2%–10%. Although the

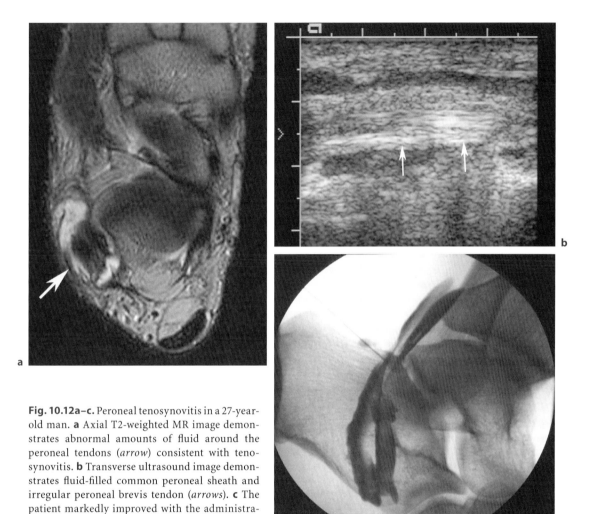

Fig. 10.12a–c. Peroneal tenosynovitis in a 27-year-old man. **a** Axial T2-weighted MR image demonstrates abnormal amounts of fluid around the peroneal tendons (*arrow*) consistent with tenosynovitis. **b** Transverse ultrasound image demonstrates fluid-filled common peroneal sheath and irregular peroneal brevis tendon (*arrows*). **c** The patient markedly improved with the administration of anesthetic and steroid using tenography

process of calcification is not fully understood, some authors propose that it begins with fibrocartilage metaplasia, the formation of chondrocytes from a tenocyte anlage (UHTHOFF and LOEHR 1997). Calcium crystals are deposited in the cartilaginous matrix and coalesce. A dormant phase of calcification occurs with minimal inflammation and symptoms, followed by a resorptive phase marked by the appearance of thin-walled vessels around the calcific deposits. This phase is characterized by local inflammation and calcium resorption, and clinical symptoms are common. Tendons subsequently heal with collagen fiber realignment and resolution of the calcium deposits.

The majority of patients are asymptomatic. Pain is likely caused by direct chemical irritation by the calcium, and local swelling of the tendon with irritation and inflammation. Patients present with point tenderness and pain that is worse at night. Pain from

associated subacromial bursitis and frozen shoulder can complicate the clinical scenario.

Percutaneous aspiration of calcium is an effective treatment for calcific tendonitis. Most studies demonstrate improvement or cure in 60%–70% of patients with intractable pain after aspiration and mechanical disruption of calcific deposits (FARIN et al. 1996). Traditionally, fluoroscopy has assisted image-guided aspiration with good results (PFISTER and GERBER 1997). Ultrasound is also very sensitive for detecting calcific tendinopathy, and is an excellent modality for percutaneous aspiration (Fig. 10.13). The use of a single 22-gauge needle with sonographic guidance has demonstrated marked benefit in patients in whom the calcified crystals are liquid (AINA et al. 2001). Frequently, however, the calcification may be solid and impossible to aspirate. If the crystals cannot be aspirated, mechanical disruption accelerates the process of spontaneous resorption with subsequent improvement in symptoms (MACK et al. 1985).

Calcific tendonitis in other locations is also amenable to percutaneous therapy. Calcific tendonitis associated with bone erosion has been described in the gluteus maximus, rectus femoris and adductor magnus insertions, among others (HAYES et al. 1987). These patients can show dramatic improvement with percutaneous aspiration and steroid injection (Fig. 10.14).

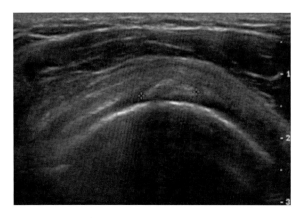

Fig. 10.13. Calcific tendonitis in a 43-year-old woman. Transverse ultrasound image shows calcific deposit near the insertion of the supraspinatus. (Image courtesy of Dr. E. Cardinal)

Lack of symptomatic improvement after percutaneous aspiration may indicate surgery. The procedure of choice is arthroscopy with aspiration of calcium under direct vision using an 18-gauge needle. Acromioplasty should also be considered as adjunctive therapy if there are symptoms of impingement.

Shoulder radiographs should be reviewed prior to the procedure. The calcification should be greater than 5 mm and stable in appearance. Calcific deposits that are decreasing in size and associated with symptom flare are likely to be resorbing spontaneously. A conservative approach is recommended in these patients. Very dense calcifications with clear margins are likely solid and not amenable to aspiration, although they can be mechanically disrupted. Striated calcifications are intratendinous and difficult to aspirate. A soft, calcific density with irregular and faint margins is likely liquid crystal and is more easily aspirated with a small-gauge needle.

Informed consent should include that there is at least a theoretical risk of clinically significant traumatic injury to the tendon, although no reported cases are known to us. The patient should also be counseled that there may be a transient increase in pain during resorption of the mechanically disrupted calcium deposits. When successful, clinical

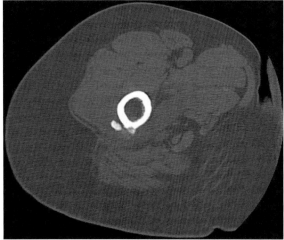

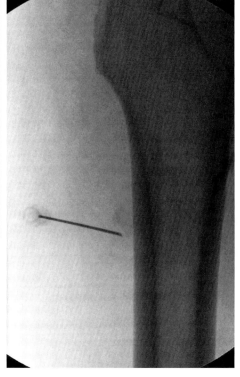

Fig. 10.14a,b. Calcific tendonitis in a 48-year-old woman. **a** Axial CT scan of the right thigh shows gluteus maximus calcific tendinosis. **b** Fluoroscopic-guided aspiration and injection of 40 mg triamcinolone led to dramatic clinical improvement

resolution of symptoms usually occurs within a few weeks of the injection.

10.4.3.3
Ultrasound Procedure

A pre-procedural diagnostic study should be performed to rule out other causes of shoulder pain, such as rotator cuff tears and paralabral cysts. Any calcific deposits are documented by size and location within the tendon. If more than one tendon is involved, the symptomatic lesion is generally associated with tendon swelling, and demonstrates point tenderness.

For supraspinatus and infraspinatus calcifications, the patient is prepped and draped in a seated position. The calcifications are interrogated using a horizontal needle approach in an anteroposterior direction under direct visualization. Subscapularis calcifications are treated in a supine position. A 22-gauge needle is adequate if the calcifications appear to have a paste-like consistency on radiographs. For more well-defined solid calcifications, an 18-gauge needle will give better results with less likelihood of needle blockage.

After the needle is placed within the calcifications, aspiration is attempted using a 10 ml syringe with 1% lidocaine and connection tubing (Fig. 10.15). Gentle mechanical disruption of the deposit is performed, with injection of lidocaine followed by aspiration. Care should be taken to hold the syringe so that calcifications will settle in the syringe and not be re-injected into the joint. If no calcium can be aspirated, the deposit should be disrupted mechanically, which should speed the

resorption process. After maximal aspiration of calcium, the needle is inserted into the subacromial bursa, and 20 mg of triamcinolone and 2 ml of 0.5% marcaine are injected.

10.4.3.4
Fluoroscopic Procedure

For supraspinatus calcifications, the patient is prepped and draped in a supine position with the arm adducted. The image intensifier may be tilted to distinguish the calcium deposit from the horizontal facet of the greater tuberosity. After preparation and local anesthetic, an 18-gauge spinal needle is placed directly within the calcific deposit. Firmness at the needle tip and patient tenderness indicate proper positioning (Fig. 10.16). Location is confirmed with maximal cephalad and caudad projections of the C-arm fluoroscopic unit. The contents are aspirated with a 10 ml syringe filled with 1% lidocaine. The syringe and connecting tube should be held so that the aspirated calcium will settle in the syringe. Syringe

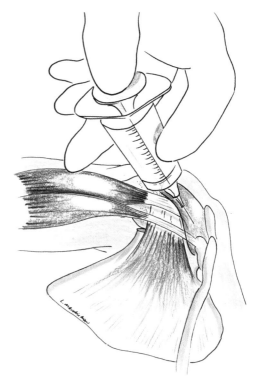

Fig. 10.16. Percutaneous treatment of supraspinatus calcifications. Patient should be in supine position for the treatment. Placement within the calcifications can be palpated by the needle and confirmed using parallax imaging with movement of the gantry

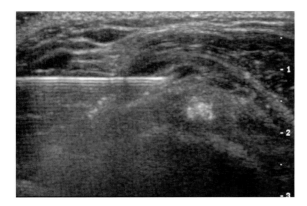

Fig. 10.15. Calcific tendonitis in a 51-year-old man. Transverse ultrasound image of the supraspinatus tendon demonstrates needle aspiration of calcifications. (Image courtesy of Dr. E. Cardinal)

contents may be switched to a sterile saline solution to prevent re-injecting aspirated calcium into the tendon. The procedure should be continued until maximal aspiration of the calcium has occurred. A second parallel needle may be helpful in cases of large, lobulated calcific deposits (Fig. 10.17). If no calcium is aspirated, the needle can be used to mechanically disrupt the mass to assist in spontaneous resorption. After aspiration and disruption of the calcific focus, 20 mg of triamcinolone and 2 ml of 0.5% marcaine are injected into the subacromial bursa.

Radiographs are obtained after the procedure to document reduction in calcium burden. Patients are instructed to keep the shoulder at rest for 5–7 days. Up to one third of patients have significant shoulder pain for 3–5 days, which is treated with ice, NSAIDS and prescription analgesics. These symptoms are generally secondary to continued calcium resorption with resolution of the calcific deposits on subsequent radiographs.

10.5
Snapping Hip

10.5.1
Rationale and Patient Selection

The most common extra-articular cause of a snapping hip occurs laterally when the gluteus medius muscle or iliotibial (IT) band catches on the greater trochanter. This syndrome is easily diagnosed clinically and seldom comes to the attention of the radiologist. The iliopsoas tendon is another cause of an extra-articular snapping hip. As the hip is flexed, the iliopsoas tendon should smoothly track medially. A sudden release and snapping sensation during movement is often noted at the level of the iliopectineal eminence. Common causes of abnormal tracking and catching of the iliopsoas tendon are osteophytes, muscular hypertrophy and tendonosis. Most patients have no associated pain. Iliopsoas

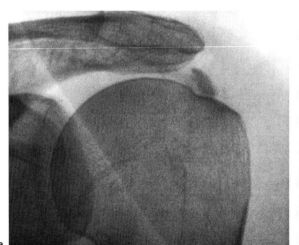

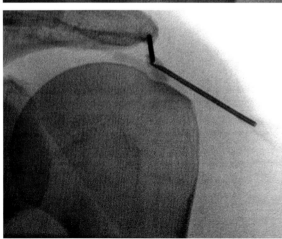

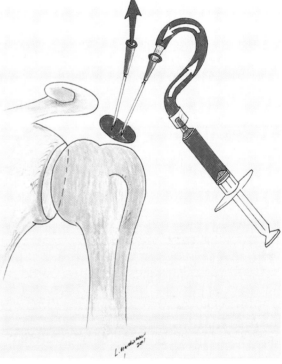

Fig. 10.17a–c. Fluoroscopic aspiration of supraspinatus calcifications in a 59-year-old man. **a** Anteroposterior fluoroscopic image shows calcific deposits within the supraspinatus tendon. **b** Diagram and (**c**) fluoroscopic image demonstrate the two-needle technique, with one needle injecting saline and the second needle aspirating

tendosis is both a cause and a result of abnormal tendon tracking, and is the most common cause of symptoms.

The combination of ultrasound and radiographs is often sufficient pre-procedural imaging for anterior extra-articular snapping hip (WUNDERBALDINGER et al. 2001). Ultrasound will confirm the diagnosis of the abnormal tendon motion. The tendon catches during flexion and suddenly snaps medially as the movement continues. The "snap" is felt at the transducer and may elicit symptoms. Ultrasound will also demonstrate thickening and heterogeneous signal change within the tendon consistent with tendinosis. Plain films and ultrasound will also often show the etiology of the snapping hip, such as osteophytes and aberrant masses in the region. MR imaging can be used for problem-solving purposes.

Diagnosis can also be made by fluoroscopy in two ways. Opacification of the iliopsoas bursa shows the tendon in relief. Its snapping motion can be seen with hip flexion under fluoroscopic vision (VACCARO et al. 1995). Injection of contrast directly into the tendon with subsequent visualization of the tendon movement has also been reported (STAPLE et al. 1988).

At our institution, the diagnosis of anterior snapping hip is usually made clinically. Patients with painful snapping hip refractory to NSAIDs and physiotherapy are referred for percutaneous treatment. Intratendinous injection with local anesthetic and steroids has been shown to relieve symptoms (VACCARO et al. 1995). Patients should be warned of the theoretical risk of injury secondary to intratendinous steroid. Percutaneous therapy sometimes fails, and some patients may require surgical treatment including bursectomy and tendon lengthening.

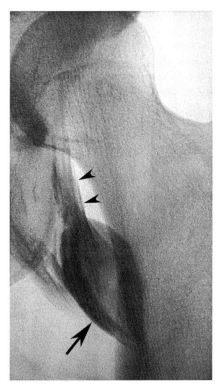

Fig. 10.18. Iliopsoas tendonitis or bursitis in a 29-year old woman. Fluoroscopic-guided injection of the iliopsoas tendon shows contrast outlining the iliopsoas tendon (*arrowheads*) and bursa (*arrow*). The patient experienced dramatic relief of symptoms

patients experience almost immediate improvement of symptoms following this procedure. This occurs despite the fact that the site of fluoroscopic injection is remote from the iliopectineal eminence.

10.5.2
Procedure

The tendon may be injected under either fluoroscopy or ultrasound. A free hand technique with a 22-gauge spinal needle is used with ultrasound. Ultrasound may also show the presence of tendinosis and associated iliopsoas bursitis. The femoral neurovascular bundle must be carefully avoided. The distal iliopsoas tendon may also be injected under fluoroscopy close to its insertion at the lesser trochanter. After confirmation of placement with intratendinous contrast, 20 mg of triamcinolone and 0.5% marcaine are injected (Fig. 10.18). In our experience, many

Muscle

10.6.1
Piriformis Syndrome

10.6.1.1
Anatomic Considerations

The piriformis is a flat triangular muscle that originates from the lateral aspect of the sacrum. It runs inferolaterally out of the greater sciatic notch to insert into the medial aspect of the greater trochanter. Its functions include external rotation during extension and abduction during flexion. The sciatic nerve runs along the pelvic surface of the piriformis and exits the pelvis inferior to the piriformis superior to the superior gemellus (Fig. 10.19).

10.6.1.2
Rationale and Patient Selection

The reported incidence of piriformis syndrome (PS) as a cause of back pain is between 0.3% and 5%. The etiology of PS is incompletely understood. Primary causes of PS relate to intrinsic abnormalities within the piriformis muscle, such as hypertrophy, myositis or post-traumatic adhesions. A history of sitting with a large wallet in the back pocket is often reported. Anatomic variants associated with PS include accessory muscles, anomalous attachments of the piriformis and an aberrant course of part or all of the sciatic nerve (Fig. 10.20) (LEE et al. 2004). Secondary causes of PS include masses near the greater sciatic notch, such as tumors, hematomas and pseudoaneurysms.

Definitive diagnosis of PS cannot be made from pre-operative imaging alone. Impingement of the sciatic nerve is often associated with specific movements, and will not be apparent on static images. In addition, piriformis hypertrophy and anatomic variants are common and often asymptomatic. The most effective method to confirm and treat PS is with a trial of local anesthetic. Transient relief of symptoms confirms the diagnosis of PS. Injection of steroids is also effective (HANANIA and KITAIN 1998). Patients may receive long-term relief from repeated injections of local anesthetic and steroids, and may

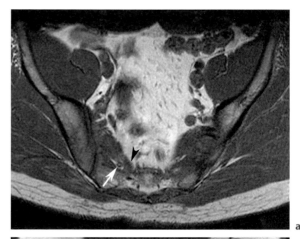
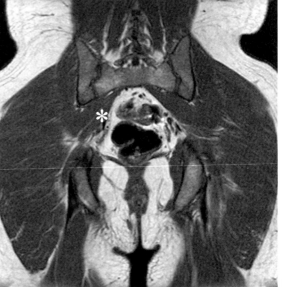

Fig. 10.20a,b. Piriformis syndrome in a 35-year-old woman. **a** Axial and (**b**) coronal T2-weighted MR images demonstrate attachment of an accessory piriformis muscle (*arrowhead*) just medial to the right S2 foramen, resulting in an intermuscular course of the S2 nerve root (*arrow*). Fat is noted between the piriformis and the accessory piriformis (*star*) on the coronal image

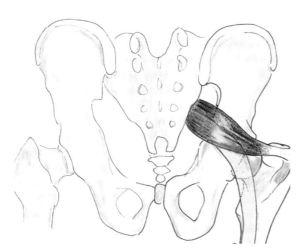

Fig. 10.19. Sciatic nerve exiting inferior to the piriformis

avoid surgery. Recurrent pain transiently relieved by local anesthetic is an indication for surgical release and reattachment of the piriformis. Successful treatment of PS with botulinum toxin has been reported (FANUCCI et al. 2001).

Sciatica caused by PS is characterized by unilateral buttock, trochanteric and posterior leg pain. These symptoms are exacerbated when lying down, sitting for long periods or rising to the standing position. Physical exam findings include pain with 60°

of hip flexion and pain with forceful internal rotation of the flexed hip in a supine patient. Imaging of the spine is prudent to rule out a disc herniation or other central causes of symptoms.

Mass lesions in the greater sciatic notch causing secondary PS on CT prior to injection require further characterization with additional imaging and surgical consultation. Percutaneous treatment is contraindicated in this circumstance. In addition to standard informed consent, the risk of transient leg numbness should be explained, as well as the theoretical possibility of nerve damage. Variations of sciatic nerve anatomy include an accessory branch of the sciatic nerve that courses within the piriformis muscle.

10.6.1.3
Procedure

Attempts to elicit pain with hip flexion and forced internal rotation of the hip should be made before and after the procedure. The patient is imaged in the prone position on CT prior to the procedure. The piriformis and greater sciatic notch should be carefully examined for masses or aberrant anatomy. A 22-gauge spinal needle is advanced into the piriformis under CT guidance. Several options for needle placement are described in the literature, including a tendinous insertion near the greater trochanter or in a perisciatic location (HANANIA and KITAIN 1998). It has been our experience that injection within the muscles of the belly is safer and

equally effective (Fig. 10.21a). After confirmation of placement with CT, 80 mg of triamcinolone and 3 ml of 0.5% marcaine are injected.

Post-injection scans are obtained to document successful muscle infiltration (Fig. 10.21b). This confirmation of intramuscular injection is a major advantage compared to blind or EMG-guided injection. The patient should be carefully evaluated for ipsilateral leg weakness and change in symptoms. Early improvement in PS is often dramatic when the diagnostic block is positive. The patient is instructed to record pain symptoms and document any changes.

10.7
Conclusion

A wide variety of diagnostic and therapeutic imaging-guided interventions are available for the treatment of musculoskeletal disorders. Percutaneous interventions involve ultrasound, fluoroscopic and CT-guided imaging techniques already in common use. With the assistance of these techniques, treatment or therapy can be delivered with extreme preciseness, maximizing the chance of a successful procedure and minimizing patient discomfort. These procedures generally give better results than blind injection or medical therapy alone, and may eliminate the need for surgery.

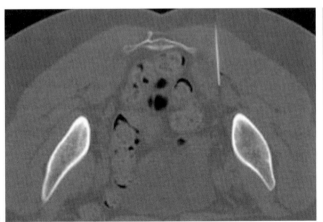 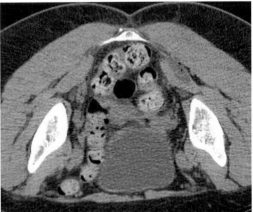

a   b

Fig. 10.21a,b. CT-guided anesthetic injection in a 50-year-old woman. **a** Axial CT scan patient in a prone position shows the needle placed in the left piriformis muscle. **b** Post-injection axial CT scan documents fluid and air within the piriformis muscle, confirming successful injection

References

Aina R, Cardinal E, Bureau NJ, Aubin B, Brassard P (2001) Calcific shoulder tendinitis: treatment with modified US-guided fine-needle technique. Radiology 221:455–461

Akgun K, Birtane M, Akarirmak U (2004) Is local subacromial corticosteroid injection beneficial in subacromial impingement syndrome? Clin Rheumatol 23:496–500

Alfredson H, Ohberg L, Forsgren S (2003) Is vasculo-neural ingrowth the cause of pain in chronic Achilles tendinosis? An investigation using ultrasonography and colour Doppler, immunohistochemistry, and diagnostic injections. Knee Surg Sports Traumatol Arthrosc 11:334–338

Blair B, Rokito AS, Cuomo F, Jarolem K, Zuckerman JD (1996) Efficacy of injections of corticosteroids for subacromial impingement syndrome. J Bone Joint Surgery Am 78:1685–1689

Cohen SP, Narvaez JC, Lebovits AH, Stojanovic MP (2005) Corticosteroid injections for trochanteric bursitis: is fluoroscopy necessary? A pilot study. Br J Anaesth 94:100–106

Edwards SG, Calandruccio JH (2003) Autologous blood injections for refractory lateral epicondylitis. J Hand Surg [Am] 28:272–278

Fanucci E, Masala S, Sodani G, Varrucciu V, Romagnoli A, Squillaci E, Simonetti G (2001) CT-guided injection of botulinic toxin for percutaneous therapy of piriformis muscle syndrome with preliminary MRI results about denervative process. Eur Radiol 11:2543–2548

Farin PU, Rasanen H, Jaroma H, Harju A (1996) Rotator cuff calcifications: treatment with ultrasound-guided percutaneous needle aspiration and lavage. Skeletal Radiol 25:551–554

Fessel DP, von Holsbeeck M (1998) Ultrasound of the foot and ankle. Sem Musc Rad 2:271–281

Hanania M, Kitain E (1998) Perisciatic injection of steroid for the treatment of sciatica due to piriformis syndrome. Reg Anesth Pain Med 23:223–228

Hayes CW, Rosenthal DI, Plata MJ, Hudson TM (1987) Calcific tendinitis in unusual sites associated with cortical bone erosion. AJR Am J Roentgenol 149:967–970

Holm PCA, Pandey SD (1973) Treatment of ganglia of the hand and wrist with aspiration and injection of hydrocortisone. Hand 5:63–68

Jaffee NW, Gilula LA, Wissman RD, Johnson JE (2001) Diagnostic and therapeutic ankle tenography: outcomes and complications. AJR Am J Roentgenol 176:365–371

Kamel M, Moghazy K, Eid H, Mansour R (2002) Ultrasonographic diagnosis of de Quervain's tenosynovitis. Ann Rheum Dis 61:1034–1035

Kleinman M, Gross AE (1983) Achilles tendon rupture following steroid injection. Report of three cases. J Bone Joint Surg Am 65:1356–1357

Koenig MJ, Torp-Pedersen S, Qvistgaard E, Terslev L, Bliddal H (2004) Preliminary results of colour Doppler-guided intratendinous glucocorticoid injection for Achilles tendonitis in five patients. Scand J Med Sci Sports 14:100–106

Lee EY, Margherita AJ, Gierada DS, Narra VR (2004) MRI of piriformis syndrome. AJR Am J Roentgenol 183:63–64

Mack LA, Matsen FA 3rd, Kilcoyne RF, Davies PK, Sickler ME (1985) US evaluation of the rotator cuff. Radiology 157:205–209

McInerney JJ, Dias J, Durham S, Evans A (2003) Randomised controlled trial of single, subacromial injection of methylprednisolone in patients with persistent, post-traumatic impingement of the shoulder. Emerg Med J 20:218–221

Naredo E, Cabero F, Beneyto, P, Cruz A, Mondejar B, Uson, J, Palop MJ, Crespo M (2004) A Randomized Comparative Study of Short Term Response to Blind Injection versus Sonographic Guided Injection of Local Corticosteroids in Patients with Painful Shoulder. J Rheumatol 31:308–314

Ohberg L, Alfredson H (2003) Sclerosing therapy in chronic Achilles tendon insertional pain-results of a pilot study. Knee Surg Sports Traumatol Arthrosc 11:339–343

Petersilge CA, Witte DH, Sewell BO, Bocsh E, Resnick D (1993) Normal Regional Anatomy of the Shoulder. MRI Clin North Am 1:1–18

Pfister J, Gerber H (1997) Chronic calcifying tendinitis of the shoulder-therapy by percutaneous needle aspiration and lavage: a prospective open study of 62 shoulders. Clin Rheumatol 16:269–274

Re LP Jr, Karzel RP (1993) Management of rotator cuff calcifications. Orthop Clin North Am 24:125–132

Schreibman KL (2004) Ankle Tenography: How what and why. Semin Roentgenol 39:95–113

Shbeeb MI, O'Duffy JD, Michet CJ Jr, O'Fallon WM, Matteson EL (1996) Evaluation of glucocorticosteroid injection for the treatment of trochanteric bursitis. J Rheumatol 23:2104–2106

Staple TW, Jung D, Mork A (1988) Snapping tendon syndrome: hip tenography with fluoroscopic monitoring. Radiology 166:873–874

Struk D, Munk PL, Lee M, Ho SG, Worsley D (2001) Imaging of Soft Tissue Infections. Radiol Clin North Am 39:277–303

Uhthoff HK, Loehr JW (1997) Calcific Tendinopathy of the Rotator Cuff: Pathogenesis, Diagnosis, and Management. J Am Acad Orthop Surg 5:183–191

Vaccaro JP, Sauser DD, Beals RK (1995) Iliopsoas bursa imaging: efficacy in depicting abnormal iliopsoas tendon motion in patients with internal snapping hip syndrome. Radiology 197:853–856

Wunderbaldinger P, Bremer C, Matuszewski L, Marten K, Turetschek K, Rand T (2001) Efficient radiological assessment of the internal snapping hip syndrome. Eur Radiol 11:1743–1747

Percutaneous Cementoplasty

Afshin Gangi, Xavier Buy, Farah Irani, Stéphane Guth, Ali Guermazi,
Jean-Pierre Imbert, and Jean-Louis Dietemann

11

CONTENTS

11.1   Introduction   *197*

11.2   **Indications and Contraindications**   *198*
11.2.1   Indications   *198*
11.2.1.1   Osteoporotic Vertebral Compression
Fractures   *198*
11.2.1.2   Osteolytic Metastases and Myeloma   *198*
11.2.1.3   Aggressive Vertebral Hemangiomas   *200*
11.2.1.4   Vertebral Osteonecrosis
(Kummel's Disease)   *200*
11.2.1.5   Traumatic Vertebral Fractures in
Young Patients   *200*
11.2.1.6   Combination with Spine Surgery and
Other Indications   *200*
11.2.2   Contraindications   *204*
11.2.2.1   Absolute Contraindications   *204*
11.2.2.2   Relative Contraindications   *204*

11.3   **Technique of Cementoplasty**   *206*
11.3.1   General Considerations   *206*
11.3.2   Imaging   *207*
11.3.3   Materials   *208*
11.3.3.1   Needles   *208*
11.3.3.2   Cement   *208*
11.3.3.3   Cement Injector   *209*
11.3.4   Image Guidance   *210*
11.3.5   Pre-Procedural Preparation   *210*
11.3.6   Cementoplasty Technique in the
Spine   *211*
11.3.6.1   Basic Mechanics of the
Beveled Needle   *211*
11.3.6.2   Lumbar Vertebroplasty   *211*
11.3.6.3   Thoracic Vertebroplasty   *216*

11.3.6.4   Cervical Vertebroplasty   *220*
11.3.6.5   Sacroplasty   *221*
11.3.7   Technique of Kyphoplasty   *225*
11.3.7.1   Equipment and Technique   *225*
11.3.7.2   Kyphoplasty Advantages and
Drawbacks   *225*
11.3.8   Cementoplasty in Other Locations   *227*
11.3.9   Cement Injection   *227*
11.3.9.1   Choice of Cement   *227*
11.3.9.2   Technique of Cement Injection   *228*
11.3.10   Post-Procedural Care   *230*

11.4   **Review of Indications, Specific Aspects
and Results**   *230*
11.4.1   Osteoporotic Vertebral Fractures   *230*
11.4.2   Bone Tumors   *232*
11.4.3   Aggressive Vertebral Hemangiomas   *232*
11.4.3.1   Therapeutic Options   *236*
11.4.3.2   Results   *237*
11.4.3.3   Treatment Strategy   *240*
11.4.4   Traumatic Vertebral Fractures in
Young Patients   *240*
11.4.5   Surgical Adjuncts and Others   *241*
11.4.6   Complications   *244*
11.4.6.1   Cement Leakage   *246*
11.4.6.2   Infection   *251*
11.4.6.3   Fracture   *252*
11.4.6.4   Allergic Reaction   *252*
11.4.6.5   Adjacent Vertebral Body Collapse   *252*
11.4.6.6   Puncture Site Bleeding   *253*
11.4.6.7   Free Fragment Retropulsion   *253*

11.5   **Conclusion**   *253*

References   *253*

A. Gangi, MD, PhD, Professor of Radiology
X. Buy, MD, Senior Radiologist
F. Irani, MD, Senior Radiologist
S. Guth, MD, Senior Radiologist
J.-P. Imbert, MD, Senior Radiologist
J.-L. Dietemann, MD, Professor
Department of Radiology B, University Hospital of Strasbourg, Pavillon Clovis Vincent BP 426, 67091 Strasbourg, France
A. Guermazi, MD, Associate Professor of Radiology
Department of Radiology, Chief Section of Musculoskeletal, Boston University School of Medicine, 88 East Newton Street, Boston, MA 02118, USA

11.1
Introduction

Percutaneous vertebroplasty is therapeutic, image guided injection of radio-opaque cement into painful, partially collapsed vertebral bodies to splint them internally, and to relieve pain and provide stability. Cement injection can also be used for consolidation and pain management in other locations with compression fractures.

Deramond and Galibert were the first to percutaneously inject acrylic cement into an aggressive vertebral hemangioma (GALIBERT et al. 1987; GANGI et al. 1994). Since then, interest in the technique has grown and many improvements have been made (HIDE and GANGI 2004). Cementoplasty has become a widely accepted procedure for the treatment of many pathological fractures and is supported by abundant peer-reviewed literature.

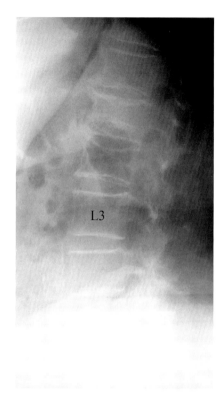

L3

Fig. 11.1. A 58-year-old man with acute pain. Lateral radiograph of the lumbar spine shows L1 and L2 compression fractures. However, it is often difficult to differentiate old from recent fractures with a radiograph. MR imaging is the most accurate imaging for planning a vertebroplasty

11.2
Indications and Contraindications

11.2.1
Indications

There are several specific indications for cementoplasty (GANGI et al. 2003):
- Osteoporotic fractures
- Painful bone tumors
- Aggressive vertebral hemangiomas
- Painful vertebral fractures associated with osteonecrosis (Kummel's disease)
- Traumatic vertebral fractures in young patients
- In combination with bone surgery and others

11.2.1.1
Osteoporotic Vertebral Compression Fractures

Vertebroplasty is now standard practice for treatment of osteoporotic fractures (Fig. 11.1) (GANGI et al. 2006; McGRAW et al. 2003). Previously it was reserved for patients in whom conservative treatment, including rest and analgesics for more than three weeks had failed, or when pain relief required narcotic dosages that produced intolerable sedation, confusion or constipation.

The greater availability of the vertebroplasty procedure and its low complication rates have resulted in more aggressive treatment of these fractures very early in the course of the disease. Early treatment stabilizes the fracture and restores vertebral body strength resulting in pain relief without narcotics or analgesics; the resulting quick return of mobility prevents decubitus complications like deep venous thrombosis, pneumonia and decubitus ulcers (MATHIS et al. 2001; ZOARSKI et al. 2002). Moreover, stopping further collapse of the vertebral body reduces abnormal mechanics of the spine.

BROWN et al. (2004) have proposed aggressive treatment with vertebroplasty of chronic osteoporotic fractures that are over a year old; these patients also benefit from the procedure though results are not as encouraging as treatment of acute fractures. It must be stressed that treatment for the underlying osteoporosis with bisphosphonates, strontium ranelate, Raloxifen and hormone replacement therapy should continue (POOLE and COMPSTON 2006).

11.2.1.2
Osteolytic Metastases and Myeloma

Osteolytic destruction of the vertebral body by metastases from cancers, multiple myeloma and lymphomas is a source of pain and disability. Due to the multifocal nature of these lesions, surgical treatment in the form of vertebrectomy and strut grafting is rarely undertaken (COTTEN et al. 1996b).

Radiation therapy does not provide consolidation, nor does it always relieve pain, and its effects are generally delayed by 1–2 weeks after therapy begins (COTTEN et al. 1998). Percutaneous vertebroplasty with injection of cement allows fast consolidation and restoration of vertebral body strength resulting in effective pain relief and stabilization of the spine. The procedure is palliative and does not stop tumor progression. It is a complement, not a replacement, to other treatment modalities for cancer (JANG and LEE 2005; WEILL et al. 1996). Only painful metastases and lesions affecting the stability of the spine should be treated (GANGI et al. 1998). For painful destruction of the vertebral body with paravertebral tumor extension, vertebroplasty can be combined with thermal ablation techniques, such as radiofrequency ablation or cryoablation, to reduce tumor mass and consolidate the vertebral body (Fig. 11.2) (GANGI et al. 2005, 2006). Vertebroplasty can also be performed at multiple levels according to the multifocal nature of the disease process. However it must be stressed that vertebroplasty is specifically indicated for management of local pain from metastatic disease and not for diffuse back pain with multiregional involvement of the spine. Cementoplasty can be used in other tumoral locations with pathological fracture, i.e. acetabulum, femoral condyles, tibial ends or talus.

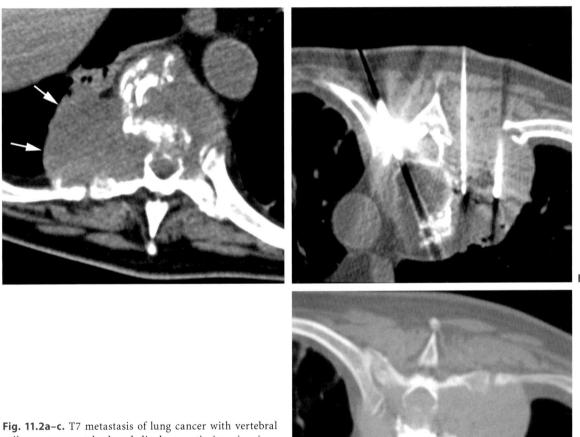

Fig. 11.2a–c. T7 metastasis of lung cancer with vertebral collapse, paravertebral and diaphragmatic invasion in a 50-year-old man, responsible for acute spinal pain with right shoulder irradiation. **a** Axial CT scan shows a large vertebral tumor with right soft tissue extension (*arrows*). **b** Axial CT scan shows bipolar radiofrequency ablation using two electrodes is applied in the right paravertebral mass to control the diaphragmatic pain and a 10-gauge vertebroplasty trocar is inserted via a left intercosto-pedicular approach. **c** Post-procedural axial CT scan shows vertebroplasty has achieved consolidation and bone pain management

11.2.1.3
Aggressive Vertebral Hemangiomas

Vertebral hemangiomas are benign vascular malformations, mainly affecting the vertebral body.
The large majority are asymptomatic and discovered incidentally (Fig. 11.3). Rarely they can be aggressive, affecting the vertebral body and posterior
elements with epidural and paravertebral extension (Figs. 11.4 and 11.5). Aggressive vertebral hemangiomas produce pain in addition to vertebral
instability and cord compression from epidural
extension. Surgery is difficult as they are highly
vascular. Vertebroplasty achieves pain relief, direct
embolization of the vascular malformation and
vertebral strengthening (COTTEN et al. 1998; IDE et
al. 1996). Deramond first described the procedure
of vertebroplasty for the treatment of an aggressive
cervical hemangioma. Patients with hemangiomas
localized to the bone only can be treated with vertebroplasty for direct vascular embolization and
stabilization. However patients with aggressive
hemangiomas, with epidural and/or paravertebral
involvement, require sclerotherapy using Ethibloc
or alcohol first, followed two weeks later by vertebroplasty to avoid secondary collapse of the vertebral body after it has been weakened by injection
of ethanol.

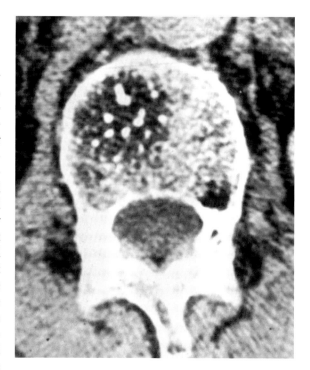

Fig. 11.3. Nonsymptomatic fatty hemangioma at L1 level in a
47-year-old woman. Axial CT scan shows a typical trabecular pattern with large fatty component with negative density
on CT. Fatty hemangiomas do not require any treatment

11.2.1.4
Vertebral Osteonecrosis (Kummel's Disease)

Kummel's disease is a delayed post-traumatic vertebral collapse that occurs several weeks or even
months after an injury. Its cause is unclear, but the
most widely accepted mechanism is osteonecrosis.
Patients are generally elderly men or women. The
typical location is the thoracolumbar junction. Imaging findings show an intravertebral horizontal
vacuum cleft which is exaggerated on hyperextension. This cleft is filled with gas in the early stage,
progressively replaced by fluid. Symptomatic Kummel's disease is an excellent indication of vertebroplasty (Figs. 11.6 and 11.7) (MATHIS 2002; McGRAW
et al. 2003).

11.2.1.5
Traumatic Vertebral Fractures in Young Patients

For traumatic vertebral fractures in the young,
kyphoplasty is the procedure of choice (MAESTRETTI
et al. 2007). It can restore vertebral body height, but

more importantly allows injection of biocompatible
calcium phosphate cement into these young, nonosteoporotic patients. It is only used for Type A1 and
some A3 spinal compression fractures (Fig. 11.8)
(MAGERL et al. 1994).

11.2.1.6
Combination with Spine Surgery and Other Indications

In surgical procedures where both anterior and posterior stabilization of the spine is required, vertebroplasty can be used to repair the vertebral body,
and avoid the more complex anterior surgical approach.

Due to the physical properties of the polymethyl-
methacrylate (PMMA) cement with high resistance
to compression forces, cementoplasty can also be
used to prevent or treat compression fractures in
extraspinal bones such as the acetabulum, femoral
condyles, tibial ends or talus.

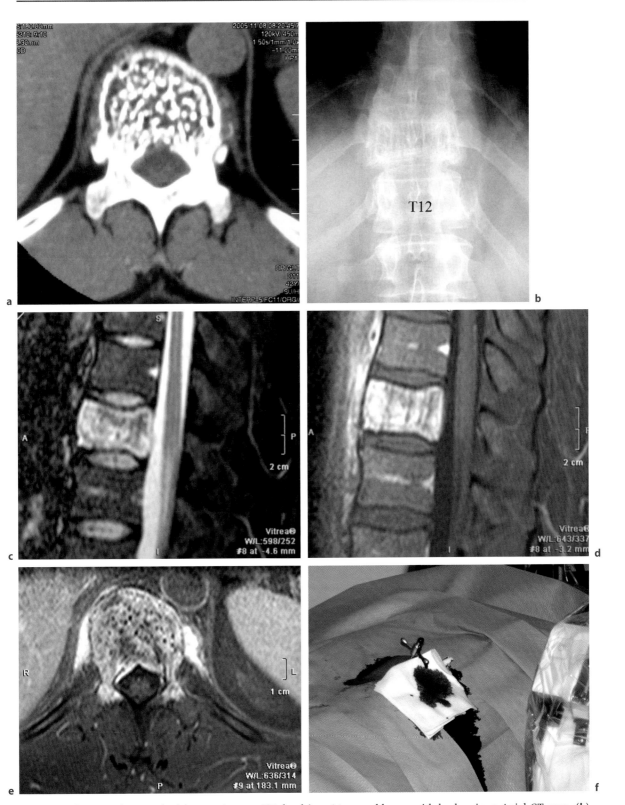

Fig. 11.4a–f. Aggressive vertebral hemangioma at T11 level in a 34-year-old man with back pain. **a** Axial CT scan, (**b**) anteroposterior radiograph, (**c**) sagittal T2 STIR, (**d**) sagittal and (**e**) axial contrast-enhanced fat-suppressed T1-weighted MR images of the thoracic spine show a vertebral hemangioma extending to the pedicles, without paravertebral extension. There is a fatty component and contrast enhancement. **f** View from the operating room shows treatment achieved by single vertebroplasty. Note typical venous bleeding in aggressive hemangiomas through the vertebroplasty trocar

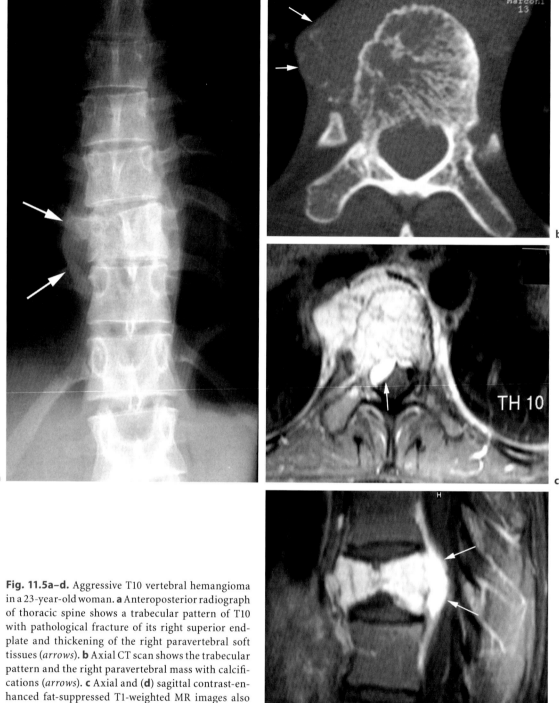

Fig. 11.5a–d. Aggressive T10 vertebral hemangioma in a 23-year-old woman. **a** Anteroposterior radiograph of thoracic spine shows a trabecular pattern of T10 with pathological fracture of its right superior endplate and thickening of the right paravertebral soft tissues (*arrows*). **b** Axial CT scan shows the trabecular pattern and the right paravertebral mass with calcifications (*arrows*). **c** Axial and (**d**) sagittal contrast-enhanced fat-suppressed T1-weighted MR images also depict a right epidural extension (*arrows*)

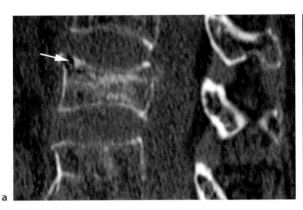

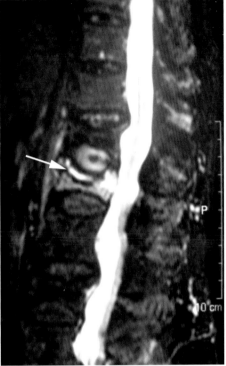

Fig. 11.6a,b. Kummel's disease or aseptic osteonecrosis at L1 level in an 80-year-old woman. **a** Sagittal CT reformatted image shows a horizontal vacuum cleft under the superior endplate filled with fluid and some gas (*arrow*) in the an-terosuperior corner. **b** Sagittal corresponding T2 STIR MR image shows high intensity fluid signal (*arrow*) within the cleft

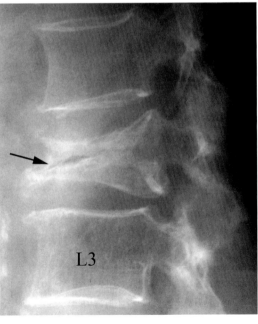

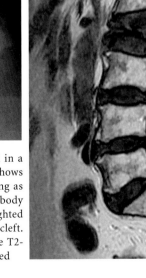

Fig. 11.7a,b. Kummel's disease or aseptic osteonecrosis at L2 level in a 74-year-old woman. **a** Lateral fluoroscopic view of lumbar spine shows the collapse and a vacuum cleft within the vertebral body appearing as a transverse radiolucent line (*arrow*) in the centre of the vertebral body or adjacent to one of its endplates. **b** Sagittal corresponding T2-weighted MR image shows no high signal intensity due to the void inside the cleft. In this particular case, even though there is no hypersignal on the T2-weighted MR image, the patient is symptomatic and should be treated

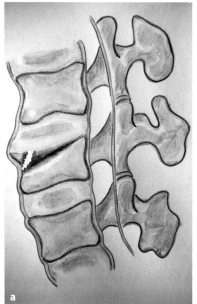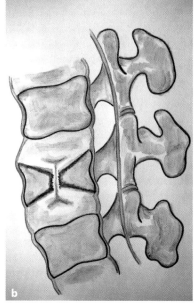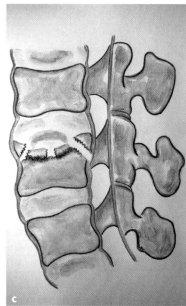

Fig. 11.8a–c. Magerl's classification of type A vertebral compression fractures. Drawings show: **a** A1 impaction fracture; **b** A2 split fracture; **c** A3 burst fracture. (Drawing courtesy of C. Kauff, RT)

11.2.2
Contraindications

11.2.2.1
Absolute Contraindications

Absolute contraindications of vertebroplasty are (GANGI et al. 2006):

- Uncorrectable coagulopathy
- Vertebral osteomyelitis or discitis
- Infection of the overlying skin
- Systemic infection
- Free posterior wall fragment with retropulsion associated with spinal canal stenosis and/or neurological symptoms (Fig. 11.9)
- Asymptomatic vertebral compression fractures and prophylaxis for osteoporosis
- Vertebral burst fractures with discoligamentous disruption following spinal trauma. Unstable spinal lesions require surgical stabilization; vertebroplasty alone is contraindicated
- Spinal tumor with rupture of the posterior wall and neurological symptoms. Non surgical patients are nevertheless treated with tumor cavitation and vertebroplasty

11.2.2.2
Relative Contraindications

Relative contraindications include:

- Vertebra plana: reduction of vertebral body height to less than one third of the original makes the procedure technically difficult. In cases where vertebral body edema is still seen on MR imaging, vertebroplasty should nevertheless be performed, but with particular caution not to insert the trocar into the disc. In Kummel's disease, positioning the patient in hyperextension and filling the cleft with cement achieve expansion of the vertebral body with some restoration of height (Fig. 11.10).
- Loss of integrity of the posterior vertebral wall (GANGI et al. 2003; WEILL et al. 1996): cement should be injected very cautiously as there is a higher incidence of epidural leak in these patients.
- Free posterior wall fragment without retropulsion and without neurological symptoms. Cement injection should be performed carefully to avoid secondary retropulsion of the fragment towards the spinal canal.

Fig. 11.9. Kummel's disease or aseptic osteonecrosis at T12 level in an 81-year-old woman. Axial CT scan shows a posterior wall free fragment retropulsed into the spinal canal. Cement injection may worsen this retropulsion

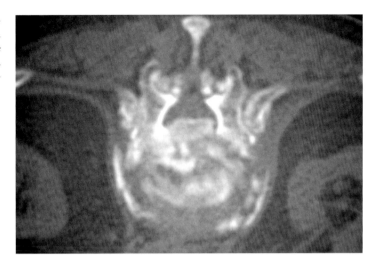

Fig. 11.10a,b. Kummel's disease or aseptic osteonecrosis at L1 level in a 78-year-old woman. **a** Sagittal unenhanced T1-weighted and (**b**) T2 STIR MR images show L1 vertebral collapse with bone marrow edema in the posterior aspect of the vertebral body

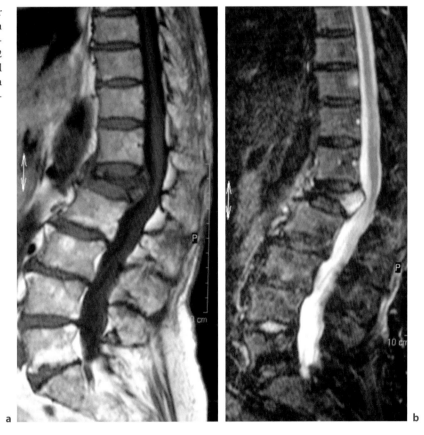

- Osteoblastic lesions: cement injection is difficult with high risk of leakage. For control of pain, thermal ablation of the lesion with radiofrequency or cryoablation will destroy the nerve endings at the tumor-bone interface, as these vertebrae do not require consolidation with cement (Fig. 11.11).

- Severe pulmonary insufficiency: use of the prone position can further compromise the pulmonary function and can produce an adverse clinical outcome.
- Lack of surgical backup and monitoring facilities (PEH and GILULA 2003).

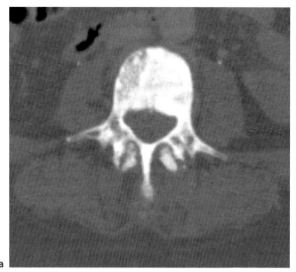

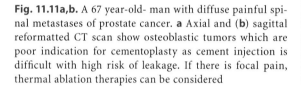

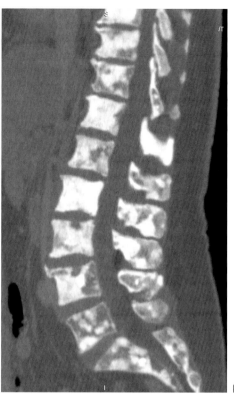

Fig. 11.11a,b. A 67 year-old- man with diffuse painful spinal metastases of prostate cancer. **a** Axial and (**b**) sagittal reformatted CT scan show osteoblastic tumors which are poor indication for cementoplasty as cement injection is difficult with high risk of leakage. If there is focal pain, thermal ablation therapies can be considered

11.3
Technique of Cementoplasty

11.3.1
General Considerations

A multidisciplinary team composed of an interventional radiologist, rheumatologist, oncologist and spine surgeon must decide which patients will benefit from the procedure. All patients must have an office visit with the treating interventional radiologist prior to the procedure. A detailed clinical examination with specific emphasis on neurological assessment must be carried out in conjunction with the imaging findings to rule out other causes of back pain like radiculopathy, degenerative spondylosis and neurological compromise. With multilevel involvement, clinical palpation of the spinous processes helps to identify the painful vertebral body (or bodies) as it results in increased midline non-radiating back pain. However manual palpation is not always accurate. Absence of pain over the involved spinous process with positive features on MR imaging does not exclude patients from treat-

ment with percutaneous vertebroplasty (GAUGHEN et al. 2002). During the office visit, the procedure, intended benefits, complications and success rate must be discussed with the patient and informed consent obtained.

Vertebroplasty can be performed under general anesthesia or sedoanalgesia using midazolam and fentanyl (MATHIS and WONG 2003; MCGRAW et al. 2003). General anesthesia is usually reserved for patients undergoing multilevel vertebroplasty in one procedure. Sedoanalgesia is very useful for patients undergoing a one or two level procedure. In our opinion, both should be administered by the anesthesiologist as most patients undergoing vertebroplasty are old with various comorbid conditions; this makes monitoring of the anesthesia or analgesia very important. During cement injection, there can be gross changes in physiological parameters as a result of pain due to increased pressure within the vertebral body. It is essential to increase the level of analgesia and sedation, at this stage of the procedure. This is better controlled by the anesthesiologist and allows the treating radiologist to concentrate on the procedure at hand.

11.3.2
Imaging

Imaging is the prerequisite for planning. MR imaging provides both anatomical and functional information and all patients undergoing percutaneous vertebroplasty should be imaged. Our MR imaging protocol consists of sagittal T1-weighted and T2 STIR images of the entire spine with axial T2-weighted images through the relevant levels. Acute, subacute and non-healed fractures are hypointense on T1-weighted images and hyperintense on T2-weighted and T2 STIR images because of marrow edema (Fig. 11.12) (MATHIS et al. 1998; STALLMEYER et al. 2003). In patients with multilevel involvement, MR imaging helps to determine accurately the levels to be treated. A collapsed vertebral body without marrow edema does not require treatment. However, in osteoporotic patients, an uncollapsed vertebral body with high signal on T2 STIR images with clinical spinous process tenderness needs treatment, as these vertebral bodies are the site of micro-fractures without collapse and the source of debilitating pain. Further, MR imaging helps to differentiate benign from malignant collapse and rules out infection (PHILLIPS 2003). In addition, a retropulsed fragment causing cord compression or abnormal cord signal can be highlighted on the MR image. In patients with malignant destruction of the vertebral body, epidural extension with cord compression and paravertebral extension are precisely delineated by contrast-enhanced MR imaging.

If multislice CT is available, we recommend thin section CT (1 mm) through the affected spinal region with multiplanar reconstructions in the sagittal and coronal planes. The higher spatial resolution of CT allows accurate delineation of the fracture, and clearly shows posterior free fragments and any compromise of the posterior vertebral wall. In malignant cases it allows accurate estimation of bone destruction, especially pedicular destruction, which helps in planning the procedure. Multiplanar reconstruction gives an accurate overview of the spine, with assessment of the degree of vertebral collapse. It also delineates sclerosis in the vertebral body (Fig. 11.11) which can interfere with cement injection and calls for a bipedicular rather than a unipedicular approach. CT also detects osteoblastic metastases which are difficult to treat with vertebroplasty.

Both MR imaging and CT help to exclude other causes of back pain like facet arthropathy, spinal canal stenosis and disc herniations.

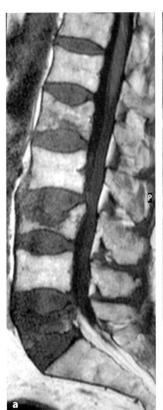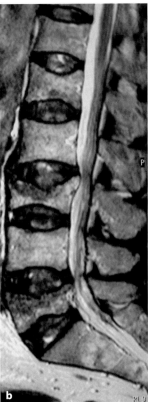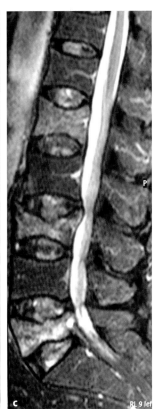

Fig. 11.12a–c.
A 67-year-old woman with acute painful osteoporotic fractures at L1, L3 and L5 levels. **a** Sagittal unenhanced T1-weighted image of the lumbar spine shows hyposignal at the three pathological levels. **b** Sagittal T2-weighted MR image shows moderate heterogeneous hyposignal. This sequence is less sensitive for the detection of acute fractures. **c** Sagittal T2 STIR MR image clearly depicts hypersignal at the three pathological levels. This sequence is the most sensitive to detect acute fractures with edema in the cancellous bone

Bone scans, which previously were advocated to determine the age of the fracture, are now only needed when clinical and imaging findings are equivocal. However, in patients in whom MR imaging is contraindicated, a bone scan is valuable to determine whether the vertebral fracture needs to be treated. Increased tracer uptake is a good predictor of a positive clinical outcome (MAYNARD et al. 2000; STALLMEYER et al. 2003).

11.3.3
Materials

11.3.3.1
Needles

Two trocar tips are available: diamond tip and beveled tip. With a diamond tip trocar, the trajectory of the needle cannot be changed after it has penetrated the bone; precise needle placement can be difficult. In contrast, the asymmetric beveled tip trocar allows some leeway to correct the needle trajectory even when deep in bone. The distribution of force moves the needle in the direction opposite the bevel face. For example, with the bevel face to the left, the needle will go to the right. This allows accurate positioning of the cementoplasty trocar, and the ability to change the cement distribution in the vertebral body by turning the bevel face during injection.

We use a beveled needle for cementoplasty (Optimed, Ettlingen, Germany) (Fig. 11.13a). The beveled edge ends in a sharp tip which lets the needle grip the bone and prevents lateral slipping off the pedicle which can result in nerve root damage. The notch on the hub indicates the side of the beveled face (Fig. 11.13b). They are available in two diameters,

10-gauge for use in the lumbar and thoracic spine and 15-gauge for the smaller vertebral bodies of the cervical spine. The distance from the skin entry point to the center of the vertebral body, seen on the axial CT or MR image, determines needle length (Fig. 11.14).

When multiple adjacent-level vertebroplasties are performed, needles of different lengths, or a contralateral approach, provide more flexibility and make attachment of the mechanical cement injector easier.

11.3.3.2
Cement

Various cements are commercially available for vertebroplasty. An ideal cement should provide sufficient mechanical strength, and be radio-dense and

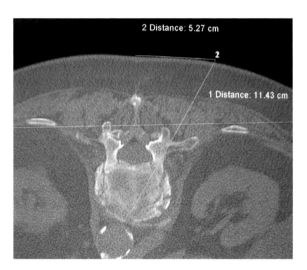

Fig. 11.14. Planning of the skin entry point in a 48-year-old woman. Axial CT scan allows precise determination of the entry point and its distance from the midline and appropriate needle length

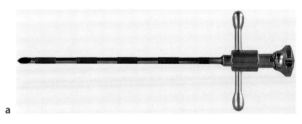

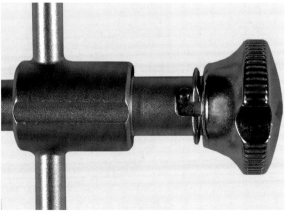

Fig. 11.13a,b. Beveled directional cementoplasty trocar. Pictures of the trocar show the notch on the hub indicating the beveled face side

viscous (DERAMOND et al. 1999). Following vertebroplasty, vertebral stiffness increases with the increase depending on the volume of cement injected. However, increased volume of cement is associated with increased risk of complications such as leaks (BELKOFF et al. 2002; HEINI and BERLEMANN 2001). Further, it has been postulated that increasing the stiffness of a particular treated vertebral body could lead to increased pressure and a higher chance of damage to adjacent, weaker, untreated vertebral bodies (HEINI et al. 2001).

Calcium phosphate (CaP) cements have been evaluated for use in percutaneous vertebroplasty. These cements are osteoconductive and biocompatible and without exothermic reaction, but are insufficiently radio-opaque, except Jectos + (Kasios, Launaguet, France). They are also difficult to inject without kyphoplasty, take time to set and provide questionable infiltration into the vertebral body (BELKOFF et al. 2002; LIM et al. 2002). In addition, experimental studies have shown that PMMA is stronger than an equal volume of CaP cement (HEINI et al. 2001). For these reasons, CaP cements are limited in our department to traumatic fractures in nonosteoporotic patients after kyphoplasty. At present PMMA is the choice of cement for percutaneous vertebroplasty as it produces significant strengthening effects with relatively small volumes.

Newer PMMA cements are inherently radio-opaque. This allows early and easy visualization of leaks, and eliminates the need for adding tungsten, zirconium or barium to provide radio-opacity. PMMA consists of a powder and a monomer which are mixed just before injection. The combination results in an exothermic polymerization reaction with formation of a hard solid. Within the first hour, 90% of the cement cures. During polymerization, the cement goes from liquid to the consistency of toothpaste to hard and solid. The cement should be injected during the paste phase when it is viscous enough to avoid venous intravasation but fluid enough to inject though the cannula. Working times vary for commercially available cements. We use Osteopal V (Heraeus, Hanau, Germany) which has an approximate working time of 8 min at room temperature (20 °C).

Why vertebroplasty relieves pain is not fully understood. Its effect on painful osteoporotic vertebral fractures is attributed to the mechanical stabilization of the fracture rather than to thermal damage of the periosteal nerves. Experimental studies have shown that the temperature is no more than 41 °C at

the posterior vertebral wall (DERAMOND et al. 1999), 42.4 °C at the cranial endplate and 41 °C at the disc level and stays above 40 °C for 1.5 min (AEBLI et al. 2006). Indeed, COTTEN et al. (1996b) in their study on vertebroplasty in malignant disease found that pain relief was not dependent on percentage of lesion fill, and postulated that the vascular, chemical and thermal forces associated with the inflammatory reaction to the heat of polymerization probably had more effect on pain relief than the mechanical forces. Other recent experimental studies have determined that vertebroplasty relieves pain by stabilizing compromised metastatic vertebrae at risk of pathological burst fracture. Vertebroplasty reduces vertebral bulge, a measure of posterior vertebral body wall motion, but the risk a burst fracture is minimized with cement posterior to the tumor, near the posterior vertebral body wall. Vertebral bulges decrease by up to 62% with 20% cement injection (TSCHIRHART et al. 2005). In experimental studies, TSCHIRHART et al. (2006) showed that vertebral stability can be restored in metastatic disease after 30% tumor ablation and injection of 1–2 mL of cement.

In clinical terms we believe that, when treating osteoporotic fractures, consolidation of the anterior two thirds of the vertebral body is necessary for good clinical outcome. In malignant disease, filling the lesion completely increases the risk of complications of epidural and foraminal leaks but without relieving pain. On the other hand, with aggressive hemangiomas, complete filling of the vascular malformation confined to the bone is necessary to avoid recurrence and spread. An effective vertebroplasty is adapted to the specific situation; it is not a "Greek sculpture" and beauty is not equal to success.

11.3.3.3
Cement Injector

Cement can be injected using 1 or 2 mL luer lock syringes, but the injection is not very well controlled and multiple syringe changes are required. Further, as the syringes are directly attached to the needle, the operator's hands are near or within the radiation field, increasing the operator dose.

We advocate the use of dedicated mechanical cement injectors with a screw system for advancing the syringe plunger (Fig. 11.15). These systems are easy to use and provide good control of the injection. If a leak is detected, the injection can be stopped immediately and the pressure relieved by reversing the screw. The 10-mL syringe allows continuous smooth

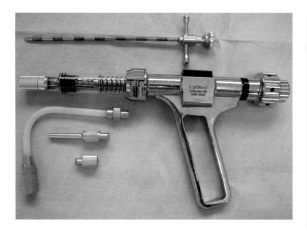

Fig. 11.15. Cementoplasty set. Screw systems allow easier and better control of cement injection, and reduce radiation exposure to the operator's hands (Optimed, Ettlingen, Germany)

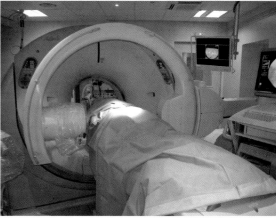

Fig. 11.16. Dual guidance using combination of CT and fluoroscopy. Picture of the operating room shows a mobile C-arm positioned between the CT table and the gantry

injection without interruption within the working time of the cement. The operator can concentrate on the fluoroscopic images and not on the amount of cement remaining in the syringes. Moreover, the operator's hands are away from the radiation field. This system is more expensive, but safer than free hand injection.

11.3.4
Image Guidance

High quality fluoroscopy is essential for vertebroplasty. Biplane fluoroscopy facilitates rapid acquisition of guidance information in two planes without complex equipment moves or projection realignments (Mathis and Wong 2003). It allows multiplanar, real-time visualization while introducing the cannula and for cement injection and distribution in the vertebral body. This configuration is particularly recommended for the inexperienced. If a biplane system is not available, adding a mobile C-arm with a fixed single-plane system creates a temporary biplane configuration. Cement injection is performed in the lateral projection and hence the higher quality image should be used for lateral projection. A single plane system is feasible so long as the operating physician recognizes the necessity of visualization in multiple planes for a safe procedure (Mathis and Wong 2003).

Dual guidance with CT and fluoroscopy (Fig. 11.16), allows precise needle placement (especially for upper thoracic vertebrae and tumor cases),

increased operator comfort and fewer complications. CT is particularly useful in difficult cases (destruction of bony landmarks, scoliosis) as it clearly differentiates the various anatomical structures (Gangi et al. 1994). A mobile C-arm is positioned in front of the CT gantry. Real-time imaging is provided by fluoroscopy in the anteroposterior (AP), lateral and oblique planes at the time of needle positioning and cement injection. Intermittent control with CT allows exact positioning of the needle in the anterior medial aspect of the vertebral body, resulting in complete vertebral fill via a unipedicular approach (Gangi et al. 2006). In certain cases, especially high thoracic levels and difficult tumors (i.e. large rupture of the posterior wall), CT fluoroscopy can prove useful for cement injection. However, we do not advocate routine use of CT fluoroscopy for vertebroplasty because of the high radiation dose to the operator.

11.3.5
Pre-Procedural Preparation

Most patients require hospitalization; however, some groups treat vertebroplasty as an outpatient procedure (Nussbaum et al. 2004). A recent normal complete blood count, coagulation profile and inflammatory marker (C-reactive protein) screen are essential.

Sedoanalgesia or general anesthesia (White 2002) is administered by the anesthesiologist, with continuous monitoring of EKG, pulse oximetry and blood pressure. Intraprocedural intravenous antibiotic cover (Cefazolin 1 mg) is recommended in immunocompromised patients, but there is no clear consensus on other patients (Gangi ct al. 2006).

The patient is prone for lumbar, thoracic and sacral levels and supine for cervical levels. For extraspinal cementoplasty, patient position depends on the location of the pathology and a safe approach that avoids nerves, vessels and visceral structures. Strict asepsis must be maintained throughout the procedure. The skin is carefully disinfected and the patient is covered with sterile drapes. The operator is sterilely dressed; the gloves are changed every 15 min.

Local anesthesia of the whole pathway is provided with 1% lidocaine through a 22-gauge spinal needle. Once the needle is in place, the cementoplasty trocar is positioned parallel to the spinal needle ("tandem technique") and introduced into the bone. A surgical hammer will control precisely the penetration of the needle, with the opposite hand acting as safety stopper. A bone biopsy can easily be performed during the same procedure if necessary, using a coaxial technique.

11.3.6
Cementoplasty Technique in the Spine

11.3.6.1
Basic Mechanics of the Beveled Needle

Large needles are stiff and their direction can only be corrected by changing the angle of the needle. Once inside the vertebral body, there is little room for trajectory correction; course corrections must be made while the needle is still within the soft

tissues. However, with beveled needles, the tip is an asymmetric wedge which facilitates directional placement, and slight trajectory modifications can be made even when the needle is deep within the vertebral body, much like a chisel in wood craft. The bevel aids the operator in needle navigation. A notch on the hub indicates the side with the bevel face; the sharp tip is opposite the notch (Fig. 11.13b). When the beveled-tip needle advances, the needle tip will tend to go in a direction slightly away from the bevel face (and the hub notch) (Fig. 11.17). For example, if the bevel faces cranially, the tip of the needle will point caudally and the needle will move in a caudal direction. The stylet of the needle should always remain entirely within the cannula when the needle is moving forward.

11.3.6.2
Lumbar Vertebroplasty

The patient is placed in prone position. Some patients cannot tolerate the prone position and are positioned three-quarter prone, with the C-arm correcting for the difference. A perfect AP projection of the involved vertebral body is needed, which may require craniocaudal angulation of the fluoroscopic tube so that the vertebral end plates are aligned. The easiest way to obtain this alignment is to begin with lateral fluoroscopy of the involved vertebrae. The vertebral body is positioned in the center of the image then the fluoroscopic tube is rotated to put the involved vertebrae upright (vertical) (Fig. 11.18). This angulation is fixed and the fluoroscope is turned to AP position. This results in visualization of the pedicle as a perfect ring in AP projection. Sometimes 5–10° of lateral rotation may be needed to fully visualize the pedicle.

Fig. 11.17a,b. Beveled needles facilitate needle placement. The bevel allows trajectory modifications, even when the needle is deep within the vertebral body. **a** Bevel faces caudally, the tip of the needle will point cranially and the needle will move in a cranial direction. **b** Bevel faces cranially, the tip of the needle will point caudally and the needle will move in a caudal direction. This is also valid for lateral trajectory modifications

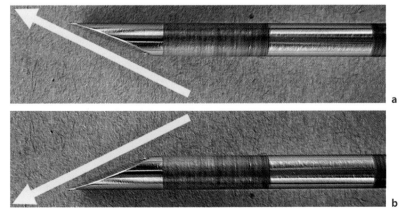

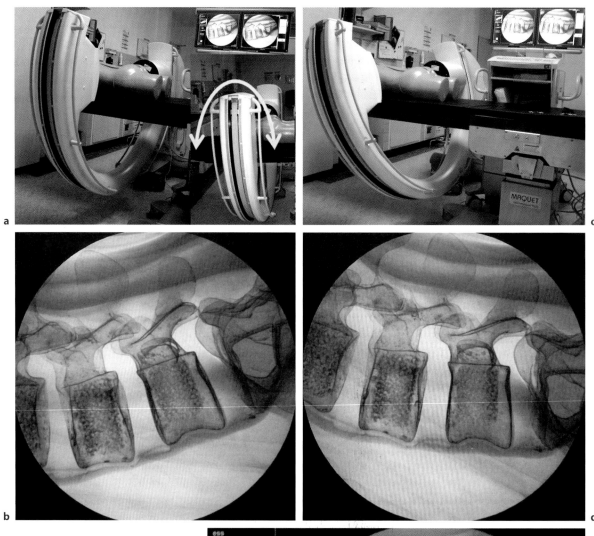

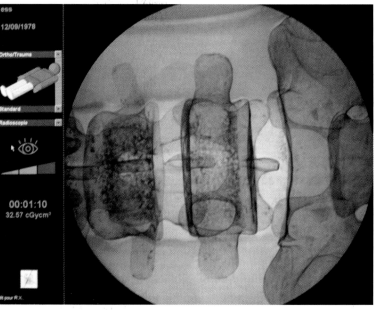

Fig. 11.18a–e. Positioning of C-arm fluoroscopy for an L5 vertebroplasty. **a** Picture and (**b**) corresponding fluoroscopic lateral view of the lumbar spine. **c** Picture and (**d**) corresponding fluoroscopic view after craniocaudal rotation of the C-arm in lateral position show the corresponding vertebral body (L5) appears vertical with both end plates parallel. Once the vertebral body is perfectly centered and in the correct axis, the angle of C-arm is blocked and the C-arm is rotated in (**e**) AP position. Keeping the predefined craniocaudal angulations, AP fluoroscopic projection shows the strict AP view of L5 with optimal visualization of the pedicles

We utilize a unipedicular approach "stay in the ring" technique which allows filling of both vertebral halves from a single puncture site (96%) with no statistically significant difference in clinical outcome from bipedicular vertebroplasty. An oblique fluoroscopic projection ("Scotty dog") is another way to determine the entry point and the puncture pathway. With this technique, the puncture is performed parallel to the X-ray beam through the pedicle (eye of the dog).

A lateral extrapedicular approach is sometimes necessary when the pedicles are too thin for the trocar. However, that raises the risk of hematoma by endangering the lumbar veins between the psoas muscle and the vertebral body.

For an optimal approach, so that the needle tip is within the anterior medial portion of the vertebral body, the entry point and its distance from the midline (spinous process) can be measured on a pre-procedural CT or MR imaging film (Fig. 11.14). If a prior CT or MR image including the skin layer is available, the lateral distance from the midline is precisely determined and marked out on the patient's skin (about 4 cm for L1 to 6 cm for L5). A paramedian line lateral and parallel to the midline is drawn, based on the measurement (Fig. 11.19). The insertion site of the needle is where the paramedian line crosses the level of the pedicle of the involved vertebral body (lateral fluoroscopy). This point is marked on the patient's skin (Fig. 11.20).

After sterile draping, local anesthesia (lidocaine 1%) is infiltrated from the skin through the soft tissue tract to the periosteum. Good infiltration of the

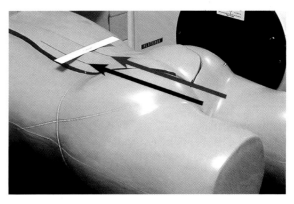

Fig. 11.19. Determining the skin entry-point. A paramedian line lateral (*black arrow*) and parallel to the midline (*blue arrow*) is drawn with the same measurement defined on a pre-procedural CT or MR images (as shown on Fig. 11.14)

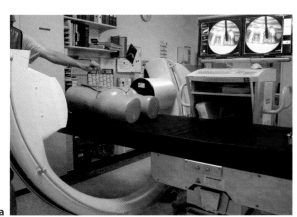

a

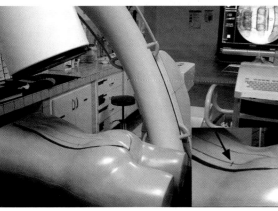

c

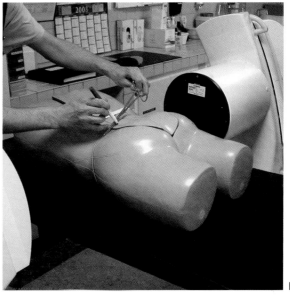

b

Fig. 11.20a–c. Determining the skin entry-point. **a** Lateral fluoroscopy with craniocaudal angulations parallel to the vertebra. The entry point is determined by a metallic long forceps on lateral view. **b** The site of insertion of the needle is the point crossing the paramedian line (as shown on Fig. 11.19) with the level of the pedicle of the involved vertebral body. **c** This point is marked on the patient's skin (*arrow*)

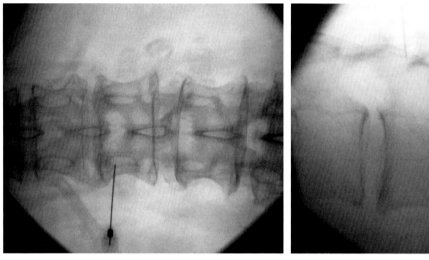
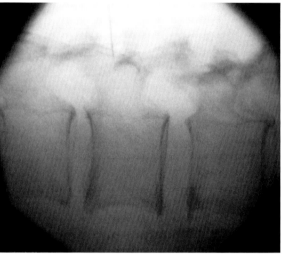

Fig. 11.21a,b. Unipedicular oblique approach for lumbar vertebroplasty in a 65-year-old man. Under fluoroscopic guidance, a 22-gauge spinal needle is positioned so that the needle tip is in contact with the upper outer quadrant of the pedicle. Positions are checked by both (**a**) AP and (**b**) lateral fluoroscopic views

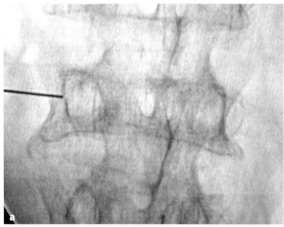

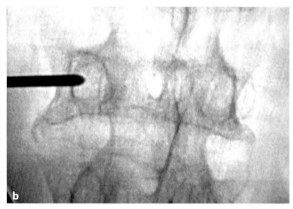

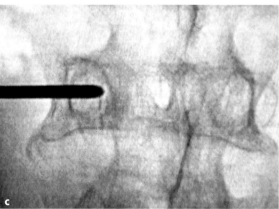

Fig. 11.22a–j. Unipedicular oblique approach for lumbar vertebroplasty in a 78-year-old woman. "Stay in the ring" technique. **a** AP fluoroscopic view shows a 22-gauge needle is positioned in contact with the upper outer quadrant of the pedicle. **b** AP fluoroscopic view shows a 10-gauge vertebroplasty trocar is inserted parallel using a tandem technique. Its bevel faces laterally. It begins to enter the pedicle which looks like a ring on AP view. **c** During penetration of the pedicle, the tip of the trocar goes closer to the inner part of the ring corresponding to the border of the spinal canal. **d** Corresponding lateral fluoroscopic view shows that the trocar is still in the pedicle and may go into the spinal canal if the angulation is not corrected. **e** Magnification at the tip of the needle before (*A*) and after 180° rotation (*B*) of the needle. **f** AP fluoroscopic view shows 180° rotation of the trocar on its axis is applied so that the bevel faces the spinal

canal. Note the increased gap between the tip of the trocar and the inner border of the pedicle. Whenever crossing the pedicle, the needle should stay in the ring. **g** Lateral fluoroscopic view shows the tip of the trocar is now beyond the posterior wall. There is no more risk for the spinal canal. **h** The trocar is inserted into the anterior third of the vertebral body. **i** AP fluoroscopic view and its corresponding (**j**) axial CT scan confirm the proper positioning on the midline

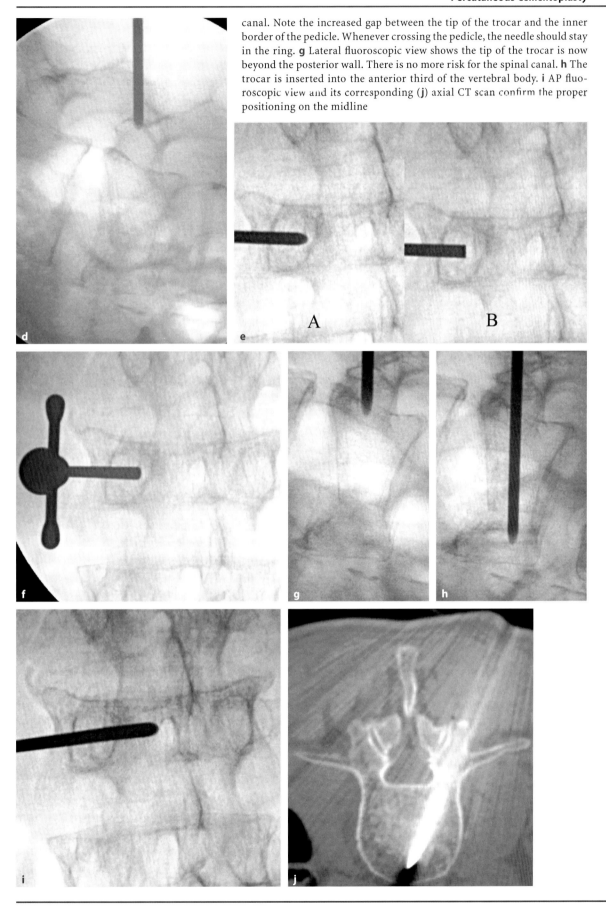

periosteum is important in patients under sedoanalgesia as the periosteum is extremely pain sensitive. Under AP fluoroscopic guidance a 22-gauge spinal needle is positioned so that the needle tip is in contact with the upper outer quadrant of the pedicle (Fig. 11.21a). In the unipedicular approach the needle tip enters the vertebral pedicle lateral to the superior articular process; in the bipedicular approach the needle enters inferolateral to the superior articular process. Lateral fluoroscopy at this point ensures that the needle tip is in contact with the pedicle and not the superior articular facet (Fig. 11.21b). Once in a satisfactory position, a 10-gauge vertebroplasty needle, with its bevel facing laterally is advanced into position utilizing the tandem needle technique, with the spinal needle providing guidance for the larger needle (Fig. 11.22a,b). On bone contact, a profile view is obtained to make sure that the needle touching the pedicle. The needle is then tapped into the bone using a mallet with intermittent AP screening. It is very important to maintain the needle tip within the ring of the pedicle on AP view till the posterior vertebral wall has been breached by the needle, as this allows safe passage of the needle through the pedicle without compromising the spinal canal. Intermittent lateral screening should be performed to view the progress of the needle through the pedicle. If the needle tip approaches the medial margin of the pedicular ring without breaching the posterior vertebral wall the direction of the needle can be changed by turning the bevel so that it faces medially (Fig. 11.22c–e). This allows the needle to progress laterally away from the spinal canal. Intermittent lateral screening should be performed again to view the progress of the needle through the pedicle. AP screening is used for passage of the needle through the pedicle. Once the posterior vertebral wall has been breached, there is a definite difference to the texture of bone especially in osteoporotic patients (Fig. 11.22f,g). In atypical cases, or if there is any doubt about the presence of malignancy, a coaxial vertebral biopsy can be performed through the outer sheath of the needle, using a 13- to 17-gauge bone biopsy needle. In patients with osteoporosis and inflammatory syndrome (raised CRP), a biopsy should be performed to rule out myeloma and underlying atypical chronic granulomatous infection like tuberculosis masquerading as osteoporosis (Fig. 11.23). At this point, further progression of the needle is monitored on lateral screening. In osteoporotic patients, the bone is extremely soft and the needle should be gently tapped into position. Using lateral fluoroscopy the needle should progress in

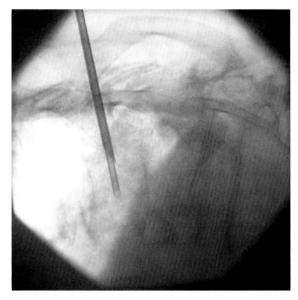

Fig. 11.23. Coaxial bone biopsy in a 64-year-old man with multiple myeloma. Sagittal fluoroscopic view shows coaxial vertebral biopsy can be performed through the outer sheath of the vertebroplasty trocar, using a 13- to 17-gauge bone biopsy needle

a medial direction (bevel facing laterally) with the shaft maintained parallel to the endplates, so that the tip comes to lie in the anterior third of the vertebral body close to the anterior margin (Fig. 11.22h). Care should be taken not to perforate the anterior cortex of the vertebral body as this could result in anterior paravertebral cement leakage. At this point AP screening should be performed to check the correct medial positioning of the needle tip, to ensure complete vertebral fill from a unipedicular approach (Fig. 11.22i). The needle tip is advanced to the anterior third of the vertebral body on a lateral view and to the midline on an AP view. These fluoroscopic projections are mandatory to appreciate the exact position and to ensure that the needle is not too oblique which may result in possible perforation of the contra-lateral vertebral body wall. If available, a CT scan is helpful at this point for visualization of the exact needle position (Fig. 11.22j). Biplane fluoroscopic equipment facilitates the rapid acquisition of guidance information (Fig. 11.24a,b).

11.3.6.3
Thoracic Vertebroplasty

Two routes have been described for thoracic vertebroplasty – the intercosto-vertebral route and the classical transpedicular route. For the transpedicu-

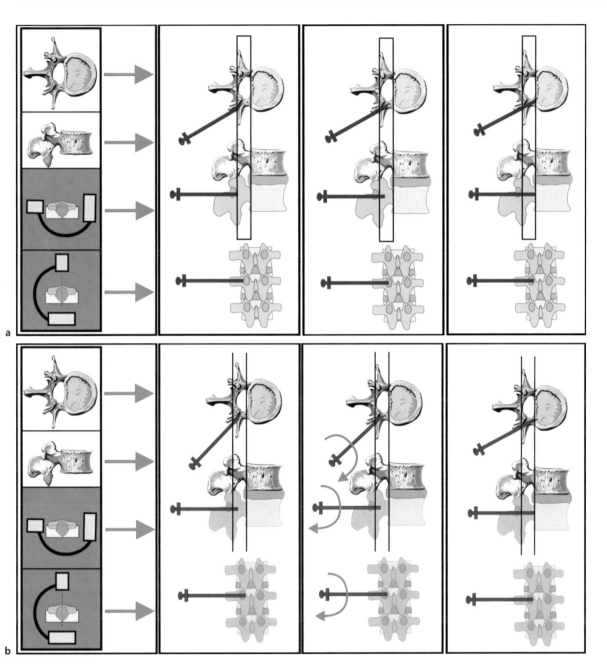

Fig. 11.24a,b. Unipedicular oblique approach for lumbar vertebroplasty. Drawings showing the "stay in the ring" technique. Three steps of the trocar insertion through the pedicle with the corresponding positions on CT, lateral and AP fluoroscopy. **a** Initial angulation of the trocar is fine and no modification of angulation is necessary. **b** Initial angulation of the trocar is too oblique. Turning the bevel towards the canal and keeping the needle more vertical allows precise advance of the trocar away from the spinal canal

lar route refer to lumbar vertebroplasty ("stay in the ring"), with the only difference being that the needle entry point is closer to the midline. The pedicles of the upper thoracic vertebrae accommodate a 15-gauge needle. We prefer the intercosto-vertebral route (Fig. 11.25) (GANGI et al. 2003, 2006).

Exclusive fluoroscopic guidance needs two fluoroscopic views to determine the exact position of the needle. The patient is positioned prone. For an optimal approach, the entry point and its distance from the midline (spinous process) can be measured on the axial CT scan or MR image. The entry point

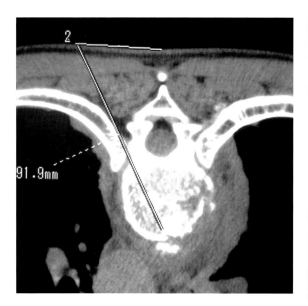

Fig. 11.25. Thoracic vertebroplasty using unilateral intercostopedicular approach in a 57-year-old man with metastatic lung cancer. Axial CT scan shows the head of the rib protects the lung. The pedicle protects the spinal canal. The tip of the vertebroplasty trocar has to be positioned in the anterior third and on the midline of the vertebral body

and angulation must allow placement of the needle tip in the midline and anterior third of the vertebral body. Vascular, visceral and neural structures must be avoided.

Using AP fluoroscopy with the necessary craniocaudal angulation, the involved vertebra is imaged so that the vertebral end plates are exactly aligned. Perfect alignment of the vertebral body in the fluoroscopic view is mandatory to avoid misplacement of the needle. The tube is then rotated 35° from the patient's sagittal plane to obtain an oblique view, so that the head of the rib and the pedicle are viewed end-on and appear as rings (Fig. 11.26).

After sterile draping, local anesthesia is performed. A 22-gauge spinal needle is advanced to the costovertebral joint in the plane of the X-rays, to reach the posterior vertebral body wall (Fig. 11.27a,b). The entire soft tissue tract is then anaesthetized including the periosteum, with the needle in contact with bone. Care must be taken not to pass anterior to the head of the rib as this would result in transgression of the pleura and pneumothorax. Utilizing the tandem needle technique, the 10-gauge vertebroplasty needle is advanced under fluoroscopy till bone contact is achieved (Fig. 11.27c–e). With a mallet, the needle is then tapped into the vertebral body under lateral screening so that the tip comes to lie close to

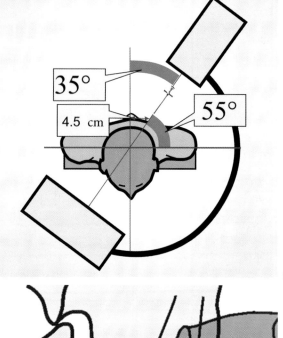

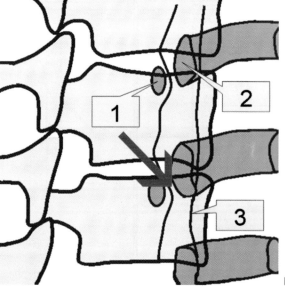

Fig. 11.26a,b. Thoracic vertebroplasty using a unilateral intercostopedicular approach under fluoroscopic-guidance. **a** Drawing shows patient lying in prone position, craniocaudal alignment first (as shown on Fig. 11.18) with the fluoroscopic tube rotated 35° laterally from the AP axis. **b** Corresponding 35° oblique fluoroscopic view shows the pedicle (1), the head of the rib (2) and the pleural line (3). The vertebroplasty trocar is inserted between the pedicle and the head of the rib, close to the upper vertebral endplate to avoid the foramen

the anterior margin. On AP screening the needle tip should lie in the midline to achieve adequate bilateral fill of the vertebral body (Fig. 11.27f,g).

Dual CT and fluoroscopy guidance increases operator comfort and safety. The procedure is the same as for fluoroscopic guidance with the needle positioning

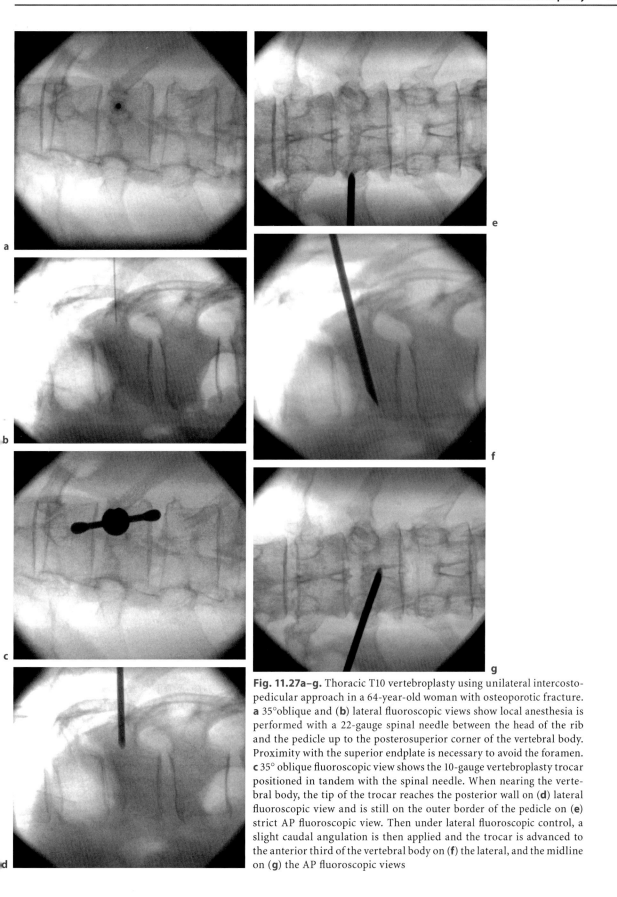

Fig. 11.27a–g. Thoracic T10 vertebroplasty using unilateral intercosto-pedicular approach in a 64-year-old woman with osteoporotic fracture. **a** 35°oblique and (**b**) lateral fluoroscopic views show local anesthesia is performed with a 22-gauge spinal needle between the head of the rib and the pedicle up to the posterosuperior corner of the vertebral body. Proximity with the superior endplate is necessary to avoid the foramen. **c** 35° oblique fluoroscopic view shows the 10-gauge vertebroplasty trocar positioned in tandem with the spinal needle. When nearing the verte-bral body, the tip of the trocar reaches the posterior wall on (**d**) lateral fluoroscopic view and is still on the outer border of the pedicle on (**e**) strict AP fluoroscopic view. Then under lateral fluoroscopic control, a slight caudal angulation is then applied and the trocar is advanced to the anterior third of the vertebral body on (**f**) the lateral, and the midline on (**g**) the AP fluoroscopic views

done under real time fluoroscopy, with CT to check the position of the needle in contact with the posterior vertebral wall, between the transverse process and the rib. This route avoids the pedicle and hence reduces the risk of transgression of the spinal canal, and is especially useful in the upper thoracic vertebral bodies where the pedicles can be very slender.

11.3.6.4
Cervical Vertebroplasty

The cervical level can be approached under fluoroscopic monitoring without CT guidance. The anterolateral approach is recommended (Fig. 11.28). For this approach the patient is supine, with a cushion under the lower neck and upper thoracic spine to hyperextend the neck. After sterile draping and local anesthesia, the carotid artery is palpated and the carotid sheath is pulled laterally and posteriorly so that the operator's fingers are in direct contact with the vertebral body and the carotid pulsations are felt

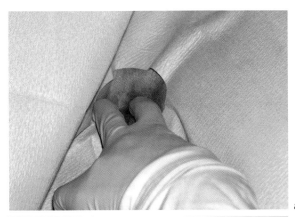

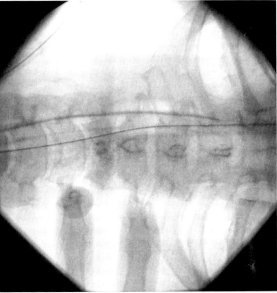

Fig. 11.29a,b. Anterolateral approach for cervical vertebroplasty in a 19-year-old women with C6 aggressive vertebral hemangioma. **a** Picture and (**b**) corresponding anterolateral fluoroscopic view show the positioning of two fingers to pull the carotid artery laterally. Keeping the fingers in contact with the vertebra, the bone trocar is inserted just between the operator's fingers

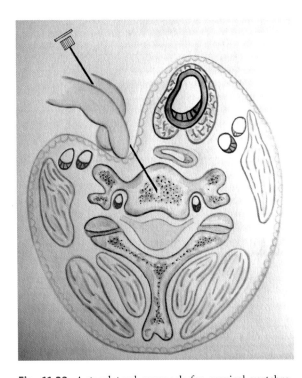

Fig. 11.28. Anterolateral approach for cervical vertebroplasty. Drawing shows the carotid artery pulled laterally so that the operator's fingers are in direct contact with the vertebral body. A 15-gauge bone trocar is inserted between operator's fingers till bone contact is achieved. The needle trajectory is between the carotid sheath laterally and the thyroid gland and the esophagus medially. (Drawing courtesy of C. Kauff, RT)

behind the palpating fingers (Fig. 11.29). A 15-gauge needle is inserted just in front of the operator's fingers till bone contact is achieved. The needle trajectory is between the carotid sheath laterally and the thyroid gland and esophagus medially. The needle is tapped into position under AP screening so that the tip lies in the midline to allow adequate fill on both sides (Fig. 11.30).

A direct transoral approach for C1 and C2 has been described; this is the most direct route which avoids neural and vascular structures (Fig. 11.31) (MARTIN et al. 2002). To avoid septic contamination

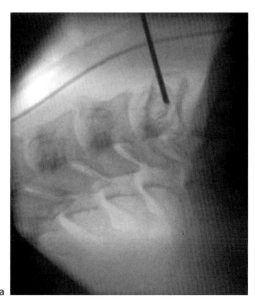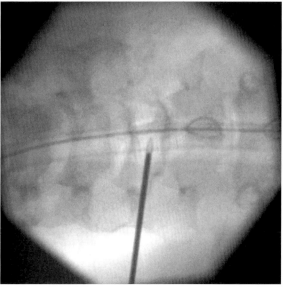

a   b

Fig. 11.30a,b. Anterolateral approach for cervical vertebroplasty in a 13-year-old girl with C6 aneurysmal bone cyst. Proper positioning in the middle of the vertebral body is checked by both (**a**) lateral and (**b**) AP fluoroscopic views

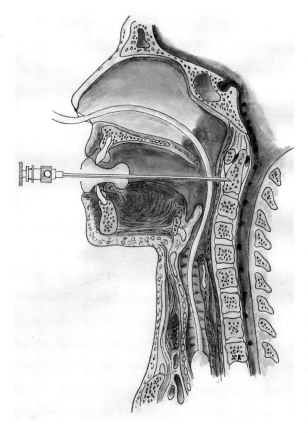

Fig. 11.31. Transoral approach for C2 puncture. Drawing shows the direct route avoids the neural and vascular structures. (Drawing courtesy of C. Kauff, RT)

of bone with oral bacterial, the tip of the bone trocar is protected in a thin sterile plastic bag (e.g. ultrasound sterile probe cover) and the bag is perforated when the needle is in direct contact with the posterior oropharyngeal wall (Fig. 11.32).

11.3.6.5
Sacroplasty

Sacral puncture is performed via a posterior approach under CT or fluoroscopic guidance. For S1 or S2 vertebral puncture, an oblique posterolateral puncture through the iliac wing is sometimes necessary (Fig. 11.33). For sacral wing cementoplasty, a straight parasagittal posterior approach is used, between the sacral foramina and the sacroiliac joint. In osteoporotic sacral insufficiency fractures, the bilateral oblique approach is preferred, but for tumor cases, the route depends upon the location of the lesion (FREY et al. 2008). Some authors describe a caudocranial angulation of 20° parallel to the long axis of the sacrum to reduce the risk of pelvic penetration by the trocar. However, the complex anatomical shape of the pelvic bone makes cement injection tricky as a single plane fluoroscopic projection cannot control the sacral foramina and the pelvis simultaneously. For this reason, we recommend the use of biplane fluoroscopy or combined CT and fluoroscopy for sacroplasty (Fig. 11.34) (MASALA et al. 2006).

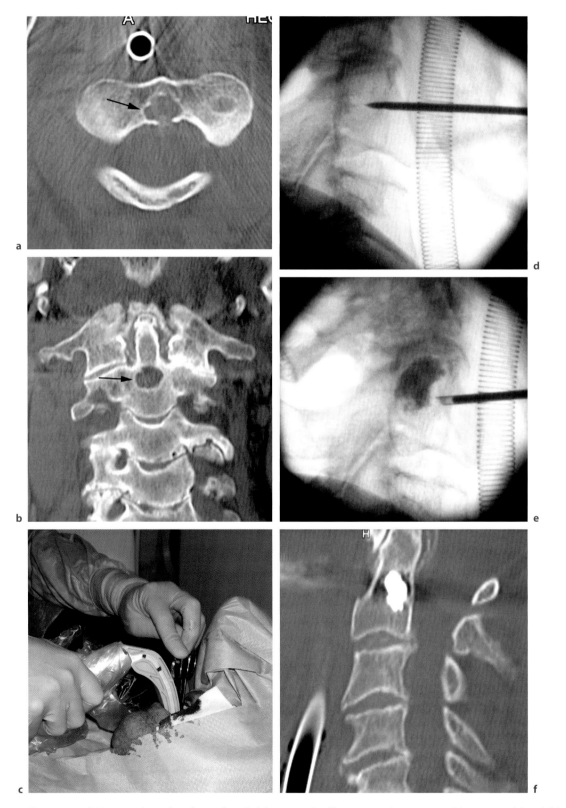

Fig. 11.32a–f. Trans-oral vertebroplasty of a painful metastasis of lung cancer in a 76-year-old man. **a** Axial and (**b**) coronal reformatted CT scans show a well defined lytic tumor (*arrow*) at the basis of the dens of C2. **c** Picture shows the direct transoral route under general anesthesia. A single use laryngoscope blade is used for better visualization. Lateral fluoroscopic views show (**d**) 15-gauge cementoplasty trocar is inserted and (**e**) cement is injected. The trocar was withdrawn after cement injection. **f** Sagittal reformatted CT image after vertebroplasty shows the cement distribution in C2. There was excellent pain relief after the procedure

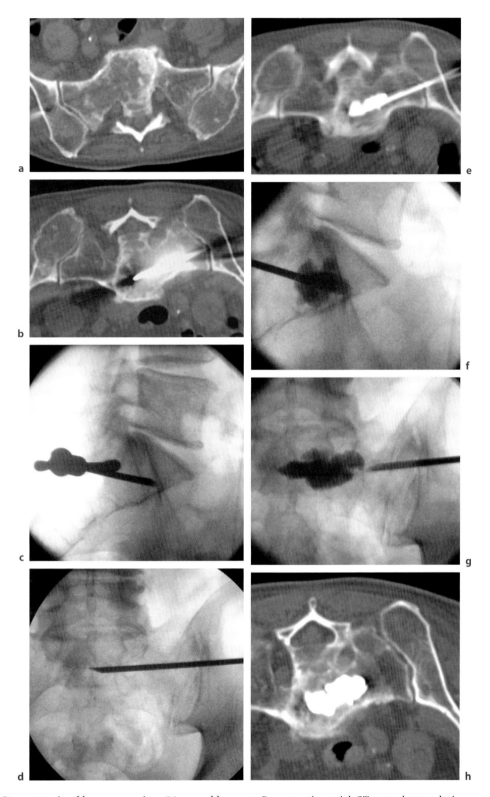

Fig. 11.33a–h. Painful S1 metastasis of lung cancer in a 56-year-old man. **a** Pre-operative axial CT scan shows a lytic tumor of the body of S1 extending to the right sacral wing. Note a lytic tumor of the posterior left iliac wing successfully treated by radiation therapy. **b** Axial CT scan shows oblique posterolateral puncture of the tumor through the right iliac wing. **c** Lateral and (**d**) AP fluoroscopic views show the cementoplasty trocar after its insertion. **e** Axial CT scan, (**f**) lateral and (**g**) AP fluoroscopic views show cement injection is performed under combined CT-fluoroscopic guidance for optimal control of the sacral foramina and the pelvis. **h** Axial CT scan after cementoplasty shows good cement filling of the sacrum. Excellent pain relief was achieved

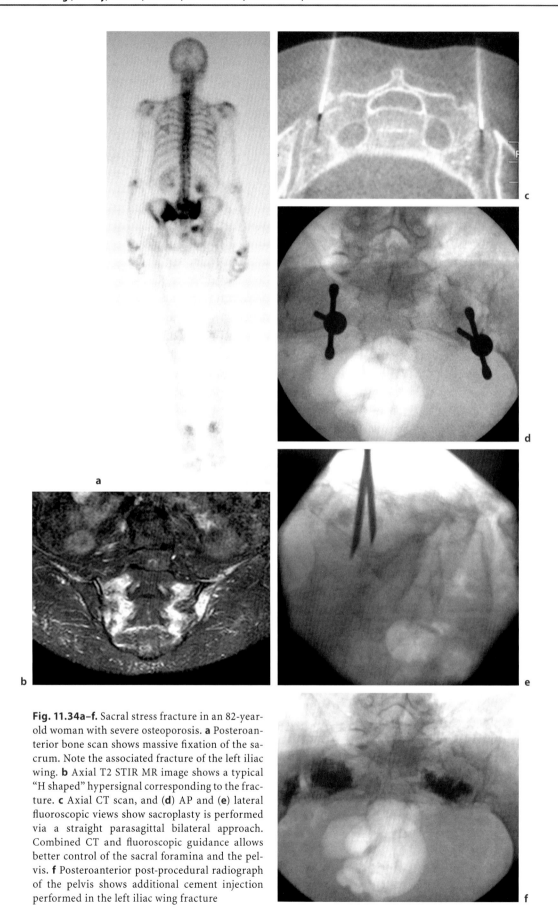

Fig. 11.34a–f. Sacral stress fracture in an 82-year-old woman with severe osteoporosis. **a** Posteroanterior bone scan shows massive fixation of the sacrum. Note the associated fracture of the left iliac wing. **b** Axial T2 STIR MR image shows a typical "H shaped" hypersignal corresponding to the fracture. **c** Axial CT scan, and (**d**) AP and (**e**) lateral fluoroscopic views show sacroplasty is performed via a straight parasagittal bilateral approach. Combined CT and fluoroscopic guidance allows better control of the sacral foramina and the pelvis. **f** Posteroanterior post-procedural radiograph of the pelvis shows additional cement injection performed in the left iliac wing fracture

11.3.7
Technique of Kyphoplasty

Kyphoplasty is a variation of vertebroplasty introduced in 2001 (LIEBERMAN et al. 2001). This technique consolidates and treats pain due to vertebral fractures, with the additional objective of restoring vertebral height, using intravertebral expansion devices, better known as "balloons", before filling the vertebral body with cement.

11.3.7.1
Equipment and Technique

The procedure is performed under strict asepsis with fluoroscopic guidance, or CT combined with fluoroscopy. Good conscious sedation or general anesthesia is required as intravertebral expansion is very painful. The approaches for lumbar and thoracic levels are similar to those described for vertebroplasty (transpedicular and intercosto-pedicular respectively). The approach is bilateral and the pathways should allow the two expanders to meet in the mid-line of the anterior portion of the vertebra.

After local anesthesia of the subcutaneous tissue up to the periosteum, a beveled bone trocar is precisely inserted into the vertebral body towards the fracture site. A Kirschner wire is inserted coaxially and the beveled trocar replaced by an 8-gauge kyphoplasty introducer (Fig. 11.35a,b). The tip of this introducer has to be positioned a few millimeters beyond the posterior wall on lateral fluoroscopic projection, so that the expandable system remains away from the spinal canal. A bone drill is advanced into the anterior vertebral body under lateral fluoroscopic control, to create a pathway for the expander.

There are two types of expanders: inflatable balloons (Kyphon Inc., Sunnyvale, CA, USA) and preformed polymer (Disc-O-Tech, Herzeliya, Israel). The former system has the advantage of expanding into the weak zones of the vertebra, while the latter is more resistant but its shape is fixed.

When using balloons a curette is also used to increase the space within the vertebra to ease inflation of the bone tamp. The pathway is also smoothed by insertion of a bone filler to prevent sharp bone fragments from rupturing the balloon. The expandable device is precisely positioned into the vertebral body, ideally facing the fracture site. When using balloons, the tamponade device is filled with half strength iodinated contrast material for visualization of the new void. Progressive inflation is achieved in increments of 50 psi to a maximum of 400 psi. Balloons often inflate asymmetrically and tend to push into the weakest areas. Unlike balloons, deployment of preformed polymer is predictable and the shape of the cavity depends only on the positioning of the polymer. Pressure is maintained until fracture reduction (Fig. 11.35c). Finally, the expandable system is removed and the cavity is filled with CaP cement under continuous lateral fluoroscopic control, using the same precautions as for conventional vertebroplasty (Fig. 11.35d,e).

11.3.7.2
Kyphoplasty Advantages and Drawbacks

When comparing conventional vertebroplasty with kyphoplasty, several points have to be emphasized:
- Restoration of height. In osteoporotic vertebral fractures where the kyphoplasty devices expand easily, the vertebral body tends to partially recollapse as soon as the expander is removed, due to the strength of the paravertebral ligaments and muscles. The absolute height restoration value on the anterior wall is about 3 mm more than with conventional vertebroplasty (DERAMOND et al. 2006; WILSON et al. 2000). Moreover, KIM al. (2006) found that height was restored with kyphoplasty, but the vertebral bodies showed significant height loss after 100,000 loading cycles. In contrast, vertebroplasty specimens had higher compression stiffness and lesser height reduction, probably due to the fact that cement seeps through cancellous bone. And yet partial restoration of height has never proved to result in additional pain relief or more improved quality of life than cement fixation alone (DERAMOND et al. 2006; MATHIS et al. 2004; MCKIERNAN et al. 2003).
- Cement leak. The overall rate of cement leaks following vertebroplasty is about 41% compared to 9% with kyphoplasty (HULME et al. 2006). However, the vast majority of leaks are into the disc and most minor venous leaks remain asymptomatic. Reported complications rates with vertebroplasty range from 1% to 6%, but comparing reports is difficult because techniques vary among institutions and depend on the choice of bone trocar, approach, cement injection, and image guidance. Also the use of injection sets is not systematic and the available acrylic cements have different viscosity and radio-opacity.

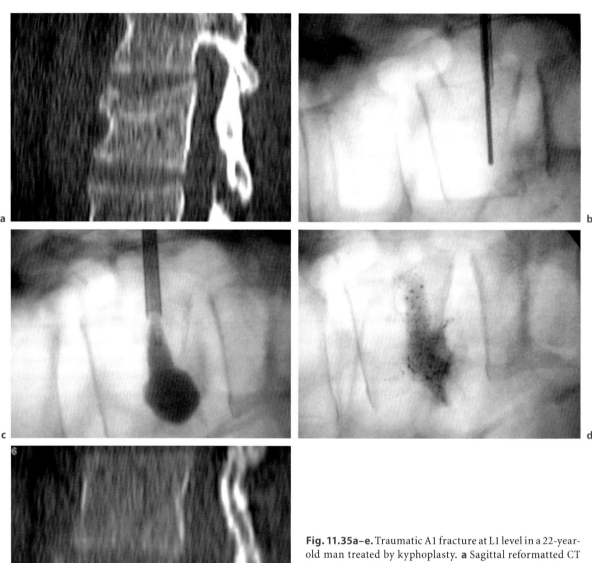

Fig. 11.35a–e. Traumatic A1 fracture at L1 level in a 22-year-old man treated by kyphoplasty. **a** Sagittal reformatted CT image shows the anterior compression fracture of the superior endplate of L1. **b** Lateral fluoroscopic view shows the 8-gauge kyphoplasty introducers are inserted over a Kirschner wire beyond the pedicle. **c** Lateral fluoroscopic view shows balloon inflation creates a cavity but no significant height restoration is achieved. **d** Lateral fluoroscopic view shows the cavity filled with calcium phosphate cement after removing the balloons. **e** Sagittal reformatted CT image shows good filling of L1 vertebra after kyphoplasty

- Efficacy of pain relief. Both techniques seem to give similar satisfactory results with success rates ranging from 70% to 90%.
- Occurrence of new fractures. New fractures of adjacent vertebrae occurred for both procedures at rates that are higher than the general osteoporotic population but approximately equivalent to the general osteoporotic population with a pre-vious vertebral fracture (ANANTHAKRISHNAN et al. 2005; HULME et al. 2006; VILLARRAGA et al. 2005).
- Cost. Kyphoplasty supplies costs about 3–4 times more than conventional vertebroplasty.
- Vertebral tumors. Inflatable systems are sometimes used with vertebral tumors to reduce the risk of cement leak before cement injection. We

do not use them, as high intratumoral pressure is associated with an increased risk of tumoral intravasation and seeding and lung emboli (SPENCE et al. 2002). For the same reason, orthopedists advocate reaming medullary bone before inserting a nail (CHOONG 2003; HEIM et al. 1995). HEIM et al. (1995) concluded that unreamed nailing of the femur with a solid rod can cause bone marrow embolization and altered pulmonary function if enough intramedullary pressure builds up during the nailing. If intratumoral cavitation is needed, radiofrequency ionization is an excellent option (c.f. Chap. 14). This low temperature bipolar radiofrequency energy is based on a sodium plasma field to break the intramolecular bonds inside the tumor, thus producing simple molecules – mainly gas evacuated through the introducer trocar. Radiofrequency ionization achieves tumoral decompression, and the cement can easily be injected inside the cavity with reduced risk of leakage.

- Traumatic compression fractures of the young patient type A1 and A3 (Fig. 11.8a,c) (MAGERL et al. 1994) are the best indications of kyphoplasty in nonosteoporotic patients (MAESTRETTI et al. 2007). This specific indication will be developed in Section 11.4.4.
- One of the major advantages of kyphoplasty is that it forms a cavity in the vertebral body, which reduces leaks. The cavity makes injecting cement easier, especially CaP cements. Cavitation can be used in other skeletal locations.

11.3.8
Cementoplasty in Other Locations

Because PMMA cement is so resistant to compression forces, cementoplasty has also been used successfully in other flat bones: acetabulum, femoral condyles, tibial ends, talus and calcaneus (Fig. 11.36) (COTTEN and DUQUESNOY 1995). The low resistance of PMMA to torsion or flexion forces makes single cementoplasty unsuitable for the diaphysis of long bones as the cement rod may break. Long bones are treated with cementoplasty only for palliative therapy, when limited strength is applied.

For the acetabulum, the approach can be anterolateral avoiding the femoral nerve and vessels, or posterior avoiding the sciatic nerve. For other bones, the pathway avoids any neurovascular structures.

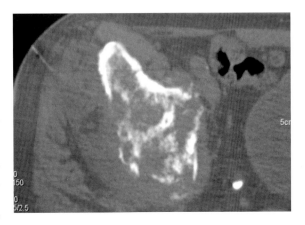

Fig. 11.36. Painful acetabular lytic tumor in a 62-year-old woman with metastatic breast cancer. Axial CT scan shows the right acetabular lytic lesion. This is an excellent indication for PMMA cementoplasty since PMMA cements have high resistance to compression forces and achieve consolidation in flat bones. The low resistance of PMMA to torsion or flexion forces makes it unsuitable for injection into diaphysis of long bones as the cement rod may break

11.3.9
Cement Injection

11.3.9.1
Choice of Cement

The ideal cement for vertebroplasty should have the following criteria:

- Proper mechanical resistance, as close as possible to healthy bone
- Viscosity that allows injection through a cannula
- Time to set between 5 and 15 min
- Sufficient radio opacity for safe injection under fluoroscopic control
- Biocompatibility and no adverse reaction

The most commonly used cement is PMMA. This low viscosity acrylic glue has a setting time of about 6–8 min. The cement is prepared by mixing powder and fluid monomer. Altering the monomer-to-powder ratio modifies the cement's mechanical properties, but slight variations due to the manner in which the cement is prepared do not seem to have clinical significance (JASPER et al. 1999). If the cement is not already radio-opaque, a radio-opacifier (zirconium, tantalum, tungsten or barium) is added to the mixture. No mechanical failure of cement has been reported in literature (JASPER et al. 2002). PMMA cements available on the market have a predefined ratio of different components to get a constant mixture. It has to be injected during its pasty polymerization phase to prevent distal venous migration. The volume to inject depends on the volume of the vertebral body and the etiology of the fracture. To achieve mechanical consolidation, cement filling in the anterior and mid columns of the vertebral body is generally sufficient. Overfilling the vertebral body may cause back pain and increases complication rates. Polymerization produces an exothermic reaction with temperatures of up to 75 °C.

In vitro tests on vertebroplasty models have found cement to be very effective, and it has been in clinical use for more than 15 years. PMMA is considered the gold standard cement despite several disadvantages. First, it is a nonbiocompatible polymer. Second, PMMA has an in vitro compressive strength of 70–100 MPa. These biomechanical properties make it too stiff and overfilling may increase strain on adjacent vertebral bodies, increasing the risk of new fracture. Third, the monomer used for the preparation of PMMA is toxic and can enter the blood stream. Several cases of anaphylactic shock have been described in the literature. Histological evaluations of vertebral bodies after PMMA injection show in the initial phase rare foci of necrosis around the cement, probably resulting from thermal injury and toxic effects of the monomer. In the late phase (after a few months), there is a very active bone formation and remodeling in the tissue adjacent to the cement, with fibrous tissue formation (KIM et al. 2004). Inflatable systems may even compress adjacent cancellous bone, thereby autografting the area around the injected cement (TOGAWA et al. 2003).

CaP cements are also available, but most are still under development. They are perfectly biocompatible and no adverse reaction has been described. They transform gradually to hydroxyapatite with little heat emission. Cadaveric studies have shown no temperature change at the bone surface, 15 min after injection (HEINI 2005). Unfortunately, CaP cements are less radio-opaque and their poor viscosity makes them difficult to inject through a cannula. Injection can be made easier: the addition of sodium citrate solution improves the viscosity. Resistance to injection can be lessened by creating a cavity with an intravertebral expansion system. Biomechanically CaP cements have less compressive strength than PMMA (about 50 MPa). In fact, their compressive strength is closer to that of normal cancellous bone (TOMITA et al. 2003). The radio-opacity of CaP

cements is low except Jectos + (Kasios, Launaguet, France), and an opacifier must be added as with PMMA. Nonetheless, their biomechanical properties and biocompatibility make CaP cements ideal for traumatic fracture in young adults.

11.3.9.2
Technique of Cement Injection

After proper placement of the needle, the stylet is removed and a fluoroscopic view is obtained and used as a reference image during cement injection, to watch for leakage. If a bone biopsy is required, it may be performed at the same time. Under fluoroscopic control, a 13–18-gauge biopsy needle is introduced coaxially through the cementoplasty trocar to obtain bone samples.

Venography is not routine before cement injection (VASCONCELOS et al. 2002). However, in hypervascular lesions with blood overflow, digital subtraction angiography with AP and lateral projections is necessary to precisely analyze the venous drainage and to anticipate a likely route for cement leakage (Fig. 11.37). In such cases, it is safer to wait until the cement is fairly thick before injecting it, to reduce the risk of intravasation. In other cases where no or minimal blood is flowing out of the cementoplasty trocar, venography is not required. Moreover, contrast medium is washed out too slowly and may interfere with the cement injection.

This phase of the procedure is controlled under strict lateral fluoroscopy, ideally biplane fluoroscopy. Fluoro-CT should not be used routinely because the radiation dose is extremely high and unseen leakage may occur if the entire vertebral volume is not visualized (TOZZI et al. 2002). To reduce the risk of cement leakage, manufacturers have developed injection sets which allow better control of pressure and speed during the procedure. A hand cranked device generates a peak intravertebral pressure of 100–220 mmHg which is 29% higher than constant rate delivery. The use of a cement pusher, i.e. stylet or blunt trocar, regardless of diameter generates an intravertebral pressure in excess of 500 mmHg. Constant slow infusion may be the single most important factor affecting intravertebral pressures. Screw injection sets are available in the market. They allow aspiration and direct injection of the cement from the same syringe in a continuous flow with minimum effort (LEE and CHEN 2004). If the cement does leak, they permit a quick release of pressure which greatly reduces the rate of complications.

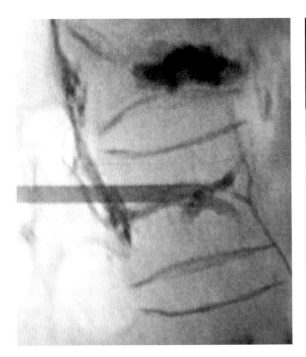

Fig. 11.37. Venography before cement injection in a 72-year-old woman with multiple myeloma. Lateral fluoroscopic view demonstrates the drainage towards the epidural veins. If there is significant bleeding after removal of the mandrin of the vertebroplasty needle, venography is performed with AP and lateral fluoroscopic projections. It helps to anticipate a potential route for cement leakage or repositioning of the needle. In such a case, the injection should be performed when the cement gets really pasty to avoid leakage

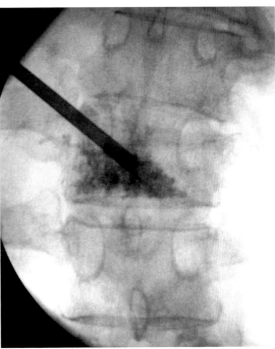

Fig. 11.38. Distribution of cement in a T9 vertebroplasty in a 70-year-old man with osteoporotic fracture. AP fluoroscopic view shows the "trabecular pattern" with the cement spreading irregularly in spongious bone. Cement injection should be slow as this distribution is associated with a higher risk of intravasation with venous leakage

The distribution of the first drops of cement has to be carefully considered. It will either spread irregularly between vertebral septa ("trabecular pattern") (Fig. 11.38), or grow slowly and homogenously around the needle tip ("chewing gum pattern") (Fig. 11.39). The trabecular pattern is associated with a higher risk of intravasation as the intravertebral vessel density is high: thus, injection should be particularly slow or even stopped for 30 s to 1 min to let the cement thicken. The chewing gum pattern occurs as the cement spreads into a cavity (osteonecrosis or after kyphoplasty); in such cases, the vessel density is low and the risk of intravasation reduced. The pasty consistency of the cement reduces the risk of leaks. However, injecting high viscosity cement requires more pressure.

Cement injection is stopped immediately whenever epidural or paravertebral opacification is observed, to prevent spinal cord compression or pulmonary embolism. A little disk leakage is common and generally asymptomatic. The needle

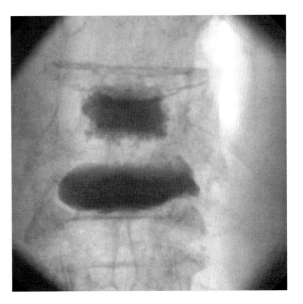

Fig. 11.39. Distribution of cement in T12 and L1 vertebroplasty in a 64-year-old man with osteoporotic fractures. AP fluoroscopic view shows the "chewing gum pattern" with the cement growing regularly and homogeneously around the needle tip, particularly at L1 level. This shape is particularly frequent in Kummel's disease with cleft (cavity) and the risk of intravasation is reduced

itself contains about 1 mL of cement, so the stylet of the needle should be completely reinserted under fluoroscopic control before the cement begins to set. The needle is removed carefully to avoid cement leakage along the pathway. Monitoring of arterial pressure is necessary during the procedure because PMMA injections can induce transient hypotension. Adding antibiotics to the cement has not proven more efficient (MORELAND et al. 2001). Total procedure time ranges from 20 to 50 min.

11.3.10
Post-Procedural Care

Overnight hospitalization is sufficient after percutaneous vertebroplasty using PMMA but this may vary depending on the general status of the patient and the level of per-procedural analgesia.

PMMA cements set within 20 min and achieve 90% of their ultimate strength within 1 h of injection. Patients can stand 6 h after the procedure. CaP cement takes up to 3 days to set and patients must be confined to bed or immobilized in a cast.

11.4
Review of Indications, Specific Aspects and Results

11.4.1
Osteoporotic Vertebral Fractures

Vertebroplasty for painful osteoporotic fractures is the leading indication of percutaneous cement injection. With the ageing population, vertebral osteoporotic fractures are common, with major socioeconomic effects. Standard conservative treatment is rest, oral painkillers and biphosphonates. If several weeks of conservative therapy fails, vertebroplasty should be considered. The ideal time to perform the procedure is much debated: it should be within 4 weeks after the trauma to avoid secondary vertebral collapse and uncontrolled pain. However, this theoretical limit varies depending upon the specific case and the morbidity secondary to prolonged bed rest. Thoracic vertebral fractures require faster treatment to prevent kyphosis which induces respiratory restriction.

Clinically, patients complain of non-radiating back pain that increases with loading. Pain is exacerbated by manual percussion of the spinous process of the pathological vertebra. Careful examination is mandatory to rule out neurological deficit due to a potential retropulsed bone fragment.

Many patients have multiple adjacent fractures, raising the problem of determining the vertebral level(s) responsible for acute pain. X-rays and CT give valuable morphological information. However, MR with sagittal T1-weighted and T2-weighted or T2 STIR sequences is ideal for pre-procedural imaging. MR imaging is highly sensitive to bone edema associated with recent fractures. It may show "pre-fractured" vertebral bodies (edema without deformity) that also require cementoplasty. It also differentiates old sclerotic fractures in which vertebroplasty is no longer necessary. If MR imaging is contraindicated, bone scan with CT is an excellent alternative (Fig. 11.40).

In case of osteonecrosis or severe vertebral collapse, axial scans should be carefully analyzed for potential posterior wall free fragments that may be pushed into the spinal canal during cement injection (Fig. 11.41).

Several vertebral fractures can be treated by cementoplasty during the same sitting, but the complication rate increases. Many of the major complications reported in the literature occurred when more than four levels were injected in one session. One hypothesis is that the cumulative dose of monomer that passes into the blood stream during several injection of PMMA may reach toxic levels. More probably, many fat emboli occur as the cement displaces bone marrow. For this reason, four levels per session should be the maximum.

The effect of cement deposition into an osteoporotic vertebral fracture on the risk of subsequent fractures at other levels remains unclear (UPPIN et al. 2003). There is an increased risk of new vertebral fractures in the vicinity of a cemented vertebra. Odds ratios for a new vertebral fracture range from 2.27 to 3.18 in the vicinity of a cemented vertebra, to 1.44 to 2.14 in the vicinity of an uncemented vertebra (GRADOS et al. 2000; LEGROUX-GEROT et al. 2004). One hypothesis to explain this risk is the excessive stiffness of PMMA. Cement injection should not exceed 30% of the vertebral body volume because of the stiffness. Significant cement leakage into the disk seems to be associated with an increased risk of new fractures in adjacent vertebral bodies. It has been reported that about 60% of vertebral bodies adjacent

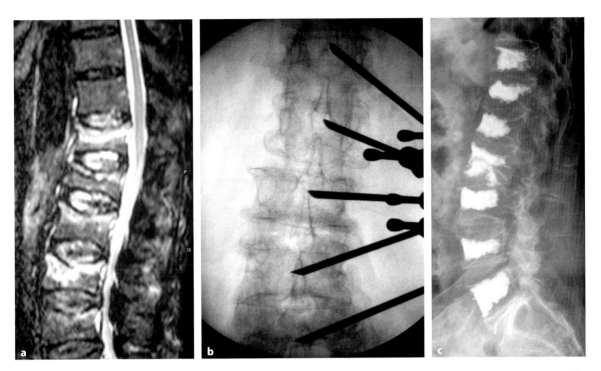

Fig. 11.40a–c. Occurrence of multiple painful adjacent vertebral fractures in a 78-year-old woman with severe osteoporosis. **a** Sagittal T2 STIR MR image shows hypersignal in all 5 lumbar vertebral bodies corresponding to recent fractures with bone marrow edema. **b** AP fluoroscopic view shows the five fractures treated by vertebroplasty. To avoid complications from microemboli of fat, the number of levels treated in a single session should be kept to a minimum. **c** Sagittal reformatted CT image shows new fractures at T11 and T12 levels were treated by a second session of vertebroplasty. Note a minor asymptomatic cement leak into the L2–L3 disk

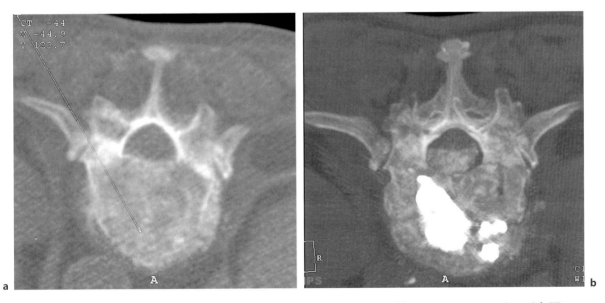

Fig. 11.41a,b. T12 painful osteonecrosis treated by vertebroplasty in a 79-year-old woman. **a** Preoperative axial CT scan shows the osteonecrosis with bilateral pedicular fracture. However, the posterior free fragment was not identified. **b** Immediate postoperative axial CT scan shows retropulsion of a large posterior wall free fragment after cement injection without any symptoms. (Image courtesy of Dr P. Brunner)

to a disk with significant cement leakage fractured during the follow-up period compared with 12% of vertebral bodies adjacent to a disk without cement leakage (Lɪɴ et al. 2004). It seems likely, however, that most new fractures are due to the progression of the disease and the distribution of previous fractures (Kᴀʟʟᴍᴇs and Jᴇɴsᴇɴ 2003).

Osteoporosis is a global bone insufficiency. Medication including vitamin D3, calcium and bisphosphonates should be prescribed to prevent new fractures.

11.4.2
Bone Tumors

Percutaneous cementoplasty is effective treatment for painful osteolytic bone metastases and myeloma (Aʟᴠᴀʀᴇᴢ et al. 2003; Sʜɪᴍᴏɴʏ et al. 2004). It treats pain and consolidates weight-bearing bone. The exothermic polymerization of PMMA can reach a temperature of up to 75 °C, but the cytotoxic effect is limited to 3 mm around the cement. The antitumoral effect is insufficient, and specific tumor therapy, i.e. chemotherapy, radiotherapy or thermal ablation, should be given in conjunction with the vertebroplasty for tumor management where appropriate (Aᴇʙʟɪ et al. 2006). Percutaneous thermal ablation using radiofrequency or cryoablation can be performed during the same procedure if tumor volume reduction is required or if a soft tissue extension also needs to be treated (c.f. Chap. 14).

Particular care has to be taken if the posterior vertebral wall is damaged, which increases the risk of epidural leak (Fig. 11.42). A posterior free fragment is usually considered contraindicatory to the percutaneous technique, as it may be pushed into the spinal canal by the anterior block of cement (Kᴀʟʟᴍᴇs 2007). Cementoplasty can also be performed in an osteosclerotic metastasis but resistance during injection is high, increasing the risk of leakage.

Acetabular osteolytic lesions may be treated with cementoplasty as this weight-bearing bone is only subject to compression forces (Fig. 11.43).

Percutaneous vertebroplasty can be performed safely and effectively with conscious sedation in patients with malignant compression fractures, i.e. metastatic disease or multiple myeloma, and epidural involvement. In such cases, several authors report an improvement in pre-vertebroplasty pain in 75%–85% patients (Aʟᴠᴀʀᴇᴢ et al. 2003; Cᴏᴛᴛᴇɴ et al. 1996b; Sʜɪᴍᴏɴʏ et al. 2004; Wᴇɪʟʟ et al. 1996; Yᴀᴍᴀᴅᴀ et al.

2004). Complications included acute increased pain or new areas of pain in 14% of patients (Sʜɪᴍᴏɴʏ et al. 2004). In a series of 21 patients treated by percutaneous vertebroplasty with PMMA, Aʟᴠᴀʀᴇᴢ et al. (2003) showed significant and early improvement in the functional status of patients with spinal metastasis. In this study, 77% of patients could walk again, and 81% were satisfied or very satisfied with the results. Improved results can be obtained by combining thermal ablation and cementoplasty in cases of large paravertebral tumor extension or extension to soft tissue (Fig. 11.44) (Bᴜʏ et al. 2006).

11.4.3
Aggressive Vertebral Hemangiomas

Vertebral hemangiomas (VH) are benign vascular malformations found in 12% of general autopsy series. Half of all bone hemangiomas are located in the spine, predominantly at the thoracic level. VH are mainly capillary and cavernous, with or without arteriovenous shunts (Cʜᴏɪ and Mᴜʀᴘʜᴇʏ 2000; Gʀᴀʏ et al. 1989; Mᴜʀᴘʜᴇʏ et al. 1995). Their nonvascular compartment includes fat, smooth muscle, fibrosis, hemosiderin and bone. The ratio of fatty and vascular component (F/V) directly correlates with the imaging features of evolution and aggressiveness (Bᴀᴜᴅʀᴇᴢ et al. 2001; Lᴀʀᴇᴅᴏ et al. 1990; Rᴏss et al. 1987) and to the clinical symptoms.

We propose a classification of the vertebral hemangiomas that accounts for the ratio of fatty and vascular components and their extension:
- Type I: Fatty hemangioma with no contrast enhancement (Fig. 11.3).
- Type II: Intermediate with a large fatty compartment and heterogeneous contrast enhancement of all abnormalities limited to the vertebrae (Fig. 11.45).
- Type III: Aggressive hemangioma (usually painful) with intense contrast enhancement limited to the vertebrae without extension to the paravertebral and epidural compartment. Paravertebral thickening can be observed. No neurological symptoms (Fig. 11.4).
- Type IV: Aggressive hemangioma with intense contrast enhancement and extension to the paravertebral and/or epidural space. Can be associated with neurological symptoms (Fig. 11.5).

Fatty VH (F>V) represent 99% of the cases (Type I). These lesions are asymptomatic, infiltrated

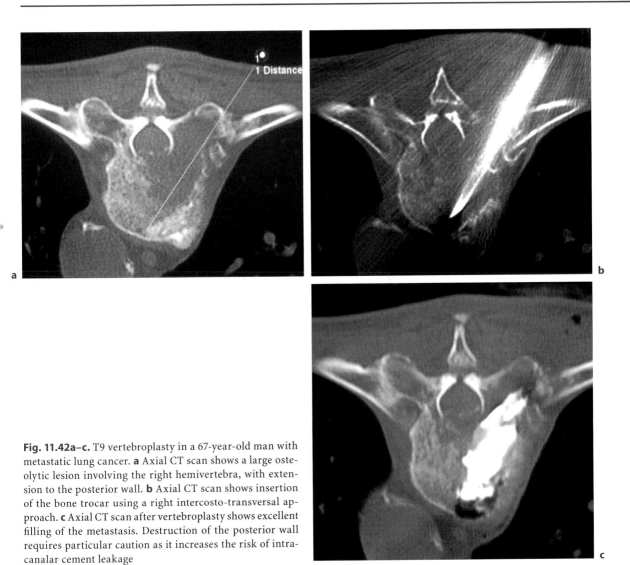

Fig. 11.42a–c. T9 vertebroplasty in a 67-year-old man with metastatic lung cancer. **a** Axial CT scan shows a large osteolytic lesion involving the right hemivertebra, with extension to the posterior wall. **b** Axial CT scan shows insertion of the bone trocar using a right intercosto-transversal approach. **c** Axial CT scan after vertebroplasty shows excellent filling of the metastasis. Destruction of the posterior wall requires particular caution as it increases the risk of intracanalar cement leakage

with fat, with negligible growth potential. They are a common incidental finding, with hyperintense signal on both T1- and T2-weighted MR imaging, due to the fat component. Contrast injection shows minimal or no enhancement. No paravertebral or epidural venous drainage can be seen. They are limited to the vertebral body. These non-aggressive VH do not require any treatment or follow-up.

Intermediate VH (F=V) (Type II) have mild vascularization. The associated symptoms are inconstant and nonspecific. Due to their unpredictable evolution, follow-up is necessary. If changes occur, treatment is required.

Aggressive VH (V>F) represent less than 1% of VH (Type III and IV). Due to their large vascular component, these lesions have a high potential for growth. They are often painful. They can extend

to the posterior arch or involve the entire vertebral body, structurally weakening it, with potential pathological fracture. They can extend to the paravertebral spaces and into the spinal canal, causing neurological compression. Pregnancy is a risk factor for quiescent VH becoming symptomatic (Castel et al. 1999; Chi et al. 2005), probably due to hemodynamic changes more than hormonal causes (Schwartz et al. 2000). On MR imaging, the signal is vascular: hypointense on T1 weighted, hyperintense on T2-weighted and intense enhancement after gadolinium administration. Treatment is always required.

Treatment options for aggressive hemangiomas (Type III and IV) include radiation therapy, decompression and reconstructive surgery, arterial embolization, vertebroplasty and intravertebral sclerotherapy. For the most complex cases, combined

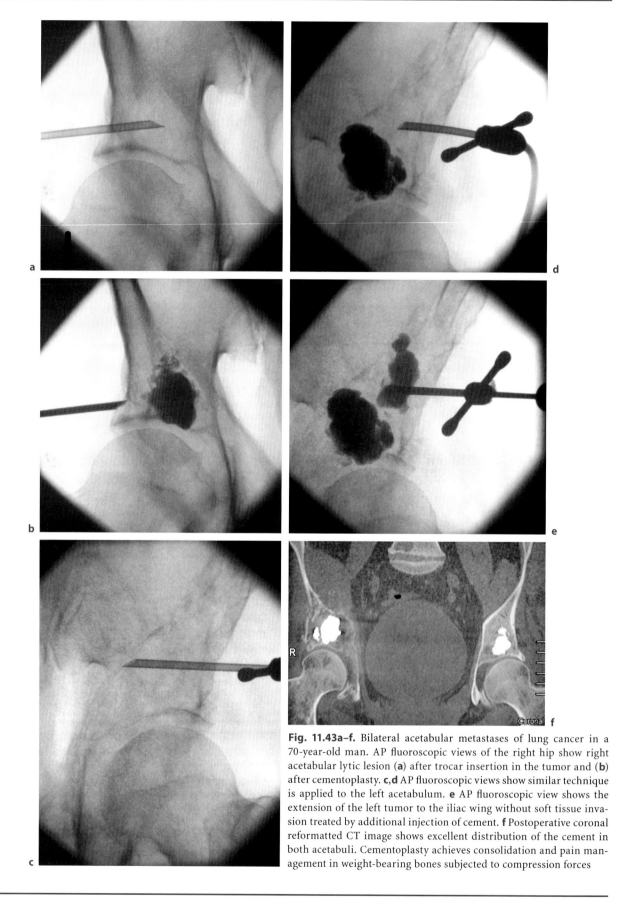

Fig. 11.43a–f. Bilateral acetabular metastases of lung cancer in a 70-year-old man. AP fluoroscopic views of the right hip show right acetabular lytic lesion (**a**) after trocar insertion in the tumor and (**b**) after cementoplasty. **c,d** AP fluoroscopic views show similar technique is applied to the left acetabulum. **e** AP fluoroscopic view shows the extension of the left tumor to the iliac wing without soft tissue invasion treated by additional injection of cement. **f** Postoperative coronal reformatted CT image shows excellent distribution of the cement in both acetabuli. Cementoplasty achieves consolidation and pain management in weight-bearing bones subjected to compression forces

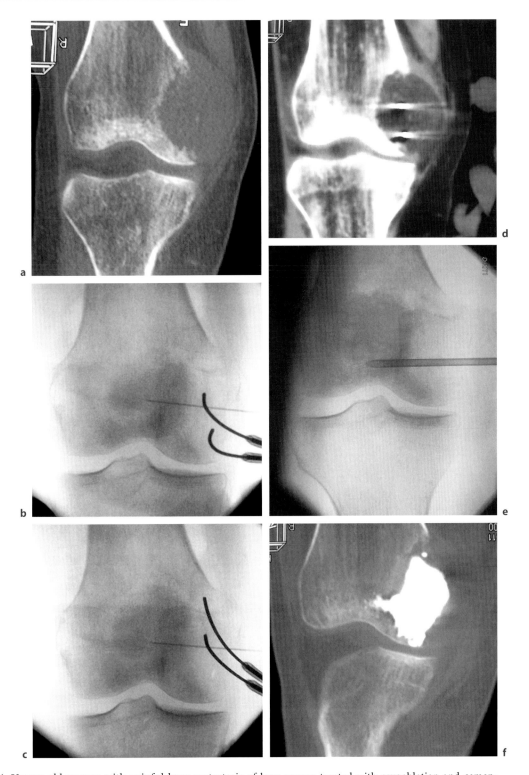

Fig. 11.44a–f. A 52-year-old woman with painful knee metastasis of lung cancer treated with cryoablation and cementoplasty. **a** Coronal reformatted CT scan shows a large osteolytic lesion of the left external femoral condyle extending to the joint and to the soft tissues. AP fluoroscopic views after positioning of two cryoprobes (**b**) in the lower part and (**c**) in the upper part of the tumor. **d** Coronal reformatted CT image shows the tumor coverage with the ice ball (hypodense). A surgical glove filled with warm fluid protects the skin from freezing. **e** AP fluoroscopic view shows a cementoplasty trocar inserted into the tumor after complete thawing. **f** Paracoronal reformatted CT image shows excellent filling of the tumor by the cement. Cementoplasty achieves bone consolidation

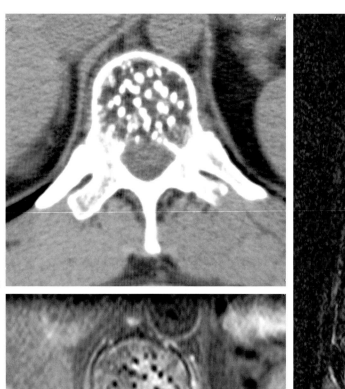

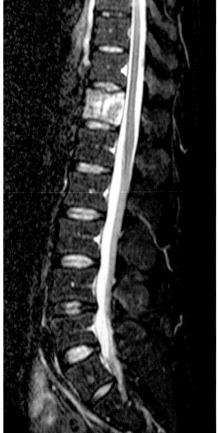

Fig. 11.45a–c. Type II intermediate vertebral hemangioma at T11 level in a 34-year-old man with moderate chronic back pain. **a** Axial CT scan, and (**b**) sagittal T2 STIR and (**c**) axial contrast-enhanced fat-suppressed T1-weighted MR images show a vertebral hemangioma limited to the vertebral body, with fatty component and moderate contrast enhancement. Follow-up is necessary and treatment is performed if symptoms or appearance change

therapies are necessary (Cortet et al. 1994; Heyd et al. 2001; Inamasu et al. 2006; Murugan et al. 2002; Nagata-Narumiya et al. 2000).

11.4.3.1
Therapeutic Options

Radiation therapy (split doses of 2 Gy, total dose of 20–40 Gy) creates vascular thrombosis by endothelial destruction (Bremnes et al. 1996; Sakata et al. 1997). Its efficacy is intermediate on pain with a reported success rate of about 70% (Faria et al. 1985). The delayed effect is unsuitable if urgent spinal cord decompression is required, nor does it

provide vertebral consolidation. Moreover, there is a risk of radiation to the spinal cord and radiation induced cancers (Obana et al. 1996; Serrano et al. 1996). Better techniques have largely replaced radiation in practice.

Surgery provides effective decompression of neurological structures and vertebral consolidation (Roy-Camille et al. 1989). The major difficulty is a high risk of massive perioperative hemorrhage; preoperative reduction of the vascular component ameliorates the risk.

Arterial embolization is rarely used alone, but is generally performed prior to surgery to reduce the risk of perioperative hemorrhage (Hernigou et al.

1994; PICARD et al. 1989; SMITH et al. 1993). Selective embolization is not always possible due to tortuous vessels or an emerging segmental anterior medullary artery. Moreover, post-capillary penetration is limited (VH is mainly a post-capillary malformation). Embolization has become uncommon since the development of direct intravertebral sclerotherapy and vertebroplasty.

Percutaneous vertebroplasty was first performed by Hervé Deramond in an aggressive VH of the axis (GALIBERT and DERAMOND 1990; GALIBERT et al. 1987). Injection of acrylic cement both obstructs the VH and consolidates the vertebra. Standard vertebroplasty techniques are used. One difference is that the rich vascularization of the hemangioma requires pre-procedural phlebography with AP and lateral projections to anticipate any risk of cement leakage. Vertebroplasty can be considered as a single treatment for aggressive VH limited to the vertebrae (Type III). Optimal filling is necessary to completely embolize the hemangioma and to avoid recurrences. However, vertebroplasty is not suitable treatment of the epidural extension of VH. Such cases require prior sclerotherapy and/or post-procedure laminectomy. Surgery following vertebroplasty is associated with reduced blood loss, and limited to laminectomy as anterior consolidation is already achieved (Fig. 11.46) (IDE et al. 1996).

Intravertebral sclerotherapy is the injection of a sclerosing agent via direct percutaneous vertebral puncture using an 18-gauge spinal needle, resulting in thrombosis of the vascular channels of the aggressive VH. Sclerotherapy is indicated to treat aggressive VH with epidural, paravertebral, foraminal or posterior arch extension, with or without neurological symptoms, i.e. type IV and rarely type III with posterior vertebral arc extension. The sclerosants are alcohol based agents. All sclerosants need to be mixed with lipiodol to make them radiopaque. Systematic AP and lateral phlebography with and without digital subtraction is required to evaluate the venous drainage of the VH and possible arterial communication. A combination of CT and fluoroscopic guidance can be useful for complex cases. The amount of sclerosant that will be needed is about the same as the amount of contrast agent needed to opacify the normally draining veins. *N*-Butyl cyanoacrylate is a rapidly polymerizing adhesive, of low viscosity which allows diffusion into the epidural component following injection into the hemangiomatous bone, and its lack of solidification does not interfere with laminectomy (COTTEN et al.

1996a). We prefer Ethibloc® (Johnson & Johnson, Brussels, Belgium), a mixture of alcohol and zein (corn protein) as its higher viscosity gives better control during injection. In addition to thrombosing vessels, alcohol based sclerosants induce a fibrous retraction, which shrinks the epidural component, and in some cases reduces neurological compression and avoids surgical decompression (GABAL 2002). However, these agents, especially Ethibloc®, induce an intense acute inflammatory reaction that may worsen neurological compression in the first 3 days (HEISS et al. 1996). Thus, for VH with epidural extension, high dose intravenous steroids are recommended (250 mg Solumedrol × 3/day) starting a day before and continuing 3 days after the procedure (Figs. 11.5 and 11.47). Fragilization induced by the sclerosants increases the risk of vertebral collapse when the vertebral body is involved (DOPPMAN et al. 2000). In such cases, consolidation is achieved by additional vertebroplasty within 15 days. Cement injection cannot be performed the same day due to the residual opacity of the sclerotic agent in the vertebra. To avoid recurrence, complete embolization of the VH is recommended, confirmed by follow-up dynamic MR imaging.

11.4.3.2
Results

In the past, aggressive hemangiomas were treated with radiotherapy and surgery. Newer treatments, vertebroplasty, sclerotherapy, embolization and decompressive surgery, alone or in combination, avoid the complications of radiation and surgery.

A surgical review of 45 patients with aggressive VH reported 75.5% favorable results based on surgery and/or radiotherapy. Mortality was 11.1% and 13 (29%) recurred (NGUYEN et al. 1989).

Radiotherapy was once widely used in the management of aggressive hemangiomas, with symptom relief in 88% of cases (YANG et al. 1985). However, the inconsistent results and the major side effects of radiation myelitis and malignant transformation (OBANA et al. 1996; SERRANO et al. 1996) have considerably reduced its use.

Hyperselective arterial embolization in 19 VH was reported by PICARD et al. (1989). In five cases, embolization was followed by surgical decompression. In two cases, embolization was not performed due to the close proximity of the artery of Adamkiewicz. Pain relief was good in 12 cases. Transarterial embolization on its own is not a promising therapeutic

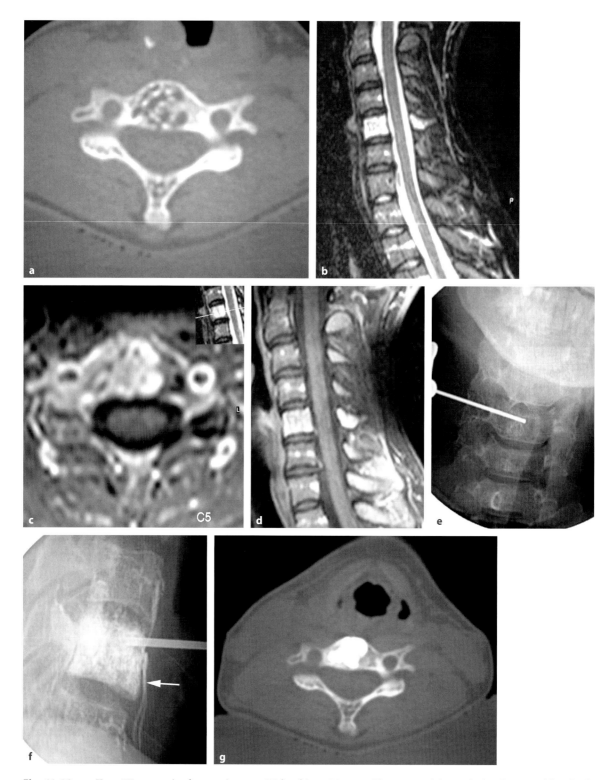

Fig. 11.46a–g. Type III aggressive hemangioma at C5 level in a 26-year-old woman with cervical pain treated by single vertebroplasty. **a** Axial CT scan, and (**b**) sagittal T2 STIR, (**c**) axial and (**d**) sagittal contrast-enhanced fat-suppressed T1-weighted MR images show an aggressive hemangioma limited to the vertebral body. **e** AP fluoroscopic view shows cementoplasty trocar after its insertion. **f** Sagittal phlebogram performed through the trocar shows the large prevertebral (*arrow*) and epidural venous drainage of the hemangioma. **g** Axial CT scan after cement injection shows optimal filling of C5. Vertebroplasty achieves excellent bone consolidation

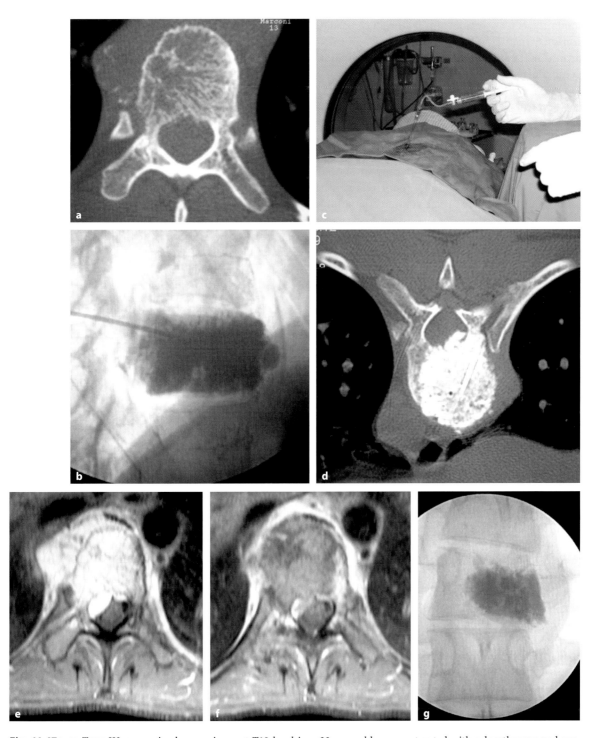

Fig. 11.47a–g. Type IV aggressive hemangioma at T10 level in a 23-year-old woman treated with sclerotherapy and vertebroplasty. **a** Axial CT scan image shows the aggressive hemangioma with right paravertebral and epidural extension, responsible for intercostal neuralgia and pathological fracture. **b** Lateral fluoroscopic view and (**c**) corresponding picture during sclerotherapy with a mixture of Ethibloc® and Lipiodol demonstrate optimal filling of the hemangioma necessary to achieve sclerosis and avoid recurrence. **d** Axial CT scan immediately after sclerotherapy confirms the optimal filling of the hemangioma and its epidural component. Axial contrast-enhanced fat-suppressed T1-weighted MR image (**e**) before and (**f**) 15 days after the procedure show the obstruction of the hemangioma and the shrinkage of its paravertebral and epidural extension. **g** AP fluoroscopic view shows cement filling after vertebroplasty performed 4 weeks after sclerotherapy to avoid secondary collapse and consolidate the vertebral body

modality as its principle aim is to reduce vascularization of the VH. It is a safe and effective adjunctive procedure to surgery as it minimizes perioperative hemorrhage (SMITH et al. 1993).

GOYAL et al. (1999) used single ethanol injection in 14 patients with symptomatic VH. They reported 86% satisfactory results. However, there were one paravertebral abscess and one secondary vertebral collapse. NIEMEYER et al. (1999) reported one Brown Sequard syndrome after sclerotherapy with ethanol in a VH. DOPPMAN et al (2000) reported two vertebral collapses following large volume ethanol injection in VH.

BRUNOT et al. (2005) reported a success rate of 90% in the short or long term in a series of 19 patients treated by single vertebroplasty for symptomatic VH. In the past 15 years, 33 aggressive VH in 32 patients (8 men, 24 women) have been treated in our institution. All patients complained of axial pain and nine had neurological symptoms (four radicular pain, five motor deficit). Single vertebroplasty was performed in 22 patients for aggressive VH limited to the vertebral body or with minimal paravertebral extension. Large paravertebral or epidural extension required combined techniques. Scheduled laminectomy was only necessary in three cases. In seven cases with paravertebral and/or epidural extension of the hemangioma, sclerotherapy was performed followed by a scheduled vertebroplasty. Significant or complete pain relief was achieved in 30 of 32 patients. Neurological symptoms were relieved in all cases. No secondary vertebral fractures were noted. Five minor cement leaks remained asymptomatic. One major recurrence occurred 10 years after initial treatment and was successfully treated with a single session of sclerotherapy with injection of 25 mL of Ethibloc®. The only major complication we encountered was a cauda equina syndrome occurring 12 h after sclerotherapy of an aggressive VH with large epidural extension. It occurred as a result of the inflammatory reaction to Ethibloc®, but the patient had not taken the high dose steroid that was prescribed. Urgent laminectomy with no perioperative blood loss led to a complete recovery.

11.4.3.3
Treatment Strategy

We advocate the following strategy for the management of aggressive vertebral hemangiomas:
- For aggressive VH limited to the vertebral body (Type III), vertebroplasty is the leading treatment

as it achieves embolization of the VH and consolidation of the vertebral body in a single session.
- For aggressive VH with large paravertebral or epidural extension (Type IV), sclerotherapy with Ethibloc® or ethanol is performed. The early inflammatory reaction is treated by high dose steroids. After 10–15 days MR imaging confirms the complete embolization of the aggressive VH, following which consolidation is achieved by additional vertebroplasty to avoid secondary collapse.
- Laminectomy is considered for major epidural extension with neurological deficit. The risk of massive perioperative hemorrhage is high if no prior treatment to reduce vascularization has been performed. Pre-operative sclerotherapy and/or arterial embolization are advocated.
- Sclerotherapy and vertebroplasty have largely replaced arterial embolization prior to laminectomy.
- Radiation therapy gives inconsistent results with delayed effects and risk of spinal cord damage. It is rarely used since the development of other techniques.

For aggressive vertebral hemangiomas, optimal embolization of the lesion is required to avoid recurrence. Clinical and imaging follow-up, i.e. MR imaging, confirm absence of further evolution.

Other vascular bone tumors or malformations such as aneurysmal bone cysts (ABC) can also be treated with cementoplasty and/or sclerotherapy. In some cases where surgery may be complex or disabling, cement injection provides an effective alternative that achieves pain control and consolidation simultaneously.

11.4.4
Traumatic Vertebral Fractures in Young Patients

One of the best indications for kyphoplasty is traumatic compression fracture in nonosteoporotic patients. Indeed, the dense trabecular bone in young patients makes cement injection extremely difficult. Moreover, creation of a prior cavity allows the use of CaP cements which are biocompatible and possess osteointegration properties that allow internal splinting in the early phase after trauma, without preventing normal bone healing. Moreover, the biomechanical properties of CaP cements are closer to normal cancellous bone than acrylic cement.

Indications include vertebral compression fracture Types A1 and A3 (MAGERL et al. 1994). In complex A3 fractures, kyphoplasty in conjunction with posterior surgical instrumentation allows for complete stabilization of the fractured vertebra without resorting to an anterior surgical approach (Figs. 11.48–11.50). The goals of kyphoplasty are rapid patient mobilization, swift relief of pain and restoration of vertebral body height. The treatment should be performed during the first 7 days after the trauma as, after the first week, height restoration becomes very difficult. Balloon expansion is difficult in nonosteoporotic bone; use of a curette before insertion is advocated. The balloon should be inflated in incremental steps. The volume of CaP cement to be injected into the vertebra correlates with the volume of contrast needed to fully inflate the balloons. The results are very promising with pain management and swift mobilization of the patients after 3 days (MAESTRETTI et al. 2007). However, restoration of vertebral body height is not reproducible. In some cases, 2–4 months after kyphoplasty, a secondary collapse is observed, probably due to the severity of the initial trauma causing secondary necrosis.

11.4.5
Surgical Adjuncts and Others

In specific cases, cementoplasty can be combined with surgery. Indeed, vertebroplasty achieves con-

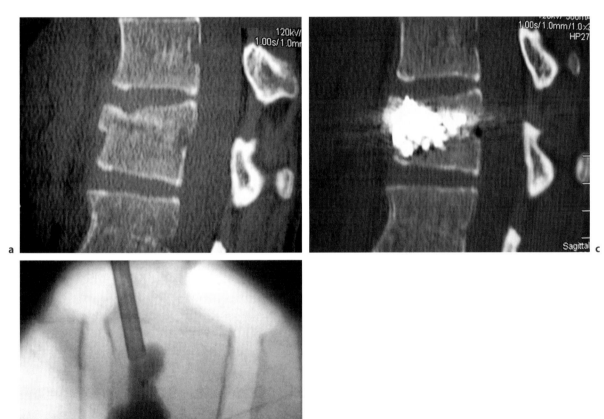

Fig. 11.48a–c. Traumatic A1 fracture at L1 level in a 21-year-old man treated by kyphoplasty. **a** Preoperative sagittal reformatted CT image shows the anterior compression fracture of the superior vertebral endplate. **b** Lateral fluoroscopic view shows kyphoplasty with balloon inflation achieves creation of a cavity and partial restoration of vertebral height. **c** Postoperative sagittal reformatted CT image after injection of calcium phosphate cement shows excellent filling of the vertebra and excellent pain relief

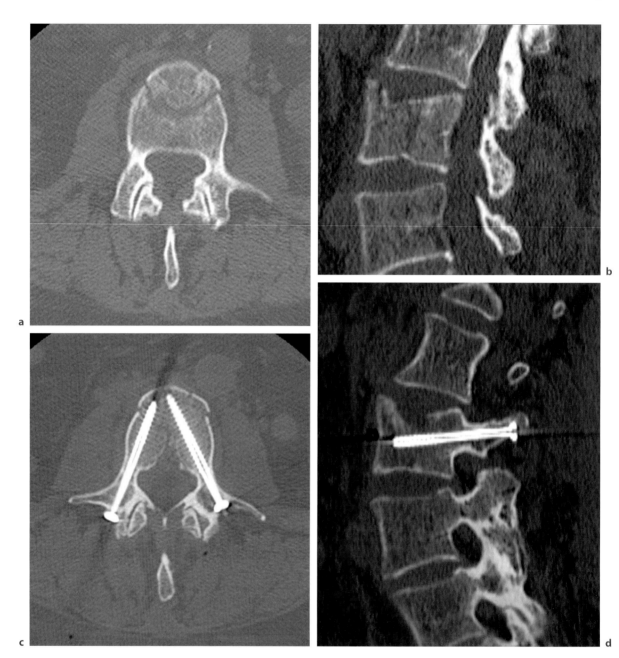

Fig. 11.49a–d. Traumatic A2 fracture at L2 level in a 32-year-old man treated by percutaneous screw fixation. **a** Preoperative axial and (**b**) sagittal reformatted CT scans show the split coronal fracture. **c** Axial and (**d**) sagittal reformatted CT scans show percutaneous bilateral transpedicular screw fixation. For this specific split fracture, a screw is more suitable than ce-mentoplasty as it pulls the anterior fragment back into contact with the posterior one. Vertebroplasty or kyphoplasty may enlarge the split and push the disk wedge into the split

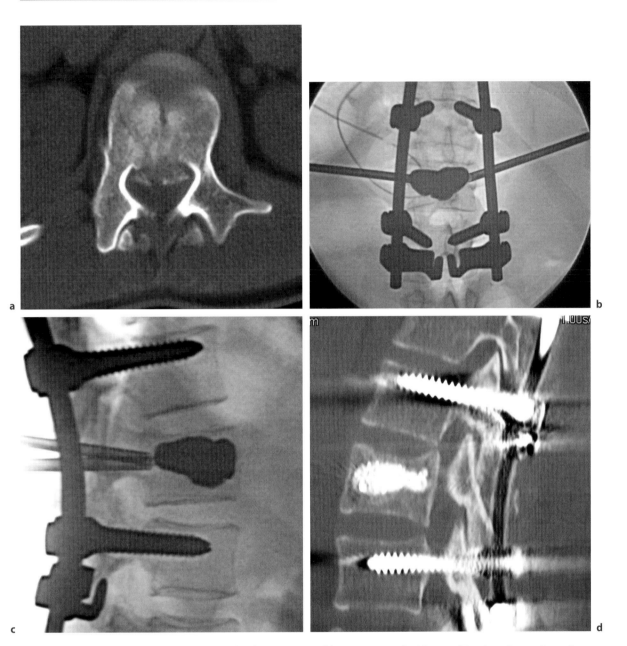

Fig. 11.50a–d. Traumatic burst fracture at L1 level in a 29-year-old woman treated with a combination of posterior arthrodesis and kyphoplasty. **a** Preoperative axial CT scan shows a rupture of the posterior wall with retropulsion into the canal. **b** AP and (**c**) lateral perioperative fluoroscopic views showing fracture reduction after posterior surgical instrumentation and kyphoplasty balloon inflation. **d** Postoperative sagittal reformatted CT image after calcium phosphate cement injection shows excellent filling of the vertebra. Anterior stabilization with cement injection avoids a complex anterior surgical approach with bone graft

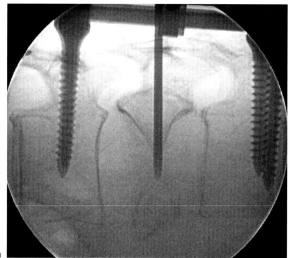

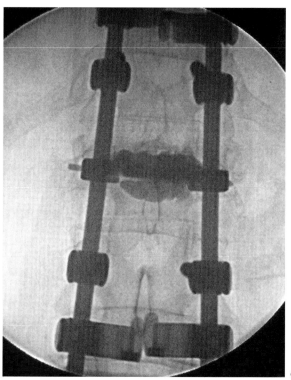

Fig. 11.51a–c. L1 vertebroplasty in a 45-year-old woman with vertebral collapse 4 months after posterior surgical fixation. **a** Lateral fluoroscopic view shows insertion of the cementoplasty trocar. **b** Lateral and (**c**) AP fluoroscopic after injection show excellent filling of the vertebra with the cement. Vertebroplasty achieves stabilization and avoids a complex anterior surgical bone graft. Excellent functional result

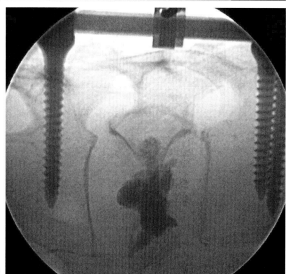

solidation of the anterior spinal column and thus can avoid complex surgical approaches. Vertebroplasty can be combined with surgery for some complex spinal fractures or performed secondarily when vertebral collapse occurs after posterior instrumentation (Fig. 11.51). In cancer patients with epidural tumor extension, posterior surgical decompression associated with vertebroplasty also avoids an anterior surgical approach (Arnold 1985). In extraspinal locations, cementoplasty or kyphoplasty can be indicated to treat symptomatic lesions or to avoid secondary compression fracture (Figs. 11.52 and 11.53).

11.4.6
Complications

Serious adverse reaction is defined as the occurrence of an unexpected or undesirable clinical event which results in surgical intervention, permanent disability or death (Gangi et al. 2003, 2006; Nussbaum et al. 2004). Minor adverse reactions are which require no immediate or delayed surgical intervention (Laredo and Hamze 2004; Zoarski et al. 2002). Published data has placed the occurrence of complications in percutaneous vertebroplasty for osteoporotic fractures at <1% and for malignant disease at <10% (McGraw et al. 2003).

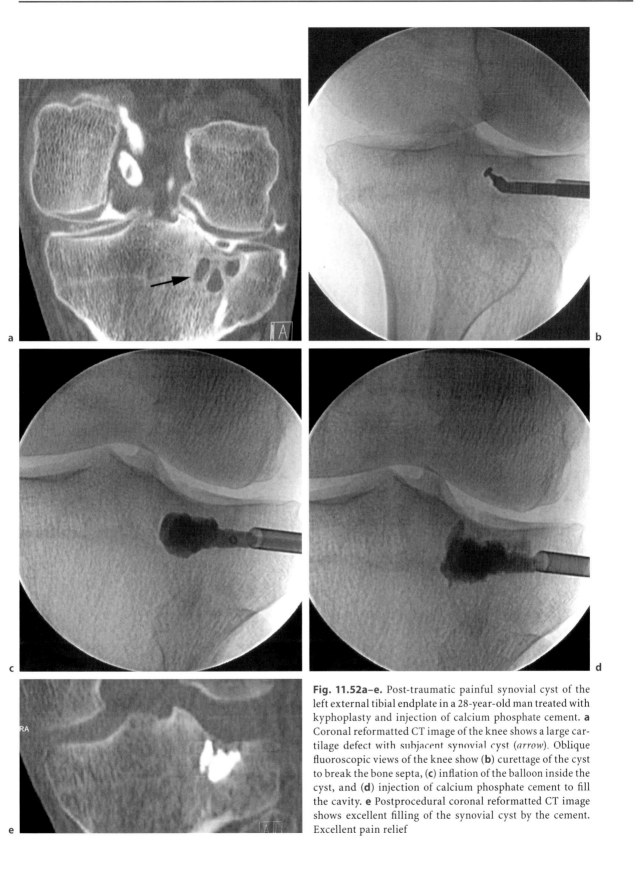

Fig. 11.52a–e. Post-traumatic painful synovial cyst of the left external tibial endplate in a 28-year-old man treated with kyphoplasty and injection of calcium phosphate cement. **a** Coronal reformatted CT image of the knee shows a large cartilage defect with subjacent synovial cyst (*arrow*). Oblique fluoroscopic views of the knee show (**b**) curettage of the cyst to break the bone septa, (**c**) inflation of the balloon inside the cyst, and (**d**) injection of calcium phosphate cement to fill the cavity. **e** Postprocedural coronal reformatted CT image shows excellent filling of the synovial cyst by the cement. Excellent pain relief

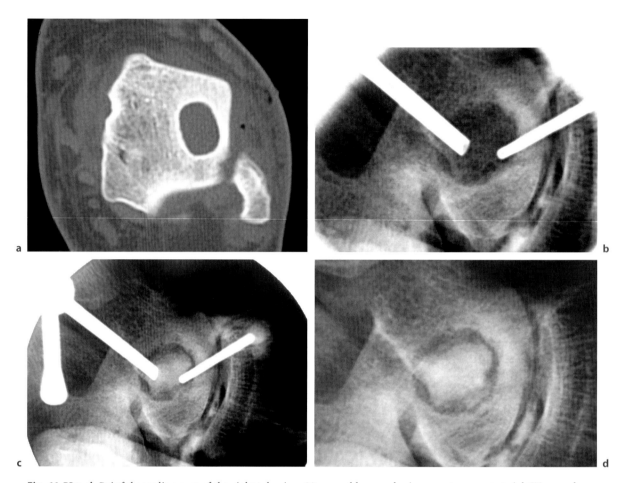

Fig. 11.53a–d. Painful ganglion cyst of the right talus in a 30-year-old man who is a paratrooper. **a** Axial CT scan shows a well circumscribed cyst. **b** Lateral fluoroscopic view of the ankle shows a 10-gauge cementoplasty trocar and a 14-gauge decompression bone trocar inserted into the cyst. Opacification of the cyst confirms delayed communication with the joint. **c** Lateral fluoroscopic view shows calcium phosphate cement injection into the cyst with expulsion of the mucoid fluid through the 14-gauge decompression trocar. **d** Postprocedural lateral radiograph of the ankle shows excellent filling of the cyst by the cement. Excellent clinical results with six-year follow-up

11.4.6.1
Cement Leakage

Cement leakage is the most frequent complication and is usually asymptomatic (NUSSBAUM et al. 2004). For osteoporotic fractures the incidence ranges from 30% to 65% and for malignant disease it is higher, 38%–72.5% (Fig. 11.54) (LAREDO and HAMZE 2004).

Transient neurological deficit persists for less than 30 days and does not require surgery. It has an incidence of 2% in osteoporotic patients and 5% in those with malignant disease. Permanent neurological sequellae last for more than 30 days and require surgery. They have not been reported in osteoporotic patients, but in patients with malignant

etiology the incidence is 2% (McGRAW et al. 2003). Cortical destruction, presence of a cortical soft tissue mass, highly vascularized lesions (Fig. 11.55) and severe vertebral collapses are likely to increase the rate of complications (LAREDO and HAMZE 2004; NUSSBAUM et al. 2004).

11.4.6.1.1
Epidural and Foraminal leaks

Epidural and foraminal leaks can produce paraplegia and radiculopathy due to cord and nerve root compression, respectively. Their incidence is higher in patients with fractures of the posterior vertebral wall and malignant disease with extensive bone destruction. Leaks can occur as a result of breaking

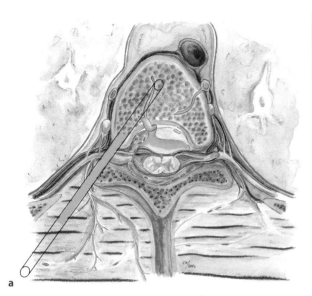

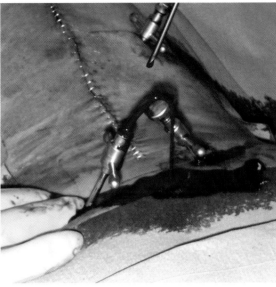

Fig. 11.55. Bilateral sacroplasty and L1 vertebroplasty in a 51-year-old woman with metastatic renal cancer. Previous arterial embolization and surgical fixation. Perioperative picture shows a highly vascular lesion with jet of blood due to intratumoral arteriovenous shunts. The risk of cement leakage is increased and cement should be injected in a very pasty phase

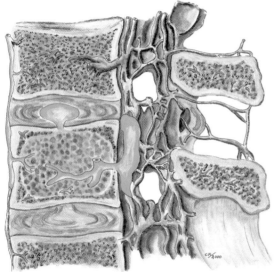

Fig. 11.54a,b. Most common cement leaks. Drawings show (**a**) intravasation of cement into the venous plexus that drains towards the epidural space, the lumbar veins, the azygos and the cava, and (**b**) disc leakage which is common but rarely symptomatic. (Drawing courtesy of C. Kauff, RT)

and arachnoid membrane fibrosis suggestive of the delayed effect of thermal injury, which can result in residual neurological deficit (TENG et al. 2003). Intradural leakage of cement has been reported but this is an extremely rare complication resulting from failure to respect the technique (LAVELLE and CHENEY 2006).

Radiculopathy is usually transient and is thought to be caused by heating of the emergent nerve root as a result of cement contact. If detected at the time of vertebroplasty, a 22-gauge spinal needle can be introduced into the foramen and the nerve root actively cooled by injecting normal saline (Fig. 11.57) (KELEKIS et al. 2003). Some patients may require a course of oral non-steroidal anti-inflammatory drugs, oral steroids or periradicular infiltration of steroid (GANGI et al. 2006). In our series of 3000 cases, we encountered 4 cases of neuralgia due to foraminal cement leakage. In two patients, the symptoms resolved spontaneously, one required a periradicular infiltration of steroid and in one patient immediate cooling of the nerve root with saline resulted in immediate resolution of symptoms.

through the medial or inferior cortex of the vertebral pedicle at the time of approach. Cement leakage into the spinal canal is usually well tolerated if there is enough residual space for the thecal sac. Paraplegia is a medical emergency and requires immediate neurosurgical decompression to avoid permanent damage to the cord (Fig. 11.56). Neurosurgical decompression shows intradural fibrosis, adhesions

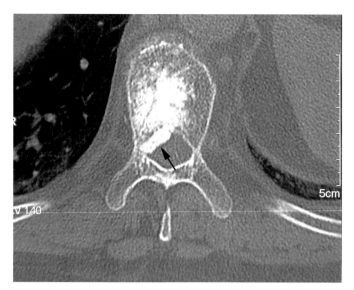

Fig. 11.56. T10 vertebroplasty in a 42-year-old woman with osteogenesis imperfecta. Axial CT scan shows right epidural cement leak (*arrow*) causing intercostal neuralgia. The needle was positioned in mid of the vertebral body and not in the anterior third. Partial relief after repeated selective steroid injections

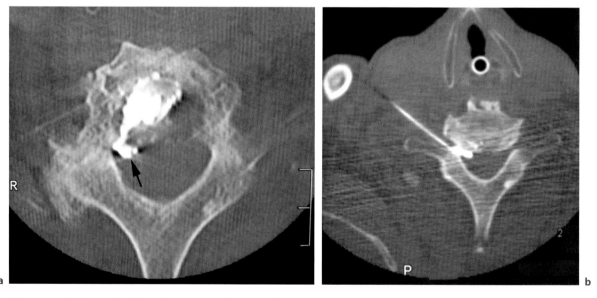

Fig. 11.57a,b. C7 vertebroplasty in a 77-year-old man with metastatic prostate cancer. **a** Axial CT scan shows a right posterolateral cement leak (*arrow*) in contact with the nerve root noticed immediately during injection. **b** Axial CT scan shows a 22-gauge spinal needle is immediately inserted into the foramen and infusion of saline to avoid thermal damage of the nerve root during polymerization of the cement. The patient experienced mild neuralgia with good relief after periradicular steroid injection

11.4.6.1.2
Perivertebral Venous Plexus Leak

Venous intravasation of cement limited to the basivertebral vein is usually asymptomatic if the operator recognizes it early and immediately stops injection (Fig. 11.58). However, failure to notice this and continued cement injection can cause filling of the epidural and paravertebral veins resulting in pulmonary embolism (Fig. 11.59). Pulmonary embolism is usually peripheral and asymptomatic (Baumann et al. 2007; Hodler et al. 2003; Scroop et al. 2002). It can present with hypotension, arrhythmia and hypocapnia. Rarely, it can be central and cause pul-

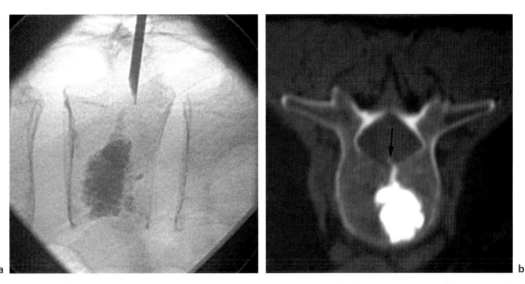

Fig. 11.58a,b. Venous intravasation of cement limited to the basivertebral vein in a 58-year-old woman with osteoporotic fracture. **a** Lateral fluoroscopic view and (**b**) corresponding axial CT scan show posterior cement intravasation into the basivertebral vein (*arrow*), without epidural extension

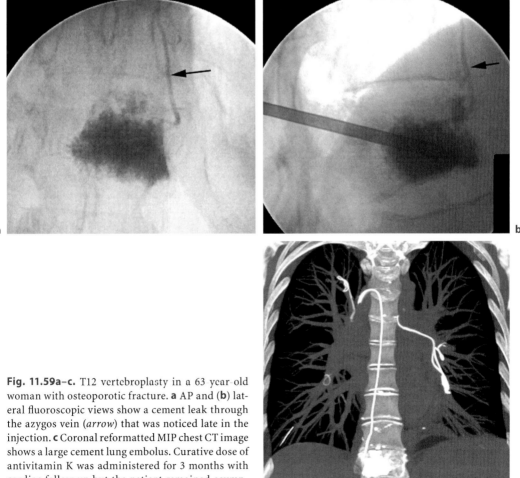

Fig. 11.59a–c. T12 vertebroplasty in a 63-year-old woman with osteoporotic fracture. **a** AP and (**b**) lateral fluoroscopic views show a cement leak through the azygos vein (*arrow*) that was noticed late in the injection. **c** Coronal reformatted MIP chest CT image shows a large cement lung embolus. Curative dose of antivitamin K was administered for 3 months with cardiac follow-up but the patient remained asymptomatic

monary infarction (FRANCOIS et al. 2003; PADOVANI et al. 1999). In our series, we observed four cases of asymptomatic pulmonary cement emboli. In one patient we observed cement lining the pulmonary veins from the heart with no symptoms.

11.4.6.1.3
Disc and Paravertebral Leak

Disc and paravertebral leaks are usually of no consequence. However, in patients with severe osteopo-

rosis, cement leaks into the anterior portion of the disc interfere with the load bearing mechanics of the vertebral column and can result in fractures of the adjacent vertebral body. Cement leaks into the middle and posterior portions of the disc are usually of no significance (Fig. 11.60) (LIN et al. 2004).

Paravertebral leaks are difficult to detect during vertebroplasty with only lateral fluoroscopy. For this reason, during cement injection, an AP view should always be used to avoid or minimize these leaks (Fig. 11.61).

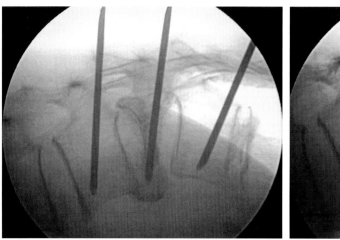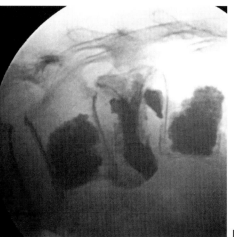

Fig. 11.60a,b. T11, T12 and L1 vertebroplasty in a 72-year-old woman with osteoporotic fracture. **a** Lateral fluoroscopic view shows the three trocars after positioning. **b** Lateral fluoroscopic view shows T11–12 disk leakage which was asymptomatic

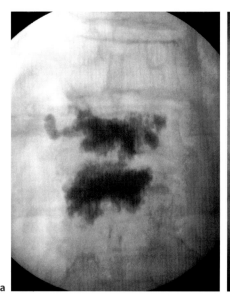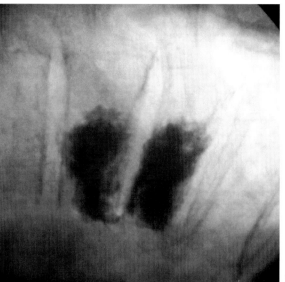

Fig. 11.61a,b. T11 and T12 vertebroplasty in a 71-year-old man treated with osteoporotic fracture. **a** AP fluoroscopic view shows cement leak in the right paravertebral soft tissues, which is not visible on (**b**) lateral fluoroscopic view

11.4.6.1.4
Cement Leakage Along the Needle Tract

Cement leakage along the needle tract is avoided by replacing the mandrin in the outer sheath before removal of the needle. If the mandrin cannot be completely inserted then the needle should be removed after several clockwise rotations within the vertebral body to cut off any cement on the needle tip. If not, removal of the needle can leave cement in the soft tissue (Fig. 11.62). If two needles are used, the needles should only be removed after completing injection through both needles; if one needle is removed before the injection is complete, cement can leak via the other needle tract (Buy et al. 2006).

11.4.6.2
Infection

Infection occurs in less than 1%. Strict asepsis must be maintained during the procedure. There are case reports in recent literature on post vertebroplasty infection with epidural abscesses resulting in neurological deficit treated with surgery and antibiotics (Alfonso Olmos et al. 2006; Mummaneni et al. 2006; Soyuncu et al. 2006; Vats and McKiernan 2006). It is essential to evaluate carefully patients with pre-procedure CRP elevation for systemic infections before the procedure. In our experience, 3 months after a vertebroplasty for an osteoporotic vertebral facture, an 82-year-old woman developed

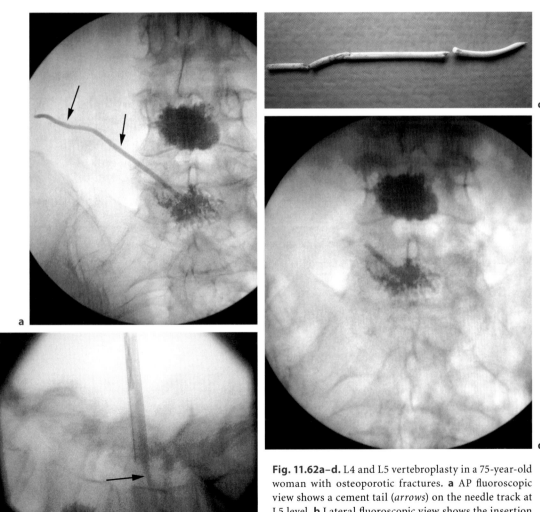

Fig. 11.62a–d. L4 and L5 vertebroplasty in a 75-year-old woman with osteoporotic fractures. **a** AP fluoroscopic view shows a cement tail (*arrows*) on the needle track at L5 level. **b** Lateral fluoroscopic view shows the insertion of a bone trocar over the cement tail (*arrow*). Its sharp tip allows it to cut the cement tail in contact with the pedicle. **c** The cement tail after removal. **d** AP fluoroscopic view shows no residual cement in the soft tissues

back pain with a posterior epidural abscess. Cyto-pathology proved it to be tuberculosis.

11.4.6.3
Fracture

Fracture of the ribs, pedicle and/or posterior elements is considered a minor adverse complication (HODLER et al. 2003), with an incidence of <1%.

11.4.6.4
Allergic Reaction

Allergic reactions to the cement are characterized by arrhythmias and hypotension. Anaphylactic reaction to PMMA resulting in death is not an insignificant risk, as has been reported to the FDA (NUSSBAUM et al. 2004).

11.4.6.5
Adjacent Vertebral Body Collapse

Collapse of the adjacent vertebral body has a reported incidence of 12.4% (UPPIN et al. 2003) and an odds ratio of 2.27 (GRADOS et al. 2000), with a relative risk 4.62 times greater than the occurrence for non-adjacent level fractures, and a tendency to occur sooner than non-adjacent level fractures (Fig. 11.63) (TROUT et al. 2006).

Treated vertebrae are stiffer than before; they act like a pillar and change the load bearing biomechanics of the spine. Due to the nondeformity of the vertebral end plates there is increased pressure in the discs, which causes increased load in the adjacent vertebra and increased risk of fracture (BAROUD and BOHNER 2006; BAROUD et al. 2003; WILCOX 2006). Further, patients on oral steroid therapy at their initial vertebroplasty are almost twice as likely as primary osteoporosis patients to have symptomatic refractures within one year of initial vertebroplasty (SYED et al. 2006).

The risk factors for the development of new compression fractures are old age, multiple levels treated at the initial vertebroplasty, less severe wedge deformity of the treated vertebra and fractures outside the thoracolumbar junction (LEE et al. 2006).

In our opinion, overfilling and disk leakage, particularly anterior leak, increase the risk of adjacent vertebral fracture in osteoporotic patients. All osteopenic patients with spontaneous spinal fracture are at high risk of new fracture, with or without vertebroplasty. These patients should receive optimal

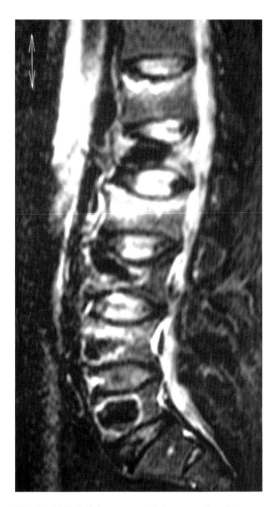

Fig. 11.63. Painful osteoporotic fractures in a 68-year-old woman. Sagittal T2 STIR MR image shows hyperintensity of T12 and L2 suggestive of acute vertebral fractures. It also shows hypointensity at L1, L3, L4 and L5 levels secondary to previous vertebroplasty. The risk of new adjacent fractures may be increased due to the excessive stiffness of PMMA. Overfilling of the vertebral body should be avoided

medical management of their osteopenia or osteoporosis, because proper medical therapy can cut the risk of new fractures by half. Second, the potential risk for new fracture should be discussed with all patients before vertebroplasty (TROUT and KALLMES 2006; TROUT et al. 2006).

11.4.6.6
Puncture Site Bleeding

Bleeding from the puncture site is associated with pain and tenderness at the puncture site and resolves in 72 h. Compression of the puncture site for 5 min following removal of the needle helps reduce this complication.

11.4.6.7
Free Fragment Retropulsion

Failure to recognize the presence of a free posterior wall fragment can result in the free fragment being pushed into the spinal canal during cement injection and causing cord compression (Fig. 11.41). It is important to recognize and respect this contraindication.

11.5
Conclusion

Percutaneous vertebroplasty has been used to treat vertebral compression fractures of diverse etiologies since 1984. Major indications are osteoporotic compression fractures and painful osteolytic metastasis. It is one of the most satisfactory techniques developed in recent years, with excellent, rapid pain control. The technique has now gained widespread acceptance and is considered a standard of care for painful osteoporotic fractures resistant to conservative medical therapy. With the number of published cases increasing in literature, the indications, technique and complications are well described. Even though simple to perform with minimal complications, for the best results the percutaneous technique should be mastered and the inclusion and exclusion criteria strictly adhered to.

Percutaneous vertebroplasty and kyphoplasty seem to provide equal pain relief and the complication rate is similar in experienced hands. Kyphoplasty allows the creation of a cavity in the vertebral body and the opportunity to restore the vertebral height. However, the benefits of kyphoplasty over vertebroplasty are unproven. The value of vertebral height restoration is uncertain and prospective randomized clinical trials are needed. In our opinion, the best indications of kyphoplasty are traumatic spinal compression fractures in nonosteoporotic patients with injection of biocompatible calcium phosphate cements.

References

Aebli N, Goss BG, Thorpe P, Williams R, Krebs J (2006) In vivo temperature profile of intervertebral discs and vertebral endplates during vertebroplasty: an experimental study in sheep. Spine 31:1674–1678; discussion 1679

Alfonso Olmos M, Silva Gonzalez A, Duart Clemente J, Villas Tome C (2006) Infected vertebroplasty due to uncommon bacteria solved surgically: a rare and threatening life complication of a common procedure: report of a case and a review of the literature. Spine 31:E770–773

Alvarez L, Perez-Higueras A, Quinones D, Calvo E, Rossi RE (2003) Vertebroplasty in the treatment of vertebral tumors: postprocedural outcome and quality of life. Eur Spine J 12:356–360

Ananthakrishnan D, Berven S, Deviren V, Cheng K, Lotz JC, Xu Z, Puttlitz CM (2005) The effect on anterior column loading due to different vertebral augmentation techniques. Clin Biomech (Bristol, Avon) 20:25–31

Arnold W (1985) Early surgical treatment of traumatic paraplegia with an external fixation device and diagonal vertebroplasty. Unfallchirurg 88:293–298

Baroud G, Bohner M (2006) Biomechanical impact of vertebroplasty. Postoperative biomechanics of vertebroplasty. Joint Bone Spine 73:144–150

Baroud G, Heini P, Nemes J, Bohner M, Ferguson S, Steffen T (2003) Biomechanical explanation of adjacent fractures following vertebroplasty. Radiology 229:606–607; author reply 607–608

Baudrez V, Galant C, Vande Berg BC (2001) Benign vertebral hemangioma: MR-histological correlation. Skeletal Radiol 30:442–446

Baumann C, Fuchs H, Kiwit J, Westphalen K, Hierholzer J (2007) Complications in percutaneous vertebroplasty associated with puncture or cement leakage. Cardiovasc Intervent Radiol 30:161–168

Belkoff SM, Mathis JM, Jasper LE (2002) Ex vivo biomechanical comparison of hydroxyapatite and polymethylmethacrylate cements for use with vertebroplasty. AJNR Am J Neuroradiol 23:1647–1651

Bremnes RM, Hauge HN, Sagsveen R (1996) Radiotherapy in the treatment of symptomatic vertebral hemangiomas: technical case report. Neurosurgery 39:1054–1058

Brown DB, Gilula LA, Sehgal M, Shimony JS (2004) Treatment of chronic symptomatic vertebral compression fractures with percutaneous vertebroplasty. AJR Am J Roentgenol 182:319–322

Brunot S, Berge J, Barreau X, Menegon P, Dousset V (2005) Long term clinical follow up of vertebral hemangiomas treated by percutaneous vertebroplasty. J Radiol 86:41–45; quiz 46–47

Buy X, Basile A, Bierry G, Cupelli J, Gangi A (2006) Saline-infused bipolar radiofrequency ablation of high-risk spinal and paraspinal neoplasms. AJR Am J Roentgenol 186:S322–326

Castel E, Lazennec JY, Chiras J, Enkaoua E, Saillant G (1999) Acute spinal cord compression due to intraspinal bleeding from a vertebral hemangioma: two case-reports. Eur Spine J 8:244–248

Chi JH, Manley GT, Chou D (2005) Pregnancy-related vertebral hemangioma. Case report, review of the literature, and management algorithm. Neurosurg Focus 19:E7

Choi JJ, Murphey MD (2000) Angiomatous skeletal lesions. Semin Musculoskelet Radiol 4:103–112

Choong PF (2003) Cardiopulmonary complications of intramedullary fixation of long bone metastases. Clin Orthop Relat Res:S245–253

Cortet B, Cotten A, Deprez X, Deramond H, Lejeune JP, Leclerc X, Chastanet P, Duquesnoy B, Delcambre B (1994) [Value of vertebroplasty combined with surgical decompression in the treatment of aggressive spinal angioma. Apropos of 3 cases]. Rev Rhum Ed Fr 61:16–22

Cotten A, Duquesnoy B (1995) Percutaneous cementoplasty for malignant osteolysis of the acetabulum. Presse Med 24:1308–1310

Cotten A, Deramond H, Cortet B, Lejeune JP, Leclerc X, Chastanet P, Clarisse J (1996a) Preoperative percutaneous injection of methyl methacrylate and N-butyl cyanoacrylate in vertebral hemangiomas. AJNR Am J Neuroradiol 17:137–142

Cotten A, Dewatre F, Cortet B, Assaker R, Leblond D, Duquesnoy B, Chastanet P, Clarisse J (1996b) Percutaneous vertebroplasty for osteolytic metastases and myeloma: effects of the percentage of lesion filling and the leakage of methyl methacrylate at clinical follow-up. Radiology 200:525–530

Cotten A, Boutry N, Cortet B, Assaker R, Demondion X, Leblond D, Chastanet P, Duquesnoy B, Deramond H (1998) Percutaneous vertebroplasty: state of the art. Radiographics 18:311–320; discussion 320–313

Deramond H, Wright NT, Belkoff SM (1999) Temperature elevation caused by bone cement polymerization during vertebroplasty. Bone 25:17S–21S

Deramond H, Saliou G, Aveillan M, Lehmann P, Vallee JN (2006) Respective contributions of vertebroplasty and kyphoplasty to the management of osteoporotic vertebral fractures. Joint Bone Spine 73:610–613

Doppman JL, Oldfield EH, Heiss JD (2000) Symptomatic vertebral hemangiomas: treatment by means of direct intralesional injection of ethanol. Radiology 214:341–348

Faria SL, Schlupp WR, Chiminazzo H Jr (1985) Radiotherapy in the treatment of vertebral hemangiomas. Int J Radiat Oncol Biol Phys 11:387–390

Francois K, Taeymans Y, Poffyn B, Van Nooten G (2003) Successful management of a large pulmonary cement embolus after percutaneous vertebroplasty: a case report. Spine 28:E424–425

Frey ME, Depalma MJ, Cifu DX, Bhagia SM, Carne W, Daitch JS (2008) Percutaneous sacroplasty for osteoporotic sacral insufficiency fractures: a prospective, multicenter, observational pilot study. Spine J 8(2):367–373

Gabal AM (2002) Percutaneous technique for sclerotherapy of vertebral hemangioma compressing spinal cord. Cardiovasc Intervent Radiol 25:494–500

Galibert P, Deramond H (1990) Percutaneous acrylic vertebroplasty as a treatment of vertebral angioma as well as painful and debilitating diseases. Chirurgie 116:326–334; discussion 335

Galibert P, Deramond H, Rosat P, Le Gars D (1987) Preliminary note on the treatment of vertebral angioma by percutaneous acrylic vertebroplasty. Neurochirurgie 33:166–168

Gangi A, Kastler BA, Dietemann JL (1994) Percutaneous vertebroplasty guided by a combination of CT and fluoroscopy. AJNR Am J Neuroradiol 15:83–86

Gangi A, Dietemann JL, Mortazavi R, Pfleger D, Kauff C, Roy C (1998) CT-guided interventional procedures for pain management in the lumbosacral spine. Radiographics 18:621–633

Gangi A, Guth S, Imbert JP, Marin H, Dietemann JL (2003) Percutaneous vertebroplasty: indications, technique, and results. Radiographics 23:e10

Gangi A, Basille A, Buy X, Alizadeh H, Sauer B, Bierry G (2005) Radiofrequency and laser ablation of spinal lesions. Semin Ultrasound CT MR 26(2):89–97

Gangi A, Sabharwal T, Irani FG, Buy X, Morales JP, Adam A (2006) Quality assurance guidelines for percutaneous vertebroplasty. Cardiovasc Intervent Radiol 29:173–178

Gaughen JR Jr, Jensen ME, Schweickert PA, Kaufmann TJ, Marx WF, Kallmes DF (2002) Lack of preoperative spinous process tenderness does not affect clinical success of percutaneous vertebroplasty. J Vasc Interv Radiol 13:1135–1138

Goyal M, Mishra NK, Sharma A, Gaikwad SB, Mohanty BK, Sharma S (1999) Alcohol ablation of symptomatic vertebral hemangiomas. AJNR Am J Neuroradiol 20:1091–1096

Grados F, Depriester C, Cayrolle G, Hardy N, Deramond H, Fardellone P (2000) Long-term observations of vertebral osteoporotic fractures treated by percutaneous vertebroplasty. Rheumatology (Oxford) 39:1410–1414

Gray F, Gherardi R, Benhaiem-Sigaux N (1989) Vertebral hemangioma. Definition, limitations, anatomopathologic aspects. Neurochirurgie 35:267–269

Heim D, Regazzoni P, Tsakiris DA, Aebi T, Schlegel U, Marbet GA, Perren SM (1995) Intramedullary nailing and pulmonary embolism: does unreamed nailing prevent embolization? An in vivo study in rabbits. J Trauma 38:899–906

Heini P (2005) The current treatment: a survey of osteoporotic fracture treatment. Osteoporotic spine fracture: the spine surgeon's perspective. Osteoporosis Intl 16(S2):85–92

Heini PF, Berlemann U (2001) Bone substitutes in vertebroplasty. Eur Spine J 10(Suppl 2):S205–213

Heini PF, Berlemann U, Kaufmann M, Lippuner K, Fankhauser C, van Landuyt P (2001) Augmentation of mechanical properties in osteoporotic vertebral bones – a biomechanical investigation of vertebroplasty efficacy with different bone cements. Eur Spine J 10:164–171

Heiss JD, Doppman JL, Oldfield EH (1996) Treatment of vertebral hemangioma by intralesional injection of absolute ethanol. N Engl J Med 334:1340

Hernigou P, Djindjian M, Ricolfi F, Dahhan P (1994) Neuroaggressive dorsal vertebral hemangioma and vertebrectomy. Apropos of 2 cases. Review of the literature. Rev Chir Orthop Reparatrice Appar Mot 80:542–550

Heyd R, Strassmann G, Filipowicz I, Borowsky K, Martin T, Zamboglou N (2001) [Radiotherapy in vertebral hemangioma]. Rontgenpraxis 53:208–220

Hide IG, Gangi A (2004) Percutaneous vertebroplasty: history, technique and current perspectives. Clin Radiol 59:461–467

Hodler J, Peck D, Gilula LA (2003) Midterm outcome after vertebroplasty: predictive value of technical and patient-related factors. Radiology 227:662–668

Hulme PA, Krebs J, Ferguson SJ, Berlemann U (2006) Vertebroplasty and kyphoplasty: a systematic review of 69 clinical studies. Spine 31:1983–2001

Ide C, Gangi A, Rimmelin A, Beaujeux R, Maitrot D, Buchheit F, Sellal F, Dietemann JL (1996) Vertebral haemangiomas with spinal cord compression: the place of preoperative percutaneous vertebroplasty with methyl methacrylate. Neuroradiology 38:585–589

Inamasu J, Nichols TA, Guiot BH (2006) Vertebral hemangioma symptomatic during pregnancy treated by posterior decompression, intraoperative vertebroplasty, and segmental fixation. J Spinal Disord Tech 19:451–454

Jang JS, Lee SH (2005) Efficacy of percutaneous vertebroplasty combined with radiotherapy in osteolytic metastatic spinal tumors. J Neurosurg Spine 2:243–248

Jasper LE, Deramond H, Mathis JM, Belkoff SM (1999) The effect of monomer-to-powder ratio on the material properties of cranioplastic. Bone 25:27S–29S

Jasper LE, Deramond H, Mathis JM, Belkoff SM (2002) Material properties of various cements for use with vertebroplasty. J Mater Sci Mater Med 13:1–5

Kallmes DF (2007) Percutaneous vertebroplasty causing an increase in retropulsion of bone fragments. J Vasc Interv Radiol 18:1333–1334

Kallmes DF, Jensen ME (2003) Percutaneous vertebroplasty. Radiology 229:27–36

Kelekis AD, Martin JB, Somon T, Wetzel SG, Dietrich PY, Ruefenacht DA (2003) Radicular pain after vertebroplasty: compression or irritation of the nerve root? Initial experience with the "cooling system". Spine 28:E265–269

Kim CW, Minocha J, Wahl CE, Garfin SR (2004) Response of fractured osteoporotic bone to polymethylacrylate after vertebroplasty: case report. Spine J 4:709–712

Kim MJ, Lindsey DP, Hannibal M, Alamin TF (2006) Vertebroplasty versus kyphoplasty: biomechanical behavior under repetitive loading conditions. Spine 31:2079–2084

Laredo JD, Hamze B (2004) Complications of percutaneous vertebroplasty and their prevention. Skeletal Radiol 33:493–505

Laredo JD, Assouline E, Gelbert F, Wybier M, Merland JJ, Tubiana JM (1990) Vertebral hemangiomas: fat content as a sign of aggressiveness. Radiology 177:467–472

Lavelle WF, Cheney R (2006) Recurrent fracture after vertebral kyphoplasty. Spine J 6:488–493

Lee ST, Chen JF (2004) A syringe compressor for vertebroplasty: technical note. Surg Neurol 61:580–584

Lee WS, Sung KH, Jeong HT, Sung YS, Hyun YI, Choi JY, Lee KS, Ok CS, Choi YW (2006) Risk factors of developing new symptomatic vertebral compression fractures after percutaneous vertebroplasty in osteoporotic patients. Eur Spine J 15:1777–1783

Legroux-Gerot I, Lormeau C, Boutry N, Cotten A, Duquesnoy B, Cortet B (2004) Long-term follow-up of vertebral osteoporotic fractures treated by percutaneous vertebroplasty. Clin Rheumatol 23:310–317

Lieberman IH, Dudeney S, Reinhardt MK, Bell G (2001) Initial outcome and efficacy of "kyphoplasty" in the treatment of painful osteoporotic vertebral compression fractures. Spine 26:1631–1638

Lim TH, Brebach GT, Renner SM, Kim WJ, Kim JG, Lee RE, Andersson GB, An HS (2002) Biomechanical evaluation of an injectable calcium phosphate cement for vertebroplasty. Spine 27:1297–1302

Lin EP, Ekholm S, Hiwatashi A, Westesson PL (2004) Vertebroplasty: cement leakage into the disc increases the risk of new fracture of adjacent vertebral body. AJNR Am J Neuroradiol 25:175–180

Maestretti G, Cremer C, Otten P, Jakob RP (2007) Prospective study of standalone balloon kyphoplasty with calcium phosphate cement augmentation in traumatic fractures. Eur Spine J 16:601–610

Magerl F, Aebi M, Gertzbein SD, Harms J, Nazarian S (1994) A comprehensive classification of thoracic and lumbar injuries. Eur Spine J 3:184–201

Martin JB, Gailloud P, Dietrich PY, Luciani ME, Somon T, Sappino PA, Rufenach DA (2002) Direct transoral approach to C2 for percutaneous vertebroplasty. Cardiovasc Intervent Radiol 25:517–519

Masala S, Konda D, Massari F, Simonetti G (2006) Sacroplasty and iliac osteoplasty under combined CT and fluoroscopic guidance. Spine 31:E667–669

Mathis JM (2002) Vertebroplasty for vertebral fractures with intravertebral clefts. AJNR Am J Neuroradiol 23:1619–1620

Mathis JM, Wong W (2003) Percutaneous vertebroplasty: technical considerations. J Vasc Interv Radiol 14:953–960

Mathis JM, Petri M, Naff N (1998) Percutaneous vertebroplasty treatment of steroid-induced osteoporotic compression fractures. Arthritis Rheum 41:171–175

Mathis JM, Barr JD, Belkoff SM, Barr MS, Jensen ME, Deramond H (2001) Percutaneous vertebroplasty: a developing standard of care for vertebral compression fractures. AJNR Am J Neuroradiol 22:373–381

Mathis JM, Ortiz AO, Zoarski GH (2004) Vertebroplasty versus kyphoplasty: a comparison and contrast. AJNR Am J Neuroradiol 25:840–845

Maynard AS, Jensen ME, Schweickert PA, Marx WF, Short JG, Kallmes DF (2000) Value of bone scan imaging in predicting pain relief from percutaneous vertebroplasty in osteoporotic vertebral fractures. AJNR Am J Neuroradiol 21:1807–1812

McGraw JK, Cardella J, Barr JD, Mathis JM, Sanchez O, Schwartzberg MS, Swan TL, Sacks D (2003) Society of Interventional Radiology quality improvement guidelines for percutaneous vertebroplasty. J Vasc Interv Radiol 14:S311–315

McKiernan F, Faciszewski T, Jensen R (2003) Reporting height restoration in vertebral compression fractures. Spine 28:2517–2521; discussion 2513

Moreland DB, Landi MK, Grand W (2001) Vertebroplasty: techniques to avoid complications. Spine J 1:66–71

Mummaneni PV, Walker DH, Mizuno J, Rodts GE (2006) Infected vertebroplasty requiring 360 degrees spinal reconstruction: long-term follow-up review. Report of two cases. J Neurosurg Spine 5:86–89

Murphey MD, Fairbairn KJ, Parman LM, Baxter KG, Parsa MB, Smith WS (1995) From the archives of the AFIP. Musculoskeletal angiomatous lesions: radiologic-pathologic correlation. Radiographics 15:893–917

Murugan L, Samson RS, Chandy MJ (2002) Management of symptomatic vertebral hemangiomas: review of 13 patients. Neurol India 50:300–305

Nagata-Narumiya T, Nagai Y, Kashiwagi H, Hama M, Takifuji K, Tanimura H (2000) Endoscopic sclerotherapy for esophageal hemangioma. Gastrointest Endosc 52:285–287

Nguyen JP, Djindjian M, Badiane S (1989) Vertebral hemangioma with neurologic signs. Clinical presentation, results of a survey by the French Society of Neurosurgery. Neurochirurgie 35:270–274, 305–308

Niemeyer T, McClellan J, Webb J, Jaspan T, Ramli N (1999) Brown-Sequard syndrome after management of vertebral hemangioma with intralesional alcohol. A case report. Spine 24:1845–1847

Nussbaum DA, Gailloud P, Murphy K (2004) A review of complications associated with vertebroplasty and kyphoplasty as reported to the food and drug administration medical device related web site. J Vasc Interv Radiol 15:1185–1192

Obana Y, Tanji K, Furuta I, Yamazumi T, Hashimoto S, Kikuchi H, Tanaka S, Ohba Y (1996) A case of malignant transformation in thoracic vertebral hemangioma following repetitive irradiation and extraction. Pathol Int 46:71–78

Padovani B, Kasriel O, Brunner P, Peretti-Viton P (1999) Pulmonary embolism caused by acrylic cement: a rare complication of percutaneous vertebroplasty. AJNR Am J Neuroradiol 20:375–377

Peh WC, Gilula LA (2003) Percutaneous vertebroplasty: indications, contraindications, and technique. Br J Radiol 76:69–75

Phillips FM (2003) Minimally invasive treatments of osteoporotic vertebral compression fractures. Spine 28:S45–53

Picard L, Bracard S, Roland J, Moreno A, Per A (1989) Embolization of vertebral hemangioma. Technic-indications-results. Neurochirurgie 35:289–293, 305–308

Poole KE, Compston JE (2006) Osteoporosis and its management. Br Med J 333:1251–1256

Ross JS, Masaryk TJ, Modic MT, Carter JR, Mapstone T, Dengel FH (1987) Vertebral hemangiomas: MR imaging. Radiology 165:165–169

Roy-Camille R, Monpierre H, Saillant G, Chiras J (1989) Role of surgical resection in the treatment of vertebral hemangioma. Neurochirurgie 35:294–295

Sakata K, Hareyama M, Oouchi A, Sido M, Nagakura H, Tamakawa M, Akiba H, Morita K (1997) Radiotherapy of vertebral hemangiomas. Acta Oncol 36:719–724

Schwartz TH, Hibshoosh H, Riedel CJ (2000) Estrogen and progesterone receptor-negative T11 vertebral hemangioma presenting as a postpartum compression fracture: case report and management. Neurosurgery 46:218–221

Scroop R, Eskridge J, Britz GW (2002) Paradoxical cerebral arterial embolization of cement during intraoperative vertebroplasty: case report. AJNR Am J Neuroradiol 23:868–870

Serrano M, Iglesias A, San Millan J (1996) Long-term response to radiotherapy of vertebral hemangioma resulting in paraplegia. Acta Oncol 35:498–499

Shimony JS, Gilula LA, Zeller AJ, Brown DB (2004) Percutaneous vertebroplasty for malignant compression fractures with epidural involvement. Radiology 232:846–853

Smith TP, Koci T, Mehringer CM, Tsai FY, Fraser KW, Dowd CF, Higashida RT, Halbach VV, Hieshima GB (1993) Transarterial embolization of vertebral hemangioma. J Vasc Interv Radiol 4:681–685

Soyuncu Y, Ozdemir H, Soyuncu S, Bigat Z, Gur S (2006) Posterior spinal epidural abscess: an unusual complication of vertebroplasty. Joint Bone Spine 73:753–755

Spence GM, Dunning MT, Cannon SR, Briggs TW (2002) The hazard of retrograde nailing in pathological fractures. Three cases involving primary musculoskeletal malignancy. Injury 33:533–538

Stallmeyer MJ, Zoarski GH, Obuchowski AM (2003) Optimizing patient selection in percutaneous vertebroplasty. J Vasc Interv Radiol 14:683–696

Syed MI, Patel NA, Jan S, Shaikh A, Grunden B, Morar K (2006) Symptomatic refractures after vertebroplasty in patients with steroid-induced osteoporosis. AJNR Am J Neuroradiol 27:1938–1943

Teng MM, Wei CJ, Wei LC, Luo CB, Lirng JF, Chang FC, Liu CL, Chang CY (2003) Kyphosis correction and height restoration effects of percutaneous vertebroplasty. AJNR Am J Neuroradiol 24:1893–1900

Togawa D, Bauer TW, Lieberman IH, Takikawa S (2003) Histologic evaluation of human vertebral bodies after vertebral augmentation with polymethyl methacrylate. Spine 28:1521–1527

Tomita S, Kin A, Yazu M, Abe M (2003) Biomechanical evaluation of kyphoplasty and vertebroplasty with calcium phosphate cement in a simulated osteoporotic compression fracture. J Orthop Sci 8:192–197

Tozzi P, Abdelmoumene Y, Corno AF, Gersbach PA, Hoogewoud HM, von Segesser LK (2002) Management of pulmonary embolism during acrylic vertebroplasty. Ann Thorac Surg 74:1706–1708

Trout AT, Kallmes DF (2006) Does vertebroplasty cause incident vertebral fractures? A review of available data. AJNR Am J Neuroradiol 27:1397–1403

Trout AT, Kallmes DF, Kaufmann TJ (2006) New fractures after vertebroplasty: adjacent fractures occur significantly sooner. AJNR Am J Neuroradiol 27:217–223

Tschirhart CE, Roth SE, Whyne CM (2005) Biomechanical assessment of stability in the metastatic spine following percutaneous vertebroplasty: effects of cement distribution patterns and volume. J Biomech 38:1582–1590

Tschirhart CE, Finkelstein JA, Whyne CM (2006) Optimization of tumor volume reduction and cement augmentation in percutaneous vertebroplasty for prophylactic treatment of spinal metastases. J Spinal Disord Tech 19:584–590

Uppin AA, Hirsch JA, Centenera LV, Pfiefer BA, Pazianos AG, Choi IS (2003) Occurrence of new vertebral body fracture after percutaneous vertebroplasty in patients with osteoporosis. Radiology 226:119–124

Vasconcelos C, Gailloud P, Beauchamp NJ, Heck DV, Murphy KJ (2002) Is percutaneous vertebroplasty without pretreatment venography safe? Evaluation of 205 consecutives procedures. AJNR Am J Neuroradiol 23:913–917

Vats HS, McKiernan FE (2006) Infected vertebroplasty: case report and review of literature. Spine 31:E859–862

Villarraga ML, Bellezza AJ, Harrigan TP, Cripton PA, Kurtz SM, Edidin AA (2005) The biomechanical effects of kyphoplasty on treated and adjacent nontreated vertebral bodies. J Spinal Disord Tech 18:84–91

Weill A, Chiras J, Simon JM, Rose M, Sola-Martinez T, Enkaoua E (1996) Spinal metastases: indications for and results of percutaneous injection of acrylic surgical cement. Radiology 199:241–247

White SM (2002) Anaesthesia for percutaneous vertebroplasty. Anaesthesia 57:1229–1230

Wilcox RK (2006) The biomechanical effect of vertebroplasty on the adjacent vertebral body: a finite element study. Proc Inst Mech Eng [H] 220:565–572

Wilson DR, Myers ER, Mathis JM, Scribner RM, Conta JA, Reiley MA, Talmadge KD, Hayes WC (2000) Effect of augmentation on the mechanics of vertebral wedge fractures. Spine 25:158–165

Yamada K, Matsumoto Y, Kita M, Yamamoto K, Kobayashi T, Takanaka T (2004) Long-term pain relief effects in four patients undergoing percutaneous vertebroplasty for metastatic vertebral tumor. J Anesth 18:292–295

Yang ZY, Zhang LJ, Chen ZX, Hu HY (1985) Hemangioma of the vertebral column. A report on twenty-three patients with special reference to functional recovery after radiation therapy. Acta Radiol Oncol 24:129–132

Zoarski GH, Snow P, Olan WJ, Stallmeyer MJ, Dick BW, Hebel JR, De Deyne M (2002) Percutaneous vertebroplasty for osteoporotic compression fractures: quantitative prospective evaluation of long-term outcomes. J Vasc Interv Radiol 13:139–148

Percutaneous Kyphoplasty in Vertebral Compression Fractures

Lotfi Hacein-Bey and **Ali Guermazi**

12

CONTENTS

12.1 Introduction 259

12.2 Indications and Contraindications 260

12.3 Technique 271

12.4 Peri-procedural Management 273

12.5 Effectiveness of Kyphoplasty 273
12.5.1 Pain Relief 273
12.5.2 Vertebral Height Restoration 274

12.6 Complications 275

12.7 Cost Considerations 278

12.8 Kyphoplasty versus Vertebroplasty: When? 279

12.9 Conclusion 279

References 279

12.1
Introduction

The principle behind the kyphoplasty procedure is to restore the height of a vertebra by inserting an inflatable bone tamp to reduce or reverse the kyphotic deformity associated with a fracture (Belkoff et al. 1999; Belkoff et al. 2000; Belkoff et al. 2001a–d; Coumans et al. 2003; Dudeney et al. 2002; Lane et al. 2000; Lane et al. 2004; Ledlie and Renfro

2003; Lieberman et al. 2001; Theodorou et al. 2002; Wong et al. 2002). The concept of inserting and inflating a balloon into a vertebral body was first developed in the mid 1980s by an orthopedic surgeon, Dr. Mark Reiley, and an engineer, Arie Scholten. It was not until 1994, ten years later, that Dr. Reiley was able to find investors interested in his "balloons in bones" idea. The newly formed Kyphon Corporation (Sunnyvale, CA, USA) had two major tasks on its hands: first, to develop a balloon capable of displacing bone, and second, to address regulatory issues. The company also provided support for Dr. Reiley to perform all initial biomechanical investigations of the balloon tamp, along with neuroradiologists who were already familiar with vertebroplasty.

The KyphX Inflatable Bone Tamp (IBT; Kyphon Inc., Sunnyvale, CA, USA) received 510(k) clearance from the United States Food and Drug Administration (FDA) in July 1998. The KyphX device was officially launched at the 2000 meeting of the National Association of Spine Surgeons (NASS), at the same time Kyphon was establishing its European branch. Initially, upon the recommendation of the FDA, a clinical trial comparing kyphoplasty to conservative medical management was started. However, soon after it was initiated the clinical trial was abandoned, primarily for lack of patient entry, and was replaced by a clinical registry designed primarily to record clinical outcomes of patients treated with kyphoplasty.

Therefore, the kyphoplasty procedure has not been formally compared to conservative medical therapy in the form of a prospective randomized clinical trial, similar in that regard to the vertebroplasty procedure. Moreover, kyphoplasty has not been evaluated in comparison to vertebroplasty. At the end of 2004, a literature search found 350 published articles on vertebroplasty, compared to only 40 articles on kyphoplasty. In addition, more than 30 of those articles were review articles on the technique, and few were peer-reviewed studies of the safety and efficacy of kyphoplasty. Considering that

L. Hacein-Bey, MD
Professor of Radiology, Radiological Associates of Sacramento Medical Group Inc., 1500 Expo Parkway, Sacramento, CA 95815, USA *and* Sutter Neuroscience Institute, 2800 L Street, Suite 630, Sacramento, CA 95816, USA
A. Guermazi, MD
Associate Professor of Radiology, Department of Radiology, Chief Section of Musculoskeletal, Boston University School of Medicine, 88 East Newton Street, Boston, MA 02118, USA

kyphoplasty was developed through commercial investment (unlike vertebroplasty, which grew slowly and steadily within academic medicine) the paucity of data is likely to raise some concern.

12.2
Indications and Contraindications

Kyphoplasty (Figs. 12.1, 12.2), like vertebroplasty, is indicated for painful vertebral compression fractures, whether related to osteoporosis (Figs. 12.3, 12.4), metastatic cancer (Fig. 12.5), multiple myeloma (Fig. 12.6) and other hematological neoplastic conditions such as lymphoma and leukemia (Fig. 12.7), or aggressive vertebral hemangiomas (Fig. 12.8) (BARR et al. 2000; BASCOULERGUE et al. 1998; DUDENEY et al. 2002; FRIBOURG et al. 2004; GAITANIS et al. 2004; GALIBERT et al. 1987; GARFIN and REILLEY 2002; HARROP et al. 2004; HEINI and ORLER 2004; HSIANG 2003; MATHIS et al. 1998; MATHIS et al. 1999; OLAN 2002; STALLMEYER 2003; TOHMEH et al. 1999; WATTS 2001; WEILL et al. 1996; WILSON et al. 2000; ZOARSKI et al. 2000b). Vertebral body fractures that are associated with compromise of the posterior wall and retropulsion, particularly if associated with neurological deficit, have been traditionally considered best treated by conventional surgical techniques, although kypho-

plasty, performed through both an open surgical (GARFIN et al. 2001; GARFIN et al. 2002; HSIANG 2003; LANE et al. 2000; LIEBERMAN et al. 2001; LIEBERMAN and REINHARDT 2003) and a percutaneous approach (HARDOUIN et al. 2002; MASALA et al. 2004; ORTIZ et al. 2002) has been successful (Figs. 12.5, 12.7).

Kyphoplasty has also been reported in the successful treatment of vertebral fracture associated with Guillain-Barré syndrome, promoting significant improvement in functional activity and neurological function by allowing the patient to enroll immediately in a rehabilitation program (MASALA et al. 2004). Extreme compression fractures (vertebra plana) make the procedure technically difficult, although not impossible if the endplates are intact (Fig. 12.7).

Traumatic fractures not associated with osteoporosis, and which cause severe recurrent pain, may be considered for kyphoplasty, particularly if the fractures are recent. However, in such patients, vertebroplasty may still be the better choice, as it may be equally effective in providing pain relief, is less invasive, and the likelihood of height recovery may be low, as the bone is significantly harder than in osteoporotic patients (Fig. 12.9).

The only absolute contraindications are the presence of systemic infection and the lack of appropriate surgical backup. Bleeding conditions may be corrected prior to the procedure in the majority of patients.

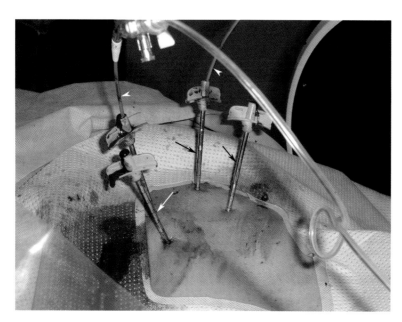

Fig. 12.1. Technique of closed percutaneous kyphoplasty in a 58-year-old woman. Peri-operative view shows the patient prone on the X-ray table. After localization of target vertebrae and sterile prepping, kyphoplasty trocars (*arrows*) are advanced into the vertebral bodies. Kyphoplasty balloons (*arrowheads*) are then navigated within the vertebra through the large trocars. Four trocars are inserted in this patient as two vertebrae are being treated

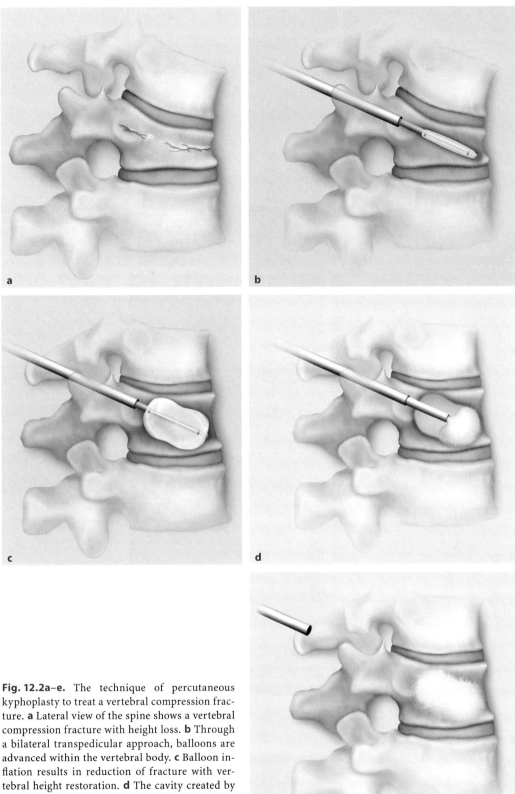

Fig. 12.2a–e. The technique of percutaneous kyphoplasty to treat a vertebral compression fracture. **a** Lateral view of the spine shows a vertebral compression fracture with height loss. **b** Through a bilateral transpedicular approach, balloons are advanced within the vertebral body. **c** Balloon inflation results in reduction of fracture with vertebral height restoration. **d** The cavity created by the balloon is gradually filled with polymethylmetacrylate. **e** The final result is a reduced vertebra which is filled with cement. (Images courtesy of Kyphon Corporation, Sunnyvale, CA, USA)

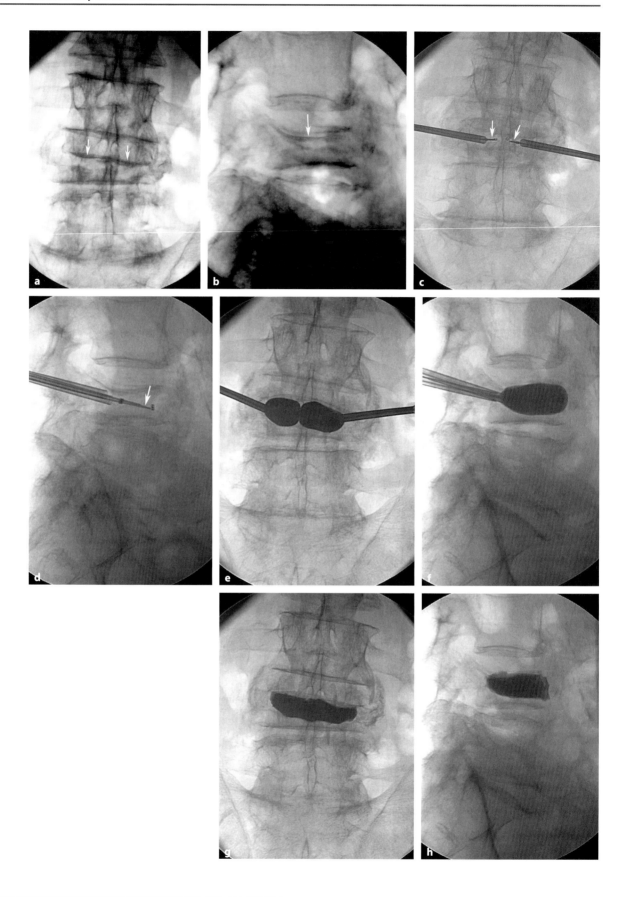

Fig. 12.3a–h. Technique of percutaneous kyphoplasty in a 91-year-old man. **a** Anteroposterior and (**b**) lateral radiographs show L4 fracture with 60%–70% height loss (*arrows*). **c** Anteroposterior radiograph shows bilateral transpedicular trocars are placed, through which uninflated balloons (*arrows*) are advanced, with their tips positioned midline and as anteriorly as possible on (**d**) lateral radiograph. **e** Anteroposterior and (**f**) lateral radiographs show the balloons are inflated, with resultant significant vertebral height recovery and bowing of the superior endplate. **g** Anteroposterior and (**h**) lateral radiographs obtained after cement delivery show an excellent vertebral filling in all dimensions

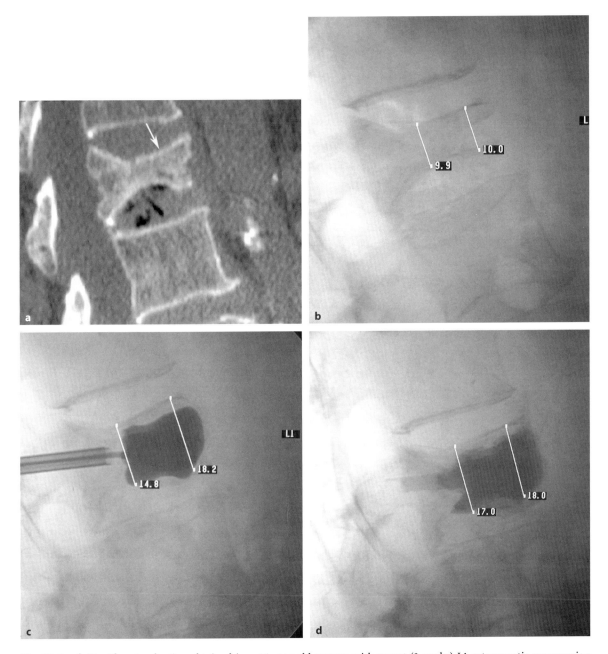

Fig. 12.4a–d. Significant reduction obtained in a 56-year-old woman with recent (3 weeks) L1 osteoporotic compression fracture. **a** Sagittal CT image reconstruction shows fracture of L1 with bowing of the endplates (arrow). **b** Lateral radiograph shows height measurements. Lateral radiographs show significant reduction (**c**) with balloon inflation, persistent (**d**) after cement injection and measured at 80%

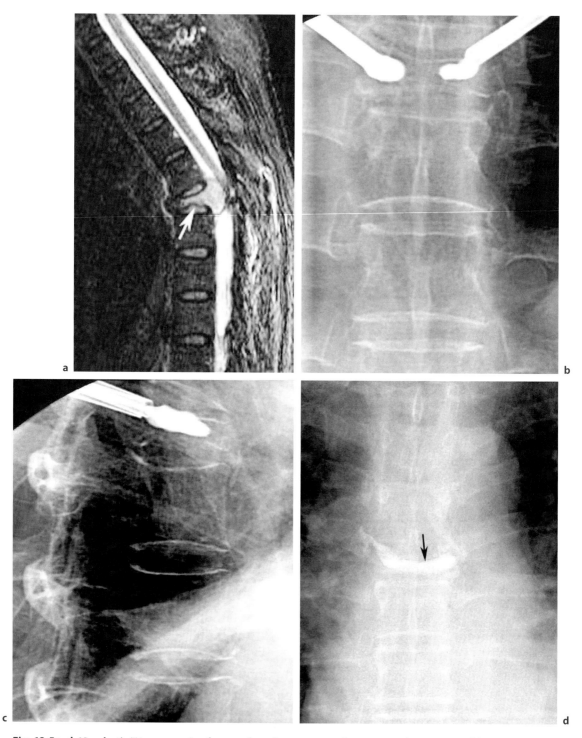

Fig. 12.5a–d. Neoplastic T6 compression fracture from lung cancer primary tumor in a 55-year-old woman causing severe pain and cord compression without neurological signs. **a** Sagittal T2-weighted MR image shows compression fracture (*arrow*) with significant retropulsion. **b** Anteroposterior and (**c**) lateral radiograph show kyphoplasty with good balloon placement. **d** Anteroposterior radiograph shows good filling of T6 with cement (*arrow*). Excellent pain relief was obtained

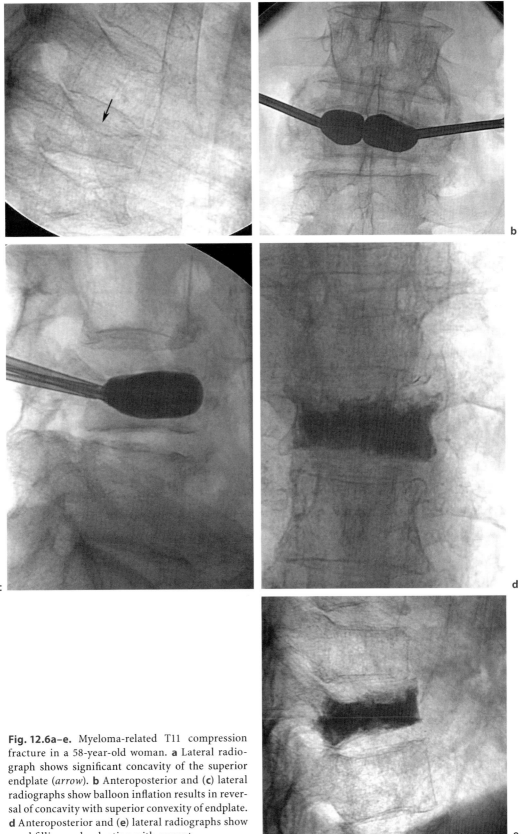

Fig. 12.6a–e. Myeloma-related T11 compression fracture in a 58-year-old woman. **a** Lateral radiograph shows significant concavity of the superior endplate (*arrow*). **b** Anteroposterior and (**c**) lateral radiographs show balloon inflation results in reversal of concavity with superior convexity of endplate. **d** Anteroposterior and (**e**) lateral radiographs show good filling and reduction with cement

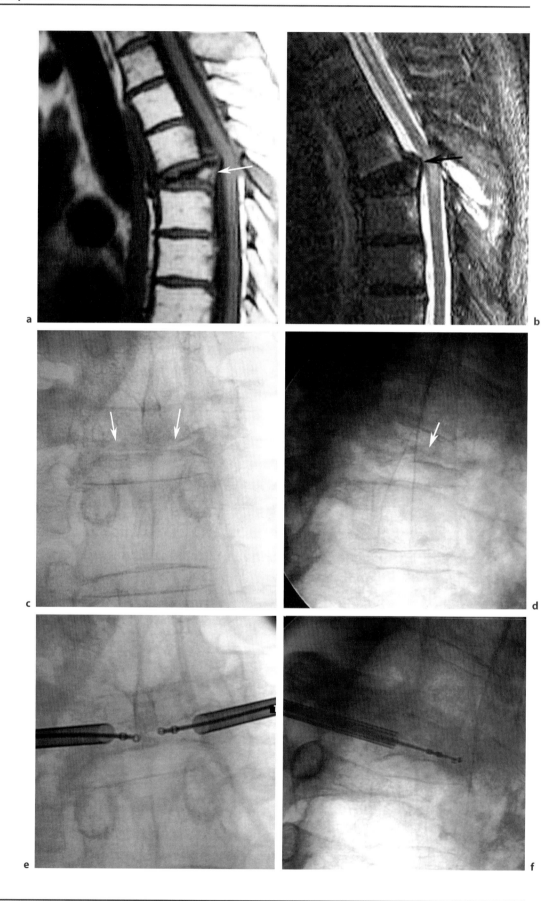

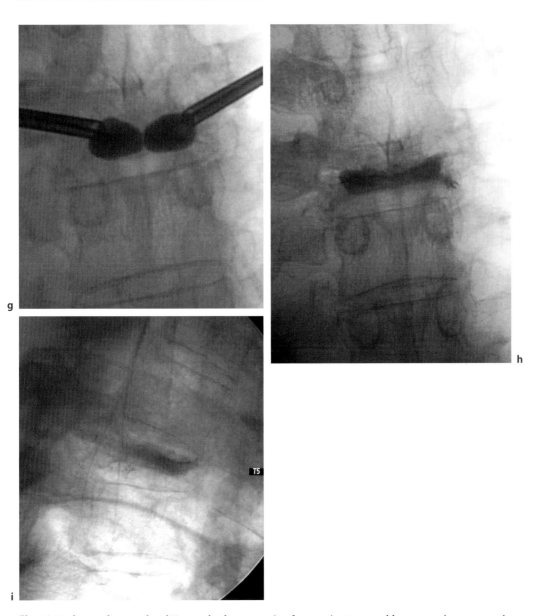

Fig. 12.7a–i. Lymphoma-related T5 vertebral compression fracture in 54-year-old man, causing severe pain and myelopathy. Sagittal (**a**) T1- and (**b**) T2-weighted MR images show important vertebral compression of T5 and T2 hyperintensity of the spinal cord related to myelopathy from retropulsed fragment (*arrow*). There is also an involvement of the spinous process of T5. **c** Anteroposterior and (**d**) lateral radiographs show severe collapse of T5 (*arrows*). **e** Anteroposterior and (**f**) lateral radiographs show careful bilateral trans-pedicular placement of small (1 cm) kyphoplasty balloons. **g** Anteroposterior radiograph shows balloon inflation results in significant height recovery. **h** Anteroposterior and (**i**) lateral radiographs show excellent filling of the vertebra with cement, resulting in total pain relief. Unexpectedly, the patient's myelopathy improved as well, presumably from vertebral stabilization

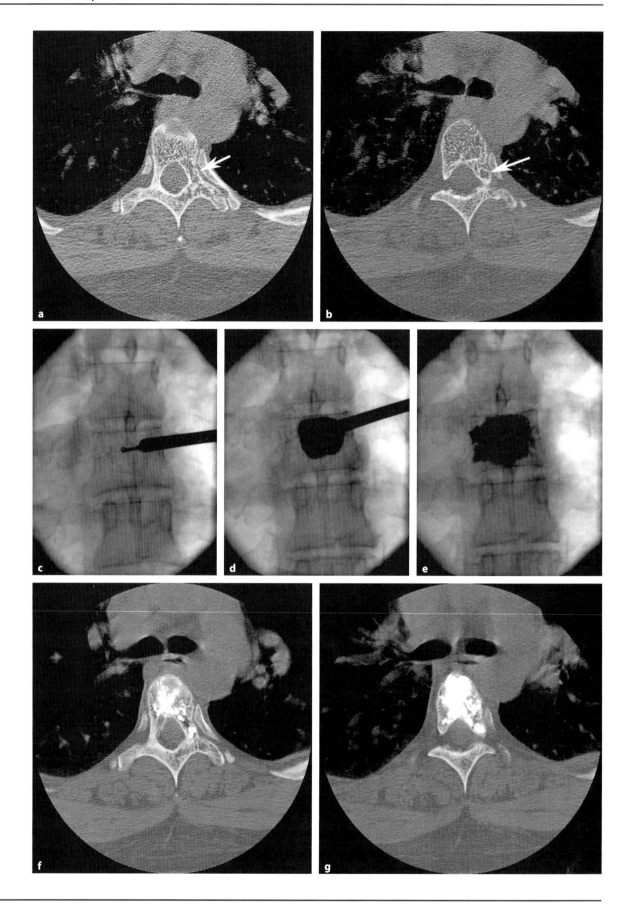

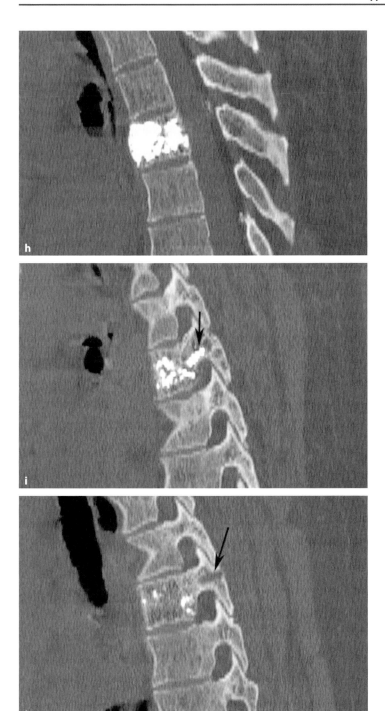

Fig. 12.8a–j. Painful hemangioma of T5 in a 30-year-old woman. This pain has been present for 20 years. **a,b** Axial CT scans of T5 show hemangioma with lucencies suggestive of fractures involving the left pedicle (*arrow*). A unilateral right transpedicular approach was planned to avoid further damage to the left pedicle. Anteroposterior radiographs show (**c**) a single uninflated balloon in place, (**d**) the balloon fully inflated, and (**e**) the T5 vertebra filled with cement. **f,g** Post-treatment axial CT scans show that the vertebra and the left pedicle are filled with cement. Sagittal CT reconstructions also demonstrate (**h**) excellent filling of the T5 vertebral body, and (**i**) the left pedicle (*arrow*); note (**j**) the right transpedicular tract (*arrow*)

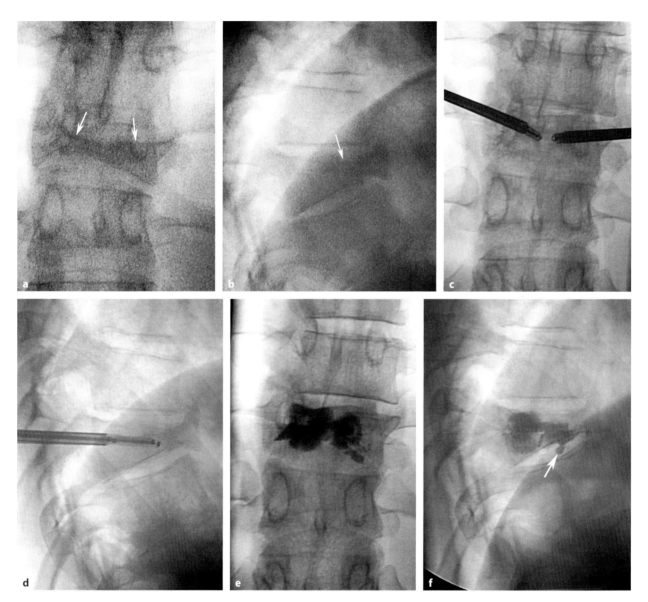

Fig. 12.9a–f. Painful fracture of T10 in an 18-year-old man. This fracture has been present for 17 months. **a** Anteroposterior and (**b**) lateral radiographs show fracture of T10 (*arrows*) with significant height loss. **c** Anteroposterior and (**d**) lateral radiographs show balloons did not expand despite excellent balloon placement and maximum pressure rates at 440 psi. **e** Anteroposterior and (**f**) lateral radiographs show good filling of the vertebra resulting in complete pain relief. There is minor leak of cement in the disc through the inferior endplate (*arrow*)

Technique

The first device developed for kyphoplasty is the KyphX balloon. Currently, Kyphon remains the sole supplier of kyphoplasty products in the United States, and the main supplier in Europe. To our knowledge, the only other vertebral reconstruction system at present is the DiscOtech-SkyBone vertebral expander device, which is marketed in Italy by Medika, Inc.

Although most kyphoplasty procedures reported so far have been performed using portable X-ray machines (C-arms) in the operating room while the patient is under general anesthesia, some patients are treated in radiology departments. With increased familiarity with the procedure, and decreased requirements for overnight patient admission, it is expected that more patients will be treated less invasively in the future.

One advantage of a radiology department setting is the common presence of high resolution fluoroscopic equipment, preferably in the biplane mode, which allows the operator to assess visualization of needle placement and cement delivery in real-time in both the lateral and frontal planes. The use of CT, along with a single plane C-arm machine, has been advocated with vertebroplasty, and may be especially useful in the small vertebrae (i.e., upper thoracic). A thorough knowledge of the spinal anatomy, and experience with needle placement, are absolute requirements.

We find that the majority of patients do not require general anesthesia, as conscious sedation is usually adequate to ensure analgesia, comfort and lack of motion during treatment. Other advantages include the ability to arouse and examine the patient if necessary, and overall shorter procedure times and less patient manipulation, possibly reducing the risk of rib and sternal fractures during the procedure.

The vertebra to be treated is first localized fluoroscopically. Access to the vertebral body is obtained via a strict transpedicular approach. First, bone needles (usually 11-gauge) are advanced in both pedicles. The accuracy of needle placement should be verified in both planes for maximum safety. Then, using sequential dilation, kyphoplasty trocars are advanced (Fig. 12.1) and positioned with their tips as anterior and as close to midline as possible (Fig. 12.3). Next, two balloons are advanced, and carefully and gradually inflated under fluoroscopic control (Figs. 12.2, 12.3). Balloon lengths currently available are 1, 1.5 and 2 cm, offering a reasonable range for the various clinical situations encountered. The balloons are then deflated and retrieved, and the newly created cavity is filled with cement (Figs. 12.2, 12.3), which is delivered with the use of bone fillers.

Cement delivery should be monitored carefully by fluoroscopy, ideally in two planes, to look for any extravasation. Leakage should prompt the operator to immediately interrupt the injection of cement.

Injection of contrast medium into the vertebra (venography) prior to cement delivery to predict the risk of leakage or passage into the venous plexus has been advocated (Mathis et al. 2001). Whether doing so adds to the safety of kyphoplasty is still uncertain, as large delivery systems permit the use of harder cement than for vertebroplasty, the cavity created by the balloon at least theoretically acts as a safer receptacle for the polymethylmetacrylate polymer, and the potential to obscure subsequent cement injection is a problem.

Although the procedure is specifically designed for a bilateral transpedicular approach, a unilateral approach may be used but requires extreme care that the trocar be advanced strictly through the pedicle (Fig. 12.10).

Exposure to radiation can be considerable during percutaneous X-ray guided procedures, and so must be kept in mind. One study evaluating the radiation risk during kyphoplasty measured a mean effective dose to patients of 8.5–12.7 mSv, and a mean gonadal dose of 0.04–16.4 mGy. It was also noted that the risk increased markedly if source-to-skin distance was less than 35 cm (Perisinakis et al. 2004). Care must be taken in the appropriate use of radioprotective measures, including the shortest possible exposure times and adequate shielding.

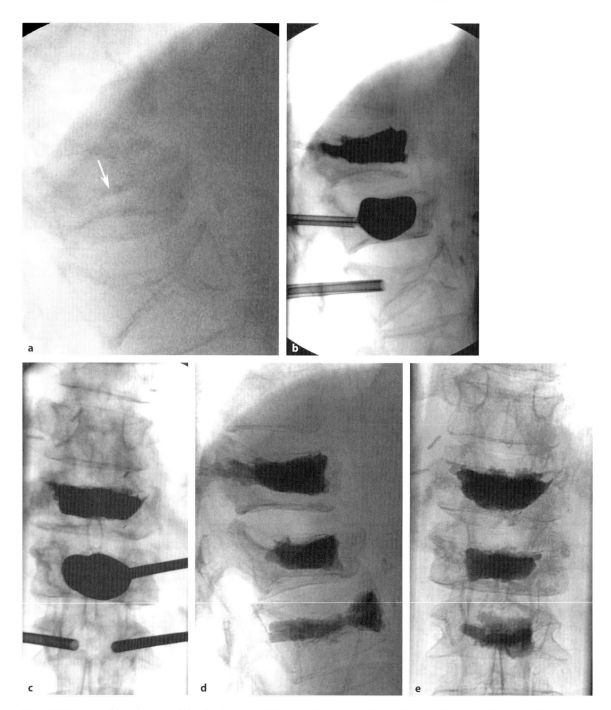

Fig. 12.10a–e. Unilateral approach kyphoplasty in a 76-year-old woman with myeloma. **a** Lateral radiograph shows severe collapse of T12 (*arrow*). **b** Anteroposterior and (**c**) lateral radiographs show unilateral right transpedicular approach was used to treat T12 with satisfactory balloon expansion. **d** Anteroposterior and (**e**) lateral radiographs show adequate cement filling similar to the levels above and below, which were treated with a bilateral approach

12.4
Peri-procedural Management

Compression fractures are usually diagnosed on plain radiographs, which allow quantification of height loss. In patients with neoplastic disease, CT scanning – including sagittal reconstruction algorithms – is particularly useful to assess the integrity of the posterior vertebral body wall. The age of the fracture is a significant indicator for kyphoplasty rather than vertebroplasty. Magnetic resonance (MR) imaging (Do 2000) and bone scanning (Maynard et al. 2000) are both useful in dating the fracture. MR imaging shows bone marrow edema present in the early stages of a fracture, while bone scanning demonstrates increased uptake of radiotracer within cortical bone resulting from inflammatory changes. Dating a fracture is particularly useful when fractures of various ages are present.

We find it best to discuss the indication in a multidisciplinary way prior to meeting with the patient. We also believe that in most cases both kyphoplasty and vertebroplasty should be discussed in detail with the patient, and that the comparative advantages and disadvantages of the procedures should be explained (Hacein-Bey et al. 2005).

A basic workup prior to treatment should identify potential medical problems that may require pre-procedural attention, such as bleeding problems or an infection.

Once the procedure is scheduled, patients are instructed to remain NPO after midnight on the day of treatment. Upon admission, patients receive intravenous fluids and their usual medications.

So far, in many (if not most) centers in the United States, kyphoplasty has been performed in operating rooms and under general anesthesia. Our practice has been to perform kyphoplasty in a radiology department, under light intravenous sedation (conscious sedation) and using high resolution biplane X-ray equipment.

Patients are gently positioned prone on the X-ray table, the same as for vertebroplasty. The level to be treated is identified both by clinical palpation and by X-ray fluoroscopy prior to prepping the patient's back in a sterile fashion, and while sedation is administered.

After the procedure, patients are typically kept for a few hours of observation in the recovery area, then discharged to home after a few minutes of gentle ambulation. Stabilization of the treated vertebra takes place rapidly after the procedure, as polymethylmetacrylate cement takes about 1 hour to reach 90% of its final strength (Belkoff et al. 1999; Belkoff et al. 2000; Belkoff et al. 2001a; Fribourg et al. 2004; Mathis et al. 2001). Although initially mandated in the United States, overnight hospitalization is no longer required for stable otherwise healthy outpatients, so that only inpatients with associated medical issues are kept in the hospital.

12.5
Effectiveness of Kyphoplasty

The overall effectiveness of kyphoplasty must be weighed against that of vertebroplasty. As current data suggest similar safety and effectiveness for both procedures, a prospective randomized comparison may be necessary in the future.

12.5.1
Pain Relief

The mechanism by which injection of cement provides pain relief is not fully understood. Most authorities believe that the relief is due to the stabilization of microfractures within the vertebral body, particularly at the level of the endplates. Other mechanisms have been proposed, however, such as thermal necrosis resulting from the exothermic reaction, which accompanies the polymerization of polymethylmetacrylate cement (temperatures of 122°C have been reported), as well as direct chemotoxicity to the pain receptors within the vertebral body. However, neither possibility is likely to play a major role in pain relief, as the relatively small doses of cement used probably do not result in marked temperature elevation, and polymer neurochemotoxicity has not been demonstrated.

Overall pain relief rates of 90% (Coumans et al. 2003; Fourney et al. 2003; Lane et al. 2000; Ledlie and Renfro 2003; Liberman et al. 2003; Nussbaum et al. 2004; Phillips et al. 2003) have been reported with kyphoplasty, similar to those provided by vertebroplasty.

In patients with cancer (myeloma and metastases of various types), Fourney et al. (2003) reported on 56 patients treated with vertebroplasty or kyphoplasty, and noted complete pain relief in 84% of patients, which persisted at one year. Gaitanis et al.

(2004) noted pain relief in 96.9% of their patients treated for osteoporosis-related fractures, mostly within 24 h, and stressed the importance of addressing associated spinal stenosis by performing laminectomies in selected patients. Overall, pain relief is consistently reported to be long-lasting, noted to persist at least one year and commonly longer after treatment (COUMANS et al. 2003; FRIBOURG et al. 2004; LEDLIE and RENFRO 2003).

The issue of new fractures after treatment must be considered. Whether the strengthening of a weak vertebra increases strain on adjacent levels, thereby causing new fractures, has been much debated. There is currently no consensus as to whether new fractures are more likely due to mechanical effects, or simply coincidental in patients with diffuse osteoporosis. With vertebroplasty, it has been reported that new fractures are diagnosed within 2 years of treatment of a first fracture in 12.4% of patients, 67% of which affect the immediately adjacent vertebra (UPPIN et al. 2003). Such fractures should be treated. With kyphoplasty, FRIBOURG et al. (2004) reported that 10 of 38 patients (26%) developed a new vertebral fracture at a follow-up of 8 months. HARROP et al. (2004) report similar numbers on a larger series of patients, with an overall incidence per patient of 22.6%, and an overall incidence per kyphoplasty procedure of 15.1%. Given such evidence, it seems likely that the onset of new fractures may be precipitated by performing a bone-strengthening and spine-straightening procedure. It is appropriate to carefully follow patients, and to be prepared to treat new fractures.

12.5.2
Vertebral Height Restoration

The restoration of vertebral height is important as it causes reduction of kyphosis, with resultant improvements in posture, functional life, pulmonary and gastro-intestinal function and survival rates. In addition, pain relief results in fewer muscle spasms and less spine pain, allowing better posture and some correction of kyphosis (THEODOROU et al. 2002). Although it is the primary benefit claimed by the technique, vertebral height restoration has not been demonstrated reliably and consistently with kyphoplasty.

The best known and most often quoted in vitro study currently available, (BELKOFF et al. 2001b), reported "significant" height recovery with kypho-plasty compared to vertebroplasty, involved only vertebrae with a maximum height loss of 25%, and also demonstrated that height recovery could be obtained with vertebroplasty alone.

A review of 66 articles on kyphoplasty published between 1998 and April 2004 in peer-reviewed journals reveals 96 patients with 133 fractures, with an average reduction of 4 mm per vertebra (NUSSBAUM et al. 2004). GAITANIS et al. (2004) report average height restorations of 4.3 mm for the anterior wall and 4.8 mm at the mid-vertebral body level. LIEBERMAN et al. (2001) reported vertebral height restoration in 70% of their patients, while GARFIN et al. (2001) reported a 46.8% rate. THEODOROU et al. (2002) reported a 62% average correction of kyphosis.

In a population of myeloma patients, LANE et al. (2000) reported excellent rates of height restoration: 91% at midvertebral body and 76% anterior vertebral body levels, with 85% pain relief overall. Indeed, in these patients the bony architecture is particularly compliant and soft, lending itself to some remodeling (Fig. 12.5). However, vertebroplasty alone has been reported to result in significant height restoration (HIWATASHI et al. 2003; MCKIERNAN et al. 2003; TENG et al. 2003), with an average reduction of 2.2 mm per vertebra (NUSSBAUM et al. 2004).

The concept of dynamic mobility of a fracture has been advanced as the most important predictor of vertebral height reconstruction (MCKIERNAN et al. 2003). Vertebral heights are measured on lateral radiographs in the standing and supine position, and differences in measurements are consistent with and proportional to the degree of dynamic instability. Most of these dynamically unstable fractures occur at the thoraco-lumbar junction. Following vertebroplasty in 65 fractures (41 patients), MCKIERNAN et al. (2003) demonstrated an average 106% increase in anterior vertebral body height (absolute increase 8.41 ± 0.4 mm), and a 40% reduction in the vertebra's kyphotic angle. Therefore the likelihood of vertebral body height restoration may be related to dynamic bone mobility rather than to the mechanism of intervention (vertebroplasty versus kyphoplasty).

For the correction of severe kyphosis, lordoplasty has been considered superior to kyphoplasty, allowing maximum vertebral height recovery and stability. With lordoplasty, the vertebrae that are adjacent to a severe fracture are reinforced first with transpedicular cannulas, which, once in place, act as a lever to obtain reduction of the collapsed vertebra (HEINI and ORLER 2004). Conceptually, lordoplasty does not rely on dynamic vertebral mobility for kyphosis reduction, and provides reinforcement of the adjacent levels (HEINI and ORLER 2004).

Overall, the superiority of vertebral height restoration provided by kyphoplasty over vertebroplasty appears to be modest. It appears that maximum height restoration is obtained in fresh fractures (< 3 weeks), particularly in dynamic fractures at the thoracolumbar junction.

12.6
Complications

In November 2004, a review was published of all complications of kyphoplasty that were reported to a special database of the FDA between 1999 (when the earliest reports were filed) and June 27, 2003 (NUSSBAUM et al. 2004). This database, the Manufacturer and User Facility Device Experience (MAUDE), was designed to record the details of medical complications occurring from the use of medical devices associated with specific procedures, and identified a total of 33 adverse events out of approximately 50,000 procedures (0.07%). Reported complications included one death, five canal intrusions (Fig. 12.11) and one epidural hematoma with permanent neurological damage, 13 canal intrusions and one epidural hematoma with transient neurological damage, one pulmonary embolism, two infections (one discitis, one osteomyelitis), one pneumothorax, one episode of blood pressure drop, and six instances of inconsequential equipment breakage. Of these 33 events, 21 were major: one death and 20 cord compressions requiring surgery, with six permanent neurological injuries. During the same period, the authors of the report noted that only three major complications had been reported in the medical literature (NUSSBAUM et al. 2004).

A prospective multicenter study (GARFIN et al. 2002) reported six major complications out of 600 cases, four of which were neurological complications (0.66%). This study further concluded that all complications were directly attributed to operator errors or breaches of technique, and therefore potentially avoidable. This study has been credited with some relevance, as it was prospective and involved multiple centers (GARFIN et al. 2002). In a different study, retrospective and involving a multicenter registry (GARFIN et al. 2001), the same authors reported a 0.2% rate of complication per fracture treated. LANE

et al. (2000) reported an overall 1% rate of severe complications with kyphoplasty, and further compared it to reported vertebroplasty complication rates of 1%–3% (for osteoporotic fractures) to 19% (for neoplastic fractures).

Pedicle fractures, although a possible cause of neurological deterioration, have been noted to heal spontaneously (HODLER et al. 2003). Other serious neurological complications related to pedicle fractures are direct spinal cord injury, epidural hematomas and cement extravasation.

Cement leaks (Fig. 12.12) have been reported in less than 10% of procedures (COUMANS et al. 2003; LEDLIE and RENFRO 2003; PHILLIPS et al. 2003). LEDLIE and RENFRO (2003) reported asymptomatic cement leaks in 9% of the vertebral bodies of their patients, though they had no device-related or procedure-related complications. PHILLIPS et al. (2003) reported asymptomatic cement leaks in 6 of 61 patients (9.8%). For vertebroplasty, HODLER et al. (2003) note that leaks are quite common and have no clinical consequence. In their report of 363 vertebrae treated in 186 consecutive patients, at least one leak was detected at 258 levels (71%). While most leaks (52.3%) were paravertebral (Fig. 12.11), there were also 22 epidural cement collections (Fig. 12.10). None of these leaks caused a clinical complication that required another intervention. They also note that 86.1% of the patients treated reported significant improvement. Cement leaks into the disc space (Fig. 12.13) are relatively common, and inconsequential.

Pulmonary embolism is a serious complication that can be fatal (ZOARSKI et al. 2002a). Asymptomatic cement emboli noted on chest X-rays were seen in 4.6% of patients in one series, all with myeloma (CHOE et al. 2004). More paravertebral leaks were also noted in these patients (CHOE et al. 2004).

Reactions to the acrylic (polymethylmethacrylate) bone cement, including hypotension and, in some cases, death, have long been known to occur, and have been considered to be anaphylactic. In fact, reactions to the cement are related to the toxicity of the free fraction of the cement monomer, which has known cardiotoxicity and can cause cardiac arrhythmias and hemodynamic instability. Because kyphoplasty uses larger delivery systems than vertebroplasty, thicker cement is used, which should limit exposure to the free cement monomer.

Noninfectious discitis (HODLER et al. 2003) has been reported following leakage of cement into the adjacent disc.

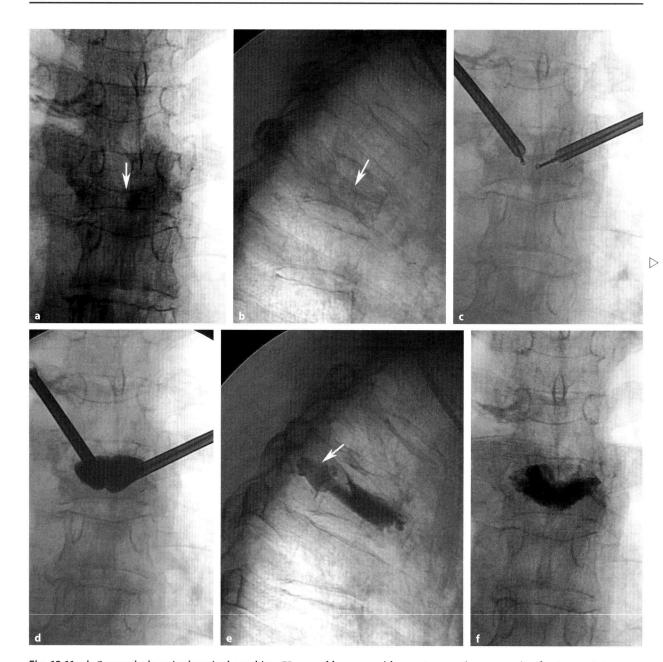

Fig. 12.11a–i. Cement leakage in the spinal canal in a 75-year-old woman with an osteoporotic compression fracture. **a** Anteroposterior and (**b**) lateral radiographs show T5 fracture with 50% height loss (*arrow*). Lateral radiographs show bilateral trocars (**c**) in place and (**d**) balloons inflated, the left side one in a more vertical position than normal. **e** Lateral post-treatment radiograph shows cement overlapping the spinal canal (*arrow*), not well appreciated on the (**f**) anteroposterior radiograph. **g** Axial CT scan shows cement collection (*arrow*) in the spinal canal, lateral to the spinal cord. **h** Coronal and (**i**) sagittal CT-myelography reconstruction images further show the degree of canal compromise. The patient was symptomatic only in the standing position, experiencing left leg paresthesias. Surgical evacuation of the cement collection resulted in full recovery

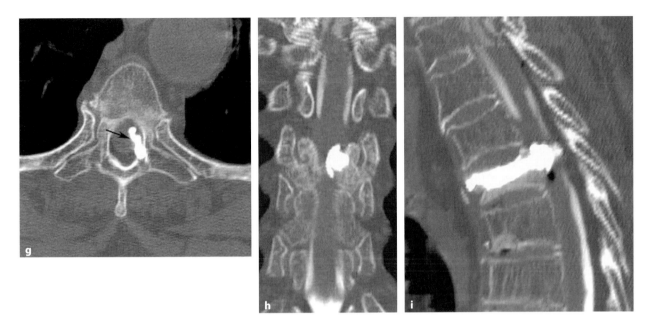

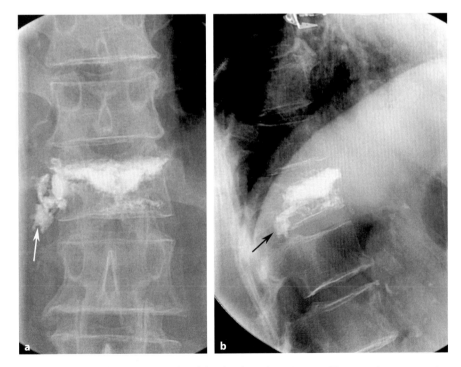

Fig. 12.12a,b. T12 fracture treated with kyphoplasty in a 78-year-old man. **a** Anteroposterior and (**b**) lateral radiographs show paravertebral cement leak (*arrow*) of no clinical consequence

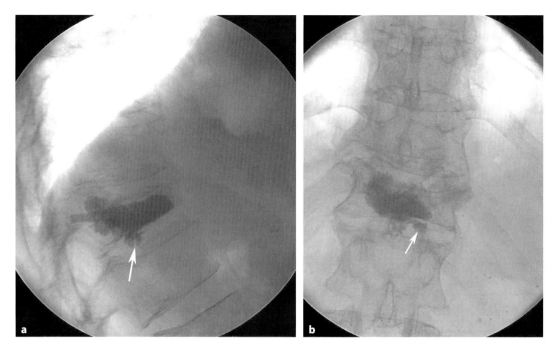

Fig. 12.13a,b. T12 fracture treated with kyphoplasty in a 56-year-old man. **a** Anteroposterior and (**b**) lateral radiographs show cement leak (*arrow*) in the T12-L1 disc of no clinical consequence

Myocardial infarction (COUMANS et al. 2003) has been reported during kyphoplasty.

Rib and sternal fractures may occur in these patients (EVANS et al. 2003; MCGRAW et al. 2002; NUSSBAUM et al. 2004) with severe osteoporosis as a result of lying prone during the procedure. It has been suggested that this risk may be higher than with vertebroplasty, as procedure times are longer (NUSSBAUM et al. 2004).

Transient post-procedural radicular pain has also been reported following kyphoplasty (EVANS et al. 2003; NUSSBAUM et al. 2004).

Overall comparisons to vertebroplasty (NUSSBAUM et al. 2004) suggest that, although both procedures are largely safe, kyphoplasty may have a higher risk of pedicle fractures and neurological injuries, while vertebroplasty may have a higher risk of cement extravasation and systemic reactions to the cement polymer.

12.7
Cost Considerations

Initially, the cost of kyphoplasty was considerably higher than that of vertebroplasty. In 2004, the cost of a standard kyphoplasty kit in the United States was $3,400, as opposed to several hundred dollars for vertebroplasty materials. In addition, in most practices, kyphoplasty procedures are performed in the operating room under general anesthesia. Also, most patients were initially admitted overnight for observation. This adds up to a differential increased cost of 10–20 times for kyphoplasty versus vertebroplasty, or a $6,000 difference in cost per treated level (Health Research Institute 2003; NUSSBAUM et al. 2004).

One study estimated that, if (as it is currently) one of every seven of the 700,000 fractures diagnosed each year in the United States were treated, and if all were treated with kyphoplasty, the cost of treatment would increase by $600 million (NUSSBAUM et al. 2004). Another study of 28 experienced orthopedic surgeons revealed that average intraservice times provided for each vertebral level were 38.9 min for vertebroplasty versus 78 min for kyphoplasty, which add considerable fluoroscopy time to the cost (DOBSON et al. 2001).

However, a more recent study of all vertebroplasty and kyphoplasty procedures performed in the United States between 1993 and 2004 showed that hospital charges for both procedures were identical, and further that average lengths-of-stay for kyphoplasty were half those of vertebroplasty (3.7

days vs. 7.3 days) (LAD et al. 2008). The same study also confirmed a steady increase in the performance of vertebroplasty and kyphoplasty procedures, estimated at 12,900% between 1993 and 2004 (LAD et al. 2008).

Between 2001 and 2002, there was a 28% increase in the number of vertebroplasties performed in the United States, from 38,000 to 48,000. During this same period, the number of kyphoplasties performed doubled from 8,300 to 16,000 (Health Research Institute 2003). As both modalities are increasingly used, the search for comparative safety and efficacy data will likely receive more attention.

12.8
Kyphoplasty versus Vertebroplasty: When?

Kyphoplasty was initially marketed as an improvement over vertebroplasty for treatment of osteoporotic fractures, advertised as a novel method designed to reduce the fracture by increasing vertebral height and reducing kyphosis and, in the process, create a void that could be filled with cement injected at a lower pressure to avoid venous extravasation of cement.

The overall current comparative experience shows an average reduction of 4 mm for kyphoplasty versus 2.2 mm for vertebroplasty (NUSSBAUM et al. 2004). As yet, there is no indication as to whether the overall minimal difference in reduction is clinically significant. As for "lower pressure" injections, although one study suggested that there were more leaks with vertebroplasty than kyphoplasty (LIEBERMAN and REINHARDT 2003) (with no discussion of which were symptomatic), another reported experimental evidence that higher pressures were noted with the use of larger systems within voids created by bone tamps (AGRIS et al. 2001).

Considering that kyphoplasty and vertebroplasty both provide similar pain relief results, have overall comparable complication rates, and the considerable cost difference between both procedures, it seems appropriate to ask the question of when kyphoplasty provides definite and superior benefits over vertebroplasty. At this time, it appears that restoration of vertebral height may be more reliable in acute (< 3 weeks) compression fractures (LIEBERMAN et al. 2001). Also, with proper experience, cement delivery in the vertebral body may be facilitated with the fill-

ing system used with kyphoplasty. Overall, kyphoplasty should not be considered at the exclusion of vertebroplasty. For the greatest benefit of patients, both options should be considered thoughtfully in the context of a multidisciplinary evaluation.

12.9
Conclusion

Kyphoplasty appears to add something to the management of patients with compression fractures, whether from osteoporosis, cancer or trauma. Although the technique is still relatively new, the ability to restore vertebral body height and spinal architecture, particularly in fresh fractures, is a considerable advantage. The role of kyphoplasty will continue to be evaluated, hopefully in the context of multidisciplinary efforts. This evaluation should not just involve comparisons with vertebroplasty, but also with standard (surgical, radiation, medical) and novel therapies. In addition to continued improvements to minimally invasive therapeutic approaches, which will likely include automated techniques, the advent of new bone cements resulting from genetic engineering research (i.e., morphogenic proteins), and concurrent developments in the understanding of the epidemiology of bone loss, should all continue to benefit patients.

References

Agris JM, Zoarski GH, Stallmeyer MJB, Ortiz O (2003) Intravertebral pressure during vertebroplasty: a study comparing multiple delivery systems. Presented at the annual meeting of the American Society of Spine Radiology, Scottsdale, AZ, February 19–23 (Abstract)

Barr JD, Barr MS, Lemley TJ, McCann RM (2000) Percutaneous vertebroplasty for pain relief and spinal stabilization. Spine 25:923–928

Bascoulergue Y, Duquesnel J, Leclercq R (1998) Percutaneous injection of methyl methacrylate in the vertebral body for the treatment of various diseases: percutaneous vertebroplasty. Radiology 169:372 (Abstract)

Belkoff SM, Mahoney M, Fenton DC, Mathis JM (1999) An in vitro biomechanical evaluation of bone cements used in percutaneous vertebroplasty. Bone 25:23S–26S

Belkoff SM, Mathis JM, Erbe EM, Fenton DC (2000) Biomechanical evaluation of a new bone cement for use in vertebroplasty. Spine 25:1061–1064

Belkoff SM, Mathis JM, Deramond H, Jasper LE (2001a) An ex vivo biomechanical evaluation of a hydroxyapatite cement for use with kyphoplasty. AJNR Am J Neuroradiol 22:1212–1216

Belkoff SM, Mathis JM, Fenton DC, Reiley ME, Talmadge K (2001b) An ex vivo biomechanical evaluation of an inflatable bone tamp used in the treatment of compression fractures. Spine 26:151–156

Belkoff SM, Mathis JM, Jasper LE, Deramond H (2001c) An ex vivo biomechanical evaluation of a hydroxyapatite cement for use with vertebroplasty. Spine 26:1542–1546

Belkoff SM, Mathis JM, Jasper LE, Deramond H (2001d) The biomechanics of vertebroplasty: the effect of cement volume on mechanical behavior. Spine 26:1537–1541

Choe DH, Marom EM, Ahrar K, Truong MT, Madewell JE (2004) Pulmonary embolism of polymethyl methacrylate during percutaneous vertebroplasty and kyphoplasty. AJR Am J Roentgenol 183:1097–1102

Cotton A, Dewatre F, Cortet B (1996) Percutaneous vertebroplasty for osteolytic metastases and myeloma. Radiology 200:525–530

Coumans JV, Reinhardt MK, Lieberman IH (2003) Kyphoplasty for vertebral compression fractures: 1-year clinical outcomes from a prospective study. J Neurosurg Spine 99:44–50

Cyteval C, Sarrabere MP, Roux JO, Thomas E, Jorgensen C, Blotman F, Sany J, Taourel P (1999) Acute osteoporotic vertebral collapse: open study on percutaneous injection of acrylic surgical cement in 20 patients. AJR Am J Roentgenol 173:1685–1690

Dobson A, DaVanzo J, Goodman C, Consunji MC (2001) A study of physician work value units for kyphoplasty. The Lewin Group, Inc.

Do HM (2000) Magnetic resonance imaging in the evaluation of patients for percutaneous vertebroplasty. Top Magn Reson Imaging 11:235–244

Dudeney S, Lieberman IH, Reinhardt MK, Hussein M (2002) Kyphoplasty in the treatment of osteolytic vertebral compression fractures as a result of multiple myeloma. J Clin Oncol 20:2382–2387

Evans AJ, Jensen ME, Kip KE, DeNardo AJ, Lawler GJ, Negin GA, Remley KB, Boutin SM, Dunnagan SA (2003) Vertebral compression fractures: pain reduction and improvement in functional mobility after percutaneous polyethylmethacrylate vertebroplasty retrospective report of 245 cases. Radiology 226:366–372

Fourney DR, Schomer DF, Nader R, Chlan-Fourney J, Suki D, Ahrar K, Rhines LD, Gokaslan ZL (2003) Percutaneous vertebroplasty and kyphoplasty for painful vertebral body fractures in cancer patients. J Neurosurg Spine 98:21–30

Franck H, Boszczyk BM, Bierschneider M, Jaksche H (2003) Interdisciplinary approach to balloon kyphoplasty in the treatment of osteoporotic vertebral compression fractures. Eur Spine J 12 Suppl 2:S163–167

Fribourg D, Tang C, Sra P, Delamarter R, Bae H (2004) Incidence of subsequent vertebral fracture after kyphoplasty. Spine 29:2270–2276

Gaitanis IN, Hadjipavlou AG, Katonis PG, Tzermiadianos MN, Pasku DS, Patwardhan AG (2004) Balloon kyphoplasty for the treatment of pathological vertebral compressive fractures. Eur Spine J 14:250–260

Galibert P, Deramond H, Rosat P (1987) Preliminary note on the treatment of vertebral angioma by percutaneous acrylic vertebroplasty. Neurochirurgie 33:166–168

Garfin S, Lin G, Lieberman IH et al. (2001) Retrospective analysis of the outcomes of balloon kyphoplasty to treat vertebral body compression fractures (VCF) refractory to medical management. Eur Spine J 10 (Suppl):S7 (Abstract)

Garfin SR, Reilley MA (2002) Minimally invasive treatment of osteoporotic vertebral body compression fractures. Spine J 2:76–80

Hacein-Bey L, Baisden JL, Wong SJ, Lemke DM, Ulmer JL, Cusick JF (2005) Treating osteoporotic and neoplastic vertebral compression fractures with vertebroplasty and kyphoplasty. J Palliat Med 8:931–938

Hardouin P, Fayada P, Leclet H, Chopin D (2002) Kyphoplasty. Joint Bone Spine 69:256–261

Harrop JS, Prpa B, Reinhardt MK, Lieberman I (2004) Primary and secondary osteoporosis' incidence of subsequent vertebral compression fractures after kyphoplasty. Spine 29:2120–2125

Health Research Institute (2003) U.S. markets for adjunctive and non-fusion spine technologies. Medtech Insights Report #103-1-US–0103

Heini PF, Orler R (2004) Kyphoplasty for treatment of osteoporotic vertebral fractures. Eur Spine J 13:184–192

Hiwatashi A, Moritani T, Numaguchi Y, Westesson PL (2003) Increase in vertebral body height after vertebroplasty. AJNR Am J Neuroradiol 24:185–189

Hodler J, Peck D, Gilula LA (2003) Midterm outcome after vertebroplasty: predictive value of technical and patient-related factors. Radiology 227:662–668

Hsiang J (2003) An unconventional indication for open kyphoplasty. Spine J 3:520–523

Jasper LE, Deramond H, Mathis JM, Belkoff SM (2002) Material properties of various cements for the use with vertebroplasty. J Mat Sci Mat Med 14:1–5

Jensen ME, Evans AJ, Mathis JM, Kallmes DF, Cloft HJ, Dion JE (1997) Percutaneous polymethylmethacrylate vertebroplasty in the treatment of osteoporotic vertebral compression fractures: technical aspects. AJNR Am J Neuroradiol 18:1897–1904

Lad SP, Patil CG, Lad EM, Hayden MG, Boakye M (2008) National trends in vertebral augmentation procedures for the treatment of vertebral compression fractures. Surg Neurol 29 May [Epub ahead of print]

Lane JM, Girardi F, Parvaianen H et al. (2000) Preliminary outcomes of the first 226 consecutive kyphoplasties for the fixation of painful osteoporotic vertebral compression fractures. Osteoporos Int (Suppl) 11:S206 (abstract)

Lane JM, Hong R, Koob J, Kiechle T, Niesvizky R, Pearse R, Siegel D, Poynton AR (2004) Kyphoplasty enhances function and structural alignment in multiple myeloma. Clin Orthop 426:49–53

Ledlie JT, Renfro M (2003) Balloon kyphoplasty: one-year outcomes in vertebral body height restoration, chronic pain, and activity levels. J Neurosurg 98 (1 Suppl):36–42

Lieberman IH, Dudeney S, Reinhardt MK, Bell G (2001) Initial outcome and efficacy of «kyphoplasty» in the treatment of painful osteoporotic vertebral compression fractures. Spine 26:1631–1638

Lieberman I, Reinhardt MK (2003) Vertebroplasty and kyphoplasty for osteolytic vertebral collapse. Clin Orthop 415 (Suppl):S176–186

Masala S, Tropepi D, Fiori R, Semprini R, Martorana A, Massari F, Bernardi G, Simonetti G (2004) Kyphoplasty: a new opportunity for rehabilitation of neurologic disabilities. Am J Phys Med Rehabil 83:810–812

Mathis JM, Barr JD, Belkoff SM, Barr MS, Jensen ME, Deramond H (2001) Percutaneous vertebroplasty: a developing standard of care for vertebral compression fractures. AJNR Am J Neuroradiology 22:373–381

Mathis JM, Eckel TS, Belkoff SM, Deramond H (1999) Percutaneous vertebroplasty: a therapeutic option for pain associated with vertebral compression fracture. J Back Musculoskel Rehab 1:11–17

Mathis JM, Petri M, Naff N (1998) Percutaneous vertebroplasty treatment of steroid-induced osteoporotic compression fractures. Arthritis Rheum 41:171–175

Maynard AS, Jensen ME, Schweickert PA, Marx WF, Short JG, Kallmes DF (2000) Value of bone scan imaging in predicting pain relief from percutaneous vertebroplasty in osteoporotic vertebral fractures. AJNR Am J Neuroradiol 21:1807–1812

McGraw JK, Lippert JA, Minkus KD, Rami PM, Davis TM, Budzik RF (2002) Prospective evaluation of pain relief in 100 patients undergoing percutaneous vertebroplasty: results and follow-up. J Vasc Interv Radiol 13 (9 Pt 1):883–886

McKiernan F, Jensen R, Faciszewski T (2003) The dynamic mobility of vertebral compression fractures. J Bone Miner Res 18:24–29

Nussbaum DA, Gailloud P, Murphy K (2004) A review of complications associated with vertebroplasty and kyphoplasty as reported to the Food and Drug Administration medical device related web site. J Vasc Interv Radiol 15:1185–1192

Olan WJ (2002) Kyphoplasty: balloon-assisted vertebroplasty. ASNR Spine Symposium. Vancouver, BC. 115-117 (Abstract)

Ortiz AO, Zoarski GH, Beckerman M (2002) Kyphoplasty. Tech Vasc Interv Radiol 5:239–249

Perisinakis K, Damilakis J, Theocharopoulos N, Papadokostakis G, Hadjipavlou A, Gourtsoyiannis N (2004) Patient exposure and associated radiation risks from fluoroscopically guided vertebroplasty or kyphoplasty. Radiology 232:701–707

Phillips FM, Ho E, Campbell-Hupp M, McNally T, Todd Wetzel F, Gupta P (2003) Early radiographic and clinical results of balloon kyphoplasty for the treatment of osteoporotic vertebral compression fractures. Spine 28:2260–2265

Stallmeyer MJ, Zoarski GH, Obuchowski AM (2003) Optimizing patient selection in percutaneous vertebroplasty. J Vasc Interv Radiol 14:683–696

Teng MM, Wei CJ, Wei LC, Luo CB, Lirng JF, Chang FC, Liu CL, Chang CY (2003) Kyphosis correction and height restoration effects of percutaneous vertebroplasty. AJNR Am J Neuroradiol 24:1893–1900

Theodorou DJ, Theodorou SJ, Duncan TD, Garfin SR, Wong WH (2002) Percutaneous balloon kyphoplasty for the correction of spinal deformity in painful vertebral body compression fractures. Clin Imaging 26:1–5

Tohmeh AG, Mathis JM, Fenton DC, Levine AM, Belkoff SM (1999) Biomechanical efficacy of unipedicular versus bipedicular vertebroplasty for the management of osteoporotic compression fractures. Spine 24:1772–1776

Uppin AA, Hirsch JA, Centenera LV, Pfiefer BA, Pazianos AG, Choi IS (2003) Occurrence of new vertebral body fracture after percutaneous vertebroplasty in patients with osteoporosis. Radiology 226:119–124

Watts NB, Harris ST, Genant HK (2001) Treatment of painful osteoporotic vertebral fractures with percutaneous vertebroplasty or kyphoplasty. Osteoporosis Int 12:429–437

Weill A, Chiras J, Simon JM (1996) Spinal metastases: indications for and results of percutaneous injection of acrylic surgical cement. Radiology 199:241–247

Wilson DR, Myers ER, Mathis JM, Scribner RM, Conta JA, Reiley MA, Talmadge KD, Hayes WC (2000) Effect of augmentation on the mechanics of vertebral wedge fractures. Spine 25:158–165

Wong WH, Olan WJ, Belkoff SM (2002) Balloon kyphoplasty. Mathis JM, Deramond H, Belkoff SM (eds) Percutaneous vertebroplasty. Springer-Verlag, New York pp 109–124

Zoarski GH, Snow P, Olan WJ, Stallmeyer MJ, Dick BW, Hebel JR, De Deyne M (2002a) Percutaneous vertebroplasty: A to Z. Tech Vasc Interv Radiol 5:223–228

Zoarski GH, Snow P, Olan WJ, Stallmeyer MJ, Dick BW, Hebel JR, De Deyne M (2002b) Percutaneous vertebroplasty for osteoporotic compression fractures: quantitative prospective evaluation of long-term outcomes. J Vasc Interv Radiol 13:139–148

Percutaneous Intraosseous Cyst Management

Josée Dubois and Laurent Garel

13

CONTENTS

13.1 Introduction 283

13.2 Vascular Anomalies 283
13.2.1 Aneurysmal Bone Cyst 283
13.2.1.1 Genetics 284
13.2.1.2 Imaging 284
13.2.1.3 Treatment 284
13.2.2 Arteriovenous Malformation 292
13.2.2.1 Imaging 292
13.2.2.2 Treatment 292

13.3 Unicameral Bone Cyst 294
13.3.1 Imaging 294
13.3.2 Treatment 294
13.3.2.1 Conservative Treatment 294
13.3.2.2 Percutaneous Treatment 295

13.4 Histiocytosis 296

13.5 Conclusion 297

References 298

13.1
Introduction

The majority of patients affected by intraosseous cysts are children or adolescents. The most commonly noted forms are vascular anomalies (including aneurysmal bone cysts), unicameral bone cysts and histiocytosis. Percutaneous treatment of intraosseous cysts is an alternative to surgical treatment. It minimizes the risk of bleeding, avoids immobilization and prevents disfiguration or dysfunc-

J. Dubois, MD
L. Garel, MD
Professors of Radiology, University of Montreal, Pediatric and Interventional Radiologists, Department of Medical Imaging, Centre Hospitalo-Universitaire Sainte-Justine, 3175 Côte Sainte-Catherine Road, Montreal, Quebec H3T 1C5, Canada

tion, particularly when the lesion is located in the head and neck region or in the pelvis.

The percutaneous approach uses imaging guidance, either fluoroscopy or CT, to guide injection of sclerosants. This chapter will describe percutaneous techniques and the various sclerosing agents used to treat the three common manifestations of intraosseous cysts noted above.

13.2
Vascular Anomalies

In the past, diagnosis and treatment of vascular anomalies were hampered by considerable confusion due to the use of inappropriate terminology. The most helpful classification based on clinical, histological and cytological features for vascular anomalies is that of MULLIKEN and GLOWACKI in 1982. They divided vascular anomalies into vascular tumors with endothelial hyperplasia and vascular malformations, both subcategorized according to the predominant channels: capillary, venous, arterial or lymphatic, and mixed. The most common intraosseous cystic lesions in these subgroups are venous malformations (aneurysmal bone cyst), arteriovenous malformations associated with intraosseous lytic lesions, and lymphatic malformations of bone.

13.2.1
Aneurysmal Bone Cyst

Aneurysmal bone cyst (ABC) was recognized and described as a distinct clinicopathological entity by JAFFE and LICHTENSTEIN in 1942. The cause and pathogenesis of ABC are unknown. None of the prevailing theories – post-therapeutic reparation, altered hemodynamics (arteriovenous fistula) or compression by another osseous lesion (KERSHISNIK and BATSAKIS 1994) – have proven valid. Considering that ABC is an expanding lesion of bone containing blood-filled spaces pathologically and radiographically, it looks very much like cavitary venous malformation.

The World Health Organization defines ABC as an expanding osteolytic lesion consisting of blood-filled spaces of variable size that are separated by connective tissue septa containing trabeculae of bone or osteoid, as well as osteoclastic giant cells (MAHNKEN et al. 2003). ABC represents approximately 3%–6% of all primary bone tumors, with 80% of patients under 20 years of age. All parts of the skeleton may be affected, with a propensity for the metaphyses of the long bones, which are involved in more than 50% of cases, and for the posterior elements of the spine, involved in 12%–30% of cases (HECHT and GEBHARDT 1998; LEITHNER et al. 1998). Clinically, patients with ABC present with local pain, tenderness, swelling or pathologic fracture.

ABC may present as a primary osteolytic lesion in 65% of cases, including solid variant (BERTONI et al. 1993), or coexisting with a preexisting lesion in 35% of cases. In adults, secondary forms are described in association with benign or malignant bone pathologies already identified histologically: fibrous dysplasia, giant-cell tumor, unicameral bone cyst, chondromyxoid fibroma, chondroblastoma, hemangioma, hemangioendothelioma, osteogenic sarcoma, chondrosarcoma or metastasis (CAMPANACCI et al. 1986). No case of malignant transformation of a primary ABC has been reported (HECHT and GEBHARDT 1998). BOLLINI et al. (1998) reported a lack of preexisting tumors in children with ABC.

13.2.1.1
Genetics

A familial pattern has been noted in three patients (LEITHNER et al. 1998, VINCENZI 1981). Recent cytogenic data have shown clonal rearrangements of chromosomal bands 16q22 and 17p13, indicating a neoplastic basis for at least some ABC (OLIVEIRA et al. 2004).

13.2.1.2
Imaging

Diagnostic features of ABC include: (1) patient under 30 years of age, (2) thinning of both bony tables (skull), (3) multiloculated expansile bony lesions,

(4) different signal intensities within the cavities (MR imaging) with fluid in one or several of these, and (5) a hypointense circular rim surrounding the entire lesion (MR imaging) (GUIDA et al. 2001).

On plain radiographs, ABC is an eccentric, well-circumscribed lytic lesion with peripheral bone expansion. A sclerotic rim is sometimes present.

CT is the best modality to outline the thin bony margins, and sometimes displays fluid–fluid levels, as well as perilesional edema (MAHNKEN et al. 2003).

On MR imaging, the presence of septa and lobulations is the most important clue to the presence of ABC. The internal septations are hypointense on all sequences separating multiple cystic components. The cystic components are hypointense on T1- and hyperintense on T2-weighted images. Heterogeneous signals can be seen secondary to the different stages of degradation of blood products. The fluid–fluid levels within the cyst are characteristic but not specific (CAKIRER et al. 2002; MAHNKEN et al. 2003), as it may be seen in giant-cell tumor, telangiectatic osteosarcoma and chondroblastoma as well (MAHNKEN et al. 2003). Contrast-enhanced MR images show an intense contrast enhancement along the peripheral capsule and internal septations.

Conventional radiography and MR imaging have respectively a sensitivity of 76.4% and 77.8%, with a specificity of 55% and 66.7%. With the combined use of both modalities, a sensitivity of 82.6% and a specificity of 70% are achieved.

13.2.1.3
Treatment

The main controversy in the management of ABC is whether or not pathologic examination is mandatory. Biopsy or curettage can overlook the primary lesion in secondary ABC (CAMPANACCI et al. 1986; SZENDROI et al. 1992). Some series have reported malignant transformation of ABC following treatment (KYRIAKOS and HARDY 1991). Two extensive curettage procedures were performed in an 11-year-old girl with histologically proven ABC. Fifty months after the onset of symptoms and 28 months after the last curettage, a highly pleomorphic osteosarcoma developed. Thirteen malignancies occurred subsequent to radiation treatment of ABC, with the sarcoma developing 2–28 years after the radiation therapy. Most were osteosarcoma or fibrosarcoma.

Fine-needle aspiration for the diagnosis of ABC is controversial due to nonspecific results and a high percentage of inadequate samples. Still, one study found that 78% of primary bone lesions were correctly diagnosed by cytology (JORDA et al. 2000).

Several elements need to be considered in the treatment of ABC. They include the relative inaccessibility of the lesion, the associated intraoperative bleeding, the proximity of the lesion to neurovascular structures and the vulnerability or integrity of the adjacent joint.

13.2.1.3.1
Surgery

Several surgical techniques have been reported: total resection (GIBBS et al. 1999), bone graft (KOSKINEN et al. 1976), phenol as an adjuvant in the control of local recurrence (CAPANNA et al. 1985), curettage and cryotherapy (SCHREUDER et al. 1997), and injection of cement (OZAKI et al. 1997).

13.2.1.3.2
Curettage

Curettage can be improved with the use of a high speed bur, saucerization and bone marrow injection (HEMMADI and COLE 1999).

The rate of recurrence after curettage with or without bone grafting varies from 18% to 59% (BOLLINI et al. 1998; CAMPANACCI et al. 1986; HECHT and GEBHARDT 1998; LEITHNER et al. 1998; OLIVEIRA et al. 2004; VINCENZI 1981). High recurrence rates after any surgical treatment of ABC have been reported, ranging from 10% to 59% and greater in children younger than 10 years. PAPAGELOPOULOS et al. (2001) reported 10 recurrences out of 35 surgical procedures: curettage in 14 and excision-curettage in 21. Six out of 35 had complications: tears of dura in two, neuropathy in one, osteomyelitis in two, and one mechanical small-bowel obstruction. MARCOVE et al. (1995) have successfully used adjuvant liquid nitrogen cryotherapy after curettage and reported an 82% cure rate after the first treatment. CAPANNA et al. (1986) used phenol to sterilize the residual cavity after curettage of benign bone tumors. The recurrence rate was 41% in patients treated with simple curettage, and 7% in those treated with curettage and phenol. OZAKI et al. (1997) packed the cavity with bone cement after extensive curettage and compared this approach with curettage and bone grafting. They found lo-

cal recurrence after curettage and cement in 17% of patients, compared to 37% after curettage and bone grafting.

RAMIREZ and STANTON (2002) reported a series of 40 patients with a minimum 2-year follow-up. The recurrence rate was 27.5%. The average time span between initial surgery and recurrence was 18.7 months (4–39 months). Complications were one physeal arrest, two fractures and one infection.

13.2.1.3.3
Selective Embolization

Selective embolization is a preoperative procedure to reduce intraoperative bleeding (DUBOIS et al. 2003; GARG et al. 2000; LECLET and ADAMSBAUM 1998). Embolization is reported to be effective after surgical failure (HEMMADI and COLE 1999) or as a single therapy (GIBBS et al. 1999; JORDA et al. 2000; KOSKINEN et al. 1976; SCHREUDER et al. 1997). Selective arterial embolization alone rarely results in radiologic cure except in the pubic bone (DE CRISTOFARO et al. 1992; KONYA and SZENDROI 1992).

Complications are related to the risk of aberrant emboli, particularly for spine lesions.

When the circulation in the ABC is under high pressure, we perform a selective embolization of the feeding artery of the ABC. The embolization is performed with materials such as gelfoam, polyvinyl alcohol or coils (Fig. 13.1).

13.2.1.3.4
Percutaneous Treatment

Sclerotherapy is safe, easy to perform, cost-effective and far less aggressive than surgery. Patients are discharged 6 h post-procedure and do not have to be immobilized.

Sclerotherapy is performed under fluoroscopic control. The puncture with an 18- or 20-gauge metallic needle (Medicut Sherwood–Davis and Geck, Gosport, UK) can be done under fluoroscopic, CT or MR guidance. The liquid is aspirated, and cytologic and bactriologic analysis must be performed. Once the lesion is accessed, it is important to move the patient to the angiographic suite to perform opacification of the cyst. It is important to assess the draining veins prior to sclerotherapy to prevent potential complications. Opacification is paramount to evaluate the pattern of the lesion, its volume and the draining veins. The amount of

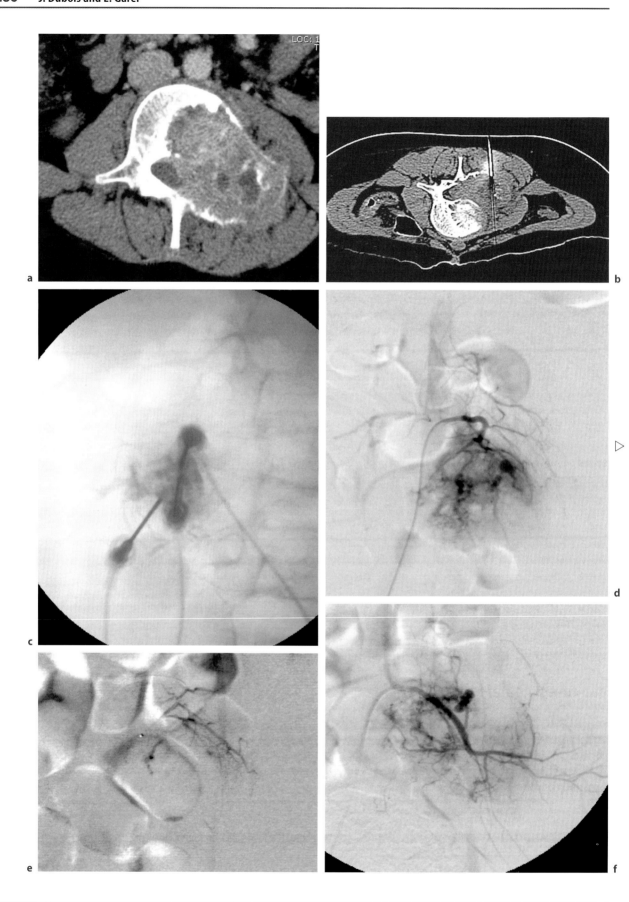

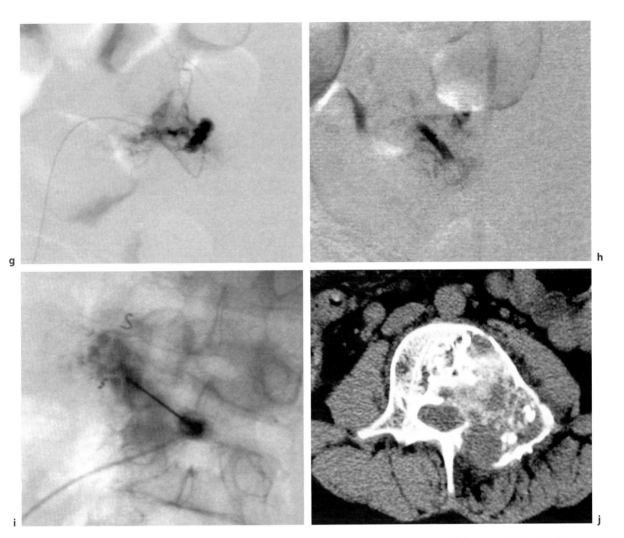

Fig. 13.1a–j. Expansile lytic bone lesion of the left pedicle and lamina of L3 in a 9-year-old boy. **a** Initial axial CT scan shows the involvement of the vertebra body. Sclerosing treatment was favored. **b** Under general anesthesia and CT guidance, a 20-gauge needle was inserted in the cyst. The patient was then transferred to the angiography suite. **c** Direct phlebography showed opacification of cavities with an important venous drainage toward the perivertebral region. Considering the pressure and the rapid wash-out, angiography was performed. **d** Angiography shows an important dilation of the second and third lumbar arteries. The selective catheterization of the second lumbar artery displays an aneurysmal dilation of the distal arteries, with stagnation of contrast in the venous phase. **e** Embolization with particles 710–1000 μm (Contour) followed by two proximal coils was performed. **f** The selective opacification of the third lumbar artery demonstrates feeding vessels. **g,h** Control postembolization arteriogram with particles 710–1000 μm (Contour) and coils. **i** Phlebography after CT-guided positioning of the needles shows the opacification of multiple cavities with less pressure and slower venous return than initially. **j** Axial CT scan performed 18 months post treatment shows significant reossification with some residual cyst. A second session of treatment is planned

sclerosing agent to be injected should be about the same as the amount of contrast medium needed to opacify the lesion before the visualization of the draining veins. Most of the time, the lesion is opacified by a single puncture because the cysts communicate. If the cysts don't communicate, a second puncture can be created. Sometimes, compression of the draining vein is necessary during the procedure to avoid pulmonary embolization (DUBOIS et al. 2003; GUIBAUD et al. 1998).

Sclerosing Agents

Direct Ethibloc injection has been proposed for the treatment of ABC (ADAMSBAUM et al. 1993). Ethibloc (Ethnor Laboratories/Ethicon, Norderstedt, Germany) contains an alcohol (60%) solution of 210 mg of zein (corn protein) per ml of alcohol, 162 mg of sodium diatrizoate per ml of alcohol (as a radiopaque marker), and 145 mg of oleum papaveris per ml of alcohol (which is added to keep the substance sterile). Ethibloc was first used with success in a series of four benign bone cysts (two UBC and two ABC) by ADAMSBAUM et al. in 1993. The sclerosing effect is due to the gigantocellular inflammatory reaction. Ethibloc has not been approved by the Food and Drug Administration (FDA).

Injection

The product is available in sterilized ready-to-inject syringes (7.5 ml). We diluted Ethibloc with 5 ml of 100% ethanol.

Mechanism

Ethibloc causes thrombus formation, local necrosis, inflammation and fibrosis. Biodegradation by enzymatic cleavage into amino acids occurs within 11–25 days. During the first few weeks following injection, Ethibloc freezes new bone formation. Later, progressive spontaneous osteogenesis reappears (LECLET and ADAMSBAUM 1998).

Results

DUBOIS et al. (2003) reported excellent regression in 94% of patients with no recurrence. GUIBAUD et al. (1998) reported total improvement in 87% of patients and partial response in 13% with no recurrence during follow-up (18 months–4 years). GARG et al. (2000) reported seven resolutions and three partial responses in ten patients. FALAPPA et al. (2002) reported a remarkable shrinkage of the cystic lesion and bone cortex thickening in 13 patients with ABC, with no complications (Figs. 13.2–13.5).

Complications

In our series of 17 cases (DUBOIS et al. 2003), we reported transitory local inflammatory reaction controlled by oral analgesics in two patients, and one patient with a sterile abscess that required drainage. Other complications of Ethibloc sclerotherapy have been described in the literature: aseptic bone necrosis (GUILBAUD et al. 1998), venous leakage in soft tissues, deep venous thrombosis, pulmonary embolism, abscess in soft tissues, fracture and epiphyseal necrosis. PERAUD et al. (2004) reported a fatal Ethibloc embolization of the vertebrobasilar system following percutaneous injection into an aneurysmal bone cyst of the second cervical vertebra.

Precautions are necessary to prevent complications: careful asepsis, preliminary injection of water soluble contrast medium, injection of embolic agent under fluoroscopic control to prevent systemic embolization, and 10 min of manual pressure on the injection site.

N-butyl cyanoacrylate (Loctite, Dublin, Republic of Ireland) is used when the ABC is in the spine or skull. This embolic agent, which is not FDA approved, is diluted with lipiodol. Histoacryl is a biological product that undergoes polymerization on contact with an ionic substance, inducing a permanent occlusion. Histoacryl is mostly used as a presurgical step, or for the treatment of arteriovenous malformations.

13.2.1.3.5
Radiation

Radiation has been found to be effective, although with a high rate of significant complications and a recurrence rate higher than 30% (GUIDA et al. 2001; CAMPANACCI et al. 1986). It is no longer recommended.

Complications include growth plate injury, gonadal damage in childhood (CAMPANACCI et al. 1986; CAPANNA et al. 1986) and development of secondary sarcoma. Radiation therapy has been used for inoperable cases.

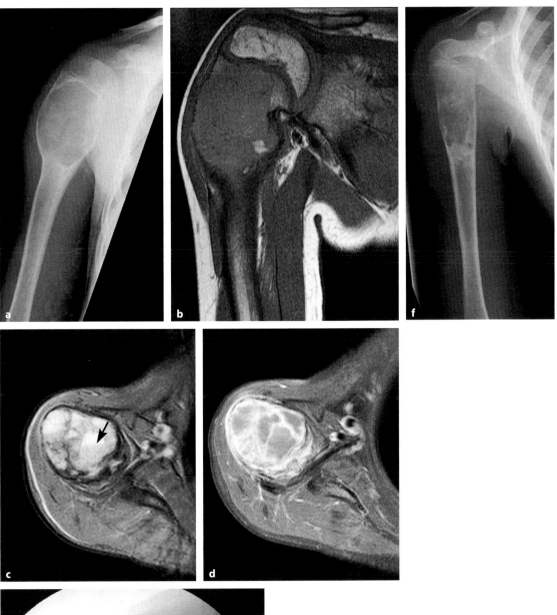

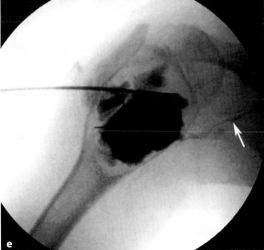

Fig. 13.2a–f. Aneurysmal bone cyst of the humerus in a 6-year-old girl. **a** Anteroposterior radiograph of the right humerus shows a lytic lesion with internal septa and lobulations. She was treated surgically without success a year later. The lesion even increased during this period. **b** Coronal T1-weighted MR image one year later demonstrates a lesion of intermediate signal intensity. **c** Axial T2-weighted gradient-echo MR image in the plane shows a fluid–fluid level (*arrow*). **d** Axial contrast-enhanced fat-suppressed T1-weighted MR image displays contrast enhancement of the septa. **e** The cyst was punctured under fluoroscopic control. Opacification outlined a draining vein (*arrow*), and Ethibloc was injected. **f** Anteroposterior radiograph performed 12 months post-Ethibloc injection shows marked improvement with few residual cysts

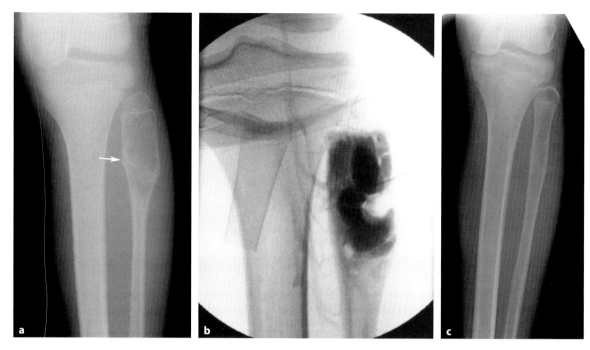

Fig. 13.3a–c. Aneurysmal bone cyst of the leg in a 14-year-old boy. **a** Anteroposterior radiograph of the left leg shows a fibular bony expansile lesion with septations, sclerotic rim and a pathological fracture (*arrow*). **b** Percutaneous puncture was performed under fluoroscopic control, showing multiple cysts with significant venous drainage. **c** Anteroposterior radiograph performed 4 years post sclerotherapy shows no recurrence

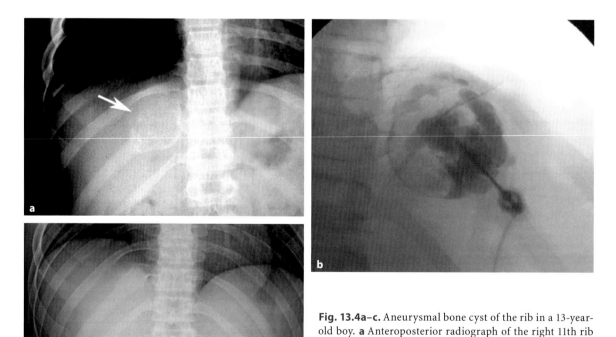

Fig. 13.4a–c. Aneurysmal bone cyst of the rib in a 13-year-old boy. **a** Anteroposterior radiograph of the right 11th rib before Ethibloc injection shows an expansile lytic lesion (*arrow*). **b** Phlebography shows multiple cavities. **c** Anteroposterior radiograph performed 4 years after two sessions of Ethibloc therapy showed excellent results

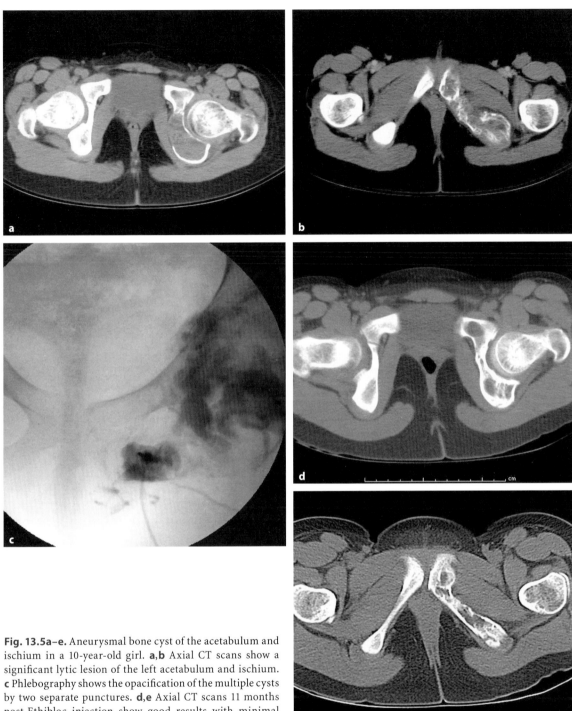

Fig. 13.5a–e. Aneurysmal bone cyst of the acetabulum and ischium in a 10-year-old girl. **a,b** Axial CT scans show a significant lytic lesion of the left acetabulum and ischium. **c** Phlebography shows the opacification of the multiple cysts by two separate punctures. **d,e** Axial CT scans 11 months post-Ethibloc injection show good results with minimal cyst

13.2.2
Arteriovenous Malformation

Arteriovenous malformation (AVM) is an abnormal communication between arteries and veins that bypasses the capillary bed. Lytic bone lesions related to AVM are uncommon. Most AVM is seen in the mandible.

The clinical presentation is a soft tissue pulsatile mass with local hyperthermia and sometimes congestive heart failure. It is important to recognize AVM to avoid a lethal loss of blood following a biopsy.

13.2.2.1
Imaging

On plain radiographs and CT, bone AVM appears as a cyst-like lesion with uni- or multilocular components. Sometimes the margins are erosive and simulate a malignant lesion.

On MR imaging, the lesion is difficult to assess because of flow voids.

Angiography is necessary to confirm the diagnosis and to assess the size and extent of the lesion. Angiography shows dilation and lengthening of afferent arteries, with early opacification of enlarged efferent veins.

13.2.2.2
Treatment

Embolization with or without surgery is mandatory. The embolization is performed by an arterial approach frequently combined with a percutaneous approach. The technique for the percutaneous approach is the same as in ABC but the embolization agents are different (Fig. 13.6). Alcohol or n-butyl isoacrylate is used for the percutaneous approach.

Ethanol (95%–98%) is the most potent and destructive agent of the vascular endothelium. Etha-

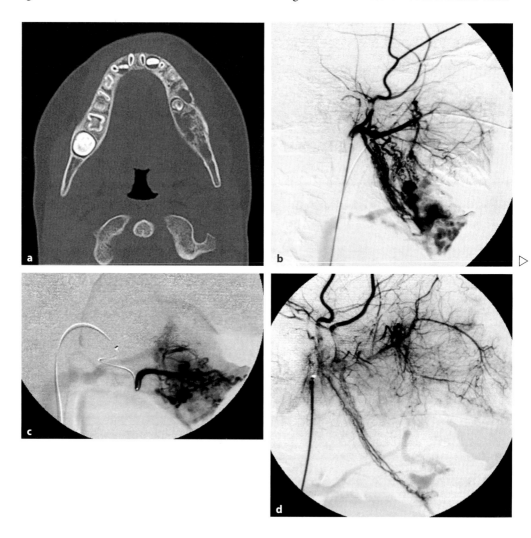

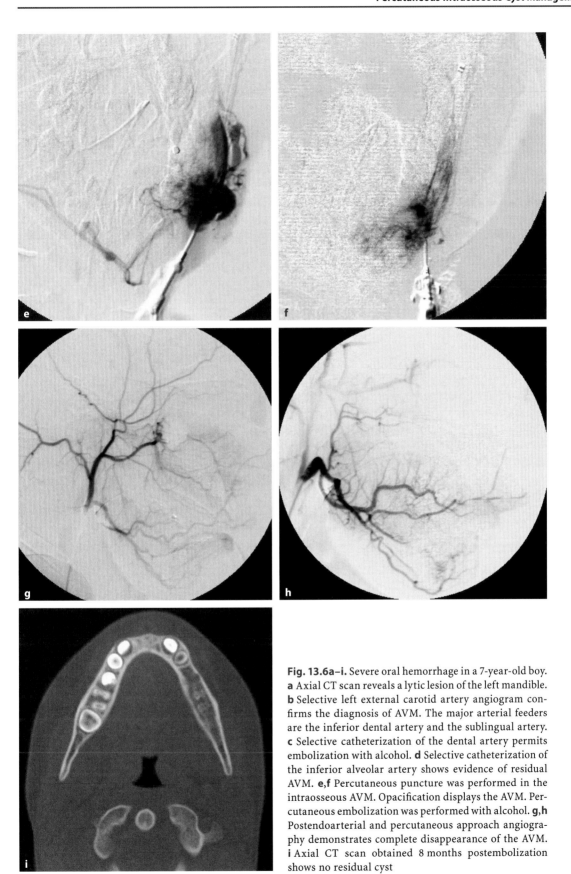

Fig. 13.6a–i. Severe oral hemorrhage in a 7-year-old boy.
a Axial CT scan reveals a lytic lesion of the left mandible.
b Selective left external carotid artery angiogram confirms the diagnosis of AVM. The major arterial feeders are the inferior dental artery and the sublingual artery.
c Selective catheterization of the dental artery permits embolization with alcohol. **d** Selective catheterization of the inferior alveolar artery shows evidence of residual AVM. **e,f** Percutaneous puncture was performed in the intraosseous AVM. Opacification displays the AVM. Percutaneous embolization was performed with alcohol. **g,h** Postendoarterial and percutaneous approach angiography demonstrates complete disappearance of the AVM. **i** Axial CT scan obtained 8 months postembolization shows no residual cyst

nol causes instant precipitation of endothelial cell proteins and rapid thrombosis.

Because of the fluidity of ethanol and its rapid absorption and circulation, we do not use this agent for ABC, although we do use it for arteriovenous malformations and venous malformations.

An undiluted form of ethanol, or ethanol opacified with oily contrast medium (9:1 or 10:2) or metrizamide powder, can be injected under fluoroscopic monitoring.

The total dose of 1 ml/kg (to a maximum of 60 cc) per session should never be exceeded (Burrows and Mason 2004). Ethanol blood levels correlate directly with the amount of injected ethanol.

Ethanol is the most effective sclerosant available for vascular anomalies, but it also results in the most serious side effects. Overall, reported complications range from 7.5%–23%. The most common complications are skin necrosis (in 10%–15% of cases) or peripheral nerve damage (in 1% of cases), cardiac arrest and pulmonary embolus. Central nervous system depression, hypoglycemia, hypertension, hyperthermia, hemolysis, pulmonary embolism, pulmonary vasospasm, cardiac arrhythmia and electromechanical dissociation have also been reported (Burrows and Mason 2004; Hanafi et al. 2001; Lee et al. 2001; Rautio et al. 2004; Yakes et al. 1993).

13.3
Unicameral Bone Cyst

Unicameral bone cysts (UBC) represent about 3% of primary bone tumors at biopsy (Lokiec and Wientroub 1998). UBC are most often seen in male patients between the ages of 3 and 15 years; the male-to-female ratio is about 2 or 2.5:1. The unicameral cyst is discovered incidentally or following a trauma. The course of UBC is related to the age of the patient. UBC is more aggressive in the first decade, with a recurrence rate four times higher than in adolescence (Lokiec and Wientroub 1998). They are most commonly found in the metaphyses of long bones, with two thirds of the lesions occurring in the proximal humerus and the remainder primarily in the proximal femur and proximal tibia. Two forms are described: inactive UBC (age greater than 10–12 years, located away from the growth plate, multilocular and with a bony wall thicker than in active cysts) (Lokiec and Wientroub 1998); and active UBC (age less than 10–12 years, located adjacent to the growth plate, unilocular and with a very thin wall).

Histologically, UBC consists of a mesothelial-lined cavity with a thin margin of reactive bone and many osteoclasts at the periphery. Small multilocular giant-cells may also be present (Robbins 1982). After pathologic fracture, foci of granulation tissue and calcium deposits can be seen (Margau et al. 2000). Analysis of the cyst fluid content shows several bone resorptive factors (e.g., prostaglandins, interleukin 1 and proteolytic enzymes) and proteins with molecular weights of 130,000; 92,000; 72,000 and less than 50,000 (Lokiec et al. 1996; Komiya et al. 1993).

13.3.1
Imaging

On plain radiographs, unicameral bone cysts appear as central, radiolucent lesions with well-defined margins, usually without septations or matrix. No periosteal reaction occurs unless there is a fracture within the lesion. After a fracture, the fallen fragment sign may be seen.

On CT, unicameral bone cysts appear as well-circumscribed lytic lesions.

On T1- and T2-weighted MR images, the fluid content of the cyst shows heterogeneous signal intensities. High signals on both imaging sequences suggest that there is either hemorrhage or colloid material in the cyst. Fluid–fluid levels can be seen in unicameral cysts secondary to intralesional hemorrhages, with internal degradation of blood products. After a fracture, septations and thick nodular peripheral enhancement are seen.

Margau et al. (2000) reported that focal nodules of homogeneous enhancement correlated with ground-glass opacity on plain film, and consolidation on follow-up.

13.3.2
Treatment

13.3.2.1
Conservative Treatment

In three different studies, spontaneous regression after a pathologic fracture was reported in 14.8%

of patients (GARCEAU and GREGORY 1954), in 6 of 8 patients (BROMS 1967), and in none of 97 patients (BOSEKER et al. 1968).

13.3.2.2
Percutaneous Treatment

13.3.2.2.1
Steroid Injection

SCAGLIETTI et al. (1979) reported on the percutaneous approach, with local injection of methylprednisolone acetate for treatment of UBC (Fig. 13.7).

Technique

The puncture is performed with an 18- or 16-gauge needle, depending on the resistance of the bone. Needle aspiration draws a clear straw-colored fluid if there has been no previous fracture or surgical treatment; the fluid becomes bloody after a fracture. The cystogram shows a single fluid-filled cavity. The injection is repeated every two months until radiological evidence of complete healing of the lesion is obtained. The Scaglietti technique is different (SCAGLIETTI et al. 1979). A single needle is introduced into the cyst with measurement of the pressure. A second needle is then inserted into the cavity to permit spontaneous escape of fluid. Opacification is performed, followed by injection of steroid.

Results

SCAGLIETTI et al. (1979, 1982) were the first to report treatment based on multiple injections of the cavity. They used 80–200 mg of methylprednisolone acetate, with no growth arrest or secondary deformity in about 90% of cases. Many authors thereafter confirmed the efficacy of methylprednisolone acetate with a recovery rate consistently over 90% (DE PALMA and SANTUCCI 1987; SCAGLIETTI et al. 1979). CAPANNA et al. (1982) reported satisfactory results in 80%, failure in 20%, and recurrence in 13.5%; although CAMPANACCI et al. (1986) reported a 15% recurrence rate, with only 50% complete healing. Local recurrence and/or no response after injection was reported to be as high as 25% (BOVILL and SKINNER 1989; CAMPANNACI et al. 1986). YU et al. (1991) showed that cortisone decreases the secretion of the synovial liquid and increases the speed of bone cell duplication.

OPPENHEIM and GALLENO (1984) compared 37 patients treated with surgery and 20 patients treated with in situ steroid injection. In the surgery group, the recurrence rate was 40%, rising to 88%

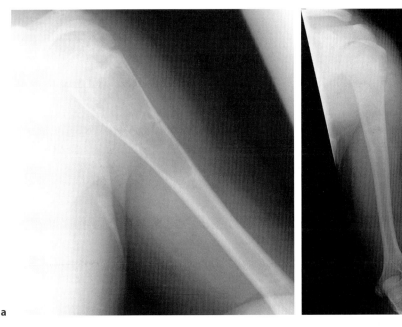

a   b

Fig. 13.7a,b. Unicameral cyst of the left humerus in a 12-year-old boy. **a** Anteroposterior radiograph at presentation shows extensive expansile lytic lesion of the proximal left humerus. **b** Anteroposterior radiograph performed 2.5 years postlesional injection of steroid shows significant bony reconstruction

in patients younger than 10 years with active cysts. Major complications were seen in 15% of cases, including infection, refracture, coxa vara, limb shortening and physeal damage.

The patients treated with steroid injection had a 5% recurrence rate, with 50% of these patients requiring more than one session. Complications were few, with a mild steroid flush in one, and extremity shortening due to a preexisting fracture in another.

13.3.2.2.2
Autologous Bone Marrow Injection

Autologous bone marrow is aspirated from the iliac crest, 6–8 ml per site. The mean volume to be injected into the UBC is 25 ml (15–60 ml).

Some series have reported excellent results following the use of percutaneously injected autologous marrow aspirate (LOKIEC et al. 1996; WIENTROUB et al. 1989). A series of 25 children (LOKIEC et al. 1996) showed complete healing after a single session of bone marrow injection in 84% of cases, satisfactory healing after two sessions in 12% of cases, and a third session needed in 4% of cases. No failure was observed in this series, with a follow-up of at least 12 months (range 12–66 months; mean: 24 months). It is known that bone marrow induces remodeling and consolidation of the bone, and this may account for the high rate of success.

13.3.2.2.3
Surgery

Surgery was the standard treatment of UBC for many years. The procedure consisted of curettage of the cyst, followed by grafting with autogenous or allogenous bone. Recurrence ranged from 25% to 50% (ROBBINS 1982). The recurrence rate for bone grafting was as high as 40% after autogenous grafting (NEER et al. 1973), and 12%–45% after allografting (SPENCE et al. 1969; SPENCE et al. 1976).

Lower recurrence rates were seen after subtotal resection (FAHEY and O'BRIEN 1973; GARTLAND and COLE 1975; MCKAY and NASON 1977). The use of adjuvant phenol after intralesional curettage was reported to be beneficial, with a recurrence rate of 20% (CAPANNA et al. 1985; SCHILLER et al. 1989).

Drilling methods were also described, but multiple operations were required and the recurrence rate was 66% (CHIGIRA et al. 1983; SHINOZAKI et al. 1996).

13.4
Histiocytosis

Langerhans cell histiocytosis (LCH) of bone is usually subcategorized into three categories: solitary bone lesion (eosinophilic granuloma), multiple bone lesions without systemic disease, and bone and systemic involvement.

Despite the profuse literature on the treatment of localized LCH, there are no widely accepted guidelines for the management of patients with this condition. The lack of guidelines can be ascribed to the absence of controlled studies, the variability in both the clinical course of the disease and the treatment and the possibility of spontaneous resolution.

From an imaging standpoint, LCH appears in the long bones as a radiolucent lesion without peripheral sclerosis, but with periosteal new bone formation; on flat bones as a radiolucent lesion with irregular margins and mild periosteal new bone formation; on the spine as vertebra plana (vertebral body involvement) or a radiolucent defect (posterior arch involvement).

Both authors agree that the diagnosis of localized bone LCH must be confirmed with operative or percutaneous biopsy, with the vertebra plana as the only exception.

The therapeutic approach remains controversial, and is dependent on institutional strategies for diagnosis confirmation and treatment. Three trends are reported in the literature: some favor surgical biopsy combined with curettage when the lesion is symptomatic and accessible (SESSA et al. 1994); others outline the value of percutaneous biopsy combined with intralesional injection of methylprednisolone (Fig. 13.8) (YASKO et al. 1998); while others report that most localized LCH bone lesions heal well without any treatment (GHANEM et al. 2003) and limit intervention to biopsy (Fig. 13.9).

Advocates of the percutaneous technique justify their approach because of its minimal invasiveness and low potential for complications. The 16-year experience of the M.D. Anderson Hospital and Tumor Institute Group (YASKO et al. 1998) has provided them with excellent results: fine-needle aspiration biopsy (18- to 22-gauge needle) and/or core-needle biopsy (Tru-Cut needle) was diagnostic for 88% of their patients, allowing concurrent in situ injection of steroids. In the rare instances (10%) of nondiagnostic percutaneous biopsy, open biopsy was performed, followed by curettage. It should be emphasized that

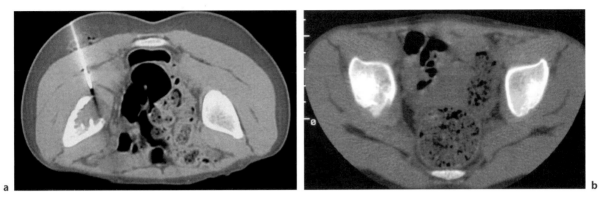

Fig. 13.8a,b. Eosinophilic granuloma of the ilion proved by biopsy in a 4-year-old boy. **a** Axial CT scan shows an ill-defined, aggressive lytic lesion of the right iliac crest. Puncture of the lesion is performed with in situ injection of 80 mg of steroid. **b** Axial CT scan 2 years later shows healing of the lesion

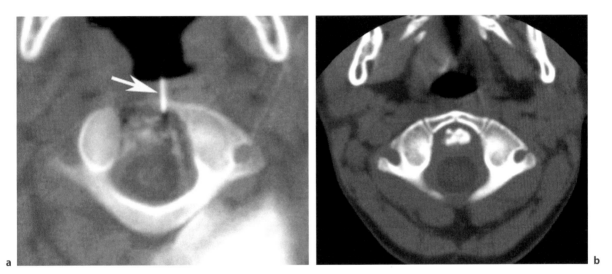

Fig. 13.9a,b. Eosinophilic granuloma of the odontoid in a 5-year-old girl. **a** Multiple biopsies were performed by transpharyngeal approach (*arrow*) under CT-guidance. As the pathology remained equivocal, there was no injection of steroid. **b** Axial CT scan 2 months later shows healing of the lesion. The healing process may have been induced by the trauma of the multiple punctures

such a protocol demands expert pathologists and cytologists on site. Finally, the mechanism of action of intralesional injection of methylprednisolone remains undefined, and definitive proof that the drug is responsible for the healing is lacking.

Whatever the institutional preferences for management, concurrent techniques should be considered: either percutaneous biopsy with or without subsequent injection of methylprednisolone, or open biopsy combined with curettage.

13.5
Conclusion

Percutaneous treatment of bony cystic lesions is a valuable alternative to surgery. Percutaneous procedures should always be performed under imaging guidance (fluoroscopy) to avoid the vascular reflux of sclerosing agents, especially in cases of ABC and AVM. Various sclerosing agents can be used successfully. Yearly follow-up is mandatory.

References

Adamsbaum C, Kalifa G, Seringe R et al. (1993) Direct Ethibloc injection in benign bone cysts: preliminary report on four patients. Skeletal Radiol 22:317–320

Bertoni F, Bacchini P, Capanna R et al. (1996) Solid variant of aneurysmal bone cyst. Cancer 71:729–734

Bollini G, Jouve JL, Cottalorda J et al. (1998) Aneurysmal bone cyst in children: analysis of twenty-seven patients. J Pediatr Orthop B 7:274–285

Boseker EH, Bickel WH, Dahlin DC (1968) A clinicopathologic study of simple unicameral bone cysts. Surg Gynecol Obstet 127:550–560

Bovill DF, Skinner HB (1989) Unicameral bone cysts. A comparison of treatment options. Orthop Rev 18:420–427

Broms JD (1967) Unicameral bone cyst: follow up study. J Bone Joint Surg Am 49:1014–1015

Burrows PE, Mason KP (2004) Percutaneous treatment of low flow vascular malformations. J Vasc Interv Radiol 15:431–445

Cakirer S, Cakirer D, Kabukcuoglu F (2002) Aneurysmal bone cyst of the orbit: a case of rare location and review of the literature. Clin Imaging 26:386–391

Campanacci M, Capanna R, Picci P (1986) Unicameral and aneurysmal bone cysts. Clin Orthop Relat Res 204:25

Capanna R, Dal Monte A, Gitelis S et al. (1982) The natural history of unicameral bone cyst after steroid injection. Clin Orthop Relat Res 166:204–211

Capanna R, Sudanese A, Baldini N et al. (1985) Phenol as an adjuvant in the control of local recurrence of benign neoplasms of bone treated by curettage. Ital J Orthop Traumatol 11:381–388

Capanna R, Bertoni F, Bettelli G et al. (1986) Aneurysmal bone cysts of the pelvis. Arch Orthop Trauma Surg 105:279–284

Capanna R, Campanacci DA, Manfrini M (1996) Unicameral and aneurysmal bone cysts. Orthop Clin North Am 27:605–614

Chigira M, Maehara S, Arita S et al. (1983) The aetiology and treatment of simple bone cysts. J Bone Joint Surg Br 65:633–637

De Cristofaro R, Biagini R, Boriani S et al. (1992) Selective arterial embolization in the treatment of aneurysmal bone cyst and angioma of bone. Skeletal Radiol 21:523–527

de Palma L, Santucci A (1987) Treatment of bone cysts with methylprednisolone acetate. A 9 to 11 year follow-up. Int Orthop 11:23–28

Dubois J, Chigot V, Grimard G et al. (2003) Sclerotherapy in aneurysmal bone cysts in children: a review of 17 cases. Pediatr Radiol 33:365–372

Fahey JJ, O'Brien ET (1973) Subtotal resection and grafting in selected cases of solitary unicameral bone cyst. J Bone Joint Surg Am 55:59–68

Falappa P, Fassari FM, Fanelli A et al. (2002) Aneurysmal bone cysts: treatment with direct percutaneous Ethibloc injection: long-term results. Cardiovasc Intervent Radiol 25:282–290

Garceau GJ, Gregory CF (1954) Solitary unicameral bone cyst. J Bone Joint Surg Am 36:267–280

Garg NK, Carty H, Walsh HP et al. (2000) Percutaneous Ethibloc injection in aneurysmal bone cysts. Skeletal Radiol 29:211–216

Gartland JJ, Cole FL (1975) Modern concepts in the treatment of unicameral bone cysts of the proximal humerus. Orthop Clin North Am 6:487–498

Ghanem I, Tolo VT, D'Ambra P et al. (2003) Langerhans cell histiocytosis of bone in children and adolescents. J Pediatr Orthop 23:124–130

Gibbs CP Jr, Hefele MC, Peabody TD et al. (1999) Aneurysmal bone cyst of the extremities. Factors related to local recurrence after curettage with a high-speed burr. J Bone Joint Surg Am 81:1671–1678

Guibaud L, Herbreteau D, Dubois J et al. (1998) Aneurysmal bone cysts: percutaneous embolization with an alcoholic solution of zein–series of 18 cases. Radiology 208:369–373

Guida F, Rapana A, Conti C et al. (2001) Cranial aneurysmal bone cyst: a diagnostic problem. With a review of the literature. Childs Nerv Syst 17:297–301

Hanafi M, Orliaguet G, Meyer P et al. (2001) Embolie pulmonaire au cours de la sclérothérapie percutanée d'un angiome veineux sous anesthésie général chez un enfant. Ann Fr Anesth Reanim 20:556–558

Hecht AC, Gebhardt MC (1998) Diagnosis and treatment of unicameral and aneurysmal bone cysts in children. Curr Opin Pediatr 10:87–94

Hemmadi SS, Cole WG (1999) Treatment of aneurysmal bone cysts with saucerization and bone marrow injection in children. J Pediatr Orthop 19:540–542

Jaffe HL, Lichtenstein L (1942) Solitary unicameral bone cyst, with emphasis on the roentgen picture, pathologic appearance and pathogenesis. Arch Surg 44:1004–1007

Jorda M, Rey L, Hanly A et al. (2000) Fine-needle aspiration cytology of bone: accuracy and pitfalls of cytodiagnosis. Cancer 90:47–54

Kershisnik M, Batsakis JG (1994) Aneurysmal bone cysts of the jaws. Ann Otol Rhinol Laryngol 103:164–165

Komiya S, Minamitani K, Sasaguri Y et al. (1993) Simple bone cyst. Treatment by trepanation and studies on bone resorptive factors in cyst fluid with a theory of its pathogenesis. Clin Orthop Relat Res 287:204–211

Konya A, Szendroi M (1992) Aneurysmal bone cysts treated by superselective embolization. Skeletal Radiol 21:167–172

Koskinen EV, Visuri TI, Holmstrom T et al. (1976) Aneurysmal bone cyst: evaluation of resection and of curettage in 20 cases. Clin Orthop Relat Res 118:136–146

Kyriakos M, Hardy D (1991) Malignant transformation of aneurysmal bone cyst, with an analysis of the literature. Cancer 68:1770–1780

Leclet H, Adamsbaum C (1998) Intraosseous cyst injection. Radiol Clin North Am 36:581–587

Lee BB, Kim DI, Huh S et al. (2001) New experiences with absolute ethanol sclerotherapy in the management of a complex form of congenital venous malformation. J Vasc Surg 33:764–772

Leithner A, Windhager R, Kainberger F et al. (1998) A case of aneurysmal bone cyst in father and son. Eur J Radiol 29:28–30

Lokiec F, Wientroub S (1998) Simple bone cyst: etiology, classification, pathology, and treatment modalities. J Pediatr Orthop B 7:262–273

Lokiec F, Ezra E, Khermosh O et al. (1996) Simple bone cysts treated by percutaneous autologous marrow grafting. A preliminary report. J Bone Joint Surg Br 78:934–937

Mahnken AH, Nolte-Ernsting CC, Wildberger JE et al. (2003) Aneurysmal bone cyst: value of MR imaging and conventional radiography. Eur Radiol 13:1118–1124

Marcove RC, Sheth DS, Takemoto S et al. (1995) The treatment of aneurysmal bone cyst. Clin Orthop Relat Res 311:157–163

Margau R, Babyn P, Cole W et al. (2000) MR imaging of simple bone cysts in children: not so simple. Pediatr Radiol 30:551–557

McKay DW, Nason SS (1977) Treatment of unicameral bone cysts by subtotal resection without grafts. J Bone Joint Surg Am 59:515–519

Mulliken JB, Glowacki J (1982) Hemangiomas and vascular malformations in infants and children: a classification based on endothelial characteristics. Plast Reconstr Surg 69:412–422

Neer CS, Francis KC, Johnston AD et al. (1973) Current concepts on the treatment of solitary unicameral bone cyst. Clin Orthop Relat Res 97:40–51

Oliveira AM, Hsi BL, Weremowicz S et al. (2004) USP6 (Tre2) fusion oncogenes in aneurysmal bone cyst. Cancer Res 64:1920–1923

Oppenheim WL, Galleno H (1984) Operative treatment versus steroid injection in the management of unicameral bone cysts. J Pediatr Orthop 4:1–7

Ozaki T, Hillmann A, Lindner N et al. (1997) Cementation of primary aneurysmal bone cysts. Clin Orthop Relat Res 337:240–248

Papagelopoulos PJ, Choudhury SN, Frassica FJ et al. (2001) Treatment of aneurismal bone cysts of the pelvis and sacrum. J Bone Joint Surg Am 83–A:1647–1681

Peraud A, Drake JM, Armstrong D et al. (2004) Fatal ethibloc embolization of vertebrobasilar system following percutaneous injection into aneurysmal bone cyst of the second cervical vertebra. AJNR Am J Neuroradiol 25:1116–1120

Ramirez AR, Stanton RP (2002) Aneurysmal bone cyst in 29 children. J Pediatr Orthop 22:533–539

Rautio R, Saarinen J, Laranne J et al. (2004) Endovascular treatment of venous malformations in extremities: results of sclerotherapy and the quality of life after treatment. Acta Radiol 45:397–403

Robbins H (1982) The treatment of unicameral or solitary bone cysts by the injection of corticosteroids. Bull Hosp Jt Dis Orthop Inst 42:1–16

Scaglietti O, Marchetti PG, Bartolozzi P (1979) Rizulati a distanza dell'azione topica dell'acetato di methylprednisolone in microcristalli in alcune lesioni dello scheletro. Arch Putti Chir Organi Mov 30:1

Scaglietti O, Marchetti PG, Bartolozzi P (1982) Final results obtained in the treatment of bone cysts with methylprednisolone acetate (depo-medrol) and a discussion of results achieved in other bone lesions. Clin Orthop Relat Res 165:33–42

Schiller C, Ritschl P, Windhager R et al. (1989) The incidence of recurrence in phenoltreated and non-phenoltreated bone cavities following intralesional resection of non-malignant bone tumors. Z Orthop Ihre Grenzgeb 127:398–401

Schreuder HW, Veth RP, Pruszczynski M et al. (1997) Aneurysmal bone cysts treated by curettage, cryotherapy and bone grafting. J Bone Joint Surg Br 79:20–25

Sessa S, Sommelet D, Lascombes P et al. (1994) Treatment of Langerhans-cell histiocytosis in children. Experience at the Children's Hospital of Nancy. J Bone Joint Surg Am 76:1513–1525

Shinozaki T, Arita S, Watanabe H et al. (1996) Simple bone cysts treated by multiple drill-holes. 23 cysts followed 2–10 years. Acta Orthop Scand 67:288–290

Spence KF, Sell KW, Brown RH (1969) Solitary bone cyst: treatment with freeze-dried cancellous bone allograft. A study of one hundred seventy-seven cases. J Bone Joint Surg Am 51:87–96

Spence KF Jr, Bright RW, Fitzgerald SP et al. (1976) Solitary unicameral bone cyst: treatment with freeze-dried crushed cortical-bone allograft. A review of one hundred and forty-four cases. J Bone Joint Surg Am 58:636–641

Szendroi M, Cser I, Konya A et al. (1992) Aneurysmal bone cyst. A review of 52 primary and 16 secondary cases. Arch Orthop Trauma Surg 111:318–322

Vincenzi G (1981) Familial incidence in two cases of aneurysmal bone cyst. Ital J Orthop Traumatol 7:251–253

Wientroub S, Goodwin D, Khermosh O et al. (1989) The clinical use of autologous marrow to improve osteogenic potential of bone grafts in pediatric orthopedics. J Pediatr Orthop 9:186–190

Yakes WF, Engelwood CO, Baker R (1993) Cardiopulmonary collapse: sequelae of ethanol embolotherapy. Radiology 189:145

Yasko AW, Fanning CV, Ayala AG et al. (1998) Percutaneous techniques for the diagnosis and treatment of localized Langerhans-cell histiocytosis (eosinophilic granuloma of bone). J Bone Joint Surg Am 80:219–228

Yu CL, D'Astous J, Finnegan M (1991) Simple bone cysts. The effects of methylprednisolone on synovial cells in culture. Clin Orthop 262:34–41

Percutaneous Bone Tumors Management

AFSHIN GANGI and XAVIER BUY

14

CONTENTS

14.1   Introduction   *301*

14.2   Cementoplasty   *302*

14.3   Chemical Ablation with Ethanol   *302*
14.3.1 Mechanism   *302*
14.3.2 Equipment   *304*
14.3.3 Patient Selection and Technique   *304*
14.3.4 Patient Outcome   *305*

14.4   Thermal Ablation   *305*
14.4.1 Laser Ablation   *305*
14.4.1.1 Mechanism   *305*
14.4.1.2 Equipment   *305*
14.4.1.3 Patient Selection and Technique   *305*
14.4.1.4 Patient Outcome   *306*
14.4.2 Radiofrequency Ablation   *309*
14.4.2.1 Mechanism   *309*
14.4.2.2 Equipment   *309*
14.4.2.3 Patient Selection and Technique   *309*
14.4.2.4 Patient Outcome   *313*
14.4.3 Cryoablation   *316*
14.4.3.1 Mechanism   *317*
14.4.3.2 Equipment   *318*
14.4.3.3 Patient Selection and Technique   *318*
14.4.3.4 Patient Outcome   *321*

14.5   Radiofrequency Ionization   *322*
14.5.1 Mechanism   *322*
14.5.2 Equipment   *322*
14.5.3 Patient Selection and Technique   *322*
14.5.4 Patient Outcome   *322*

14.6   Thermal Protection and Insulation   *324*

14.7   Treatment Strategy   *325*
14.7.1 Curative Treatment   *326*
14.7.2 Palliative Treatment   *326*

14.8   Conclusion   *326*

        References   *326*

14.1
Introduction

Image-guided tumor management is a minimally invasive treatment for localized bone tumors. Compared to other modalities, minimally invasive procedures require fewer resources, less time, recovery, and cost, and often reduced morbidity and mortality. Many percutaneous techniques are available. Some aim to treat pain and consolidate bone, i.e. cementoplasty. Others ablate or reduce the tumor, i.e. chemical and thermal ablation techniques. Bone tumor management generally falls into two categories: curative, and far more frequently, palliative.

Few patients with secondary bone tumors qualify for open surgery. However, percutaneous curative ablation is highly effective for treating some benign or malignant localized bone tumors. Pain management in terminally ill patients with tumors involving bone can be challenging. Conventional therapeutic options for pain control include radiation therapy and/or chemotherapy, surgery, and the use of opioids and other analgesics.

In this chapter, existing image-guided techniques for the treatment of primary and secondary bone tumors, ethanol ablation, cementoplasty, radiofrequency ablation, laser photocoagulation, radiofrequency ionization, and cryoablation will be reviewed and discussed. Each has its advantages and drawbacks. Ablation reduces tumor size and relieves pain. Cementoplasty consolidates bone and treats pain. The details of each technique including mechanism of action, equipment, patient selection, treatment technique, and recent patient outcome are presented.

A. GANGI, MD, PhD, Professor of Radiology
X. Buy, MD, Senior Radiologist
Department of Radiology B, University Hospital of Strasbourg, Pavillon Clovis Vincent BP 426, 67091 Strasbourg, France

14.2
Cementoplasty

Percutaneous injection of methylmethacrylate, i.e. cementoplasty, provides notable pain relief and bone strengthening in patients with malignant vertebral tumor and acetabular osteolytic metastasis (GANGI et al. 1996, 2003).

The cement is highly resistant to compression forces but susceptible to torsion forces, and is therefore used to treat and prevent compression fractures. The mechanical properties of bone cement also strengthen bone, stabilize microfractures and reduce mechanical forces. Consequently, injection of methylmethacrylate is also indicated when the object is to improve mobility in patients with osteolysis involving the weight-bearing part of the vertebral body (Fig. 14.1), acetabulum (Fig. 14.2), and in any bones subject to compression forces only. The pain-reducing effect of cement cannot be explained by consolidation of the pathologic bone alone. In fact, good pain relief is obtained after injection of only 2 mL of cement into a metastasis. Radiation therapy can provide partial or complete pain relief, and it may prevent tumor growth. Most patients experience some relief within 10–14 days. Unfortunately, for some patients the relief may be insufficient or local tumors may recur but further therapy cannot be tolerated. Moreover, radiation therapy

results in only minimal and delayed (2–4 months) bone strengthening; it does not allow patients with extensive lytic lesions of the weight-bearing part of the acetabulum to stand (cf. to Chap. 11 for the indications, technique and results).

14.3
Chemical Ablation with Ethanol

Worldwide, ethanol ablation is probably the most accepted minimally invasive method for treating primary malignant hepatic tumors. Ethanol is also widely used in pain management (neurolysis) and ablation of osteolytic bone metastases (GANGI et al. 1994b). If conventional anticancer therapy including radiotherapy is insufficient and high doses of opiodes are necessary to control pain, alcoholization is an alternative therapy.

14.3.1
Mechanism

Within cells, ethanol causes dehydration of the cytoplasm and subsequent coagulation necrosis, followed by fibrous reaction. Within vessels, ethanol induces necrosis of endothelial cells and platelet aggregation, causing thrombosis and tissue ischemia.

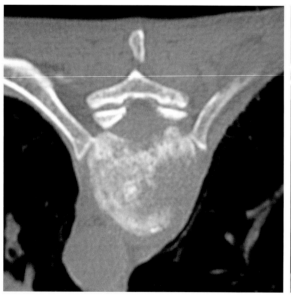 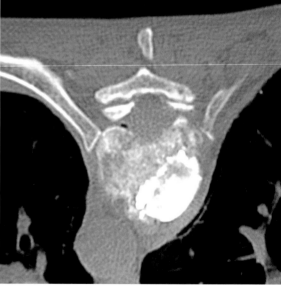

a   b

Fig. 14.1a,b. Painful T10 metastasis in a 54-year-old man with lung cancer. **a** Axial CT scan shows lytic metastasis limited to the vertebral body. **b** Axial CT scan shows single vertebroplasty achieved excellent pain management and consolidation

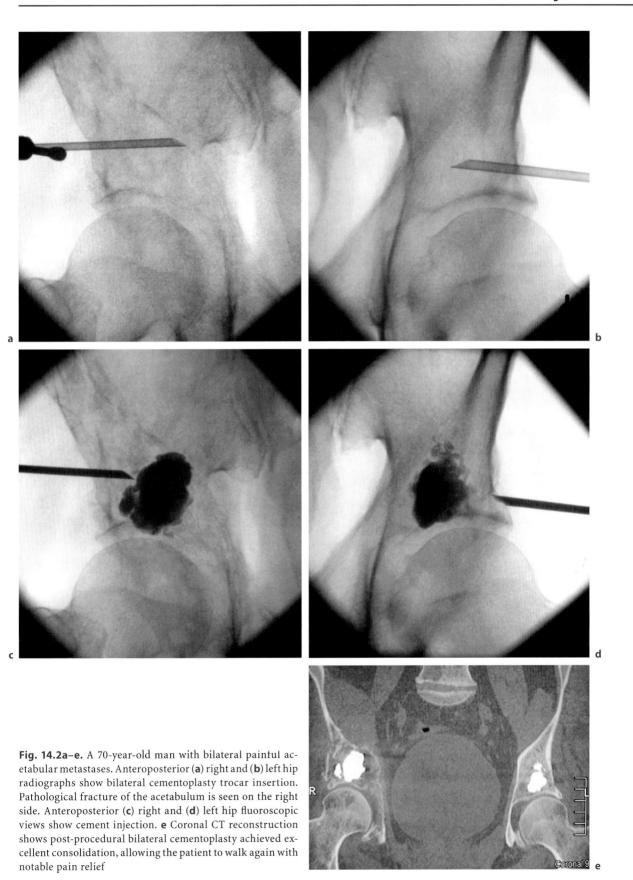

Fig. 14.2a–e. A 70-year-old man with bilateral painful acetabular metastases. Anteroposterior (**a**) right and (**b**) left hip radiographs show bilateral cementoplasty trocar insertion. Pathological fracture of the acetabulum is seen on the right side. Anteroposterior (**c**) right and (**d**) left hip fluoroscopic views show cement injection. **e** Coronal CT reconstruction shows post-procedural bilateral cementoplasty achieved excellent consolidation, allowing the patient to walk again with notable pain relief

14.3.2
Equipment

The procedure is performed under CT guidance. Equipment consists of a syringe, sterile 95% ethanol, a 22-gauge spinal needle, a connecting tube, contrast media and lidocaine.

14.3.3
Patient Selection and Technique

Chemical ablation is useful for palliation of painful osteolytic bone tumors without risk of fracture, when conventional therapies have failed (GANGI et al. 1996). After delineation of tumor location and size on contiguous pre-contrast and post-contrast CT scans, the optimal puncture site and angle are defined. Contrast-enhanced CT determines which part of the tumor is necrotic.

Ethanol injection in bone is very painful and alcohol instillation requires neuroleptanalgesia. According to the size, number of lesions, and amount of pain, alcoholization can be performed in one session or several. Following local anesthesia using lidocaine 1%, a 22-gauge needle is placed in the nonnecrotic part of the tumor. Contrast medium 25% diluted is injected into the lesion first to predict the distribution (Fig. 14.3). If the contrast medium diffuses beyond the tumor boundaries, particularly if it reaches contiguous neurological structures, the procedure must not proceed.

Depending on its size, 3–25 mL of 95% ethanol are instilled into the tumor. In large tumors, alcohol is selectively instilled into regions considered responsible for pain, usually the periphery of the metastasis and osteolytic areas. After injection of 3 mL of alcohol, control CT evaluates the distribution inside the tumor. If the ethanol is unevenly distributed within the tumor, particularly in large metastases, the needle is repositioned in regions of poor diffusion and the injection is repeated.

The size and shape of the induced necrosis with ethanol vary with the degree of vascularization, necrosis and tissue consistency. They are not always reproducible. One reason thermal ablation techniques are now preferred is that they provide much more predictable ablation volumes.

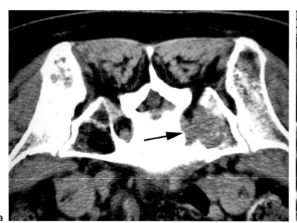
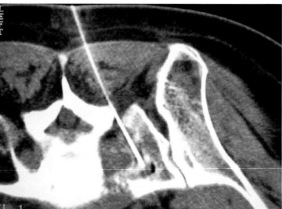
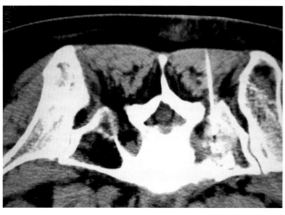

Fig. 14.3a–c. Painful metastasis of the right sacral wing in a 45-year-old woman with metastatic breast cancer. **a** Axial CT scan of the pelvis demonstrates the right lytic sacral metastasis (*arrow*). **b** Axial CT scans shows a 22-gauge spinal needle inserted into the tumor with iodine contrast administration to check for contrast distribution. **c** Axial CT scan shows heterogeneous distribution of the injected 5 mL of 95% ethanol. Good pain relief was achieved

14.3.4
Patient Outcome

Another major advantage of alcoholization of bone metastases, compared to radiotherapy or chemotherapy, is rapid pain relief within 24 h. In 74% pain relief is satisfactory. In 26% tumor size is reduced; in 18.5% tumor size increases. Duration of pain relief ranges from 10 to 27 weeks. The best results are with small metastases, i.e. tumors ranging from 3 to 6 cm in diameter. Patients experience low grade fever and hyperuricemia in the first 3 days when massive tumor necrosis follows large ethanol injections.

14.4
Thermal Ablation

14.4.1
Laser Ablation

Experimental studies have shown that a reproducible thermal injury can be produced with near-infrared wavelength lasers, i.e. neodymium yttrium aluminum garnet (Nd:YAG), diode laser 800–1000 nanometer wavelength. Nd:YAG lasers have been used to treat tumors of the esophagus, stomach, colon, and pulmonary bronchus. Laser ablation of bone tumors started in the 1990s (GANGI et al. 1997b, 2007).

14.4.1.1
Mechanism

Laser energy, with its powerful and precise ability to ablate, coagulate, and vaporize dense tissues as well as its transmissibility in optical fiber, is an ideal tool for use in percutaneous ablations. Interstitial laser ablation (ILA) consists of percutaneous insertion of optical fibers into the tumor. The tumor is coagulated and destroyed by direct heating. From a single, bare 400-mm laser fiber, light at optical or near-infrared wavelengths will scatter within tissue and be converted into heat. Light energy of 2.0 W will produce a spherical ablation volume of 1.6 cm diameter in bone. Higher power results in charring and vaporization around the fiber tip. For larger volumes of necrosis (>1.6 cm), several bare fibers 1.5–2 cm apart spread through the lesion are necessary (GANGI et al. 1997a).

14.4.1.2
Equipment

Infrared lasers are the most common. Compact solid-state diode lasers are now available (wavelength around 800 nm) with power outputs up to 60 W. This energy can be delivered through fibers over 10 m in length with the great advantage of being fully compatible with MR imaging.

14.4.1.3
Patient Selection and Technique

Because of the small amount of ablation with a bare tip fiber without cooling, laser is used in small tumors or when metallic implants, for example, contraindicate radiofrequency (RF) ablation (Fig. 14.4). Large tumors require several fibers. With a low-power laser technique, a well defined coagulation volume of predictable size and shape can be obtained in bone tissue. However, the small size of the ablation limits it to small tumors.

Osteoid osteomas are usually less than 1 cm in diameter and are ideal for laser ablation. The laser fiber (400–600 µm) is inserted coaxially into the tumor under CT guidance (1 mm collimation). In tumors surrounded by thick cortical bone, a drill needle is used (14-gauge Bonopty® Penetration Set, RADI Medical Systems, Uppsala, Sweden) for coaxial insertion of the fiber (Fig. 14.5). The access route is crucial and should avoid all neurovascular structures. Moreover, heat diffusion must be taken into account to avoid complications. Insulating techniques can protect adjacent vulnerable structures (Figs. 14.6 and 14.7). For subperiosteal tumors, an 18-gauge spinal needle is used to insert the fiber. Pain during penetration of the nidus is typical of osteoid osteoma and the procedure should be performed under general anesthesia or regional block. A biopsy should be performed before ablation, especially in doubtful cases. Then, the fiber is positioned in the center of the nidus. To confirm the precise central position of the fiber, a short CT volume acquisition scan with multiplanar reconstructions can be helpful (Fig. 14.7). Optimal positioning is the key point for success. For ablation, 2 W power is applied for 6–10 min depending on the tumor's size. At the end of the ablation, 5–10 mL of rupivacaine 2 mg/mL are injected (strictly extravascularly) in contact with the periosteum to reduce post-procedural pain.

Large painful bone metastases can be treated by inserting up to eight simultaneously energized bare fibers into the tumor with less then 2 cm spacing.

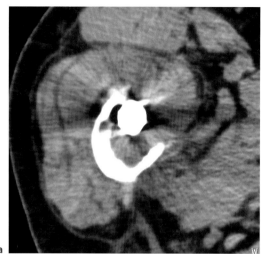

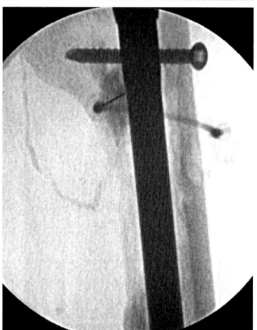

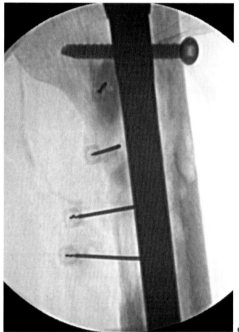

Fig. 14.4a–c. Painful femoral metastasis previously consolidated with a surgical nail in a 65-year-old man with renal cancer. **a** Axial CT scan shows the tumor surrounding the nail, with a large cortical rupture. The metallic nail is a contraindication for RF ablation. **b** Anteroposterior femoral radiograph shows insertion of a spinal needle into the tumor. Contrast injection shows venous drainage towards the pelvis which contraindicates ethanol injection. **c** Anteroposterior femoral radiograph shows 4 18-gauge spinal needles are finally inserted and laser ablation is performed. Good pain relief was achieved

14.4.1.4
Patient Outcome

The success rate is excellent and similar to RF ablation (ROSENTHAL et al. 2003; WITT et al. 2000). Over 170 osteoid osteomas have been treated with laser ablation in the past 14 years in our institution. Successful treatment in a single session was achieved in 95% of cases. Post-procedural pain was systematically controlled with non-steroidal anti-inflammatory drugs (NSAIDs) and analgesics beginning while the anesthesia was still in effect and for 12 h after the procedure. Major complications such as neurological damage were avoided by insulation techniques and thermal monitoring discussed at the end of this chapter. The only notable complications were two cases of neurodystrophia of the wrist. We advocate regional block for ablation of nidi in the extremities. We also had 5% recurrences, mainly intra-articular lesions, all of which were successfully treated by a second session (GANGI et al. 2007).

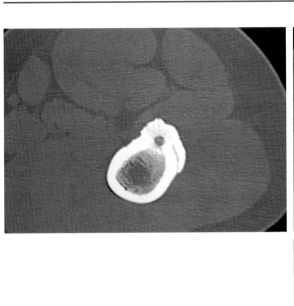

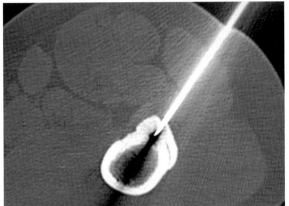

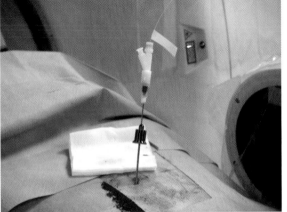

Fig. 14.5a–c. An 18-year-old man with femoral osteoid osteoma treated with laser ablation. **a** Axial CT scan shows the nidus surrounded by dense sclerotic reaction. **b** Axial CT scan demonstrates the 14-gauge bone penetration set with a drill used to reach the nidus. **c** Photo from the CT room (different case) shows an 18-gauge spinal needle protecting the optical fiber is inserted coaxially so that only the active tip of the fiber remains in the nidus

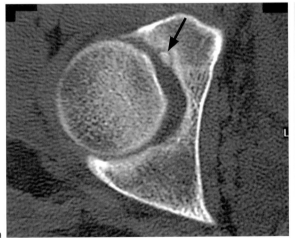

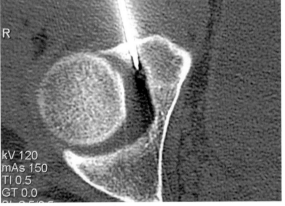

Fig. 14.6a–c. A 23-year-old man with acetabular osteoid osteoma treated with laser ablation. **a** Axial CT scan shows the right acetabular intra-articular nidus (*arrow*). **b** Axial CT scan demonstrates the 14-gauge bone penetration set used to reach the nidus. The optical fiber protected by an 18-gauge spinal needle is inserted coaxially. **c** Axial CT scan shows simultaneous intra-articular injection of 10 mL of saline to protect the cartilage from thermal injury

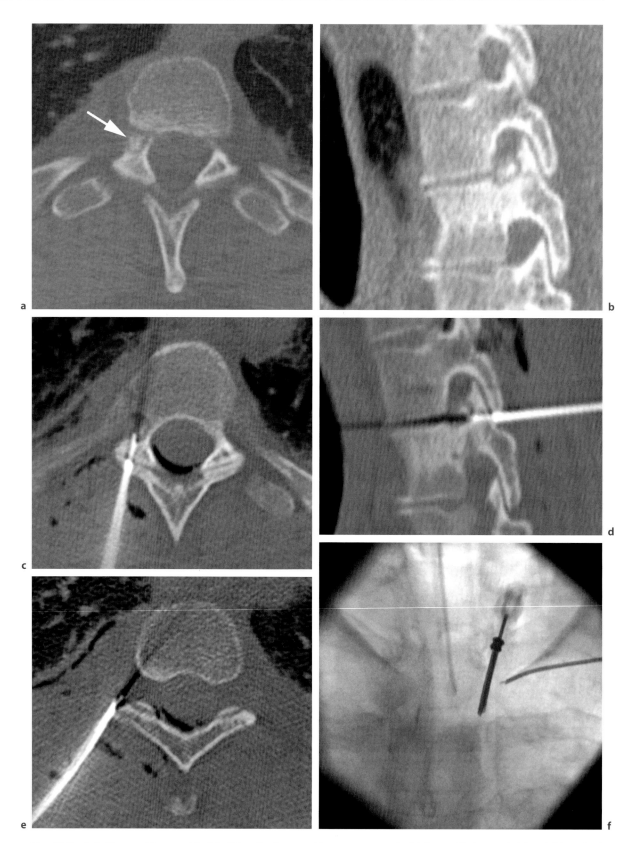

Fig. 14.7a–f. A 29-year-old man with right T3 pedicular osteoid osteoma treated with laser ablation. **a** Axial and (**b**) sagittal reformat CT scans show the right pedicular T3 nidus (*arrow*) in contact with the T2 nerve root in the foramen, without cortical interposition. **c** Axial and (**d**) sagittal reformat CT scans demonstrate the proper positioning of the14-gauge bone penetration set with the optical fiber coaxially inserted into the nidus. **e** Axial CT scan and (**f**) anteroposterior fluoroscopic view of the thoracic spine show thermal protection of the T2 nerve root by an 18-gauge spinal needle positioned in the foramen allowing coaxial insertion of a thermocouple for continuous thermal monitoring, and neural insulation by epidural injection of 10 mL of CO_2

14.4.2
Radiofrequency Ablation

Radiofrequency (RF) ablation is one of the most promising thermal techniques for the treatment of localized tumors. RF ablation started in the early 1990s with hepatic tumors. Its major advantage over chemical ablation (ethanol) is better control of the ablation zone without risk of leaking. The major disadvantage of RF ablation is possible thermal damage to vulnerable surrounding structures, particularly nerve roots, and sometimes, penetration of the lesion. As much as 5 mm or more of cortical bone will provide adequate insulation. However, the less bone the less insulation, and thin (≤1 mm) or ruptured cortical bone provides little insulation and makes the procedure hazardous to nearby structures (Dupuy et al. 2000). The surrounding soft tissue temperature during RF ablation depends directly on the thickness of the cortical bone lamella and the distance from the periosteum (Bitsch et al. 2006).

In these cases the ablation should be performed very carefully; protection of the surrounding structures and monitoring of the temperature is mandatory. Temperature mapping with MR imaging is very promising (Okuda et al. 2004; Seror et al. 2006).

14.4.2.1
Mechanism

Alternating electric current in the RF range can produce focal thermal injury in living tissue. Shielded needle electrodes are used to concentrate the energy in the selected tissue. The tip of the electrode conducts the current, which causes local ionic agitation and subsequent frictional heat leading to ablation. RF refers not to the emitted wave but rather to the alternating electric current that oscillates in the range of high frequency (200–1200 kHz). Schematically, a closed-loop circuit is created. The conventional "monopolar" technique uses a single electrode directly inserted into the tumor and large dispersive ground pads to close the electrical loop (Fig. 14.8). However, with monopolar RF ablation, the current density drops off as the inverse square of the distance from the electrode and heating drops off as the inverse of the fourth power of the distance. This limits the volume that can be ablated.

To increase RF-induced coagulation necrosis, several investigators have proposed bipolar RF ablation. In the bipolar mode, a second electrode is used instead of the dispersive plate, and there is a high and constant electric field gradient between the two electrodes. Bipolar RF ablation gives larger, faster and more predictable results than the monopolar mode (Buy et al. 2006).

For the bipolar technique, no ground pad is necessary; the electrical loop is enclosed between the two electrodes (Fig. 14.9) which bracket the tumor on either side. This closed electrical loop between the two electrodes produces much better delimitation of the ablation with protection of surrounding tissue (Fig. 14.10). However, if the ablation exceeds 10 min, even with the bipolar technique thermal diffusion can still injure adjacent tissue ("hot potato effect").

A variation of bipolar RF ablation uses a unique electrode with two different polarities on the same electrode. This bipolar method creates large well defined oval areas of coagulative necrosis and is less dependent on local tissue inhomogeneities.

To increase the size of the ablation, newer machines combine multipolar techniques with conventional monopolar and bipolar techniques.

14.4.2.2
Equipment

An RF device consists of an electrical generator, electrode, and ground pad. The generators used in our department are all impedance-based systems. Each manufacturer has a different electrode design. The most difficult part of bone ablation is penetrating the tumor. Needle-shape probes are easier to insert than expandable electrodes with several tines. However, in lytic tumors, any type of probe can be used (multi-tined, perfusion, internally cooled). If the tumor is surrounded by cortical bone, a dedicated bone trocar and sometimes a drill are required for coaxial insertion of the RF electrode.

14.4.2.3
Patient Selection and Technique

As yet there is no consensus on when RF ablation is indicated for oncological use, despite the widespread proliferation of the technology. Image-guided local tumor treatment relies on the assumption that local disease control may improve survival (Wood et al. 2002). RF ablation in bone can be curative or palliative (Gangi et al. 2005).

The major use of bone RF ablation is to palliate pain in bone metastases that have resisted conventional therapies (Fig. 14.11). For complete ablation, the tumor size should be less than 5 cm in diameter.

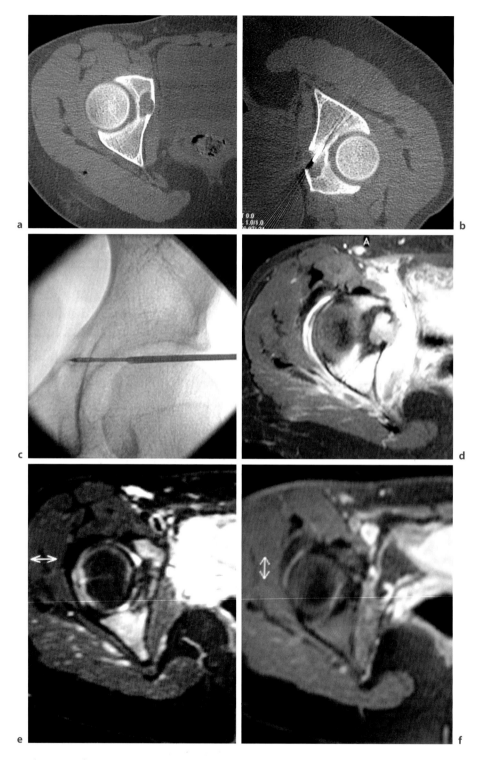

Fig. 14.8a–f. A 15-year-old girl with painful osteoblastoma of the right acetabulum. **a** Axial CT scan shows an 18-mm lytic lesion of the right acetabulum. **b** Axial CT scan shows puncture of the tumor via a posterior approach, avoiding the sciatic nerve. **c** Anteroposterior fluoroscopic view of the right hip shows the RF electrode is inserted coaxially through the bone trocar. The bone trocar is then withdrawn to avoid any conductivity along the track. The patient experienced leg pain and fever two days after the procedure. **d** Axial contrast-enhanced fat-suppressed T1-weighted MR image shows a large post ablative soft tissue inflammation. Axial (**e**) T2 STIR and (**f**) contrast-enhanced fat-suppressed T1-weighted MR images performed 1 week later show the complete necrosis of the bone tumor and the resolution of the edema with NSAIDs

Fig. 14.9. Bipolar RF mode. Diagram illustrates the two electrodes (*2* and *3*) are inserted together in parallel, bracketing the tumor (*1*). The closed electrical loop achieves larger, faster and more predictable lesions

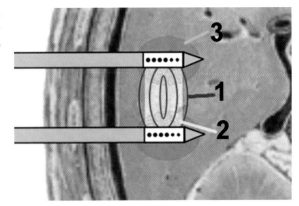

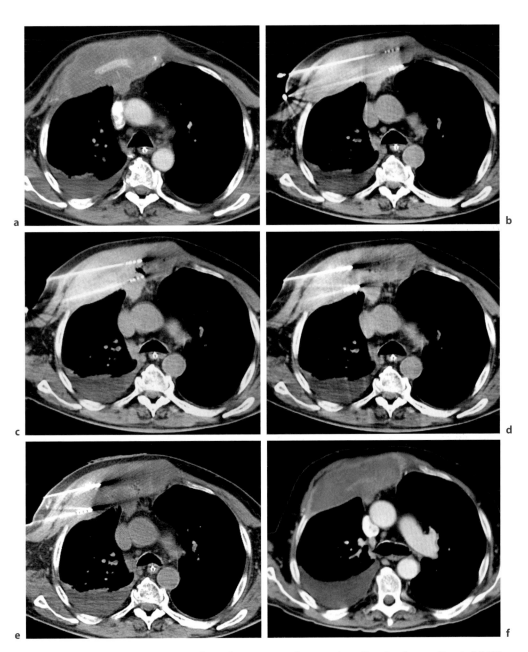

Fig. 14.10a–f. A 63-year-old man with excruciating pain due to large metastatic tumor invading the chest wall. **a** Axial CT scan shows the chest tumor wall before ablation. **b–e** Axial CT scans show bipolar RF ablation is performed in four different positions. **f** Axial contrast-enhanced CT scan performed one month after the procedure shows large necrotic area within the tumor. Excellent pain relief was achieved

Large bone metastases from thyroid cancer in association with 131 iodine therapy, for example, can also benefit from this technique. The curative indications of bone RF ablation are primary or secondary bone tumors when there are contraindications for surgery or the patient refuses surgery. Osteoid osteoma and osteoblastoma are ideally suited to curative percutaneous ablation (Fig. 14.8).

Ablation protocols vary with the size of the lesion. Assuming a 3-cm thermal injury, tumors less than 2 cm in diameter can be treated with one ablation, while tumors greater than 3 cm require 4–10 overlapping ablations with the monopolar technique. The length of the procedure depends on the number of ablations performed.

The best guidance system for bone tumor ablation is CT, although adding fluoroscopy is useful in some locations, e.g. the spine, or when cementoplasty is to follow the ablation (GANGI et al. 1994a). Bone RF ablation is a painful procedure which requires regional block or often general anesthesia. At the end of the ablation, 5–10 mL of rupivacaine 2 mg/mL are injected strictly extravascularly in contact with the periosteum. NSAIDs and analgesics together are systematically prescribed during the first 12 h to reduce post-procedural pain. The drugs are administered before the anesthesia wears off.

In osteoid osteomas, the RF ablation technique is similar to laser ablation. The small size of this nidus doesn't require large ablation with perfusion or internally cooled electrodes. A 1-cm active tip electrode is used to reach a temperature of 90 °C maintained for 6–10 min. The success rate is similar to laser ablation, over 85% (ROSENTHAL et al. 1995, 2003). Recurrence is 5%–10%.

A bone biopsy needle is necessary to pass through cortical bone. The electrode is then coaxially inserted into the lesion. Because the bone needle is not insulated, it should not touch the active part of the RF electrode. For this reason, after the insertion of the electrode, the bone needle is pulled back to avoid electrical conduction along the needle track. As usual, the ablation protocol begins with low power and increases progressively. To avoid rapid increases of impedance, the electrode tip should not be directly in contact with mineralized bone. The "oven effect" is particularly marked when the tumor is surrounded by cortical bone. If impedance increases too quickly, power should be reduced.

For tumors in close proximity to neurological structures or other organs, thermal protection techniques are required (Figs. 14.12 and 14.13). They are based on continuous thermal monitoring of adjacent vulnerable structures with one or more thermocouples (temperature sensors) and on organ displacement or insulation using hydrodissection, CO_2 injection or balloon interposition.

To ablate large tumors involving weight-bearing bones, additional consolidation with cementoplasty or surgery should be considered to prevent secondary fracture (Figs. 14.14 and 14.15) (TOYOTA et al. 2005). To avoid too fast setting of cement, the injection is delayed until the temperature of the tumor has fallen to normal level.

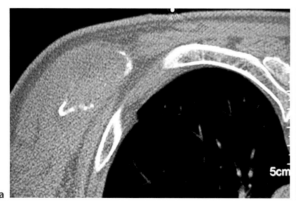
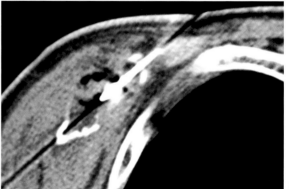

Fig. 14.11a,b. Painful right scapular metastasis in a 70-year-old man with lung cancer. **a** Axial CT scan shows the right osteolytic scapular lesion. **b** Axial CT scan shows monopolar RF ablation is performed with puncture in the long axis of the tumor. Excellent pain relief was achieved after 24 h

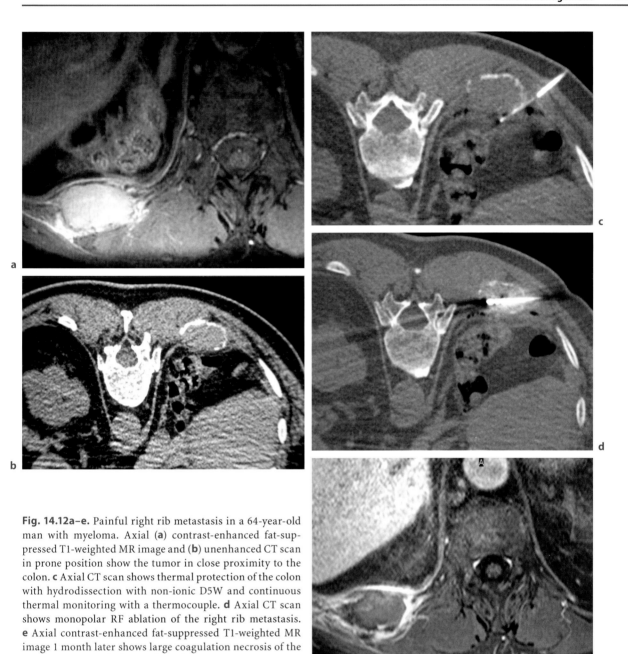

Fig. 14.12a–e. Painful right rib metastasis in a 64-year-old man with myeloma. Axial (**a**) contrast-enhanced fat-suppressed T1-weighted MR image and (**b**) unenhanced CT scan in prone position show the tumor in close proximity to the colon. **c** Axial CT scan shows thermal protection of the colon with hydrodissection with non-ionic D5W and continuous thermal monitoring with a thermocouple. **d** Axial CT scan shows monopolar RF ablation of the right rib metastasis. **e** Axial contrast-enhanced fat-suppressed T1-weighted MR image 1 month later shows large coagulation necrosis of the mass. Fast pain relief was achieved

14.4.2.4
Patient Outcome

For osteoid osteomas, the success rate of bone RF ablation is similar to laser (>85%). For painful malignant bone tumors, significant and rapid pain relief is achieved in 78% with substantial decrease of medication. We follow up with MR imaging 1 month after the procedure. The ablation zone appears hypo- or non-enhancing. Complete necrosis is associated with no enhancement inside the tumor best seen on dynamic

sequences with subtraction. During the first 6–24 h patients experience substantial amounts of local pain which is well controlled with narcotics and NSAIDs. With block anesthesia, post procedural pain is easier to control. In our series of 147 patients treated for a maximum of three bone metastases, satisfactory results with notable decrease of visual analog score (VAS) and reduction of analgesics were obtained in 87% of patients. Advanced disease makes recurrence of pain in relation to other metastases common, but the large majority of patients remain pain free at the ablated area.

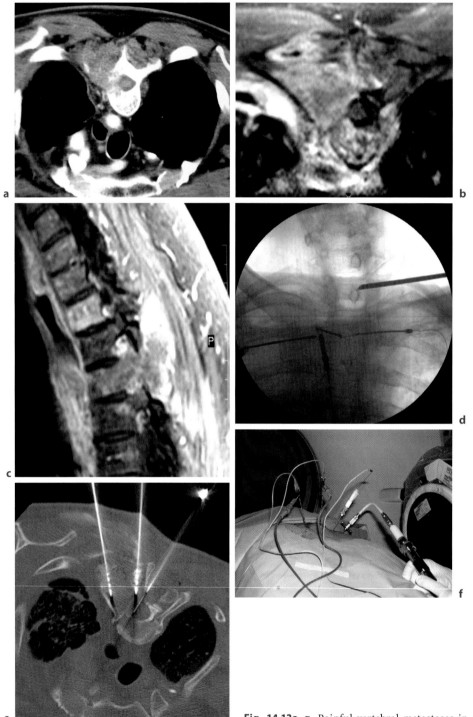

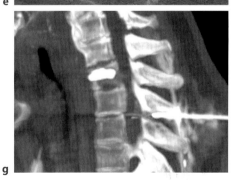

Fig. 14.13a–g. Painful vertebral metastases in a 66-year-old man with lung cancer. **a** Axial CT scan, (**b**) axial and (**c**) sagittal contrast-enhanced fat-suppressed T1-weighted MR images show T3 metastasis involving the right pedicle and the transverse process. There is also a metastasis limited to T1 vertebral body. **d** Anteroposterior fluoroscopic view, (**e**) axial CT scan, (**f**) operating room view, and (**g**) sagittal CT scan reformat show bipolar RF ablation of T3 metastasis with thermal monitoring of the epidural space. Monitoring was required because of the rupture in the cortical wall. The epidural temperature should not exceed 45 °C. No consolidation was necessary for this level, as the vertebral body was preserved. On the other hand, only a single vertebroplasty was needed to achieve consolidation of T1 and pain relief since the tumor was limited to the vertebral body. Excellent pain relief was achieved 24 h later

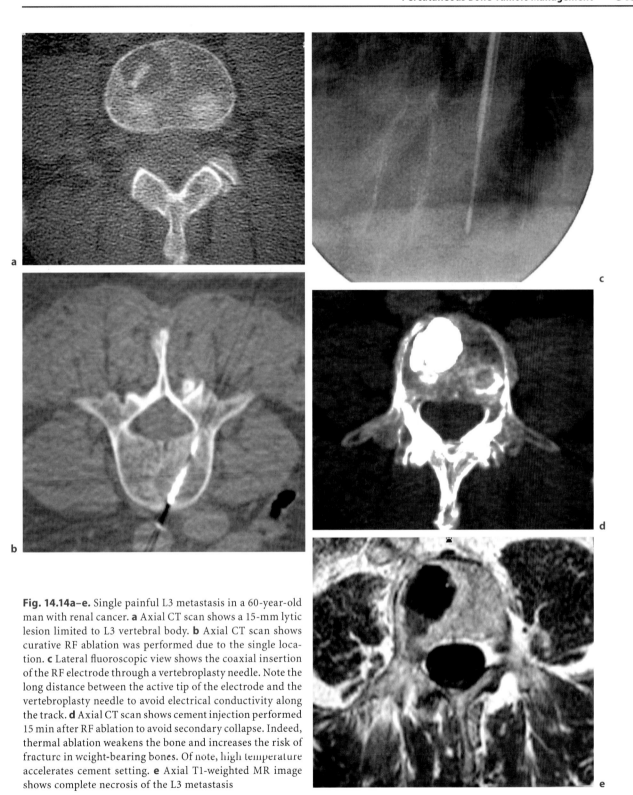

Fig. 14.14a–e. Single painful L3 metastasis in a 60-year-old man with renal cancer. **a** Axial CT scan shows a 15-mm lytic lesion limited to L3 vertebral body. **b** Axial CT scan shows curative RF ablation was performed due to the single location. **c** Lateral fluoroscopic view shows the coaxial insertion of the RF electrode through a vertebroplasty needle. Note the long distance between the active tip of the electrode and the vertebroplasty needle to avoid electrical conductivity along the track. **d** Axial CT scan shows cement injection performed 15 min after RF ablation to avoid secondary collapse. Indeed, thermal ablation weakens the bone and increases the risk of fracture in weight-bearing bones. Of note, high temperature accelerates cement setting. **e** Axial T1-weighted MR image shows complete necrosis of the L3 metastasis

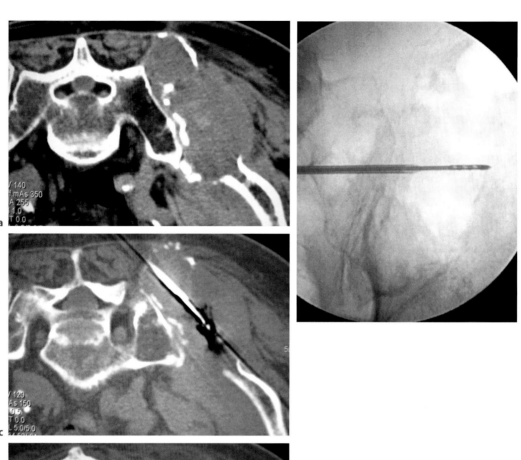

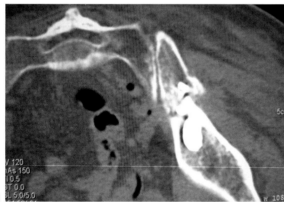

Fig. 14.15a–d. A 53-year-old man with excruciating pain and confined to bed due to a large left iliac metastasis with pathological acetabular fracture. **a** Axial CT scan shows the left iliac lytic lesion. **b** Anteroposterior fluoroscopic view and (**c**) axial CT scan show RF ablation is performed in the superior part of the metastasis involving the iliac bone. **d** Axial CT scan shows additional cementoplasty was performed to achieve consolidation of the acetabular fracture. The patient was able to walk the next day

14.4.3
Cryoablation

Cryoablation is the application of extreme cold to destroy diseased tissue, including cancer cells. Research has demonstrated that the critical temperature range to kill cells is between –20 °C and –40 °C. Temperatures higher than this result in supercooling of the tissues, but no intracellular ice formation (HOFFMANN and BISCHOF 2002). Cryoablation has been used to destroy skin lesions since the 1960s,

and with improved imaging techniques and the development of percutaneous cryoprobes, it is now applied to prostate, liver, bone, kidney and cervical cancer (ADAMS et al. 1968; BAHN et al. 1995; BLAND et al. 2007; CALLSTROM et al. 2006; CLARKE et al. 2007; COOPER AJ et al. 1978; DE LA TAILLE et al. 2000; GAGE and BAUST 2007; LEZOCHE et al. 1998; LONG and FALLER 1999; PATEL et al. 1996; PERMPONGKOSOL et al. 2006; SEWELL et al. 2001). First-generation devices were limited to intraoperative use. Indeed, the use of liquid nitrogen for tissue cooling, the lack of well-insulated probes and the large diameter of the cryoprobe require laparoscopic interventions. The percutaneous cryoprobes deliver argon gas through a segmentally insulated probe; the gas expands in the sealed probe tip and the temperature drops to –100 °C within a few seconds. The resulting ball of ice within the cell is thawed by replacing the argon gas with helium, which warms when it expands.

14.4.3.1
Mechanism

The latest generation cryoablation equipment offers advantages over previous designs. These machines rely on argon for freezing but also use helium to warm probes and accelerate the treatment process, and they offer additional safety by being able to rapidly stop the ice ball formation. This fundamental advance involves the application of the Joule-Thomson effect (Fig. 14.16). In some gases, such as argon, the atoms stick to each other (attraction; sticky marmalade); in others, such as helium, the atoms repel each other (repulsion; pushing rubber). Increasing the volume of a gas drains energy from the environment. For attractive gases like argon, this results in a temperature drop. Other gases such as helium, are repulsive, and the temperature rises when they expand. Cryoablation cleverly applies these Joule-Thomson behaviors to freeze or thaw

tissues easily in a clinical setting (BAUST and GAGE 2005; THEODORESCU 2004).

The destructive effects of cryoablation fall into two groups: cellular injury and vascular injury.

14.4.3.1.1
Direct Cell Injury

The damaging effects of low temperature on cells begin gradually as the temperature drops. If continued long enough, cell death results, even without exposure to freezing temperatures (THEODORESCU 2004). As the temperature falls to less than 0 °C, water crystallizes. This results in more significant damage than mere prolonged cooling.

Crystal formation occurs first in the extracellular spaces, which withdraws water and creates a hyperosmotic extracellular environment. This in turn draws water from the cells. Effective "cellular dehydration" occurs predominantly between 0 °C and –20 °C. Given enough time in this dehydrated state, the increased intracellular electrolyte concentration is often sufficient to destroy the cells. However, this effect might not be lethal to all cells. In these situations, the formation of intracellular ice, which begins at temperatures below –20 °C, is almost always lethal (BAUST and CHANG 1995; MAZUR 1977). Many cells might contain ice crystals by –15 °C, but to be certain of intracellular ice formation the tem-

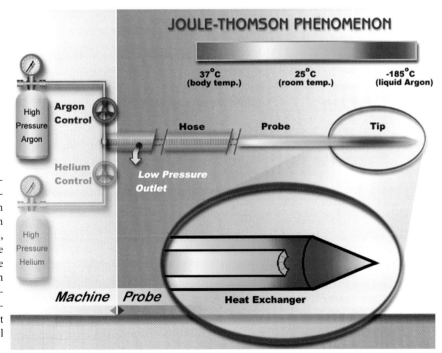

Fig. 14.16. Principle of cryoablation based on Thompson-Joules phenomenon. Diagram illustrates fast decompression of argon gas is endothermic, allowing drop of temperature below –186 °C at the tip of the cryoprobe. In contrast helium gas decompression is exothermic with increase of temperature up to 33 °C, allowing fast thawing. (Courtesy of Galil Medical, Yokneam, Israel)

perature must drop to less than –40 °C (BAUST and CHANG 1995). From the clinical perspective, it is important to note that intracellular ice crystal formation is more efficient at rapid cooling rates; slower rates of cooling will result in cellular dehydration as described above. During thawing, ice crystals fuse to form larger crystals, a process called recrystallization, which occurs at temperatures warmer than –40 °C. In tissues with closely packed cells, these large crystals are disruptive to cell membranes and cause additional cell damage (THEODORESCU 2004). It is important to remember that the temperature of the edge of the ice ball is 0 °C, which is not sufficient for systematic cell death. Therefore ice ball should extend 5 mm beyond the tumor borders.

14.4.3.1.2
Vascular Injury

Loss of circulation resulting in cellular anoxia and hypoxia is considered the main mechanism of injury in cryosurgery. During the initial freeze cycle, the tissue responds with vasoconstriction, with a resultant decrease in blood flow that eventually ceases when freezing is complete. During thawing, the circulation returns with a compensatory vasodilatation. However, the endothelial damage from cryoablation results in increased permeability of the capillary walls, edema, platelet aggregation, and microthrombus formation. Progressive circulatory stagnation results over the ensuing hours. Many small blood vessels become completely thrombosed 3–4 h after thawing. Larger arterioles might remain open for up to 24 h. Together, these effects culminate in tissue necrosis, except at the periphery of the previously frozen volume of tissue (COOPER IS 1964; THEODORESCU 2004).

14.4.3.2
Equipment

Currently available equipment relies on the Joule-Thomson effects of argon and helium gases to freeze and heat the probes and accelerate the treatment process. They also offer additional safety by being able to stop ice ball formation rapidly. Metallurgic advances have led to the development of thinner probes (17-gauge), which have been easily adapted to percutaneous interventions (THEODORESCU 2004).

One of the major advantages of these new systems is the possibility of inserting multiple probes (up to 25) to use simultaneously (Fig. 14.17). There is evidence to suggest that when a given volume of tumor is subjected to lethal temperatures by three smaller probes, rather than one larger probe, the affected volume is greater. Different cryoprobes are available to make various sizes and shapes of ice ball (Fig. 14.18).

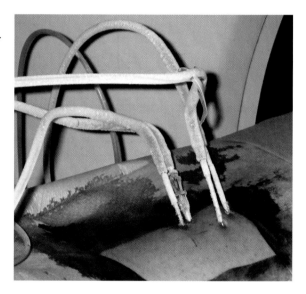

Fig. 14.17. Cryoablation of large metastasis in a 50-year-old woman. View from the CT room shows the procedure required the insertion of four cryoprobes. Note that up to 25 cryoprobes can be used simultaneously

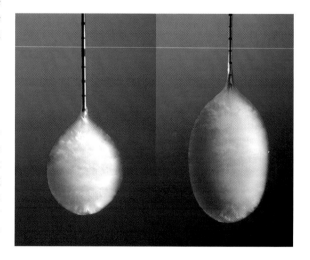

Fig. 14.18. The shape and the size of the ice ball can vary with the cryoprobe type. (Courtesy of Galil Medical, Yokneam, Israel)

14.4.3.3
Patient Selection and Technique

Indications and the procedure are very similar to RF ablation. Planning is the same. However, up to 25 cryoprobes can be used simultaneously. The learning phase for the operator is shorter but the danger of damage to surrounding tissue still exists. Insulation with fluid should be avoided. CO_2 is best for tissue insulation and protection of surrounding organs (Fig. 14.19).

The procedure is performed under sedation or general anesthesia. Percutaneous cryoablation appears to require less analgesia than RF ablation. Prospective trials with validated pain scales are needed to examine this further (ALLAF et al. 2005). Cryoablation of skeletal metastases is a time-consuming procedure. Two 10-min freeze cycles, each separated by 8 min of passive thawing, are performed per position. Spiral CT with multiplanar reconstruction is used intermittently to monitor the ice ball (Fig. 14.20).

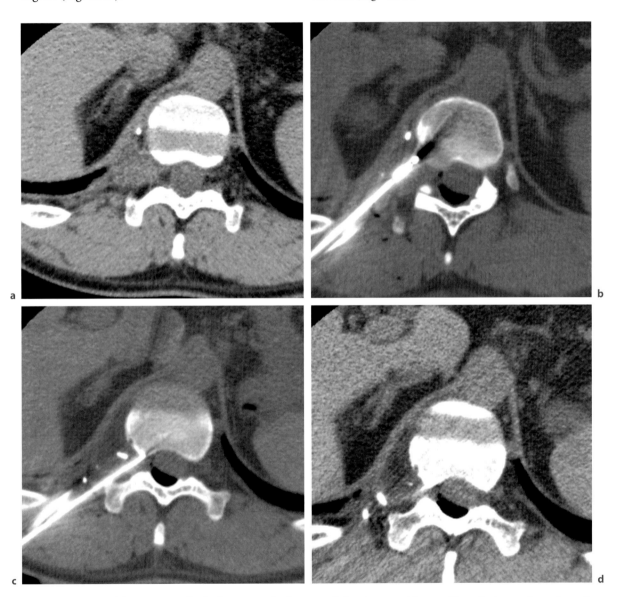

Fig. 14.19a–d. Painful recurrence of a single paravertebral metastasis in a 24-year-old man with testicular carcinoembryonic tumor and previous retroperitoneal lymphadenectomy. **a** Axial CT scan shows the right paravertebral tumor with foraminal extension. **b** Axial CT scan demonstrates the ice seed cryoprobe inserted in the tumor. Note epidural injection of CO_2 for thermal insulation of the neurological structures. **c** Axial CT scan shows the position of the thermocouple in the foramen for continuous thermal monitoring of the nerve root. **d** Axial CT scan shows hypodense ice ball fully covering the tumor

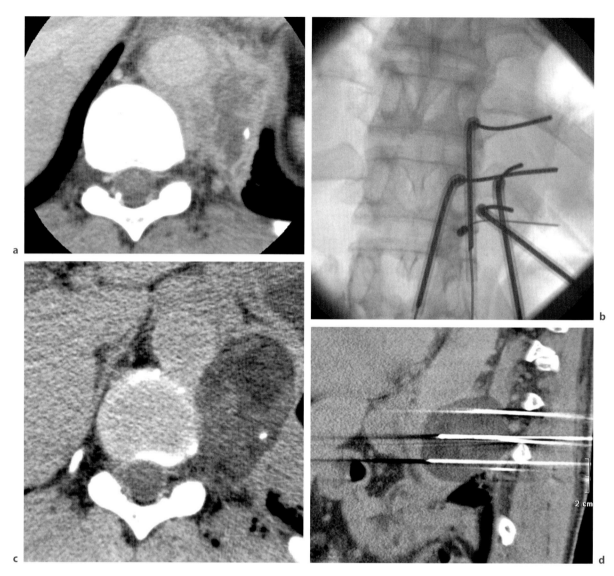

Fig. 14.20a–d. A 45-year-old man with painful paravertebral recurrence of carcinoembryonic tumor. **a** Axial CT scan shows large tumor in the left paravertebral space at T11–12 level with periaortic extension. Embolization was not possible due to Adamkiewicz artery supplying the tumor at T10 level. **b** Anteroposterior fluoroscopic view demonstrates four ice rod cryoprobes inserted into the tumor. **c** Axial and (**d**) sagittal reformat CT scans show the precise margins of the ice ball which should not extend to T10 level. In case of palliative treatment, complete ablation of the tumor is not needed

An "ice ball" forms at the tip of the probe which has a predictable geometry based on the length and diameter of the expansion room at the tip of the probe. To ensure complete cell death and ablation of the tumor, it is important to extend the margins of the ice ball a minimum 5 mm beyond the tumor margins. The ice ball can be visualized by ultrasound, CT and MR imaging. Ultrasound, though very practical for certain applications, visualizes the superficial side of the ice ball only. Most centers do not have the ability to employ MR imaging during treatment, which

leaves CT as the most practical and widely employed modality for this purpose (Fig. 14.21).

Compared to other forms of percutaneous ablation, cryotherapy offers the additional advantages of direct visualization of the ice ball and less postprocedural pain (BELAND et al. 2005; CALLSTROM et al. 2006). Cryoablation is also efficient in painful sclerotic bone metastases since the ice ball extends through sclerotic bone.

Successful cryoablation tissue destruction depends on four criteria: excellent monitoring of the

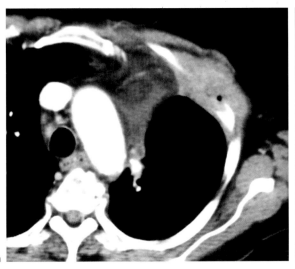

a

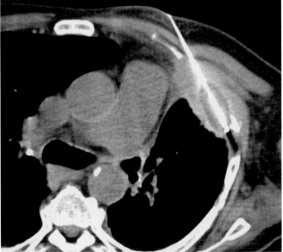

b

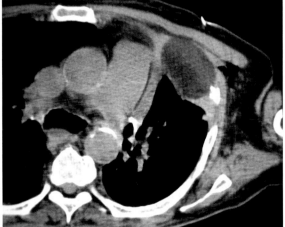

c

Fig. 14.21a–c. A 57-year-old man with metastatic lung cancer. **a** Axial CT scan shows the metastasis of the left chest wall, refractory to radiation therapy. **b** Axial CT scan demonstrates two ice rod cryoprobes inserted in the long axis of the tumor under conscious sedation. Note the hypodense ice ball surrounding the cryoprobe after 3 min of freezing. **c** Axial CT scan after second phase of freezing shows the ice ball's margins are clearly seen. Complete pain relief was achieved 24 h after ablation

process; fast cooling to a lethal temperature; slow thawing; and repetition of the freeze-thaw cycle (two cycles minimum). Meeting these criteria depends on imaging to visualize precisely the ice ball, the size of the probe, and the arrangement of the probes, with 2 cm being the best gap between probes (BAUST and GAGE 2004; CLARKE et al. 2007; GAGE and BAUST 1998; HOFFMANN and BISCHOF 2002; LITTRUP et al. 2007; THEODORESCU 2004). Repetition of the treatment cycle is associated with more extensive and more certain tissue destruction, because cells are subjected to additional deleterious physicochemical changes after they are already weakened by damage sustained in the first cycle (GAGE and BAUST 1998).

The longer it takes for the ice ball to thaw, the greater the damage to the cells; current data suggest that slow thawing is a more important mechanism of cell death than rapid cooling (GAGE and BAUST 1998; THEODORESCU 2004).

14.4.3.4
Patient Outcome

Percutaneous cryoablation seems to be safe and effective for palliation of pain due to metastatic disease and to treat small primary tumors involving bone (CALLSTROM et al. 2006).

Careful monitoring of the cryoablation is mandatory to avoid freezing any nearby neurovascular structures or the skin. Large vessels may act as a cold sink protecting both themselves and adjacent structures. If nerves are inadvertently incorporated into the periphery of the ice ball, with a temperature less than –20 °C, a temporary neuropraxia may develop, which should resolve with time. If nerves are somehow in the center of the ice ball, where temperatures of –40 °C or lower predominate, permanent neurological damage may result (KORPAN 2001).

To prevent pathological fractures, consolidation is necessary particularly in long bones (BICKELS et al. 2004). In spinal or acetabular tumors, percutaneous cementoplasty should be combined with cryoablation to avoid compression fractures. The cement is injected after complete thawing of the ice ball or the day after the cryotherapy.

A syndrome of multiorgan failure, severe coagulopathy, and disseminated intravascular coagulation following hepatic cryoablation has been described and referred to as the "cryoshock phenomenon" (BAGEACU et al. 2007; SEIFERT et al. 2002; SEIFERT and MORRIS 1999).

14.5
Radiofrequency Ionization

Radiofrequency ionization is a low temperature bipolar technique producing a plasma field at the tip of the electrode. The plasma breaks the intramolecular bonds causing cavitation inside the tissue and subsequent decompression. RF ionization is widely used in ENT surgery, cardiac surgery, arthroplasty and spine nucleotomy, and has recently been introduced for bone tumor decompression; the first bone treatment at our institution was in 2004.

14.5.1
Mechanism

RF ionization is based on Coblation® (controlled or cold ablation) technology. This non-thermal technique uses a bipolar RF electrode to excite a conductive medium (saline solution), creating a focused high energy plasma (BELOV 2004). This plasma, acting like a condenser, has sufficient energy to break the intramolecular bonds inside the tumor. Complex molecules disintegrate into simple molecules, mainly gas that escapes through the introducer needle. This process is achieved at relatively low temperatures (40–70 °C), compared to conventional thermal ablation RF devices. The ionization process consumes most of the heat and no radiofrequency current passes directly through the target tissue. The result is volumetric removal of the tumor with minimal damage to surrounding tissue.

14.5.2
Equipment

RF ionization inside bone requires a dedicated RF generator and a 16-gauge bipolar electrode (Cavity SpineWand®) (Arthrocare®, Sunnyvale, CA, USA). A bone trocar allows tumoral access and coaxial insertion of the RF electrode. A side arm catheter is connected to the electrode to slowly inject saline solution for activation of the plasma field. The bent tip of the electrode allows digging several channels inside the tumor by rotating the electrode on its axis. These maneuvers are monitored under fluoroscopic guidance. If there is any risk at all of neurological damage, CT-fluoroscopic monitoring is mandatory.

14.5.3
Patient Selection and Technique

The best candidates for this technique are non-surgical painful spinal tumors with intracanalar extension, or rupture of the vertebral posterior wall with risk of retropulsion of the tumor after vertebroplasty (Fig. 14.22). In these cases, reducing volume reduces pressure. After cavitation in spinal lesions, acrylic cement is injected into the cavity for consolidation.

Rupture of the posterior wall of the vertebral body with high risk of a cement leak or a shift of the tumor in the canal with neurological consequences are indications for coblation. In spinal tumors cavitation before vertebroplasty is advocated by some authors to reduce the risk of leakage. Unlike intravertebral expandable systems that increase the intratumoral pressure, cavitation creates a void without increasing the pressure and moving the tumor.

14.5.4
Patient Outcome

The epidural temperature does not increase during cavitation. The tip of the electrode is at 70 °C. The cavitation can be visualized on CT scan with intratumoral gas but it is not usually necessary. Cementoplasty is easier and safer after cavitation. The cement fills the cavity evenly reducing the risk of leakage and retropulsion of the tumor (GEORGY and WONG 2007). No major complications were reported; in two cases we observed reduced neuralgia due to tumor decompression.

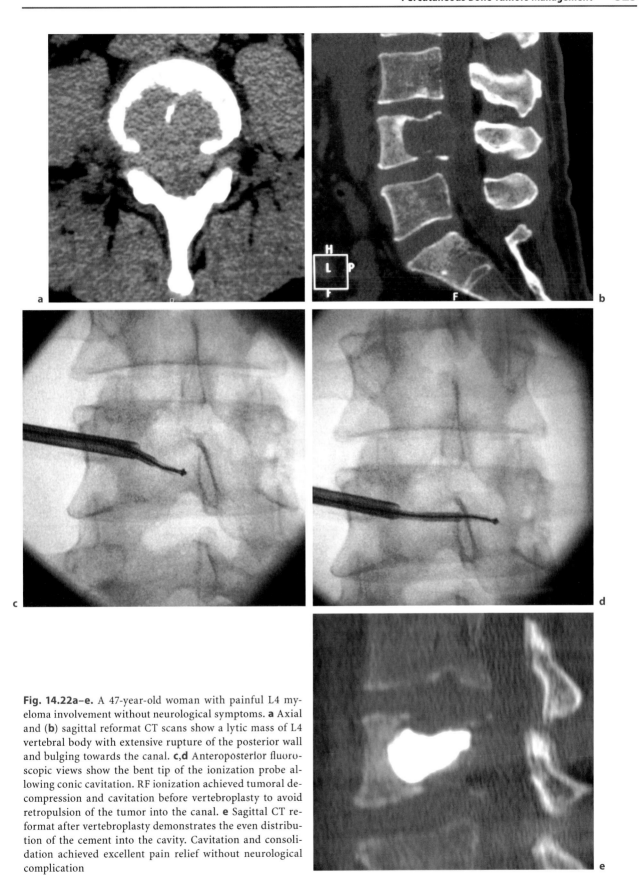

Fig. 14.22a–e. A 47-year-old woman with painful L4 myeloma involvement without neurological symptoms. **a** Axial and (**b**) sagittal reformat CT scans show a lytic mass of L4 vertebral body with extensive rupture of the posterior wall and bulging towards the canal. **c,d** Anteroposterior fluoroscopic views show the bent tip of the ionization probe allowing conic cavitation. RF ionization achieved tumoral decompression and cavitation before vertebroplasty to avoid retropulsion of the tumor into the canal. **e** Sagittal CT reformat after vertebroplasty demonstrates the even distribution of the cement into the cavity. Cavitation and consolidation achieved excellent pain relief without neurological complication

14.6
Thermal Protection and Insulation

Percutaneous image-guided thermal ablation is considered minimally invasive, but there is a potential risk of thermal injury to adjacent vulnerable structures, such as the bowel, gall bladder, urinary tract and nerves. Several methods have been reported to circumvent this problem, mainly by interposing fluid, gas or balloons between the ablation zone and adjacent structures (DIEHN et al. 2003; GANGI et al. 2007; KAM et al. 2004; LAESEKE et al. 2006). A thermocouple adjacent to the non-target vulnerable structures provides continuous monitoring of the surrounding temperature and allows precise regulation of the cooling or heating regimens (Fig. 14.13). RF heating at 45 °C is neurotoxic to the spinal cord and the peripheral nerves; thus maximum precautions should be taken when there is no intact insulating cortex between the tumor and the neurological structures (DUPUY et al. 2000). Bone does insulate, but the degree of protection depends on the thickness of the bone lamella. BITSCH et al. (2006) investigated heat conduction and dissipation in cortical bone during RF ablation and found temperatures of 50–70 °C directly at the periosteum for several minutes, which would imply significant damage to nearby nerve tissue and adjacent structures. Temperatures were at or above 45 °C within a 10 mm circumference of the periosteum in all specimens without perfusion. Only the 5 mm lamella thickness group was below this mark 5 mm from the periosteum.

DUPUY et al. (2000) underline the difference between thermal diffusion in bone and soft tissue. In their experiment, the generated temperatures were consistently lower within the vertebral body than in the paraspinal muscle for similar treatments. For example, at 10 min the maximum temperatures observed in bone were 48, 41, and 39 °C at a distance from the RF electrode of 5, 10 and 15 mm, respectively, compared with a maximum of 84, 62, and 58 °C, in paraspinal muscles.

Non-target structures need protection. There are several methods for providing insulation that can be used alone or in combination.

Hydrodissection is commonly used (Fig. 14.12). Saline is not a suitable solution for hydrodissection when RF is involved, because of its high electrical conductivity. Dextrose (5%) in distilled water or sterile water has been advocated. However, large amounts of fluid may be necessary to provide an adequate thermal insulator blanket and this can induce fluid overload. In diabetic patients, use of D5W can result in significantly increased serum glucose levels which require monitoring both during and after the ablation procedure. We do not use fluid in cryoablation, as the fluid can easily freeze in contact with the ice ball and increase the risk of damage to adjacent organs.

CO_2 is a natural by-product of human metabolism. It has been used in medicine for decades. Its lack of renal and hepatic toxicity, non-allergic nature, high solubility and ability to be injected in a cohesive bolus make it a useful alternative contrast medium in angiography for patients with renal insufficiency and allergy to iodinated contrast. It is not advocated in supra-diaphragmatic or coronary angiography for fear of cerebral embolism when injected in large boluses.

CO_2 is highly soluble in blood and fairly innocuous to the peritoneum. It is eliminated by respiration. However, when large amounts of CO_2 are injected to induce pneumoperitoneum during laparoscopic procedures, abdominal cramping and post-procedural discomfort have been reported.

CO_2 has lower thermal conductivity (14.65 mW/mK at 0 °C) than water or air (23.94 mW/mK). It displaces the non-target structures away from the treatment zone, creating an excellent thermal insulator blanket. In our experience, using the dedicated CO_2 injection syringe allows precise control of the volume of gas insufflated under positive pressure (1.326 atm or 1.3 bar). Less CO_2 is injected compared to KAM et al. (2004) which eliminates, or at least reduces, post-procedural discomfort. The presence of a special filter on the injector syringe prevents contamination with room air. Room air is less soluble than CO_2 and may create a fatal air embolism, especially when used in large amounts in the peritoneal cavity. Moreover, air has a slightly higher thermal conductivity than CO_2.

Thermal insulation by CO_2 dissection cannot be used in ultrasound-guided interventions as the ring down artifact from gas completely degrades the image. Further, sound waves are unable to penetrate adequately the ice ball created by cryoablation and hence complete lesion coverage is not possible by ultrasound. CT on the other hand exquisitely delineates gas from the surrounding soft tissue structures and allows excellent visualization of the ice ball. CT allows monitoring of the progress of the ice ball and completeness of lesion coverage in cryoablation; it also monitors the CO_2 thermal insulator blanket, which may require repeated injections.

CO_2 insulation with thermal monitoring increases the safety of the procedure. The thermocouples can be inserted coaxially through an 18-gauge spinal needle (Fig. 14.23). A side arm fitting is used to fix the thermocouple inside the spinal needle; the side arm allows injection of D5W or CO_2 for cooling or insulation of vulnerable structures (Figs. 14.7, 14.12, 14.13, and 14.19). The number of thermocouples depends on whether the structure is less than 3 cm from the tumor with no intervening bone. Using thermocouples with RF ablation requires some caution. The tip of the metal-based thermocouple should never be too close to the RF electrode, as this can lead to arcing and electrical conductivity. Laser thermosensors are more suitable.

In our experience, carbon dioxide dissection with dedicated CO_2 injector is a safe and simple method to provide thermal insulation. CO_2 can be easily and precisely injected via 22-gauge spinal needles to displace non-target organs away from the treatment zone, It provides adequate neural protection and creates a well defined thermal insulator blanket. Combining CO_2 dissection with continuous temperature monitoring of adjacent vulnerable structures provides greater safety during thermal ablation procedures. Under CT guidance, the displaced organs can be clearly visualized and the margins of the ablated zone better monitored particularly when

controlling the ice ball created by cryoablation. CO_2 dissection increases the success rate and the safety of percutaneous CT-guided thermal ablation procedures and reduces complications.

Gas insulation efficiently protects surrounding organs unless the temperature of the organ will exceed 43 °C, in which case gas is insufficient and liquid is necessary (FROESE et al. 1991). In fact, gas is optimal for insulation, but fluid provides much better cooling.

14.7
Treatment Strategy

Management of patients with bone tumors requires consideration of many factors:
- Histology of the tumor, with differentiation of benign and malignant tumors
- Careful evaluation of the patient's general condition
- An understanding of the disease process
- An appreciation of the degree of bone destruction (consolidation)
- A working knowledge of available treatment options
- Always – the goal of the treatment: curative or palliative?

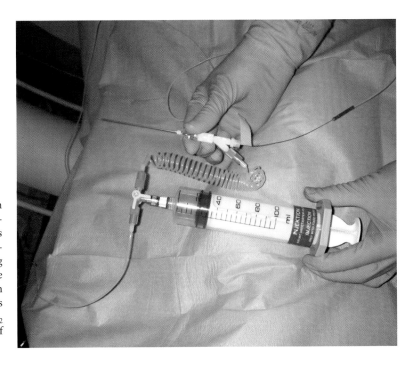

Fig. 14.23. Thermal protection with CO_2 and thermocouple. The CO_2 injection set includes a dedicated gas filter and a graduated syringe (Optimed, Ettlingen, Germany) allowing injection of 10–100 mL of CO_2. Note the side arm fitting connected to an 18-gauge spinal needle which allows simultaneous connection of the CO_2 injection set and coaxial insertion of the thermocouple

14.7.1
Curative Treatment

Benign lesions such as osteoid osteomas or osteoblastomas do not usually exceed 3 cm and a single ablation technique is sufficient.

For malignant non-surgical patients, a multidisciplinary decision is mandatory. In slow growing cancers with less than three proven localizations and less than 5 cm size, curative percutaneous ablation can be considered. Thermal ablation further weakens the involved medullary bone. If weight bearing bone is involved and there is a risk of pathological fracture, consolidation with cementoplasty or surgery is necessary. However, cementoplasty is limited to flat bones subject to compression forces.

14.7.2
Palliative Treatment

For palliative treatment of painful bone tumors (metastases), the therapeutic goal is not complete ablation of the tumor but one or more of the following:

- Tumor reduction
- Pain management
- Prevention of pathological fractures
- In some cases, decompression of spinal tumors extending towards the spinal canal or prevention of intracanalar tumoral retropulsion after vertebroplasty

A precise clinical evaluation of the patient is mandatory: origin, location and intensity of pain, previous treatment, tolerance of anesthesia, and life expectancy. Whole body imaging is necessary to precisely analyze the lesions and their relationship to surrounding structures. A multidisciplinary decision is required to choose the most efficient and least disabling technique:

1. For painful tumors involving flat weight bearing bone without invasion of surrounding tissues, associated with risk of compression fracture, cementoplasty is best.
2. For painful bone tumors with extension to surrounding soft tissues, thermal ablation is required to reduce the tumoral volume and control the pain from soft tissue and periosteum invasion. In this cases, thermal ablation should particularly target the periphery of the tumor. However, if there is a risk of pathological fracture, an additional con-

solidation technique is required (cementoplasty for flat bones or surgery for long bones).
3. For non-surgical spinal tumors extending towards the canal with rupture of the posterior wall and epidural extension, percutaneous tumor decompression with RF ionization is the best technique. After tumor decompression, the resulting cavity is filled with cement.

14.8
Conclusion

Management of bone tumors has been made easier by the development of numerous percutaneous techniques; consolidation (cementoplasty), tumor ablation (ethanol, laser ablation, RF ablation, cryoablation) and tumor decompression (RF ionization). Moreover, these percutaneous techniques may be performed prior to radiation therapy, which complements their action due to similar but delayed effects on pain. They may also be used if radiation therapy has failed to relieve pain or in local recurrences. The main advantage of thermal ablation techniques is the ability to create a well-controlled focal thermal injury with minimal morbidity and mortality.

The choice of treatment requires multidisciplinary team work. Excellent knowledge of the different techniques and their indications is essential. Careful patient selection helps to determine the therapeutic intent: curative or palliative, and which technique is most suitable. More complex cases often require combined therapies. However, the less disabling technique should always be considered first.

References

Adams DA, Rand RW, Roth NH, Dashe AM, Heuser G, Hanley J, Parker M (1968) Cryoablation of the pituitary in the treatment of progressive diabetic retinopathy. Diabetes 17:634–640

Allaf ME, Varkarakis IM, Bhayani SB, Inagaki T, Kavoussi LR, Solomon SB (2005) Pain control requirements for percutaneous ablation of renal tumors: cryoablation versus radiofrequency ablation – initial observations. Radiology 237:366–370

Bageacu S, Kaczmarek D, Lacroix M, Dubois J, Forest J, Porcheron J (2007) Cryosurgery for resectable and unresectable hepatic metastases from colorectal cancer. Eur J Surg Oncol 33:590–596

Bahn DK, Lee F, Solomon MH, Gontina H, Klionsky DL, Lee FT Jr (1995) Prostate cancer: US-guided percutaneous cryoablation. Work in progress. Radiology 194:551–556

Baust J, Chang Z (1995) Underlying mechanisms of damage and new concepts in cryosurgical instrumentation. International Institute of Refrigeration, Paris, France

Baust JG, Gage AA (2004) Progress toward optimization of cryosurgery. Technol Cancer Res Treat 3:95–101

Baust JG, Gage AA (2005) The molecular basis of cryosurgery. BJU Int 95:1187–1191

Beland MD, Dupuy DE, Mayo-Smith WW (2005) Percutaneous cryoablation of symptomatic extraabdominal metastatic disease: preliminary results. AJR Am J Roentgenol 184:926–930

Belov SV (2004) The technology of high-frequency cold-hot plasma ablation for small invasive electrosurgery. Med Tekh 25–30

Bickels J, Kollender Y, Merimsky O, Isaakov J, Petyan-Brand R, Meller I (2004) Closed argon-based cryoablation of bone tumours. J Bone Joint Surg Br 86:714–718

Bitsch RG, Rupp R, Bernd L, Ludwig K (2006) Osteoid osteoma in an ex vivo animal model: temperature changes in surrounding soft tissue during CT-guided radiofrequency ablation. Radiology 238:107–112

Bland KL, Gass J, Klimberg VS (2007) Radiofrequency, cryoablation, and other modalities for breast cancer ablation. Surg Clin North Am 87:539–550

Buy X, Basile A, Bierry G, Cupelli J, Gangi A (2006) Saline-infused bipolar radiofrequency ablation of high-risk spinal and paraspinal neoplasms. AJR Am J Roentgenol 186:S322–326

Callstrom MR, Atwell TD, Charboneau JW, Farrell MA, Goetz MP, Rubin J, Sloan JA, Novotny PJ, Welch TJ, Maus TP, Wong GY, Brown KJ (2006) Painful metastases involving bone: percutaneous image-guided cryoablation – prospective trial interim analysis. Radiology 241:572–580

Clarke DM, Robilotto AT, Rhee E, VanBuskirk RG, Baust JG, Gage AA, Baust JM (2007) Cryoablation of renal cancer: variables involved in freezing-induced cell death. Technol Cancer Res Treat 6:69–79

Cooper AJ, Fraser JD, MacIver A (1978) Host responses to cryoablation of normal kidney and liver tissue. Br J Exp Pathol 59:97–104

Cooper IS (1964) Cryobiology as viewed by the surgeon. Cryobiology 51:44–51

De La Taille A, Benson MC, Bagiella E, Burchardt M, Shabsigh A, Olsson CA, Katz AE (2000) Cryoablation for clinically localized prostate cancer using an argon-based system: complication rates and biochemical recurrence. BJU Int 85:281–286

Diehn FE, Neeman Z, Hvizda JL, Wood BJ (2003) Remote thermometry to avoid complications in radiofrequency ablation. J Vasc Interv Radiol 14:1569–1576

Dupuy DE, Hong R, Oliver B, Goldberg SN (2000) Radiofrequency ablation of spinal tumors: temperature distribution in the spinal canal. AJR Am J Roentgenol 175:1263–1266

Froese G, Das RM, Dunscombe PB (1991) The sensitivity of the thoracolumbar spinal cord of the mouse to hyperthermia. Radiat Res 125:173–180

Gage AA, Baust J (1998) Mechanisms of tissue injury in cryosurgery. Cryobiology 37:171–186

Gage AA, Baust JG (2007) Cryosurgery for tumors. J Am Coll Surg 205:342–356

Gangi A, Kastler BA, Dietemann JL (1994a) Percutaneous vertebroplasty guided by a combination of CT and fluoroscopy. AJNR Am J Neuroradiol 15:83–86

Gangi A, Kastler B, Klinkert A, Dietemann JL (1994b) Injection of alcohol into bone metastases under CT guidance. J Comput Assist Tomogr 18:932–935

Gangi A, Dietemann JL, Schultz A, Mortazavi R, Jeung MY, Roy C (1996) Interventional radiologic procedures with CT guidance in cancer pain management. Radiographics 16:1289–1304; discussion 1304–1306

Gangi A, Gasser B, De Unamuno S, Fogarrassy E, Fuchs C, Siffert P, Dietemann JL, Roy C (1997a) New trends in interstitial laser photocoagulation of bones. Semin Musculoskelet Radiol 1:331–338

Gangi A, Dietemann JL, Gasser B, Mortazavi R, Brunner P, Mourou MY, Dosch JC, Durckel J, Marescaux J, Roy C (1997b) Interstitial laser photocoagulation of osteoid osteomas with use of CT guidance. Radiology 203:843–848

Gangi A, Guth S, Imbert JP, Marin H, Dietemann JL (2003) Percutaneous vertebroplasty: indications, technique, and results. Radiographics 23:e10

Gangi A, Basile A, Buy X, Alizadeh H, Sauer B, Bierry G (2005) Radiofrequency and laser ablation of spinal lesions. Semin Ultrasound CT MR 26:89–97

Gangi A, Alizadeh H, Wong L, Buy X, Dietemann JL, Roy C (2007) Osteoid osteoma: percutaneous laser ablation and follow-up in 114 patients. Radiology 242:293–301

Georgy BA, Wong W (2007) Plasma-mediated radiofrequency ablation assisted percutaneous cement injection for treating advanced malignant vertebral compression fractures. AJNR Am J Neuroradiol 28:700–705

Hoffmann NE, Bischof JC (2002) The cryobiology of cryosurgical injury. Urology 60:40–49

Kam AW, Littrup PJ, Walther MM, Hvizda J, Wood BJ (2004) Thermal protection during percutaneous thermal ablation of renal cell carcinoma. J Vasc Interv Radiol 15:753–758

Korpan N (2001) Basics of cryosurgery. Springer, Berlin Heidelberg New York

Laeseke PF, Sampson LA, Brace CL, Winter TC III, Fine JP, Lee FT Jr (2006) Unintended thermal injuries from radiofrequency ablation: protection with 5% dextrose in water. AJR Am J Roentgenol 186:S249–254

Lezoche E, Paganini AM, Feliciotti F, Guerrieri M, Lugnani F, Tamburini A (1998) Ultrasound-guided laparoscopic cryoablation of hepatic tumors: preliminary report. World J Surg 22:829–835; discussion 835–836

Littrup PJ, Ahmed A, Aoun HD, Noujaim DL, Harb T, Nakat S, Abdallah K, Adam BA, Venkatramanamoorthy R, Sakr W, Pontes JE, Heilbrun LK (2007) CT-guided percutaneous cryotherapy of renal masses. J Vasc Interv Radiol 18:383–392

Long JP, Faller GT (1999) Percutaneous cryoablation of the kidney in a porcine model. Cryobiology 38:89–93

Mazur P (1977) The role of intracellular freezing in the death of cells cooled at supraoptimal rates. Cryobiology 14:251–272

Okuda S, Kuroda K, Kainuma O, Oshio K, Fujiwara H, Kuribayashi S (2004) Accuracy of MR temperature measurement based on chemical shift change for radiofrequency ablation using hook-shaped electrodes. Magn Reson Med Sci 3:95–100

Patel BG, Parsons CL, Bidair M, Schmidt JD (1996) Cryoablation for carcinoma of the prostate. J Surg Oncol 63:256–264

Permpongkosol S, Nielsen ME, Solomon SB (2006) Percutaneous renal cryoablation. Urology 68:19–25

Rosenthal DI, Springfield DS, Gebhardt MC, Rosenberg AE, Mankin HJ (1995) Osteoid osteoma: percutaneous radiofrequency ablation. Radiology 197:451–454

Rosenthal DI, Hornicek FJ, Torriani M, Gebhardt MC, Mankin HJ (2003) Osteoid osteoma: percutaneous treatment with radiofrequency energy. Radiology 229:171–175

Seifert JK, Morris DL (1999) World survey on the complications of hepatic and prostate cryotherapy. World J Surg 23:109–113; discussion 113–114

Seifert JK, France MP, Zhao J, Bolton EJ, Finlay I, Junginger T, Morris DL (2002) Large volume hepatic freezing: association with significant release of the cytokines interleukin-6 and tumor necrosis factor a in a rat model. World J Surg 26:1333–1341

Seror O, Lepetit-Coiffe M, Quesson B, Trillaud H, Moonen CT (2006) Quantitative magnetic resonance temperature mapping for real-time monitoring of radiofrequency ablation of the liver: an ex vivo study. Eur Radiol 16:2265–2274

Sewell PE, Arriola RM, Robinette L, Cowan BD (2001) Real-time I-MR-imaging – guided cryoablation of uterine fibroids. J Vasc Interv Radiol 12:891–893

Theodorescu D (2004) Cancer cryotherapy: evolution and biology. Rev Urol 6(Suppl 4):S9–S19

Toyota N, Naito A, Kakizawa H, Hieda M, Hirai N, Tachikake T, Kimura T, Fukuda H, Ito K (2005) Radiofrequency ablation therapy combined with cementoplasty for painful bone metastases: initial experience. Cardiovasc Intervent Radiol 28:578–583

Witt JD, Hall-Craggs MA, Ripley P, Cobb JP, Bown SG (2000) Interstitial laser photocoagulation for the treatment of osteoid osteoma. J Bone Joint Surg Br 82:1125–1128

Wood BJ, Ramkaransingh JR, Fojo T, Walther MM, Libutti SK (2002) Percutaneous tumor ablation with radiofrequency. Cancer 94:443–451

Percutaneous Management of Painful Shoulder

15

Caroline Parlier-Cuau, Marc Wybier, Bassam Hamze, and Jean-Denis Laredo

CONTENTS

15.1   Introduction   *329*

15.2   **Aspiration of Calcific Tendinitis**   *329*
15.2.1   Background   *329*
15.2.2   Indications   *330*
15.2.3   Technique   *332*
15.2.4   Results and Discussion   *336*

15.3   **Brisement Procedure for
        Adhesive Capsulitis**   *337*
15.3.1   Background   *337*
15.3.2   Technique   *338*
15.3.3   Results   *340*
15.3.3.1 Our Experience   *340*
15.3.3.2 Discussion   *340*

15.4   **Conclusion**   *341*

        References   *341*

15.1
Introduction

Two different painful conditions of the shoulder may be treated with simple percutaneous procedures. In pain related to calcific deposits within the rotator cuff tendons, dramatic pain relief may be obtained by needle aspiration of the calcification, followed by in situ injection of steroids. In frozen shoulder syndrome, distension arthrography and associated intra-articular injection of steroids provides pain relief and some improvement in joint motion in 90% of patients. In this chapter, the techniques of these procedures are detailed, and their results discussed.

15.2
Aspiration of Calcific Tendinitis

15.2.1
Background

Calcific tendinitis results from the deposition of calcium hydroxyapatite crystals in or around tendons, mostly in periarticular locations. The shoulder is the most frequent location of calcific tendinitis (Fig. 15.1). However, calcific tendinitis may be encountered in a variety of anatomical locations, such as the hip, wrist, foot and cervical spine. Some patients have a single joint involved, while many others have bilateral involvement of the shoulders or involvement of several different joints (calcium hydroxyapatite deposition disease).

Apatite deposits may be symptomatic. In such cases, pain may be related to the inflammation process caused by the presence of the calcification (Bosworth 1941). The aim of needle aspiration in calcified deposits (NACD) is to decrease pain by removing a significant part of the calcification. Partial removal of the calcification by needle aspiration is

C. Parlier-Cuau, MD, Assistant Professor
M. Wybier, MD, Consultant Radiologist
B. Hamze, MD, Consultant Radiologist
J.-D. Laredo, MD, Professor and Chairman
Department of Musculoskeletal Radiology, Lariboisière University Hospital, 2 rue Ambroise Paré, 75010 Paris, France

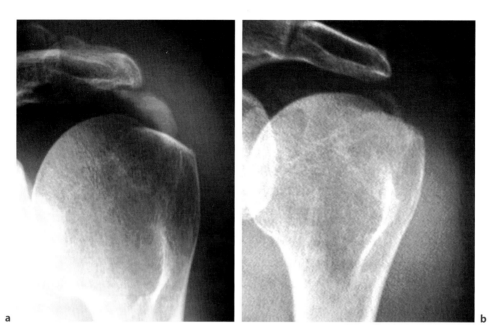

Fig. 15.1a,b. Aspiration of calcific tendinitis in a 45-year-old woman. **a** Anteroposterior radiograph of the left shoulder shows a supraspinatus calcific deposit with faint, milky appearance and fuzzy contours, which normally indicate that the deposit is liquid and will be easily aspirated. **b** Antero-posterior radiograph of the left shoulder after needle aspiration shows hardly any residual deposit

usually followed by spontaneous resorption of the remaining calcium (Comfort and Arafiles 1978). This is probably facilitated by the opening of the calcium-containing cavity in the course of the needle aspiration (Farin et al. 1995; Laredo et al. 1994; Normandin et al. 1988). NACD is mostly indicated for calcified tendinitis of the shoulder; however, it may be occasionally performed in other locations.

15.2.2
Indications

The procedure has three goals: (1) evacuation of a maximum of calcium, (2) opening of the calcium-containing cavity and fragmentation of the residual calcific deposits to facilitate resorption during the following weeks, and (3) reduction of inflammation secondary to the presence and migration of residual calcific deposits by in situ injection of corticosteroids.

The most important clinical selection criteria for NACD is exacerbation of pain at night (Simon 1975; Welfing 1964). Conversely, absence of pain at night, pain caused by a specific kind of motion within a given arc, and limitation of a specific motion suggest

that pain is related to an impingement syndrome rather than to calcific deposits. Prior studies have shown that, in most cases, no cuff tear is associated with calcified tendinitis (Normandin et al. 1988; Jim et al. 1993; Matsen et al. 1985). Careful radiologic evaluation is necessary prior to NACD. The structure of the calcific deposits and their relation to the rotator cuff tendons (Fig. 15.2) and subacromial bursa must be determined (Bosworth 1941; Welfing 1964). Other features to evaluate are number, size, density, contours, homogeneity of the calcific deposits (Figs. 15.3–15.5) and their tendency to evacuate into the subacromial bursa (Laredo et al. 1994; Normandin et al. 1988). The absence of changes on successive X-rays is an indication for needle aspiration. The calcification must be larger than 5 mm in diameter. The composition of the deposit will determine the success or failure of the aspiration. Faint milky calcifications with fuzzy contours are usually liquid and easily aspirated (Fig. 15.1), while very dense calcifications with clearly defined margins are often very hard and cannot be aspirated (Fig. 15.5). Irregular striated calcifications are usually located within tendon fibers (Figs. 15.3a, 15.4, 15.6). They usually correspond to degenerative tendinitis and cannot be aspirated.

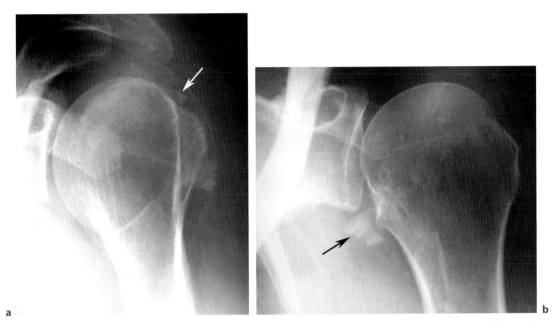

Fig. 15.2a,b. Calcific tendinitis in a 70-year-old woman. Anteroposterior radiographs of the left shoulder with good localization of the calcific deposits at (**a**) external rotation for the supraspinatus tendon (*arrow*) and (**b**) internal rotation for the subscapularis tendon (*arrow*)

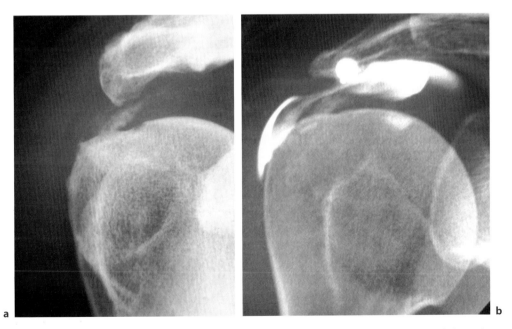

Fig. 15.3a,b. Calcific tendinitis in a 55-year-old woman. **a** Anteroposterior radiograph of the right shoulder shows supraspinatus calcific deposits with striated appearance. This calcification is usually located within the tendon fibers and cannot be significantly evacuated by needle aspiration. **b** Bursography of the subacromial bursa under fluoroscopic guidance with subsequent injection of steroid into the bursa under fluoroscopy. This may improve the clinical outcome of this type of calcific tendinitis

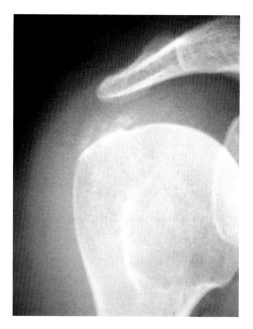

Fig. 15.4. Calcific tendinitis in a 65-year-old woman. Anteroposterior radiograph of the right shoulder shows calcific deposits with striated appearance. These deposits are usually located within the tendon fibers and cannot be significantly evacuated by needle aspiration

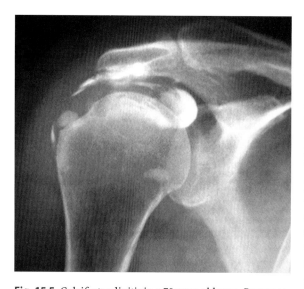

Fig. 15 5. Calcific tendinitis in a 70-year-old man. Bursography of the right subacromial bursa under fluoroscopic guidance shows a very dense calcification with clearly defined margins. This calcification is often very difficult to aspirate. Injection into the bursa of steroid may help good clinical outcome

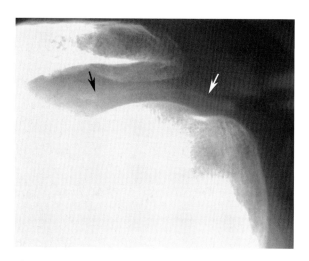

Fig. 15.6. Calcific tendinitis in a 60-year-old man. Anteroposterior radiograph of the left shoulder shows linear calcifications (*arrows*) usually located within the tendon fibers corresponding to degenerative tendinitis and which cannot be aspirated

15.2.3
Technique

The technique described here is performed under fluoroscopic guidance and concerns the shoulder, which is the most frequent site of tendinous calcific deposits. Recently, ultrasound has also been shown to reliably detect and localize rotator cuff calcifications (FARIN 1996). NACD under ultrasound guidance has also been reported by two different teams (FARIN et al. 1995; FARIN 1996; FARIN et al. 1996; AINA et al. 2001). A direct anteroposterior approach under fluoroscopic guidance is used. The patient is placed in a supine position on the radiographic table. The X-ray beam is centered vertically to the shoulder, or slightly tilted if it allows better separation of the calcium deposit from the underlying bone on the image intensifier screen. The arm is positioned according to the location of the calcification within the rotator cuff. Aseptic conditions are mandatory. The skin and superficial planes are anesthetized with 1% lidocaine. A 19-gauge needle is vertically advanced under fluoroscopic guidance to the center of the calcification following a direction parallel to the X-ray beam (Figs. 15.7, 15.8). During the entire approach the needle appears on the image intensifier screen as a single point in the center of the calcification (Figs. 15.7, 15.8). At any time during the procedure, the X-ray beam can be successively tilted cranially and caudally to confirm on the screen

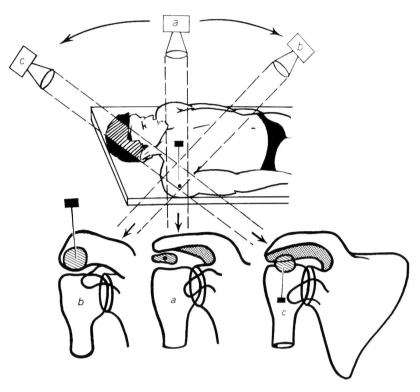

Fig. 15.7a–c. Fluoroscopic procedure to check that the needle tip is within the calcific deposits. **a** The X-ray beam is directed along the needle axis, and the needle appears as a dot in the center of the calcification. **b** and (**c**) show the X-ray beam successively tilted in maximal cephalad and caudad directions. If correctly placed, the needle tip will remain within the calcification. [With permission from NORMANDIN et al. 1988]

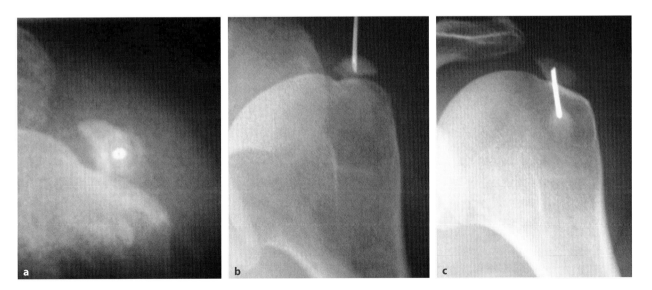

Fig. 15.8a–c. Fluoroscopic procedure to check the correct position of the needle tip in a 45-year-old man. **a** The needle is advanced parallel to the X-ray beam and appears on the screen as a single point in the center of the left supraspinatus calcific deposits. The X-ray beam is successively tilted in maximal (**b**) cephalad and (**c**) caudad directions, with the needle tip always appearing within the calcification

that the needle is actually within the calcification (Figs. 15.7, 15.8). Firmness at the needle tip indicates that the calcification has been reached. The calcium is aspirated first with a syringe containing lidocaine and then containing sterile water or saline solution (1–2 ml), alternately injecting the solution and with-

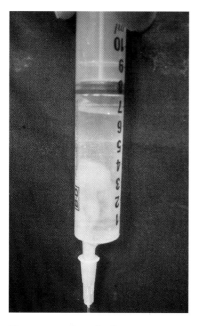

Fig. 15.9. Aspirated calcium appears as a white cloudy return in the syringe

drawing the aspirate. Aspirated calcium appears in the syringe as a white cloudy return (Fig. 15.9). The procedure is repeated until maximal aspiration of calcium has been obtained (Figs. 15.1, 15.10). In large and lobulated calcific deposits, insertion of two needles may be necessary (Fig. 15.11). The amount of calcium aspirated at the end of the procedure is variable and never complete (10%–80%) (Figs. 15.11, 15.12). In some cases, the calcification is hard and no calcium can be aspirated. However, disruption of the calcific deposit with the needle may in itself accelerate the process of spontaneous resorption (Comfort and Arafiles 1978; Laredo et al. 1994; Normandin et al. 1988; Moutounet et al. 1984) and is as important as aspiration. Once the maximum calcium has been aspirated, 2–3 ml of prednisolone acetate (50–75 mg) are injected in situ (Moutounet et al. 1984) or into the subacromial bursa under fluoroscopy (Figs. 15.3b, 15.5).

Radiographs are performed at the end of the procedure to document evacuation of the deposits (Fig. 15.13). In the majority of cases, the procedure is well-tolerated and painless.

Keeping the shoulder at rest for 5 or 6 days is recommended. One third of patients have a painful reaction rarely lasting more than 2–4 days. This is managed with intermittent application of ice, prescription pain medication and nonsteroidal anti-

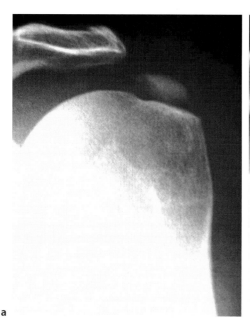
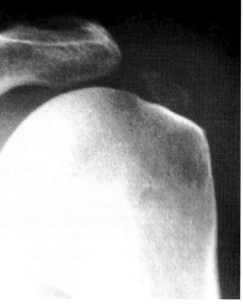

a   b

Fig. 15.10a,b. Aspiration of calcific tendinitis in a 65-year-old woman. Anteroposterior radiographs of the left shoulder show supraspinatus calcific deposits (**a**) before and (**b**) after needle aspiration. The calcification is fragmented and faint

Fig. 15.11. Aspiration of calcific tendinitis in a 54-year-old man. Anteroposterior radiograph of the right shoulder shows a large and lobulated calcific deposit of the supraspinatus tendon. Two needles are necessary to obtain a maximal aspiration of calcium

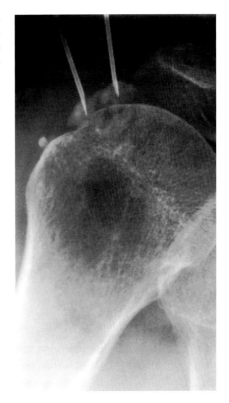

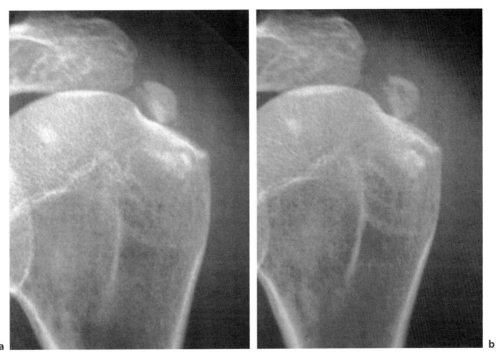

Fig. 15.12a,b. Aspiration of calcific tendinitis in a 60-year-old woman. **a** Anteroposterior radiograph of the left shoulder shows infraspinatus tendon calcific deposits. **b** Most of the calcification cannot be aspirated, but creating an opening between the cavity and surrounding vascularized tissues may cause local inflammation and hyperemia, which accelerates resorption

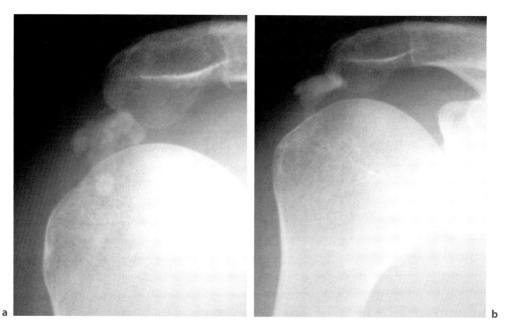

Fig. 15.13a,b. Calcific tendinitis in a 49-year-old woman. **a** Anteroposterior radiograph of the right shoulder shows infraspinatus tendon calcific deposits. **b** Anteroposterior radiograph is obtained at the end of the procedure to document decreased density of the deposits

inflammatory agents (MOUTOUNET et al. 1984). This painful crisis is usually accompanied by an almost complete resorption of the remaining calcification.

15.2.4
Results and Discussion

Although aspiration of calcific deposits is conventionally done under fluoroscopy, it can also be performed quickly and efficiently with ultrasound. Usually, rotator cuff calcifications appear under ultrasound as bright echogenic images with posterior acoustic shadowing (FARIN et al. 1995; FARIN et al. 1996). In this case it is easy to localize the calcific deposits. Ultrasound is a valuable tool for guiding aspiration, and does not involve ionizing radiation. Its real-time capabilities permit continuous monitoring of the needle position relative to the target and surrounding structures. In a few cases calcifications appear without posterior acoustic shadowing (FARIN et al. 1995) and ultrasound guidance could therefore be more difficult than fluoroscopic guidance. Either ultrasound or fluoroscopic guidance can be used, but they both require proper training.

According to several studies, good and excellent results are achieved in 61% (NORMANDIN et al. 1988) to 74% (FARIN et al. 1996) of cases. COMFORT

and ARAFILES (1978) first described this technique and reported nine cases followed for an average of 9 years. Good-to-excellent results were obtained with needle irrigation and aspiration, and follow-up on plain radiographs showed no residual deposits. In 1989, NORMANDIN et al. reported 69 cases of calcific tendinitis treated by needle aspiration. The clinical results were good in 60.9% of cases at 11–45 months (mean, 24 months) of follow-up. Aspiration of large amounts of calcium and secondary resorption of residual deposits on plain radiographs in the following weeks were significantly associated with good results. By contrast, when the calcification was hard or stone-like encrusted within the tendon fibers, no significant calcium was aspirated and the results were poor. In 1994, PFISTER and GERBER reported on 212 patients with calcific tendinitis of the shoulder treated with needle aspiration. At 5-year follow-up 60% of the patients were free of pain, 34% had a marked pain relief and 6% were unchanged. These results, however, were not compared to the untreated outcome of shoulder calcific tendinitis, which is often favorable. In 1996, FARIN et al. reported 61 patients with rotator cuff calcifications treated by needle aspiration and lavage under ultrasound guidance. Clinical results were good in 74% of cases, and moderate or poor in 26%. Clinical results were compared to the changes in the calcification on plain radiographs at 1-year follow-up. In cases with a good result, the calcification decreased in size in 86% of cases, and was unchanged in 14%. In cases with a moderate or poor result, the calcification decreased in size in 37% of cases, while no change was seen in 63%.

Surgical excision of calcifications of the rotator cuff gives prompt, complete and permanent relief of symptoms (McLaughlin 1963). At present, surgical excision of calcifications is mostly performed through arthroscopy (Ark et al. 1992; Jerosch et al. 1998). There are, however, many objections to the use of surgery as the primary procedure in rotator cuff calcifications, mainly the prolonged period of disability and potential complications of surgery, especially the risk of secondary reflex sympathetic dystrophy. Therefore, NACD should always be attempted first since it is minimally invasive and provides good results in at least two thirds of patients (Comfort and Arafiles 1978; Normandin et al. 1988; Farin et al. 1996; Pfister and Gerber 1994). In our experience, there have been no technical failures resulting from difficulty in locating the calcification with the needle under fluoroscopic guidance. With NACD, as with arthroscopic treatment of calcific tendinitis (Ark et al. 1992), it does not seem essential to remove the deposit completely. If the size of calcification is unchanged after the procedure, however, it is important to decrease the density of the calcification. The good results in such cases can be explained by the opening of the calcium-containing cavity and the creation of an opening between the cavity and surrounding vascularized tissues (Fig. 15.12). This may cause local inflammation and hyperemia, which in turn accelerate the process of resorption.

Extracorporeal shock wave therapy (ESWT) in the treatment of shoulder calcific tendinitis has been described recently (Haake et al. 2002; Rompe et al. 1998; Rompe et al. 2001; Loew et al 1999; Charrin and Noel 2001). It may offer a new and safer nonsurgical treatment of chronic calcific tendinitis of the shoulder. Good and excellent results were obtained in 55%–64% of cases (Charrin 2001; Rompe et al. 1998; Rompe et al. 2001). Charrin and Noel (2001) reported a series of 32 patients treated with ESWT. Lessened pain was noted in 55.1% of the patients after 24 weeks. In another series of 21 patients, 62% were significantly improved at 12-week-follow-up (Loew et al. 1999). In a series of 50 patients treated with ESWT, Rompe et al. (2001) had 60% good and excellent results after one year, and 64% good and

excellent results after 2 years. A significant factor in these results is the use of exact focusing of ESWT (Haake et al. 2002; Charrin and Noel 2001) and high-energy shock waves (Rompe et al. 1998; Rompe et al. 2001; Loew et al. 1999). All these reports, however, are noncontrolled studies with an open format. Ebenbichler et al. (1999) have conducted a randomized, double-blind study in patients with symptomatic calcific tendinitis. Results showed that ESWT helps resolve calcifications and is associated with short-term (6 weeks) clinical improvement. But at 9 months, the difference between the two groups was no longer significant.

15.3
Brisement Procedure for Adhesive Capsulitis

15.3.1
Background

Frozen shoulder syndrome (FSS) is still an enigma. It is characterized by the spontaneous onset of pain in the shoulder with insidious progressive restriction of both active and passive motion in every direction, especially external rotation and anterior elevation. Pain is often very severe and disturbs sleep. After several weeks and months, the painful phase gradually abates and is followed by a period of stiffness. This period of stiffness without improvement lasts between 4 and 12 months (Reeves 1975). Spontaneous gradual recovery of motion then follows over a period of several months. The total duration of FSS may be difficult to evaluate since the exact times of onset and resolution are frequently questionable (Reeves 1975; Blockley et al. 1954; Sany et al. 1982; Shaffer et al. 1992). The initial pain may be confused with that of a shoulder tendinitis or trauma that, not infrequently, precedes FSS. Complete recovery from FSS is also difficult to define. Some patients who consider their range of motion still restricted show no restriction on objective testing at long-term follow-up, and other patients who regard their range of motion as normal have significant restriction at clinical examination (Reeves 1975; Blockley et al. 1954; Sany et al. 1982; Shaffer et al. 1992). Distention arthrography (DA), which is one of the treatments of FSS, consists of injection of contrast media, steroids, lidocaine and a large volume of fluid into the joint to obtain joint distension.

15.3.2
Technique

Distention arthrography is an outpatient procedure. The patient is in the supine position, with the arm at the side and the palm up as much as possible to hold an external rotation of the shoulder, which facilitates needle placement into the anterior aspect of the glenohumeral joint. The X-ray beam is oriented vertically over the joint. The skin is prepped with an iodine solution. Skin and superficial planes are anesthetized with 1% lidocaine. A 20-gauge 9-cm needle is inserted vertically under fluoroscopic control into the anterior aspect of the joint through the anesthetized skin.

First, 2–3 ml of contrast material (meglumine loxaglate) are injected and immediately outline the glenohumeral space, confirming the correct intra-articular needle position. The joint capacity must be measured and is usually dramatically reduced (REEVES 1975; SHAFFER et al. 1992; BINDER et al. 1984; CORBEIL et al. 1992; EKELUND and RYDELL 1992; FAREED and GALLIVAN 1989; MULCAHY et al. 1994; OZAKI et al. 1989). In most patients, joint space volume is no more than 2–3 ml, and there is a loss of distensibility of the capsule. In most cases, the arthrogram is very suggestive of adhesive capsulitis (Fig. 15.14, 15.15a, 15.16a), with a marked reduction in size of all joint recesses, including the inferior (axillary) and internal (subcoracoid and subscapularis) recesses. The bicipital tendon sheath is inconsistently opacified. In addition, the synovial pouch around the humeral head is "tight looking" and has an irregular indented outline. Early lymphatic filling is not uncommon. However, arthrography may be surprisingly normal in some patients with full clinical criteria of FSS (SHAFFER et al. 1992; BINDER et al. 1984). A rotator cuff tear is present in 10%–31.3% of cases (REEVES 1975; SANY et al. 1982; BINDER et al. 1984; EKELUND and RYDELL 1992; MULCAHY et al. 1994).

Second, 3 ml of 2% lidocaine and 1.5 ml of cortivazol are injected intra-articularly. Injection of fluids immediately causes a severe exacerbation of shoulder pain. Characteristically, releasing the plunger of the syringe leads to immediate return

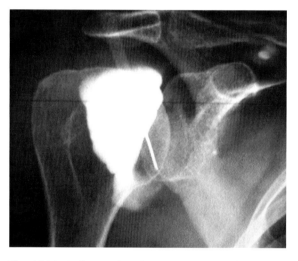

Fig. 15.14. Arthrography of FSS in a 48-year-old woman. Anteroposterior arthrogram of the right shoulder shows internal joint recesses are not filling

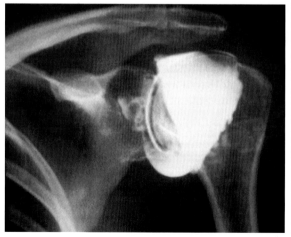
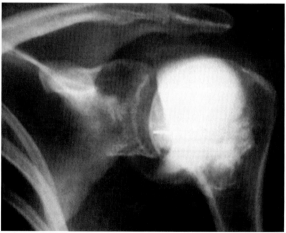

a   b

Fig 15.15a,b. Distention arthrography of FSS in a 40-year-old woman. **a** Anteroposterior arthrogram of the left shoulder shows internal joint recesses are not filling. **b** Distention arthrography was obtained with 39 ml of chilled sterile saline solution

the procedure is to distend the joint with the largest possible volume of fluid (usually up to 40–50 ml) (Figs. 15.15b, 15.16b, 15.17) without fluid extravasation. Fluid extravasation may occur at the subscapular recess or the bicipital tendon sheath, causing a sudden drop in resistance to distension (Fig. 15.18). Further injection would be ineffective and the procedure should be stopped.

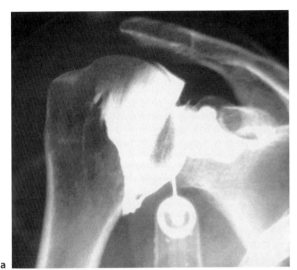

a

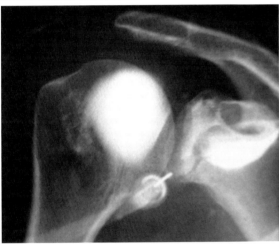

b

Fig. 15.16a,b. Distention arthrography of FSS in a 51-year-old woman. **a** Anteroposterior arthrogram of the right shoulder shows internal and inferior joint recesses are filling insufficiently. **b** Arthrogram of distended shoulder after injection of 40 ml of fluid

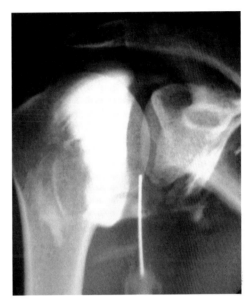

Fig. 15.17. Distention arthrography of FSS in a 48-year-old woman. Anteroposterior arthrogram of the right shoulder shows distended shoulder after injection of a large amount of fluid (26 ml)

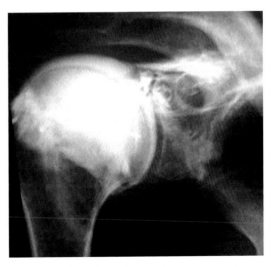

Fig. 15.18. Distention arthrography of FSS in a 55-year-old man. Anteroposterior arthrogram of the right shoulder shows distended shoulder with fluid extravasation at the subscapular recess and at the bicipital tendon sheath

of fluid into the syringe and immediate decrease of shoulder pain.

Third, distension of the capsule is performed using 30–40 ml of chilled sterile saline solution according to Fareed and Gallivan's technique (FAREED and GALLIVAN 1989). The maximum volume injected depends on the distensibility of the joint capsule. Joint distension (the "brisement procedure") (ANDREN and LUNBERG 1965), requires slow, graduate, intermittent injection of a larger and larger volume of chilled sterile saline solution. To avoid excessive fluid efflux from the needle while settling a new syringe of saline solution, a lockable three-way stopcock can be placed over the needle. The aim of

Arthrographic distension is immediately followed by active assisted range of motion exercises under the supervision of a physical therapist. The patient should perform physical therapy exercises at home for several days.

15.3.3
Results

15.3.3.1
Our Experience

Our experience is a noncontrolled study of 30 glenohumeral joints in 29 patients with FSS (17 women and 12 men; age range 41–65 years; mean age 49 years) treated with DA. Patients were assessed for pain (Huskisson visual analog scale) and shoulder range of motion in internal and external rotations, anterior and posterior elevations and abduction, first before AD and then at 15 and 45 days after treatment. At 15 days, 80% of patients considered their results very good (53%) or good (27%). At 45 days, 90% of patients considered their results very good (80%) or good (10%); all of the patients reported benefiting from the procedure at 45 days.

15.3.3.2
Discussion

A wide variety of treatments for FSS have been investigated. Physiotherapy is recommended in most of the published reports, including home exercise consisting of pendulum and resistance exercises several times daily. Oral (Blockley et al. 1954) and local (Bulgen et al. 1984) steroids are also frequently prescribed. Manipulation of the shoulder under general anesthesia (Sharma et al. 1993) or under interscalenic brachial plexus block anesthesia (Pollock et al. 1994; Dodenhoff et al. 2000) has also been proposed. More recently, arthroscopic release (Pollock et al. 1994; Andersen et al. 1998; Pearsall et al. 1999; Klinger et al. 2002; Holloway et al. 2001) or surgical excision of the coracohumeral ligament (Ozaki et al. 1989; Bunker and Anthony 1995) has been reported to be highly effective in patients who did not respond to conservative therapy. Contracture of the coracohumeral ligament due to the chronic fibrotic thickening present in FSS restrains external rotation of the shoulder with the arm at the side (Ozaki et al. 1989; Bunker and Anthony 1995) and acts as a check against external rotation, resulting in loss of both active and passive movement (Bunker and Anthony 1995).

The therapeutic value of DA has been widely studied (Corbeil et al. 1992; Ekelund and Rydell 1992; Fareed and Gallivan 1989; Mulcahy et al. 1994; Sharma et al. 1993; Hsu and Chan 1991; Jacobs et al. 1991; Rizk et al. 1994; Gam et al. 1998; Laroche et al. 1998; Noel et al. 2000) since Andren and Lunberg (1965) first reported that joint distension during DA could treat shoulder restriction effectively. Most studies evaluating DA were noncontrolled series (Ekelund and Rydell 1992; Fareed and Gallivan 1989; Mulcahy et al. 1994; Sharma et al. 1993; Rizk et al. 1994; Laroche et al. 1998). Satisfactory (good and excellent) results were obtained in 68 to 96% of cases. Data provided by controlled studies (Corbeil et al. 1992; Jacobs et al. 1991; Gam et al. 1998) are more limited and their results less clear. Corbeil et al. (1992) found no statistical difference in range of motion at 3-month follow-up between patients having a nondistensive arthrography with intra-articular injection of steroids and those having additional intra-articular injection of 20 ml of lidocaine. In addition, Jacobs et al. (1991) reported no statistical difference in range of motion after 16 weeks between patients treated with intra-articular injection of steroids only and those treated with intra-articular steroids and distension. However, in the later group, distension consisted of intra-articular injection of only 6 ml of lidocaine plus 3 ml of air. Gam et al. (1998) reported significant improvement in range of motion after 12 weeks for patients treated with intra-articular steroids and distension. Certainly, further controlled studies are necessary to confirm the value of DA in FSS. DA should be combined with other treatments: intra-articular glucocorticoids, gentle mobilization under local anesthesia, sedation or general anesthesia (Laroche et al. 1998).

Regarding the specific technique used in DA, Rizk et al. (1994) found, in an open trial including 16 patients, that good results were achieved only when the capsule was ruptured during the procedure; our experience does not confirm this result, as capsular rupture did not occur during joint filling in most of our patients.

As mentioned above, physiotherapy is widely recommended as an early therapy either alone or in association with other treatments including DA. The goal of physiotherapy is to relieve pain, improve motion and restore function. Physiotherapy is widely used and generally held to be beneficial. Nevertheless, no convincing evidence of efficacy has been found in well-designed studies (NOEL et al. 2000). However, to our knowledge, the advantage of physiotherapy in association with DA over DA alone has not been studied. In contrast, several reports showed that DA is effective in patients who did not respond to physiotherapy (EKELUND and RYDELL 1992; FAREED and GALLIVAN 1989, SHARMA et al. 1993), suggesting that DA has advantages over physiotherapy alone in treating FSS. In our institution, patients recently treated with DA received no assistance from a physical therapist and were asked to perform regular home physical therapy exercises by themselves in the days following the procedure.

Finally, assessing the results of treatment in FSS is challenging since FSS is a self-limiting condition with spontaneous recovery after several months or years. BULGEN et al. (1984) reported that various treatment regimens, including intra-articular injection of steroids, ice therapy and mobilizations, have few long-term advantages over no treatment in FSS. However the aim of procedures such as DA in FSS is not to modify the whole course of the disease but simply to shorten its most disabling phase.

15.4
Conclusion

In the case of calcific tendinitis, needle aspiration of tendinous calcific deposits is a well-tolerated conservative procedure that should be attempted after failure of medical treatment in chronically painful shoulders associated with rotator cuff deposits. Excellent and good results vary from 61%–74% of patients. In these patients, dramatic and durable improvement is obtained without surgery. Therefore, surgery should be reserved for failures of NACD. Extracorporeal shock wave therapy for calcific tendinitis appears to be an effective therapy in 55%–64% of cases, but additional controlled studies are necessary to confirm the value of this technique.

In frozen shoulder syndrome, DA, which includes intra-articular injection of steroids followed by hydraulic distension, provides good and excellent results in 90% of patients. DA provides rapid improvement in pain and joint stiffness, and shortens the disabling period. But only noncontrolled studies can be found in the literature, and the role of intra-articular injection of steroids and hydraulic distension in the achievement of good results is not well established. Their usefulness remains to be examined in controlled studies.

References

Aina R, Cardinal E, Bureau NJ, Aubin B, Brassard P (2001) Calcific shoulder tendinitis: treatment with modified US-guided fine-needle technique. Radiology 221:455–461

Andersen NH, Sojbjerg JO, Johannsen HV, Sneppen O (1998) Frozen shoulder: arthroscopy and manipulation under general anesthesia and early passive motion. J Shoulder Elbow Surg 7:218–222

Andren L, Lundberg BJ (1965) Treatment of rigid shoulder by joint distension during arthrography. Acta Orthop Scand 36:45–53

Ark JW, Flock TJ, Flatow EL, Bigliani LU (1992) Arthroscopic treatment of calcific tendinitis of the shoulder. Arthroscopy 8:183–188

Binder AI, Bulgen DY, Hazleman BL, Tudor J, Wraight P (1984) Frozen shoulder: an arthrographic and radionuclear scan assessment. Ann Rheum Dis 43:365–369

Bosworth BM (1941) Calcium deposits in the shoulder and subacromial bursitis. A survey of 122 shoulders. JAMA 116:2477

Bulgen DY, Binder AI, Hazleman BL, Dutton J, Roberts S (1984) Frozen shoulder: prospective clinical study with an evaluation of three treatment regimens. Ann Rheum Dis 43:353–360

Bunker TD, Anthony PP (1995) The pathology of frozen shoulder. A Dupuytren-like disease. J Bone Joint Surg Br 77:677–683

Charrin JE, Noel ER (2001) Shockwave therapy under ultrasonographic guidance in rotator cuff calcific tendinitis. Joint Bone Spine 68:241–244

Comfort TH, Arafiles RP (1978) Barbotage of the shoulder with image-intensified fluoroscopic control of needle placement for calcific tendinitis. Clin Orthop 135:171–178

Corbeil V, Dussault RG, Leduc BE, Fleury J (1992) Adhesive capsulitis of the shoulder: a comparative study of arthrography with intra-articular corticotherapy and with or without capsular distension. Can Ass Radiol J 43:127–130

Dodenhoff RM, Levy O, Wilson A, Copeland SA (2000) Manipulation under anesthesia for primary frozen shoulder on early recovery and return to activity. J Shoulder Elbow Surg 9:23–26

Ebenbichler GR, Erdogmus CB, Resch KL et al. (1999) Ultrasound therapy for calcific tendinitis of the shoulder. N Engl J Med 340:1533–1538

Ekelund AL, Rydell N (1992) Combination treatment for adhesive capsulitis of the shoulder. Clin Orthop Relat Res 282:105–109

Fareed DO, Gallivan WR Jr (1989) Office management of frozen shoulder syndrome. Treatment with hydraulic distension under local anesthesia. Clin Ortho Relat Res 242:177–183

Farin PU (1996) Consistency of rotator cuff calcifications.

Observations on plain radiography, sonography, computed tomography, and at needle treatment. Invest Radiol 31:300–304

Farin PU, Jaroma H, Soimakallio S (1995) Rotator cuff calcifications: treatment with US-guided technique. Radiology 195:841–843

Farin PU, Rasanen H, Jaroma H, Harju A (1996) Rotator cuff calcifications: treatment with ultrasound-guided percutaneous needle aspiration and lavage. Skeletal Radiol 25:551–554

Gam AN, Schydlowsky P, Rossel I, Remvig L, Jensen EM (1998) Treatment of "frozen shoulder" with distension and glucorticoid compared with glucorticoid alone. A randomised controlled trial. Scand J Rheumatol 27:425–430

Haake M, Deike B, Thon A, Schmitt J (2002) Exact focusing of extracorporeal shock wave therapy for calcifying tendinopathy. Clin Orthop 397:323–331

Holloway GB, Schenk T, Williams GR, Ramsey ML, Iannotti JP (2001) Arthroscopic capsular release for the treatment of refractory postoperative or post-fracture shoulder stiffness. J Bone Joint Surg Am 83:1682–1687

Hsu SY, Chan KM (1991) Arthroscopic distension in the management of frozen shoulder. Int Orthop 15:79–83

Jacobs LG, Barton MA, Wallace WA, Ferrousis J, Dunn NA, Bossingham DH (1991) Intra-articular distension and steroids in the management of capsulitis of the shoulder. Br Med J 302:1498–1501

Jerosch J, Strauss JM, Schmiel S (1998) Arthroscopic treatment of calcific tendinitis of the shoulder. J Shoulder Elbow Surg 7:30–37

Jim YF, Hsu HC, Chang CY, Wu JJ, Chang T (1993) Coexistence of calcific tendinitis and rotator cuff tear: an arthrographic study. Skeletal Radiol 22:183–185

Klinger HM, Otte S, Baums M, Haerer T (2002) Early arthroscopic release in refractory shoulder stiffness. Arch Orthop Trauma Surg 122:200–203

Laredo JD, Bellaiche L, Hamze B, Naouri JF, Bondeville JM, Tubiana JM (1994) Current status of musculoskeletal interventional radiology. Radiol Clin North Am 32:377–398

Laroche M, Ighilahriz O, Moulinier L, Constantin A, Cantagrel A, Mazieres B (1998) Adhesive capsulitis of the shoulder: an open study of 40 cases treated by joint distention during arthrography followed by an intraarticular corticosteroid injection and immediate physical therapy. Rev Rhum Engl Ed 65:313–319

Loew M, Daecke W, Kusnierczak D, Rahmanzadeh M, Ewerbeck V (1999) Shock-wave therapy is effective for chronic calcifying tendinitis of the shoulder. J Bone Joint Surg Br 81:863–867

McLaughlin HL (1963) The selection of calcium deposits for operation: the technique and results of operation. Surg Clin North Am 43:1501–1504

Matsen ML, Kilcoyne RF, Davies PK, Sickler ME (1985) US evaluation of the rotator cuff. Radiology 157:205–209

Moutounet J, Chevrot A, Godefroy D, Horreard P, Zenny JC, Auberge T, Laoussadi S (1984) Radioguided puncture-infiltration in the treatment of refractory calcifying periarthritis of shoulders. J Radiol 65:569–572

Mulcahy KA, Baxter AD, Oni OO, Finlay D (1994) The value of shoulder distension arthrography with intra-articular injection of steroid and local anaesthetic: a follow-up study. Br J Radiol 67:263–266

Noel E, Thomas T, Schaeverbeke T, Thomas P, Bonjean M, Revel M (2000) Frozen shoulder. Joint Bone Spine 67:393–400

Normandin C, Seban E, Laredo JD et al. (1988) Aspiration of tendinous calcific deposits. In: Bard M, Laredo JD (eds) Interventional radiology in bone and joints. Springer-Verlag, Wien New York, p 285

Ozaki J, Nakagawa Y, Sakurai G, Tamai S (1989) Recalcitrant chronic adhesive capsulitis of the shoulder. Role of contracture of the coracohumeral ligament and rotator interval in pathogenesis and treatment. J Bone Joint Surg Am 71:1511–1515

Pfister J, Gerber H (1994) Treatment of calcific humeroscapular periarthropathy using needle irrigation of the shoulder: retrospective study. Z Orthop Ihre Grenzgeb 132:300–305

Pearsall AW, Osbahr DC, Speer KP (1999) An arthroscopic technique for treating patients with frozen shoulder. Arthroscopy 15:2–11

Pollock RG, Duralde XA, Flatow EL, Bigliani LU (1994) The use of arthroscopy in the treatment of resistant frozen shoulder. Clin Orthop 304:30–36

Reeves B (1975) The natural history of the frozen shoulder syndrome. Scand J Rheumatol 4:193–196

Rizk TE, Gavant ML, Pinals RS (1994) Treatment of adhesive capsulitis (frozen shoulder) with arthrographic capsular distension and rupture. Arch Phys Med Rehabil 75:803–807

Rompe JD, Burger R, Hopf C, Eysel P (1998) Shoulder function after extracorporal shock wave therapy for calcific tendinitis. J Shoulder Elbow Surg 7:505–509

Rompe JD, Zoellner J, Nafe B (2001) Shock wave therapy versus conventional surgery in the treatment of calcifying tendinitis of the shoulder. Clin Orthop 387:72–78

Sany J, Caillens JP, Rousseau JR (1982) Remote development of capsular retraction of the shoulder. Rev Rhum Engl Ed 49:815–819

Shaffer B, Tibone JE, Kerlan RK (1992) Frozen shoulder. A long-term follow-up. J Bone Joint Surg Am 74:738–746

Sharma RK, Bajekal RA, Bhan S (1993) Frozen shoulder syndrome. A comparison of hydraulic distension and manipulation. Int Orthop 17:275–278

Simon WH (1975) Soft tissue disorders of the shoulder: frozen shoulder, calcific tendinitis and bicipital tendinitis. Orthop Clin North Am 6:521–539

Welfing J (1964) Les calcifications de l'épaule. Diagnostic clinique. Rev Rhum Engl Ed 1:265–270

Closed Reduction and Percutaneous Fixation of Pelvic Fractures

16

Rolf Huegli, Thomas Gross, Augustinus L. Jacob, and Peter Messmer

CONTENTS

16.1   **Introduction**   *343*

16.2   **Epidemiology**   *344*

16.3   **General Work-Up**   *344*

16.4   **Radiological Assessment**   *344*

16.5   **Biomechanics and Classification**   *344*
16.5.1   Pelvic Ring Fractures   *344*
16.5.1.1   AO/ASIF-Classification   *345*
16.5.2   Acetabular Fractures   *347*

16.6   **Conventional Surgery Principles**   *348*
16.6.1   Posterior Pelvic Ring Fractures   *348*
16.6.2   Acetabular Fractures   *349*

16.7   **Minimally Invasive Reduction Methods**   *349*
16.7.1   Closed Reduction   *350*
16.7.2   Percutaneous Reduction   *351*
16.7.3   Open or Limited Access Reduction   *351*

16.8   **Minimally Invasive Fixation Methods**   *352*
16.8.1   Principles of Image-Guided Fixation   *352*
16.8.2   Restoration of Stability   *352*
16.8.3   Hardware   *352*

16.9   **Combinations of Minimally Invasive Reduction and Fixation Methods**   *353*

16.10   **Image Guidance Methods**   *353*
16.10.1   Online Guidance   *353*
16.10.2   Offline Guidance   *354*
16.10.2.1   Fluoroscopy Based Navigation   *355*
16.10.2.2   CT and MR-Based Navigation   *355*

16.10.3   Robotic Assistance   *356*
16.10.4   Placement and Immobilization   *356*

16.11   **Typical Minimally Invasive Procedures**   *356*
16.11.1   External Fixation of the Anterior Pelvic Ring   *357*
16.11.2   Superior Pubic Ramus Screw   *357*
16.11.3   Iliosacral Screws   *357*
16.11.4   Acetabular Roof or Iliac Wing Screw   *360*
16.11.5   Other Access Paths   *360*

16.12   **Quality Criteria**   *360*
16.12.1   Clinical Criteria   *360*
16.12.2   Imaging Criteria   *360*

16.13   **Results**   *362*

16.14   **Indications for Minimally-Invasive Therapy**   *364*
16.14.1   Superior Pubic Ramus   *364*
16.14.2   Sacrum, Ilium and Sacroiliac Joint   *364*
16.14.2.1   Fractures and Fracture-Dislocations   *364*
16.14.2.2   Other Indications   *364*
16.14.3   Acetabulum   *364*

16.15   **Conclusion**   *364*

       References   *365*

R. HUEGLI, MD
Head, Institute of Radiology, Cantonal Hospital Bruderholz, Batteriestrasse 1, 4101 Bruderholz, Switzerland
T. GROSS, MD
Head, Division of Traumatology, Ospedale Regionale di Lugano, Via Tesserete 46, 6900 Lugano, Switzerland
A. L. JACOB, MD
Head, Division of Interventional Radiology, University Hospital Basel, Petersgraben 4, 4031 Basel, Switzerland
P. MESSMER, MD
Consultant Surgeon, Ortho Trauma Center, Rashid Hospital, DOHMS, P.O. Box 4545, Dubai, United Arab Emirates

16.1
Introduction

This chapter on minimally-invasive percutaneous screw fixation of acetabular and sacral fractures will try to guide the reader through the process of understanding the biomechanics and classification of the specific injury he or she is investigating, recognizing and weighing the different conservative, minimally-invasive and open treatment options and explaining how to perform some of the minimally-invasive techniques. Close collaboration between orthopedic surgeon and radiologist is strongly advised to provide the best possible service to your patients. The literature on fluoroscopic, CT-based and navigated techniques is discussed and illustrated with examples from our own experience.

16.2
Epidemiology

Pelvic fractures account for about 0.3%–8% of all fractures (GANSSLEN et al. 1996; SENST and BIDA 2000) and are mostly high impact traumas. In multiple trauma, pelvic ring injury is present in about 20% of cases (GANSSLEN et al. 1996). The injury itself is potentially life-threatening (KELLAM et al. 1987) as are the associated lesions (head, chest, abdomen and limbs) (POOLE and WARD 1994). The mortality rate ranges between 10% and 31% (BEN-MENACHEM et al. 1991; HUNTER et al. 1997; POHLEMANN et al. 1994). The morbidity may be high in survivors (TILE 2003). Pelvic ring lesions remain a clinical challenge.

16.3
General Work-Up

Thorough clinical examination and conventional X-rays are the first instruments to detect important pelvic dislocations and instabilities that need emergency treatment of bleeding. In the further stabilized patient, detailed analysis with computed tomography (CT) is needed for the planning of definitive pelvic trauma treatment. If a multi-slice CT is readily available near or in the emergency room it will probably replace conventional pelvic imaging altogether.

16.4
Radiological Assessment

Radiological assessment is crucial in the diagnosis of pelvic trauma. An anteroposterior pelvic radiograph continues to be recommended by the advanced trauma life support (ATLS) protocol (VAN OLDEN et al. 2004) as an early diagnostic adjunct in the resuscitation of blunt trauma patients. However, because of the complexity of pelvic and acetabular fractures, exact pathological anatomy is not easily detected by routine radiographs and in many cases details or fractures are not visible at all (FALCHI and ROLLANDI 2004). The false negative

rate for pelvic fractures in conventional anterior posterior views is up to 32%. In up to 55% of cases where a fracture can be detected on plain film, CT reveals additional fractures or an upgrade in the fracture classification (GUILLAMONDEGUI et al. 2002).

Spiral and increasingly multi-slice CT provides information regarding the extent of fractures and is clearly superior to radiography for evaluation of the spatial fracture fragments. It is an effective tool for the comprehension of complex fracture types, particularly in combination with multiple two-dimensional or three-dimensional reconstructions. Additionally CT scans allow a detailed analysis of ligamentous and – by adding contrast media – vascular injuries. Given these striking advantages over conventional radiography, CT has emerged as the gold standard for pelvic fracture assessment (WEDEGARTNER et al. 2003).

16.5
Biomechanics and Classification

The main function of the pelvic ring is to transmit forces from the lower extremities to the spine (ISLER and GANZ 1996). Correspondingly, the main task of therapy is to restore this ability and not high-precision anatomical reconstruction. The acetabular joint, besides load bearing, has the additional function of allowing free movement of the femoral head. Acetabular fractures therefore need minute anatomic reduction and fixation of the articular surface to avoid or minimize post-traumatic osteoarthritis or at least prepare the joint for later replacement (STARR et al. 2001). These different biomechanical functions necessarily lead to different classifications. Fractures of the acetabulum and the posterior pelvic ring must therefore be classified separately.

16.5.1
Pelvic Ring Fractures

Pelvic fractures involve one or more bones of the pelvis and may include the ligamentous structures between these bones. Since the pelvic ring is a relatively rigid structure, an injury to the posterior ring (ilium, sacroiliac joint, sacrum) rarely occurs without a concomitant interruption of the anterior ring (symphysis, obturator rings, acetabula). Only in cases of direct trauma can isolated fractures of the affected bone be observed.

16.5.1.1
AO/ASIF-Classification

There are several classifications for pelvic ring disruptions. TILE (1996) modified the pioneering classification of Pennal from the late 1950s (PENNAL et al. 1980) which was based purely on force direction and included an anteroposterior compression type, a lateral compression type, and vertical shear injuries. The Association for the Study of Internal Fixation (AO/ASIF) classification is based on the integrity of the osseous and ligamentous posterior sacroiliac ring segment and its ability or inability to transmit forces from the lower extremities to the spine.

The AO/ASIF classification groups fractures according to increasing severity. Injuries are classified as stable, rotationally unstable but vertically stable, or rotationally and vertically unstable. 'A' is the least complicated type with preserved posterior stability, 'B' with partial posterior stability, and type 'C' is the most complicated with complete loss of posterior stability (Fig. 16.1) (ISLER and GANZ 1996; TILE 1996, 2003):

● Stable 'A' injuries can resist gradual load bearing without any further treatment. Anatomically these are isolated fractures of the anterior pelvic ring.
● Rotationally unstable 'B' fractures are unable to withstand forces acting inward and/or outward on the anterior pelvic structures (Fig. 16.2). Anatomically they are complete anterior plus partial posterior disruptions, e.g. a symphyseal rupture combined with a complete tear of the anterior sacroiliac ligamentous structure.
● Rotationally and vertically unstable 'C' fractures are additionally unstable against vertical loading that will lead to a cranial displacement of the affected side (Fig. 16.3).

An unsolved clinical problem is the lack of an instrument to assess pelvic stability. Especially in big or obese patients, pathological mobility and movement of the fragments may be almost impossible to appreciate even under fluoroscopy. When negative, the clinical examination for instability is not reliable. Radiographically a spontaneously reduced unstable C fracture may be indistinguishable from a partially stable B fracture. In our practice we classify these injuries as transitional B/C fractures. Even if we consider all additional information from the history of the accident sometimes only a secondary dislocation will reveal under-classification and consequently under-treatment (ORANSKY and TORTORA 2007).

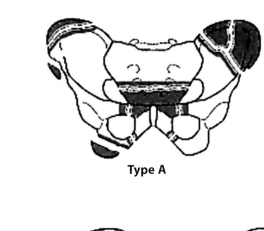

Type A

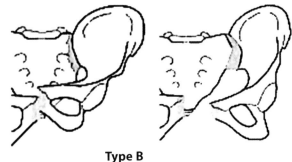

Type B

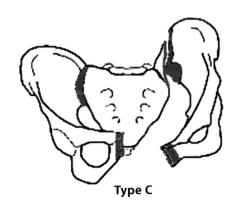

Type C

Fig. 16.1. AO classification of pelvic ring fractures: principal types A to C

Type B. Pelvic ring unstable in rotation and stable in vertical translation

B 1   Unilateral outward rotation injury ('open book') = symphyseal disruption

B 1.1 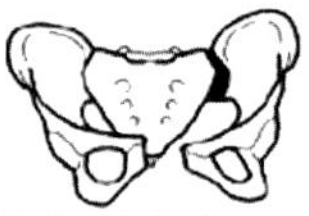   Incomplete disruption of dorsal pelvic ring with unilateral external rotation given an anterior disruption of SI-joint

B 1.2 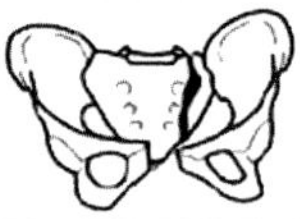   Incomplete disruption of dorsal pelvic ring with unilateral external rotation given a sacral fracture

B 2   Lateral compression injury with unilateral inward rotational dislocation

B 2.1 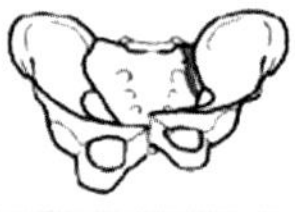   Incomplete unilateral disruption of dorsal pelvic ring given an anterior sacral compression fracture

B 2.2 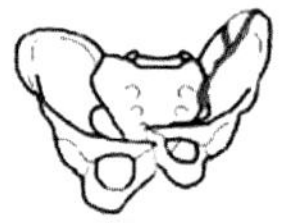   Incomplete unilateral disruption of dorsal pelvic ring given a partial SI-joint disruption

B 2.3 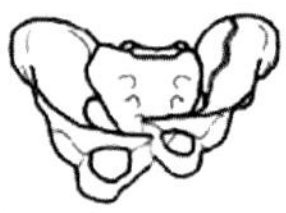   Incomplete unilateral disruption of dorsal pelvic ring given an incomplete fracture of the dorsal part of the ilium

B 3   Bilateral Type B injuries

B 3.1 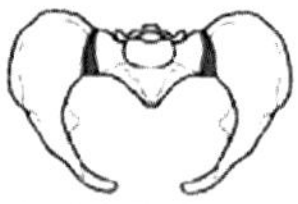   Incomplete bilateral disruption of dorsal pelvic ring given a bilateral fracture of the ilium

B 3.2 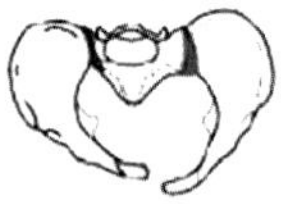   Incomplete bilateral disruption of dorsal pelvic ring combined with a B 1 or B 2 injury

B 3.3 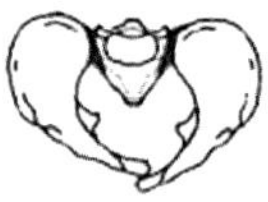   Incomplete bilateral disruption of dorsal pelvic ring given a bilateral B 2 injury

Fig. 16.2. AO classification of pelvic ring fractures: features of different B-type fractures

In major trauma centers 50%–60% of pelvic ring fractures are type A, 20%–30% type B and only about 10%–20% are vertically or translationally unstable (Type C) (TILE 1996). The most frequent isolated pelvic lesions are fractures of the ischiopubic bones (transpubic instability), injuries involving the sacroiliac joint (transiliosacral instability), and sacral fractures (transsacral instability). More than 90% of type A lesions are treated conservatively (GANSSLEN et al. 1996). In sharp contrast, conservative therapy of unstable type B and C lesions has a much worse long term outcome with 50%–75% of patients showing insufficient results (FELL et al. 1995). Adequate reduction and operative fixation of these unstable lesions is mandatory.

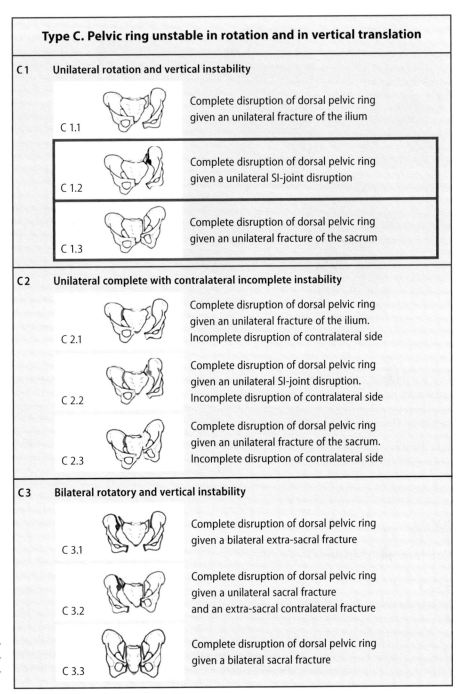

Fig. 16.3. AO classification of pelvic ring fractures: features of different C-type fractures

16.5.2
Acetabular Fractures

Acetabular fractures occur mainly in a young active population as a result of high energy trauma. Cartilaginous defects and particularly displaced fractures, especially those that heal in an unreduced position, promote posttraumatic osteoarthritis.

The most frequently used classification for acetabular fractures is the AO/ASIF classification that follows the fundamental work of LETOURNEL (1981). Sixteen fractures are divided into five simple and five associated fracture types. The simple types are fractures of the posterior wall (A), posterior column (B), anterior wall (C), anterior column (D), and transverse fractures (E) (Fig. 16.4); the associated types

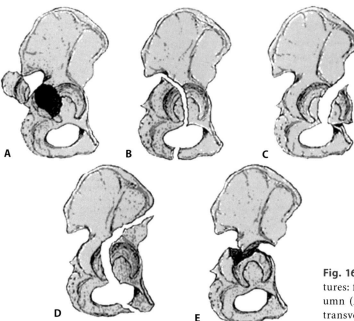

Fig. 16.4. Letournel/AO classification acetabular fractures: fractures of the posterior wall (*A*), posterior column (*B*), anterior wall (*C*), anterior column (*D*), and transverse fractures (*E*)

are combinations of simple types. The accepted treatment is open surgical reduction of the fracture and internal fixation with metallic screws and plates. In selected cases minimally-invasive therapy is possible (Gay et al. 1992; Gross et al. 2004; Jacob et al. 2000b; Starr et al. 1998).

16.6

Conventional Surgery Principles

16.6.1
Posterior Pelvic Ring Fractures

Operative treatment of displaced posterior pelvic ring disruptions remains controversial. Accurate posterior pelvic reductions and stable fixations have been shown to correlate with improved functional results (Slatis and Huittinen 1972). Stable fixation of the posterior pelvis has been achieved by using a variety of techniques including sacral bars, tension band plates, and others, each with its own problems.

- *Type A fractures* of the pelvic girdle rarely undergo surgery. Muscle avulsion fractures, fragment dislocation as well as persistent pain and slow rehabilitation, may be indications for open or percutaneous surgery in selected patients.

- *Type B fractures* remain a domain of conservative therapy (Tile 2003). However, there are certain type B fractures, e.g. open book lesions with symphyseal disruption of more than 2–3 cm (classified as B2.2), which frequently undergo surgery because of partial but disabling functional pelvic ring instability. Other indications for surgical approaches are early functional instability after treatment and potentially unstable type B/C lesions to prevent later dislocations and malunions.

- *Type C fractures* by definition are all unstable and are treated surgically.

- *Transitional Type B/C fractures.* As outlined above these lie in a gray area between the B and C categories. Only secondary dislocation, anterior ring implant failure, posterior ring non-union and bad functional outcome will disclose when a 'C' fracture has received 'B' under-treatment with conservative therapy or anterior stabilization only (Oransky and Tortora 2007). On the other hand, open surgery of the posterior pelvic ring for all fractures in this gray zone clearly incurs too much surgical morbidity. Minimally invasive fixation of the posterior pelvic ring is much less aggressive than open surgery and carries a very low risk of complications. In our practice minimally invasive percutaneous fixation is performed in all type B/C fractures.

16.6.2
Acetabular Fractures

The treatment objective is the restitution of joint surface integrity. An insufficient reduction of the acetabular joint congruency leads to posttraumatic osteoarthritis in a third of patients, while radiologically anatomical reduction does so in only about 10% (Letournel 1993). Since the early works of Letournel (1993), open reduction and internal fixation (ORIF) of displaced or unstable acetabular fractures has evolved as the gold standard (Judet et al. 1964; Qureshi et al. 2004).

The choice of surgical approach is based on the fracture pattern, fragment displacement direction, skin conditions at the surgical incision site, and time elapsed since the injury (Letournel 1993; Matta et al. 1986). Acetabular fracture surgery often requires extensive exposure, frequently resulting in major blood loss, and in associated significant complications (Kaempffe et al. 1991; Letournel 1981; Reinert et al. 1988). After anterior or posterior open surgical approaches the incidence of iatrogenic injuries to the femoral neurovascular bundle (Gruson and Moed 2003), the sciatic nerve and the gluteal vessels (Haidukewych et al. 2002), or to the lateral femoral cutaneous nerve ranges from 0.3%–57% (Kloen et al. 2002).

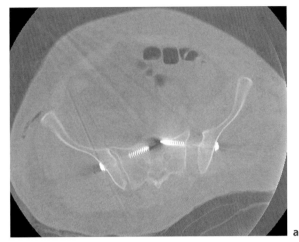

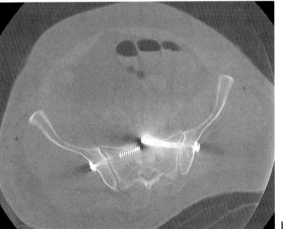

Fig. 16.5a,b. Closure of rupture gap of sacroiliac joints by screw fixation in a 31-year-old man with bilateral sacroiliac joint rupture from a motor vehicle accident. **a** Axial CT scan during the procedure shows widely dehiscent left sacroiliac joint with iliosacral screw head already at the iliac cortex. **b** Axial CT scan at the end of the procedure shows the left sacroiliac joint is now closed after carefully tightening both iliosacral screws alternately to prevent sinking the screw heads

16.7
Minimally Invasive Reduction Methods

The ability to produce a satisfactory reduction is the prerequisite for fixation. Several types of dislocation identified through imaging have to be addressed during the reduction process (Wedegartner et al. 2003):

- Fracture or luxation gap: This is the simplest and most trivial form of dislocation shared even by "non-displaced" fractures where ideally all points on one fragment have the same distance to their corresponding points on the other fragment. Reduction is achieved by the very step of fixation, preferably perpendicular to the gap plane (Fig. 16.5).
- *Translation* comes in dorsoventral, laterolateral and craniocaudal flavors and in combinations thereof. While all of these can be approached by external manipulation, craniocaudal dislocation often is additionally treated by extension.

- Rotation of one fragment vs another is often tried by percutaneously inserting a guide pin or Schanz screw and using these as a handle.
- An acetabular *joint step* is generally difficult to reduce by minimally invasive means.

For good results, a decent reduction must be achieved and maintained in pelvic ring injuries and an anatomical reduction in acetabular fractures. Open reduction using posterior surgical exposures can be complicated by wound problems (Goldstein et al. 1986; Kellam et al. 1987). Closed reduction is possible in several ways depending on type and amount of dislocation, fracture age, involvement of joint surfaces and/or neural structures. Reduction should be attempted as early as possible to forestall consolidation of hematomas and soft tissue fibrosis that may render reduction impossible within 2 days. The following minimally invasive types of reduction can be applied (Gansslen et al. 2006; Gay et al. 1992; Gross et al. 2004; Jacob et al. 1997, 2000c):

- Closed reduction (CR) is the least invasive method and is preferred whenever success is possible
- Percutaneous reduction (PR) is the next more invasive variant; it uses percutaneously attached handles
- Open or limited access reduction (OR, LAR) requires formal though small incisions and exposure and is only chosen when CR and PR are not feasible

16.7.1
Closed Reduction

In contrast to percutaneous fixation (PF) where simple geometrics can be applied, CR is more of a craft than a technical science. CR may be difficult or impossible especially in fractures that are more than about 2 days old. In these cases open reduction has to be performed in combination with percutaneous or internal fixation (IF). CR usually has to be judged by control imaging. Imaging quality, time and radiation dose may impose a practical limit on the number of repetitive efforts towards CR. Means of CR include the following:

- *Placement or reduction by gravity* is the simplest measure in dislocations. A wide open left sacro-iliac rupture will usually close by a substantial amount if the patient is rotated from supine to right lateral position. Should the same patient be placed in prone position for percutaneous fixation the gap will most probably not close (Fig. 16.6).
- *External manipulation* is possible by pushing or pulling. The posterior and lateral aspect of the iliac crest, the posterior surface of the sacrum, the superior pubic ramus and the femur can be used as handles of external manipulation. Normally the two main fragments of the pelvis are pushed in opposite directions to decrease the dislocation.
- *Extension* is a special variant of external manipulation, where a longitudinal mechanical pull of about 50–150 Newton is applied to one leg for a period of time (minutes to days) to reduce a cranial dislocation of a hemipelvis. The reduction resembles more a slow plastic flow of the soft tissues than an abrupt change of position. Extension has to be maintained during surgery until fixation is achieved (Fig. 16.7) (Jacob et al. 2000a).

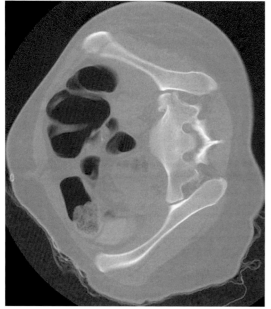
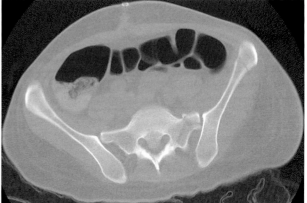

Fig. 16.6 a,b. Reduction by placement in a 24-year-old woman who sustained a high impact compression injury. **a** Axial CT scan with patient in lateral decubitus shows substantial overlap of anterior fragment in lateral compression fracture. **b** Axial CT scan shows partial decompression by simple change of placement to supine position

16.7.2
Percutaneous Reduction

Percutaneous reduction is performed by first percutaneously attaching handles to fragments and then working on the handles. The handles used most often are Schanz screws. Devices especially designed for the task of PR have still to be developed. These methods are in routine clinical use:

- A pelvic clamp is usually applied in the emergency room primarily to stop pelvic hemorrhage by closing a gaping posterior pelvic ring, thereby reducing the internal pelvic volume and assisting spontaneous tamponade.
- Schanz screws can be placed anywhere on the pelvis deemed suited for force transmission with due respect for neurovascular structures. Most often they are inserted into the anterior superior iliac spine or the iliac crest. Screw insertion into deep structures like the sacrum may itself necessitate image guidance.
- External fixators take the handle concept one step further offering a mechanical advantage, precise movements and the ability to retain the reduction once achieved (Fig. 16.8) (KELLAM 1989).

16.7.3
Open or Limited Access Reduction

This is done using standard surgical techniques. Examples are limited access reduction of a posterior sacral dislocation or of an acetabular fracture followed by percutaneous screw fixation.

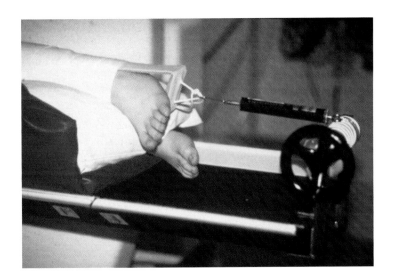

Fig. 16.7. Extension device for continued traction on CT table

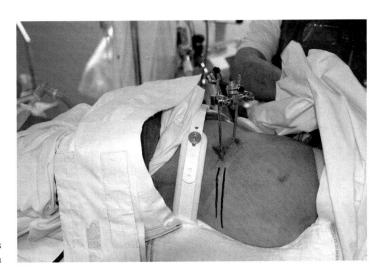

Fig. 16.8. External fixator for percutaneous manipulation and preliminary stabilization

16.8
Minimally Invasive Fixation Methods

The fixation methods described here are very basic and can be described as image guided linear actions where a planned trajectory is to be reproduced as closely as possible. Essentially we are talking about precisely placing compression and positioning screws.

16.8.1
Principles of Image-Guided Fixation

Percutaneous fixation is done in a way familiar to interventional radiologists:

- It is normally performed in a linear fashion following a trajectory dictated by the intended placement of the screws.
- There is a total disregard of anything like surgical access anatomy or dissection planes. The target path nonchalantly crosses through skin, fat, fascia, muscle and other structures. The only condition is avoidance of critical structures which may actually enforce a biomechanically less than optimal approach or a limited access fixation.
- PF is divided into a targeting step where a relatively innocuous guide wire is placed and a fixation step where the active element, normally a cannulated screw, is slid safely down the guide wire through all intervening tissues.

16.8.2
Restoration of Stability

The following rules can be established regarding the restoration of stability in the different degrees of instability outlined in Section 16.5.1.1:

- *Stable injuries* are normally treated *conservatively* with partial load bearing using crutches.
- *Rotationally unstable fractures* are typically addressed with an *anterior stabilization only* that together with the intact posterior sacroiliac ligament complex will suffice to restore stability. In simple non-displaced fractures this can be accomplished either by antegrade or retrograde superior pubic ramus screws. Reconstruction

plates are typically used in displaced, comminuted and/or complex cases. The stability of both constructs is essentially equivalent (Simonian et al. 1994b).
- In *rotationally and vertically unstable fractures* both the anterior plus the posterior pelvic ring stability have to be restored. In our patients this is normally done in a single stage approach with anterior plating first which mostly also reduces the posterior pelvic ring for subsequent percutaneous iliosacral screw fixation.

16.8.3
Hardware

So far there is no hardware yet designed especially for the percutaneous mode of operation. Percutaneous reduction and fixation relies on standard surgical hardware like Schanz screws, external fixators, guide wires, cannulated screws and others. Several points may be worth mentioning:

- We use *2.8-mm AO/ASIF guide wires* (Synthes Inc., Solothurn, Switzerland) that are both rigid and sharp. Rigidity is especially important when navigation is employed where only the outer end of the guide wire is held and the tip is extrapolated assuming a perfect linearity. Acuity helps to avoid the guide pin sliding off a bone entry site when there is an obtuse angle between guide and cortex.
- We mostly use *self-cutting self-tapping AO/ASIF 7.3-mm* set position and lag screws (Synthes Inc., Solothurn, Switzerland) that obviate the need for separate drilling and tapping steps. They can be employed immediately after correct placement of the guide wires is verified.
- Fully threaded *set position screws* are employed only when compression is unwanted or dangerous, e.g. in severe foraminal comminution, to fix the fragments in their current relative position. Since they do not compress the fracture they are biomechanically not as strong as lag screws. *Lag screws* that are only threaded a certain distance from their tip backwards exercise strong compression on the fracture and are used in all other cases. The length of threaded portion is chosen so that it lies entirely in the far fragment. Sometimes a lag screw is inserted first to achieve controlled compression that is than held with an additional set position screw.

Combinations of Minimally Invasive Reduction and Fixation Methods

The reduction and fixation methods outlined above can be used together in a variety of possible combinations as given in Table 16.1.

Image Guidance Methods

The main objective of percutaneous fixation is to place precisely an implant that is equally precisely adapted to the respective morphology. The main risks of percutaneous fixation are neurological injuries resulting from penetration of the intervertebral root or the vertebral canal. They and other vital structures like iliac and pelvic vessels or the sciatic nerve have to be safeguarded using image guidance.

16.10.1
Online Guidance

Online guidance denotes guidance through imaging or fluoroscopy while actually working on the patient:

- *2D-fluoroscopy* is a well established method in orthopedic surgery. Its drawbacks are poor depiction in obese or osteopenic persons or when gastrointestinal contrast media has been applied, operator dependence, 2D visualization only and potentially substantial radiation dose for patient and personnel. Inlet and outlet views are used to guide iliosacral screw fixation. Combined obturator–outlet views are helpful for acetabular roof screws. Intra-operative 2D-fluoroscopy is normally preceded by pre-operative CT to understand better the fracture and to detect 'dysmorphisms' (ROUTT et al. 2005) that may complicate or even preclude 2D-fluoroscopic guidance. Implant position is controlled by postoperative CT either routinely or on individual indication.
- *3D-fluoroscopy* using fan beam CT like the Iso-C3D (Siemens Medical Solutions, Erlangen, Germany) (KONIG et al. 2005) is the next generation of fluoroscopic devices. Currently the field of view of these systems is restricted to a cube of about 12 cm edge length, the soft tissue contrast resolution is lower and the noise substantially higher compared to a standard CT scanner.
- *Intra-operative CT* provides the most precise and most expensive guiding method. Guidance is performed like a standard CT or CT fluoroscopy-guided procedure. A striking advantage is that by the end of the procedure the post-operative control is already done. In strictly percutaneous procedures a normal CT suite may be sufficient from a hygienic point of view even when this has to be approved by the competent local authorities. A sterile operating room is a prerequisite for any open or hybrid procedure (JACOB et al. 2000b).

Table 16.1. Possible combinations of minimally invasive reduction and fixation methods

Procedure	Typical situation
Open or limited access reduction and internal fixation (ORIF/LARIF)	Standard or less invasive surgery
Open or limited access reduction and percutaneous fixation (ORPF/LARPF)	– When percutaneous fixation is possible after open reduction – Open release of neural compression combined with percutaneous fixation
Closed or percutaneous reduction and percutaneous fixation (CRPF/PRPF)	Standard minimally invasive technique in non-displaced or externally reducible fractures
Closed or percutaneous reduction and limited access fixation (CRLAF/PRLAF)	Limited surgical access for guided insertion of an implant when a vital structure is in the biomechanically optimal path

16.10.2
Offline Guidance

Offline guidance with medical navigation systems (MNS) provides simulation of continuous image guidance with the imager switched off (MESSMER et al. 2001). In this way it spares dose in X-ray dependent procedures and eventually the intraoperative imaging modality itself. Working with pre-scanned CT images may to a certain extent obviate intraoperative CT. MNS can offer guiding views that are not available during online imaging like multiplanar reconstructions or maximum intensity projections.

MNS are to minimally invasive technique what a global positioning system (GPS) is to car driving: They show the therapist where he or she is working in patient anatomy. There are three important elements to an MNS: The body in which to navigate, the map or image of that body and the instrument whose movements are followed with tracking and then displayed in the map.

There is also a very important disadvantage to every off-line MNS: It may not show you the truth. What you see on screen may not be what you actually get in instrument placement in the patient. A distance or difference between virtual and real world is called the "virtual-real mismatch". The operator has to be aware of this phenomenon and how to detect it with simple verification steps. There are two principle ways this mismatch may occur (MESSMER et al. 2001):

- The relation between map (imaging anatomy) and road (patient anatomy) has been lost. In the automotive world this could happen by the GPS not seeing enough satellites. In the operation room, an unperceived displacement of a reference base in regard to the piece of anatomy referenced, e.g. a vertebra may occur. This may unfortunately go undetected both by the MNS and by the operator.
- The road has changed but the map has not. This may happen when patient anatomy is altered by the procedure itself, like in a reduction process or even in a resection. If not all pieces of the anatomic puzzle are referenced and followed by the MNS this again will go undetected by the MNS rendering the display meaningless. The only way out is acquiring a new map, either by intraoperative imaging or by complex numerical methods elastically matching the old map to the new road (METZNER et al. 2006).

There exists a relatively wide variety of MNS that can be discerned from one another by the following criteria (Table 16.2):

- *Method of map acquisition and type of map produced.* This may be an imaging map produced by ultrasound, X-Ray, CT or MR imaging, or functional information gathered by kinematic measurements, e.g. the center of rotation of the femoral head. The latter obviously is only pos-

Table 16.2. Characteristics of navigation systems

Acquisition method	Type of map	Acquisition time	Registration necessary	Additional imaging necessary	Denomination	Remarks
Kinematic tracking of joint motion	Mechanical model	Pre-or Intra-procedural	No	No	Kinematic navigation (CT-less navigation)	
2D-fluoroscopy	2D-projectional	Intra-procedural	No	No	Fluoroscopy based navigation	
3D-fluoroscopy	3D	Intra-procedural	No	No	3D-Fluoroscopy based navigation	3D-map limited to field of view of fluoroscope
CT	3D	Pre-procedural	Yes	Yes/no	CT-based navigation	
CT	3D	Intra-procedural	No	No	CT-modality based navigation	
MRI	3D	Pre-procedural	Yes	Yes/no	MRI-based navigation	
CT	3D	Intra-procedural	No	No	MRI-modality based navigation	

sible in joints. The map may be 2D-projectional, 2D-tomographic or 3D (TAYLOR 1996).

- *Time of map acquisition.* This may be pre-operatively in a two-stage or intra-operatively in a single-stage approach. There are important implications to this. For a single-stage procedure you need the image modality of your choice in the therapy suite. In a two-stage procedure the concordance between map and anatomy is lost as soon as the patient moves after image acquisition, e.g. to go back to the ward. At the time of procedure you need to bring the map into agreement with the anatomy again by a process called registration. In a one-stage procedure the alignment between both worlds never gets lost (TAYLOR 1996).
- *Necessity of registration and accessory imaging.* Registration is done by identifying a sufficient number of common features in map and road to be able to calculate a transform between both worlds. Identifying the common features or landmarks is normally done by the therapist, the subsequent calculation by the MNS-software. In these procedures it may be necessary to do pre-operative imaging in addition to diagnostic imaging just for the purposes of registration and navigation which may defeat the concept of sparing dose by navigation altogether (SCHAEREN et al. 2002).
- *Type of tracking mechanism.* Most tracking systems today use passive or active optical markers that are localized by a 3D optical digitizer. Magnetic localizers are still limited in field of view and

accuracy, but do not depend on an unobstructed optical path between markers and localizer like the optical systems.

16.10.2.1
Fluoroscopy Based Navigation

In the last decade, fluoroscopy-based navigation systems have been widely introduced into surgical trauma applications. The use of computerized fluoroscopic navigation systems enables the simultaneous use of several radiographic projections. In navigated procedures several C-arm projections can be displayed simultaneously on the navigation screen (STOCKLE et al. 2004). With conventional fluoroscopy control for pelvic fracture treatment substantial fluoroscopy times are needed whereas in navigated procedures this time can be decreased markedly although at the expense of total procedure time (SUHM et al. 2004). Three-dimensional-fluoroscopy-based navigation is the newest incarnation of this method offering 3D-tomographic image maps.

16.10.2.2
CT and MR-Based Navigation

CT- and MR-based navigation has been used mostly in two stages and more rarely in single stage procedures. This is due to the fact that only very few institutions maintain a CT or an MR imaging machine with associated navigation capabilities in a sterile environment fit for open surgery (Figs. 16.9 and 16.10) (JACOB et al. 2000b; SUHM et al. 2004).

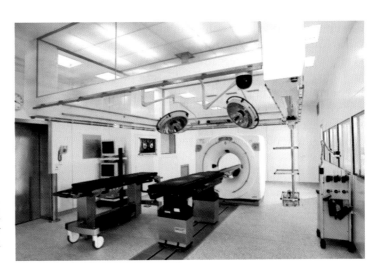

Fig. 16.9. The multifunctional image-guided therapy suite (MIGTS) in Basel University Hospital. Note large laminar air flow inlet cassette at the ceiling and CT in background

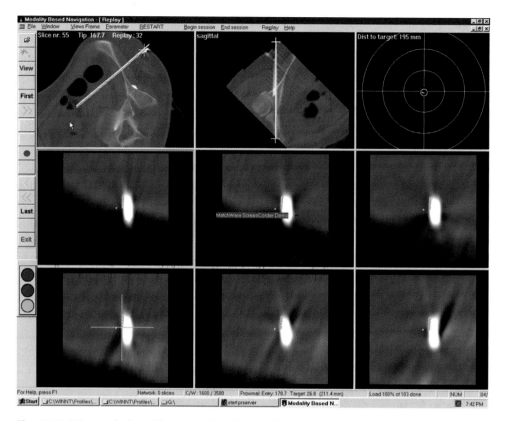

Fig. 16.10. CT-control after midway insertion of antegrade superior ramus screw with homebuilt navigation system in MIGTS. The control images have in turn been fed to the navigation system for a replay of the navigation process. First two images in upper row show current direction of guide pin in two planes with yellow lines. Third image in upper row presents an artificial horizon perpendicular to the target trajectory. If the yellow line is within the inner circle, guide pin closely follows planned trajectory. Last six images are sequential bird's eye views perpendicular to the target trajectory. Note that the guide pin lies nicely along the planned path

16.10.3
Robotic Assistance

Robotics has gone through some ups and especially downs in the last decade. Big ambitious projects failed (GLAUSER et al. 1995; SCHRADER 2005; SIEBERT et al. 2002). A more conservative approach not using an "active" robot actually performing the procedure but robotic assist devices like the Innomotion (Innomedic, Herxheim, Germany) that leave the proper medical act to the physician is probably more promising (Fig. 16.11) (CLEARY et al. 2006).

16.10.4
Placement and Immobilization

In most circumstances, and certainly with navigation and assist devices, it is necessary to immobilize the patient. We routinely use a vacuum mattress and broad adhesive tape for this purpose. Furthermore, in our experience it is most helpful to optimally present the injured side in such a way that the screw trajectories are 'as orthogonal as possible' – either vertically or horizontally (Fig. 16.12).

16.11
Typical Minimally Invasive Procedures

These include all methods that are less invasive than standard open reduction and internal fixation using the classical ilioinguinal or Kocher-Langebeck approaches. There are a relatively small number of typical access paths that are commonly used in pelvic and acetabular fractures.

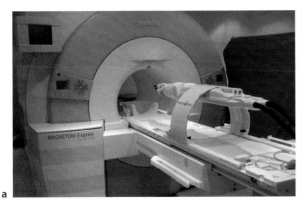

a

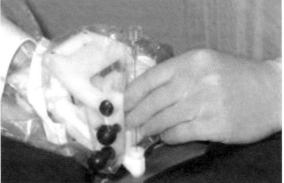

b

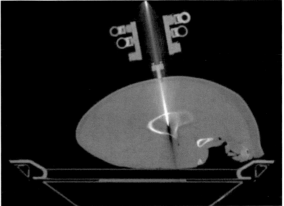

c

Fig. 16.11a–c. Innomotion assist device for MR and CT. **a** Setup with Siemens Espree Magnet. **b** Needle insertion through guide bush. **c** In vitro guide pin insertion under CT-control. Note the circular markers used to detect position of robotic arm

16.11.1
External Fixation of the Anterior Pelvic Ring

External fixation of the anterior pelvic ring is a viable alternative when there is substantial displacement and open reduction is not advisable from local or general contraindications. In our hands it is only used as a bridging maneuver. The fixator is applied using standard surgical techniques and a 2D-fluoroscope (MÜLLER et al. 1991).

16.11.2
Superior Pubic Ramus Screw

The retrograde superior pubic ramus screw was described first by ROUTT et al. (1995b). It is useful in non-displaced and non-comminuted fractures of the anterior acetabular pillar or the midportion of the superior pubic ramus. In these cases it can replace an anterior reconstruction plate fitted either through a formal or reduced ilioinguinal approach. It can also be introduced in a craniodorsal to caudoventral or antegrade fashion instead of the retrograde direction starting near the pubic symphysis.

The antegrade way is very demanding in terms of a long trajectory that requires very high targeting precision while the retrograde approach can fail because of interference with the genitals. The relatively big 7.3 mm cannulated screws are not an ideal implant for this technique especially because of the very narrow isthmic portion above and in front of the hip joint. Once inserted, though, they provide a firm fixation.

16.11.3
Iliosacral Screws

Iliosacral screws inserted from the lateral ilium across the sacroiliac joint and into the upper sacral vertebral body have become a popular form of posterior pelvic internal fixation in sacroiliac joint disruptions and sacral fractures (NELSON and DUWELIUS 1991; ROUTT et al. 1995a; SIMONIAN et al. 1994a). Numerous techniques for iliosacral screw insertion have been described using fluoroscopy, CT, and direct visual guidance. Iliosacral screws can be inserted with the patient in the supine, prone, or lateral position Fig. 16.13) (EBRAHEIM et al. 1987;

Fig. 16.12a–d. A 52-year-old woman with disruption of right sacroiliac joint. **a** Immobilization of the patient with broad adhesive tape on vacuum mattress. **b** Axial CT scan with patient in left lateral decubitus shows stable position as a result of good immobilization. Note perfect spontaneous reduction of right sacroiliac joint. **c** Axial CT scan at the end of the procedure shows the screw is positioned across the right sacroiliac joint. **d** Axial CT scan after subtraction of figures (**b**) and (**c**) shows almost perfect subtraction with only the screw remaining

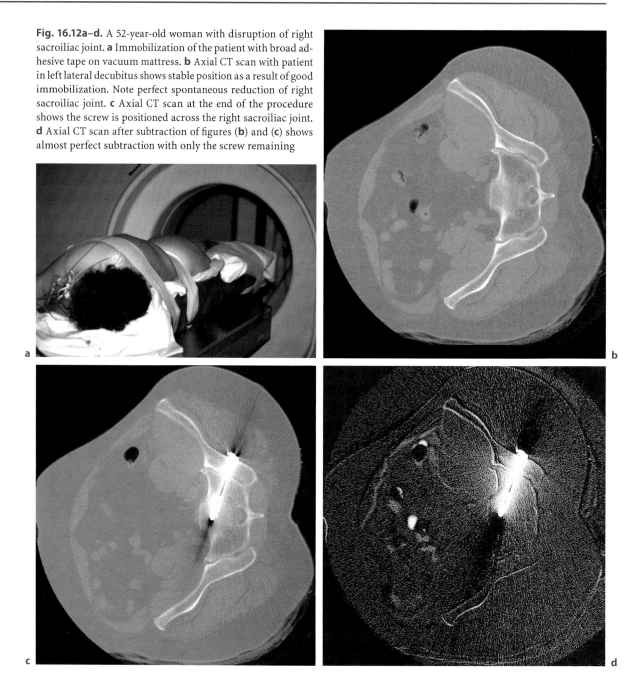

Fig. 16.13a–f. Planning of iliosacral compression screw in a 73-year-old woman with transforaminal fracture of the right sacral ala. **a** Axial CT scan with patient immobilized in lateral decubitus position shows open anterior reduction and fixation has already been performed with small residual dislocation. The first line is drawn from the target in the first sacral body to the skin entry to produce an approximate right angle between the trajectory and the fracture line (for best compression) as well as the outer cortex (to prevent slippage of the guide pin). Other factors are central position in both the near and far fragments, length of path within far fragment and avoidance of critical structures (sacral root, intravertrebral disk). **b** Axial CT scan demonstrates extrapolation of final position of guide pin. Guide pin has been placed at the outer cortex according to plan. Position is checked and extrapolated along the guide pin trajectory. **c** Axial CT scan shows outer end of rubber band measurement is advanced to the tip of the guide pin, thus indicating the remaining insertion depth for guide pin. **d** Axial CT scan shows final determination of screw length. Guide pin has been drilled to the final position. Intraosseous length is

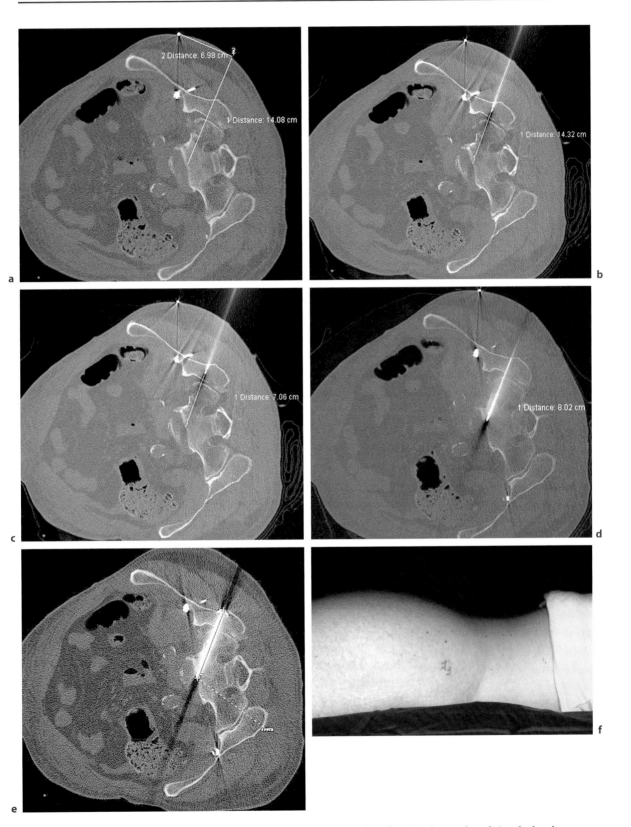

measured which corresponds to free screw length without screw head and washer. Total screw length is calculated as measured length plus approximately 5 mm for head and washer minus expected compression in cases of a substantial fracture gap. **e** Axial CT scan shows screw in place. **f** Clinical appearance of skin entry sites 2 months after procedure

Matta and Saucedo 1989; Routt et al. 1995a). The complications of iliosacral screw usage include fixation failures, misplaced screws, nerve injuries, infections, and poor posterior pelvic reduction, among others (Keating et al. 1999; Routt et al. 1995a).

We usually place and immobilize the patient on the contralateral side to achieve reduction by gravity and a nice target path. This approach may necessitate two placements in bilateral pathologies. Supine and prone positions both offer bilateral access. Iliosacral screw fixation in supine position may be difficult because the dorsolateral to ventrolateral trajectory of the guide pins may interfere with the operating room table and draping as well as imaging. Prone placement nicely presents both sides but may be associated with ventilation problems and tends to externally rotate the iliac wings if anterior fixation is not yet performed.

Iliosacral screws form a very strong construct that is biomechanically equal or superior to sacral bars and open or local plating (Pohlemann et al. 1993). Biomechanically, double iliosacral screw fixation achieves the strongest fixation in posterior pelvic ring disruptions (Yinger et al. 2003). In severely comminuted transforaminal fractures we employ set position screws to avoid further compression of the sacral foramina.

16.11.4
Acetabular Roof or Iliac Wing Screw

Gay (1992) described a series of six patients in which CT was used to guide percutaneous placement of cannulated 6.5-mm screws. The procedure was done in the CT suite under sterile conditions. Starr et al. (1998; 2001) fluoroscopically guided percutaneous screws to stabilize nondisplaced or minimally displaced acetabular fractures. The fluoroscopic technique is also useful for supplemental fixation combined with open reduction and internal fixation of complex acetabular fractures.

In cases of acetabular fractures without substantial steps or comminution the acetabular roof screw is a very nice tool to close the fracture gap and restore mechanical stability. We usually employ two screws, one close to the joint and one a little bit more cranially. The trajectory of the screws is dictated by the exact orientation of the fracture line and may sometimes require limited access to pull aside vital structures like the femoral nerve (Gross et al. 2004).

Generally we use an anterior approach (Fig. 16.14) as opposed to others that propose a posterior access where the sciatic nerve often precludes an optimal path of the screw (Jacob et al. 2000c).

16.11.5
Other Access Paths

In selected cases, we and others employed additional access paths like a "bottom-up" screw in transverse fractures of the posterior acetabular pillar (Fig. 16.15) or an iliac wing screw to close a gaping iliac crest. These paths are chosen according to the situation at hand.

16.12
Quality Criteria

The following quality criteria are taken from the literature and from our own experience. If these criteria are fulfilled a decent morphological and clinical result as well as a minimum of complications can be expected.

16.12.1
Clinical Criteria

- Good indication adapted to the individual situation
- Infection rate <1%
- Pain
- Function
- Rehabilitation and return to work

16.12.2
Imaging Criteria

All patients with surgically treated fractures of the pelvis and acetabulum at our institution undergo postoperative CT-control where the following observations are made (Jacob et al. 1997; Müller 1991):
- Screws should lie as close to perpendicular to the fracture gap as anatomically and/or technically possible.
- With lag screws, the threads should in their entirety lie in the distant fragment.

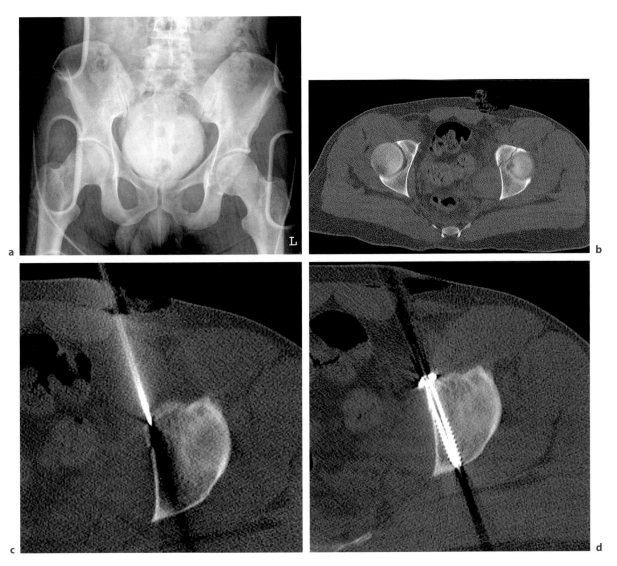

Fig. 16.14a–d. Left-sided acetabular fracture in a 19-year-old man who suffered a motor bike accident. **a** Anteroposterior X-ray of the pelvis shows a transverse fracture of the posterior column plus bilateral pubic and ischial fractures. **b** Axial CT scan of the left acetabulum demonstrates additional paracoronal fracture of anterior pillar not visible on the pelvic X-ray. **c** Axial CT scan of the pelvis shows limited access CT-guided screw fixation of anterior pillar through anterior approach with incision immediately lateral to the rectus muscle as planned on diagnostic CT. Surgical access to the anterior pillar is gained and the femoral neurovascular bundle is safely held to the side. A 2.8-mm guide pin is initially placed under direct side. Corrections and final placement are done under CT guidance. **d** Axial CT shows post procedure screw placement. The screw and thread length were determined by CT measurements

- With set position screws there should be no additional compression compared to the original images.
- In posterior ring fractures, the maximum offset in any direction (right-left, ventrodorsal, craniocaudal) should be less than 10 mm.
- Superior pubic ramus screws should splint both fragments centrally a sufficient distance. The residual dislocation must therefore be just large enough to allow passage of the screw in the marrow canal.
- If the load bearing articular surface of the hip joint is affected, residual gaps should be ≤3 mm and steps ≤1 mm.
- No perforation of hardware into the hip joint should be visible.

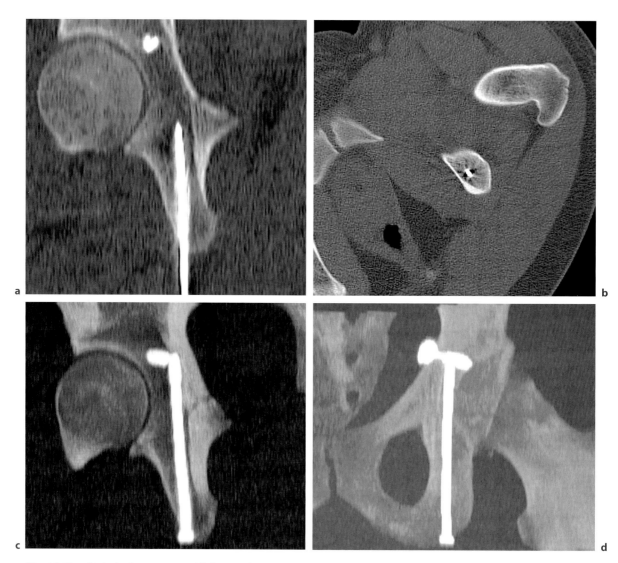

Fig. 16.15a–d. Limited access CT-guided screw fixation of posterior pillar through "bottom-up" approach in a 26-year-old man injured when a wall collapsed on him. Patient is placed in contralateral decubitus with as much flexion in the ipsilateral hip joint as possible while still allowing the patient to pass through the CT gantry. Incision is then done over the tip of the ischial bone which should be easily palpable. Again, the ischial bone is exposed while taking care not to damage the sciatic nerve and a 2.8-mm guide pin is placed by hand under direct sight. **a** Coronal 2D CT reconstruction shows subsequent placement of guide pin and screw again performed under CT guidance. **b** Axial CT scan shows single slice CT is of almost no help in cases where the main direction of the implant is axial. This situation requires the use of multiplanar reconstructions based on spiral CT. A navigation system or robotic-assistance can help to keep the necessary control scans to a minimum. **c** Coronal 2D CT reconstruction shows final position of bottom-up screw across the transverse fracture of the posterior acetabular column. Note compression of fracture, short 16 mm thread fully within contralateral fragment and close proximity of screw tip to the previously inserted acetabular roof screw. **d** 3D maximum intensity projection CT shows final position of the screw across the fracture

Table 16.3. Reported results in the literature of iliosacral screw fixation

Author	van den Bosch et al.	Peng et al.	Arand et al.[a]	Stöckle et al.	Grützner et al.	Jacob et al.	Keating et al.
Year	2002	2006	2004	2004	2002	1997	1999
N patients.	88	18	9	28 screws	7 pts	13	38
N screws	285		9	28 screws	7 pts		85
Implant	7.3-mm cannulated screws			7.3-mm cannulated screws			
Patient position							22 prone, 16 supine
Guidance method	2D-fluoroscopy	Single-plane vs biplane 2D-fluoroscopy	2D-fluoroscopy based navigation	2D-fluoroscopy based navigation		CT-navigation	
Procedure times		45.0 vs 16.0 min	44 min				
'Dose'		5.7 vs 4.5 min fluoroscopy time					
Malpositioned screws @ postoperative imaging modality	7% (15/220) @ CT 44% (4/9) in pts with neurologic complaints)	0/? @ radiography	5% (1/22) @ CT due to bending of guide wire	1/28 @ CT	0-2/14	0/27	13% (5/38) pts @ radiography
Early complications	Neurologic complications in 8% (7/88 pts) necessitating re-operation.19% (6/31 pts) with screw in second sacral body had neurologic complications	1/18 superficial wound infection		1 malreduction of the posterior pelvic ring noticed in the postoperative X-ray			13% (5/38) pulmonary embolism 14% (3/22) deep infection in pts with ORIF, 0% (0/16) in pts with CRPF
Follow-up	11.6 mos						?
Non-union							44% (15/34) malunions 57% (4/7) malunions in pts without anterior fixation
Functional result							85% (22/26) troublesome pain
Late complications							26% (10/38) 'gradual loss of reduction' @ 2 mos

[a] Relative migration of the iliac and sacral bone structures between CT scans taken preoperatively and intraoperative navigation may result in an intolerable inaccuracy of computer guidance

16.13
Results

Table 16.3 provides an overview of published results of minimally invasive pelvic surgery. In a recent report of 2D-fluoroscopy guidance in B-type fractures up to 8% (7/88) of all patients and 19% (6/31) of the subgroup with a screw in the second sacral body exhibited neurological complaints and needed reoperation for iliosacral screw fixation. There were 7% (15/220) malpositioned screws in all the patients who underwent postoperative CT and 44% (4/9) in the subgroup with neurologic complaints (VAN DEN BOSCH et al. 2003). This is in contrast to better results reported earlier. It also demonstrates the obvious fact that patients with malpositioned screws are at much higher risk for iatrogenic neurologic injury.

Excellent results have been published for acetabular fractures with 2D-fluoroscopy guidance by STARR et al. (1998, 2001). Very precise results have been obtained for CT-guidance by several groups for iliosacral as well as acetabular screw fixation. Excellent results have been reported for both 2D-fluoroscopy and CT-based navigation systems.

KEATING et al. (1999) reported surprisingly high rates of pulmonary embolism, deep infection, late loss of reduction and pain. It is of note, though, that 58% (22/38) of their patients actually underwent open reduction and internal fixation and not closed reduction and percutaneous fixation.

16.14
Indications for Minimally-Invasive Therapy

This is our resume of the literature and our own experience. Other opinions may exist.

16.14.1
Superior Pubic Ramus

The percutaneous antegrade or retrograde superior pubic ramus screw is indicated as the anterior component of unstable pelvic ring fracture stabilization if a straight and sufficiently wide trajectory for the passage of the screw within the superior pubic ramus and clear of the hip joint can be found. This assumes either a small primary displacement or a good reduction (ROUTT et al. 1995b).

16.14.2
Sacrum, Ilium and Sacroiliac Joint

16.14.2.1
Fractures and Fracture-Dislocations

- Percutaneous iliosacral screws are indicated as the posterior component of unstable pelvic ring fracture stabilization if there is either a small primary displacement or a good reduction could be achieved.
- In comminuted sacral fractures involving the foramina or the canal set position screws should be used either exclusively or after controlled compression with a lag screw. This control can be performed intraoperatively either visually by CT or functionally by somatosensory evoked potentials (MOED et al. 1998).

16.14.2.2
Other Indications

There are reports about the use of iliosacral screws in sacroiliac joint arthritis and metastatic destruction (EBRAHEIM and BIYANI 2003) as well as postpartum pelvic pain and sacral nonunion (HUEGLI et al. 2003; VAN DEN BOSCH et al. 2002). All of these indications must still be considered experimental.

16.14.3
Acetabulum

In our hands we minimally-invasively treat acetabular fractures which exhibit all of the following criteria (GAY et al. 1992; GROSS et al. 2004; JACOB et al. 2000c):
- Two or at least very few fragments of the load bearing portion
- Far fragment big enough to accommodate threaded portion of lag screw
- No intra-articular fragments
- No or very small articular step-off or impression

16.15
Conclusion

Minimally-invasive percutaneous screw fixation of the pelvic ring in combination with closed, minimal-access or open reduction can be successfully applied to a variety of sacral, iliac and pubic fractures and combinations thereof. Iliosacral and superior pubic ramus screws are the most prominent and widely used examples of this technique.

The same holds true for acetabular fractures with the restriction that a minute reduction of joint surfaces has to be achieved before percutaneous fixation is attempted to prevent premature osteoarthritis.

A rational interdisciplinary selection of the best treatment modality – be it open, hybrid, or closed – is of paramount importance and often is the most difficult part of the process. High quality pre-operative and intra-operative imaging, image-guidance, navigation or robotic-assistance are all essential for an equally high quality of surgical results.

References

Arand M, Kinzl L, Gebhard F (2004) Computer-guidance in percutaneous screw stabilization of the iliosacral joint. Clin Orthop Relat Res 422:201–207

Ben-Menachem Y, Coldwell DM, Young JW, Burgess AR (1991) Hemorrhage associated with pelvic fractures: causes, diagnosis, and emergent management. AJR Am J Roentgenol 157:1005–1014

Cleary K, Melzer A, Watson V, Kronreif G, Stoianovici D (2006) Interventional robotic systems: applications and technology state-of-the-art. Minim Invasive Ther Allied Technol 15:101–113

Ebraheim NA, Biyani A (2003) Percutaneous computed tomographic stabilization of the pathologic sacroiliac joint. Clin Orthop Relat Res 408:252–255

Ebraheim NA, Rusin JJ, Coombs RJ, Jackson WT, Holiday B (1987) Percutaneous computed-tomography-stabilization of pelvic fractures: preliminary report. J Orthop Trauma 1:197–204

Falchi M, Rollandi GA (2004) CT of pelvic fractures. Eur J Radiol 50:96–105

Fell M, Meissner A, Rahmanzadeh R (1995) Long-term outcome after conservative treatment of pelvic ring injuries and conclusions for current management. Zentralbl Chir 120:899-904

Gansslen A, Pohlemann T, Paul C, Lobenhoffer P, Tscherne H (1996) Epidemiology of pelvic ring injuries. Injury 27(Suppl 1): S-A13–20

Gansslen A, Hufner T, Krettek C (2006) Percutaneous iliosacral screw fixation of unstable pelvic injuries by conventional fluoroscopy. Oper Orthop Traumatol 18:225–244

Gay SB, Sistrom C, Wang GJ, Kahler DA, Boman T, McHugh N, Goitz HT (1992) Percutaneous screw fixation of acetabular fractures with CT guidance: preliminary results of a new technique. AJR Am J Roentgenol 158:819–822

Glauser D, Fankhauser H, Epitaux M, Hefti JL, Jaccottet A (1995) Neurosurgical robot Minerva: first results and current developments. J Image Guid Surg 1:266–272

Goldstein A, Phillips T, Sclafani SJ, Scalea T, Duncan A, Goldstein J, Panetta T, Shaftan G (1986) Early open reduction and internal fixation of the disrupted pelvic ring. J Trauma 26:325–333

Gross T, Jacob AL, Messmer P, Regazzoni P, Steinbrich W, Huegli RW (2004) Transverse acetabular fracture: hybrid minimal access and percutaneous CT-navigated fixation. AJR Am J Roentgenol 183:1000–1002

Grützner PA, Rose E, Vock B, Holz F, Nolte LP, Wentzensen A (2002) Computerassisted screw osteosynthesis of the posterior pelvic ring. Initial experiences with an image reconstruction based optoelectronic navigation system. [German] Unfallchirurgie 105:254–260

Gruson KI, Moed BR (2003) Injury of the femoral nerve associated with acetabular fracture. J Bone joint Surg 85-A:428–431

Guillamondegui OD, Pryor JP, Gracias VH, Gupta R, Reilly PM, Schwab CW (2002) Pelvic radiography in blunt trauma resuscitation: a diminishing role. J Trauma 53:1043–1047

Haidukewych GJ, Scaduto J, Herscovici D, Sanders RW, DiPasquale T (2002) Iatrogenic nerve injury in acetabular fracture surgery: a comparison of monitored and unmonitored procedures. J Orthop Trauma 16:297–301

Huegli RW, Messmer P, Jacob AL, Regazzoni P, Styger S, Gross T (2003) Delayed union of a sacral fracture: percutaneous navigated autologous cancellous bone grafting and screw fixation. Cardiovasc Intervent Radiol 26:502–505

Hunter JC, Brandser EA, Tran KA (1997) Pelvic and acetabular trauma. Radiol Clin North Am 35:559–590

Isler B, Ganz R (1996) Classification of pelvic ring injuries. Injury 27(Suppl 1): S-A3-12

Jacob AL, Messmer P, Stock KW, Suhm N, Baumann B, Regazzoni P, Steinbrich W (1997) Posterior pelvic ring fractures: closed reduction and percutaneous CT-guided sacroiliac screw fixation. Cardiovasc Intervent Radiol 20:285–294

Jacob AL, Kaim A, Baumann B, Suhm N, Messmer P (2000a) A simple device for continuous leg extension during CT-guided interventions. AJR Am J Roentgenol 174:1687–1688

Jacob AL, Regazzoni P, Steinbrich W, Messmer P (2000b) The multifunctional therapy room of the future: image guidance, interdisciplinarity, integration and impact on patient pathways. Eur Radiol 10:1763–1769

Jacob AL, Suhm N, Kaim A, Regazzoni P, Steinbrich W, Messmer P (2000c) Coronal acetabular fractures: the anterior approach in computed tomography-navigated minimally invasive percutaneous fixation. Cardiovasc Intervent Radiol 23:327–331

Judet R, Judet J, Letournel E (1964) Fractures of the acetabulum: classification and surgical approaches for open reduction. Preliminary report. J Bone Joint Surg Am 46:1615–1646

Kaempffe FA, Bone LB, Border JR (1991) Open reduction and internal fixation of acetabular fractures: heterotopic ossification and other complications of treatment. J Orthop Trauma 5:439–445

Keating JF, Werier J, Blachut P, Broekhuyse H, Meek RN, O'Brien PJ (1999) Early fixation of the vertically unstable pelvis: the role of iliosacral screw fixation of the posterior lesion. J Orthop Trauma 13:107–113

Kellam JF (1989) The role of external fixation in pelvic disruptions. Clin Orthop Relat Res 241:66–82

Kellam JF, McMurtry RY, Paley D, Tile M (1987) The unstable pelvic fracture. Operative treatment. Orthop Clin North Am 18:25–41

Kloen P, Siebenrock KA, Ganz R (2002) Modification of the ilioinguinal approach. J Orthop Trauma 16:586–593

Konig B, Erdmenger U, Schroder RJ, Wienas G, Schaefer J, Pech M, Stockle U (2005) Evaluation of image quality of the Iso C3D image processor in comparison to computer tomography. Use in the pelvic area. Unfallchirurg 108:378–385

Letournel E (1981) Surgical treatment of fractures of the acetabulum: results over a twenty-five year period. Chirurgie 107:229–236

Letournel E (1993) The treatment of acetabular fractures through the ilioinguinal approach. Clin Orthop Relat Res 292:62–76

Matta JM, Saucedo T (1989) Internal fixation of pelvic ring fractures. Clin Orthop Relat Res 242:83–97

Matta JM, Letournel E, Browner BD (1986) Surgical management of acetabular fractures. Instr Course Lect 35:382–397

Messmer P, Baumann B, Suhm N, Jacob AL (2001) Navigation systems for image-guided therapy: a review. RoFo 173:777–784

Metzner R, Eisenmann U, Wirtz CR, Dickhaus H (2006) Pre- and intraoperative processing and integration of various anatomical and functional data in neurosurgery. Stud Health Technol Inform 124:989–994

Moed BR, Ahmad BK, Craig JG, Jacobson GP, Anders MJ (1998) Intraoperative monitoring with stimulus-evoked electromyography during placement of iliosacral screws. An initial clinical study. J Bone Joint Surg 80:537–546

Müller ME, Perren SM, Allgöwer M (1991) Manual of internal fixation: techniques recommended by the AO-ASIF Group, 3rd edn. Springer, Berlin Heidelberg New York

Nelson DW, Duwelius PJ (1991) CT-guided fixation of sacral fractures and sacroiliac joint disruptions. Radiology 180:527–532

Oransky M, Tortora M (2007) Nonunions and malunions after pelvic fractures: why they occur and what can be done? Injury 38:489–496

Peng KT, Huang KC, Chen MC, Li YY, Hsu RW (2006) Percutaneous placement of iliosacral screws for unstable pelvic ring injuries: comparison between one and two C-arm fluoroscopic techniques. Trauma 60:602–608

Pennal GF, Tile M, Waddell JP, Garside H (1980) Pelvic disruption: assessment and classification. Clin Orthop Relat Res 151:12–21

Pohlemann T, Angst M, Schneider E, Ganz R, Tscherne H (1993) Fixation of transforaminal sacrum fractures: a biomechanical study. J Orthop Trauma 7:107–117

Pohlemann T, Bosch U, Gansslen A, Tscherne H (1994) The Hannover experience in management of pelvic fractures. Clin Orthop Relat Res 305:69–80

Poole GV, Ward EF (1994) Causes of mortality in patients with pelvic fractures. Orthopedics 17:691–696

Qureshi AA, Archdeacon MT, Jenkins MA, Infante A, DiPasquale T, Bolhofner BR (2004) Infrapectineal plating for acetabular fractures: a technical adjunct to internal fixation. J Orthop Trauma 18:175–178

Reinert CM, Bosse MJ, Poka A, Schacherer T, Brumback RJ, Burgess AR (1988) A modified extensile exposure for the treatment of complex or malunited acetabular fractures. J Bone Joint Surg 70:329–337

Routt ML, Kregor PJ, Simonian PT, Mayo KA (1995a) Early results of percutaneous iliosacral screws placed with the patient in the supine position. J Orthop Trauma 9:207–214

Routt ML, Simonian PT, Grujic L (1995b) The retrograde medullary superior pubic ramus screw for the treatment of anterior pelvic ring disruptions: a new technique. J Orthop Trauma 9:35–44

Routt ML, Nork SE, Mills WJ (2005) Percutaneous fixation of pelvic ring disruptions. Clin Orthop Relat Res 415:15–29

Schaeren S, Roth J, Dick W (2002) Effective in vivo radiation dose with image reconstruction controlled pedicle instrumentation vs. CT-based navigation. Orthopade 31:392–396

Schrader P (2005) Technique evaluation for orthopedic use of Robodoc. Z Orthop Ihre Grenzgeb 143:329–336

Senst W, Bida B (2000) Expert assessment of pelvic injuries. Zentralbl Chir 125:737–743

Siebert W, Mai S, Kober R, Heeckt PF (2002) Technique and first clinical results of robot-assisted total knee replacement. Knee 9:173–180

Simonian PT, Routt ML, Harrington RM, Mayo KA, Tencer AF (1994a) Biomechanical simulation of the anteroposterior compression injury of the pelvis. An understanding of instability and fixation. Clin Orthop Relat Res 309:245–256

Simonian PT, Routt ML, Harrington RM, Tencer AF (1994b) Internal fixation of the unstable anterior pelvic ring: a biomechanical comparison of standard plating techniques and the retrograde medullary superior pubic ramus screw. J Orthop Trauma 8:476–482

Slatis P, Huittinen VM (1972) Double vertical fractures of the pelvis. A report on 163 patients. Acta Chir Scand 138:799–807

Starr AJ, Reinert CM, Jones AL (1998) Percutaneous fixation of the columns of the acetabulum: a new technique. J Orthop Trauma 12:51–58

Starr AJ, Jones AL, Reinert CM, Borer DS (2001) Preliminary results and complications following limited open reduction and percutaneous screw fixation of displaced fractures of the acetabulum. Injury 32(Suppl 1):SA45–50

Stockle U, Krettek C, Pohlemann T, Messmer P (2004) Clinical applications–pelvis. Injury 35(Suppl 1):S-A46–56

Suhm N, Messmer P, Zuna I, Jacob LA, Regazzoni P (2004) Fluoroscopic guidance versus surgical navigation for distal locking of intramedullary implants. A prospective, controlled clinical study. Injury 35:567–574

Taylor RH (1996) Computer-integrated surgery: technology and clinical applications. MIT Press, Cambridge

Tile M (1996) Acute pelvic fractures: I. Causation and classification. J Am Acad Orthop Surg 4:143–151

Tile M (2003) Fractures of the pelvis and acetabulum, 3rd edn. Williams & Wilkins, Baltimore

van den Bosch EW, van Zwienen CM, van Vugt AB (2002) Fluoroscopic positioning of sacroiliac screws in 88 patients. J Trauma 53:44–48

van den Bosch EW, van Zwienen CM, Hoek van Dijke GA, Snijders CJ, van Vugt AB (2003) Sacroiliac screw fixation for tile B fractures. J Trauma 55:962–965

van Olden GD, Meeuwis JD, Bolhuis HW, Boxma H, Goris RJ (2004) Advanced trauma life support study: quality of diagnostic and therapeutic procedures. J Trauma 57:381–384

Wedegartner U, Gatzka C, Rueger JM, Adam G (2003) Multislice CT (MSCT) in the detection and classification of pelvic and acetabular fractures. RoFo 175:105–111

Yinger K, Scalise J, Olson SA, Bay BK, Finkemeier CG (2003) Biomechanical comparison of posterior pelvic ring fixation. J Orthop Trauma 17:481–487

Interventional Vascular Radiology in Musculoskeletal Lesions

17

PAULA KLURFAN, KAREL G. TERBRUGGE, KONGTENG TAN, and MARTIN E. SIMONS

CONTENTS

17.1   Introduction   367

17.2   Vascular Malformations   368
17.2.1 Classification   368
17.2.2 Clinical Diagnosis of
       Vascular Malformation   368

17.3   Arteriovenous Shunts   368
17.3.1 Intramuscular Arteriovenous Shunts   369
17.3.2 Cutaneous Arteriovenous Shunts   369
17.3.3 Intraosseous Arteriovenous Shunts   370
17.3.4 Treatment of Arteriovenous Shunts   370

17.4   Arteriolar-Capillary Malformations   372

17.5   Capillary-Venous Malformations and
       Venous Vascular Malformations   373
17.5.1 Venous Vascular Malformations   374

17.6   Lymphatic Malformations   378
17.6.1 Macrocystic and Microcystic
       Malformations   378
17.6.2 Mixed Vascular Malformations   378

17.7   Metameric Arteriovenous Shunts   379

17.8   Klippel-Trenaunay and Parkes Weber
       Syndromes   379

17.9   Endovascular Management of
       Musculoskeletal Tumors   379

17.10 Conclusion   382

       References   383

P. KLURFAN, MD, Clinical Fellow in Interventional Neuro-
radiology
K. G. TERBRUGGE, MD, FRCP, Professor of Radiology and
Surgery, Head, Division of Neuroradiology
M. E. SIMONS, BSc, MD, FRCPC, Assistant Professor of
Medical Imaging
Department of Radiology, Toronto Western Hospital,
University of Toronto, 399 Bathurst Street, 3-East Wing,
Toronto, ON M5T 2S8, Canada
K. TAN, MD, FRCS, FRCR, Assistant Professor
Department of Radiology, University Health Network,
University of Toronto, NCSB, 1C563, 585 University Avenue,
Toronto, ON M5G 2N2, Canada

17.1 Introduction

Vascular malformations are errors of vascular morphogenesis (FISHMAN and MULLIKEN 1993; MULLIKEN and GLOWACKI 1982). Although generally considered to be present at birth, they are usually not apparent, and become evident or symptomatic only later in life. They grow in proportion to the growth of the affected child, but may increase in size secondary to specific triggering factors, including hemodynamic or rheological changes such as increased blood flow, resulting in vessel elongation and dilation, obstruction or thrombosis. The development of individual lesions, especially high-flow lesions, may be stimulated by various factors, including endocrine (puberty, pregnancy), trauma and iatrogenic insults such as incomplete surgery, proximal embolization and infection. Most vascular malformations are not visible at birth and only become apparent over time. A quiescent preexisting defect must be postulated, as well as the influence of revealing triggers. Vascular malformations may correspond to a defective remodeling process.

Although curative management would be ideal, the price to achieve this may not justify the risk, and therefore a less ideal and less aggressive intervention (closing a high flow arteriovenous fistula, reducing the venous hypertension, etc.) may palliate the symptoms or slow the evolution of the disease.

In children under 10 years of age with symptomatic vascular lesions involving the musculoskeletal system, additional problems arise that do not occur in adults, such as the natural growth and maturation of the skeleton, and the potential for growth of the lesion with stimulation and induction of angiogenesis, which interferes with bone growth. However, early intervention can arrest and even reverse such changes.

Endovascular management of musculoskeletal tumors has become useful and effective in recent years. Highly vascular lesions such as benign (aneurysmal bone cyst, giant-cell tumor, hemangioma, osteoid osteoma and osteoblastoma) and malignant lesions (chondrosarcoma, osteosarcoma and metastases) can now be safely treated endovascularly to reduce their size, lowering risk and facilitating surgical resection, or for palliative purposes.

17.2
Vascular Malformations

17.2.1
Classification

Vascular malformations are classified according to the particular segment or segments of the vascular tree that are affected by the malformation (Burrows et al. 1983; Jackson et al. 1993; Mulliken and Glowacki 1982; Bhattacharya et al. 2001).
Accordingly we can distinguish:

- Arteriovenous vascular malformations (fistulas, nidi)
- Arteriolar-capillary vascular malformations
- Capillary vascular malformations
- Capillary-venous vascular malformations
- Venous vascular malformations
- Veno-lymphatic vascular malformations
- Lymphatic vascular malformations
- Metameric vascular malformations

17.2.2
Clinical Diagnosis of Vascular Malformation

The diagnosis of a vascular malformation is usually made clinically, from the patient's history and physical examination. Judicial use of cross sectional non-invasive imaging is helpful to determine the extent of the lesion and to demonstrate associated lesions or multifocality of involvement. Rarely is there a need for any invasive procedures to establish the diagnosis and the type of malformation involved.
Magnetic resonance (MR) imaging is the most useful single imaging modality in the investigation of vascular malformations. The combination of multiplanar spin echo imaging and flow-sensitive sequences permits characterization of the nature and extent of most lesions. Computed tomography (CT) is less helpful in defining flow characteristics and the extent of vascular malformations, but has a role in demonstrating the nature and extent of bony

involvement, and the presence of phleboliths, which are pathognomonic of venous malformations. Ultrasound, including Doppler techniques, can determine tissue and flow characteristics in superficial lesions, and may be helpful in guiding the direct puncture of venous malformations. Plain radiographs are useful mainly to document bony changes. Angiography is reserved for intervention and may be necessary to confirm the diagnosis and to demonstrate the angioarchitecture of the soft tissue capillary or arteriovenous malformations or fistulas.

17.3
Arteriovenous Shunts

An arteriovenous shunt consists of a network of abnormal vascular channels (nidus) or a direct communicating channel (fistula) (Fig. 17.1) interposed between feeding arteries and draining veins. Except for the extremely rare high-flow lesions, which can present with cardiac overload in infancy, most soft tissue arteriovenous shunts are usually asymptomatic during the first two decades of life. They often manifest as a cutaneous blush, with or without underlying soft tissue hypertrophy. Clinical findings include local hyperthermia, pulsations, thrill and bruit. The high flow of arteriovenous shunts may lead to increased cardiac output, which can be symptomatic. The symptomatic evolution of these lesions often seems to be precipitated by hormonal factors (puberty, pregnancy, and hormonal therapy), trauma, infection or iatrogenic factors (surgery, embolization). Venous hypertension may result in tissue ischemia, ultimately leading to pain and skin ulceration, often associated with severe bleeding.

17.3.1
Intramuscular Arteriovenous Shunts

Intramuscular arteriovenous malformations may be associated with pain. These arteriovenous lesions are rarely limited to a single muscle. Some lesions are small (micro arteriovenous malformations) and clinically difficult to detect. They appear as recurrent hematomas, particularly in the muscle where the lysed hematoma may be diagnosed as a cystic lesion that bled secondarily. Surgical exploration of these lesions demonstrates small malformations on the wall of the cavity.

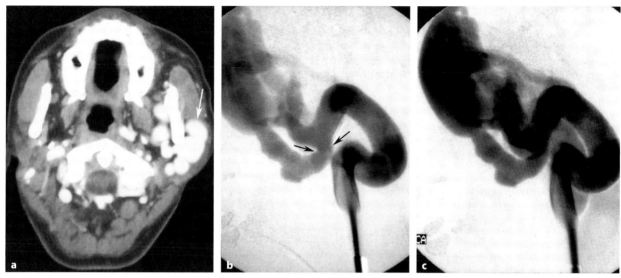

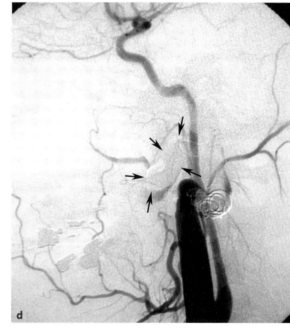

Fig. 17.1a–d. Slowly enlarging pulsatile-mass lesion involving the left cheek in a 12-year-old boy due to a facial arteriovenous shunt. **a** Axial contrast-enhanced CT scans demonstrate prominent vascular channels (*arrow*) in the left preauricular area. Left lateral external carotid angiograms in (**b**) early and (**c**) late arterial phase demonstrate a single hole fistulous communication (*arrows*) between the proximal internal maxillary artery and an adjacent facial vein. Transarterial single balloon detachment was performed at the site of the fistula, resulting in immediate and complete obliteration of the fistula; several coils were deposited in the proximal external carotid artery for added protection. **d** Post embolization left lateral common carotid angiogram demonstrates closure of the arteriovenous fistula. Note the cast of the single balloon (*arrows*) and the discrepancy between the grossly enlarged proximal trunk of the external carotid artery and the size of the internal carotid artery

17.3.2
Cutaneous Arteriovenous Shunts

Cutaneous arteriovenous shunts initially demonstrate a superficial blush and warmth. As they develop, the color intensifies and tortuous, tense veins may appear. Dystrophic changes, ulceration, bleeding and persistent pain may follow. MR imaging confirms the diagnosis of an arteriovenous malformation and will demonstrate its extent, although it is often difficult to distinguish between the actual nidus and the feeding and draining ves-

sels. Trauma is a frequent source of lesional growth with hemorrhagic complications, particularly in children.

17.3.3
Intraosseous Arteriovenous Shunts

Intraosseous arteriovenous shunts are rare and have been over-diagnosed in most instances. The misdiagnosis results from an erroneous interpretation of associated features caused by a superficial soft tissue arteriovenous malformation. The associated bone hypertrophy results from the indirect consequences of venous and lymphatic interference by the adjacent subcutaneous or muscular lesion, and must be distinguished from truly intraosseous vascular malformations (Lum and TerBrugge 2002). Throughout the years many authors have advocated various treatment strategies for intraosseous vascular malformations of the bony skeleton, including embolization, surgical resection and combined treatments. Immediate results usually have been successful regardless of the methods employed; however, long-term outcomes are disappointing, with "recurrence" of the malformations and occasionally progression of disease. Proximal vessel ligation by surgery or embolization does little to decrease blood flow since recruitment of new feeding vessels quickly reestablishes blood supply to the lesion, and the reactive nonsprouting angiogenesis may become indistinguishable from the nidus, which should be avoided at all costs. Only complete "removal", either by surgical resection or embolic devascularization of the vascular malformation, results in a "cure". "Cure" is defined as the complete eradication of disease resulting in permanent resolution of symptoms.

17.3.4
Treatment of Arteriovenous Shunts

Management of extremity arteriovenous malformations is problematic due to the rarity of the condition, which makes it difficult for clinicians to gain sufficient experience to provide optimum treatment. Upton et al. (1999), White et al. (2000), Sofocleous et al. (2001) and Tan et al. (2004) noted this problem when they presented the results of their long-term studies. Our experience with noncentral nervous system head and neck, as well as limb and body, arteriovenous shunts includes 121 patients since 1985. We have been using tissue adhesive (glue, N-butyl-cyanoacrylate [NBCA]) almost exclusively for endovascular treatment, occasionally supplemented with or replaced by polyvinyl alcohol if the nidal angioarchitecture is "angiomatous" and of the slow-flow type. Single hole arteriovenous fistulas can be treated efficiently with either detachable balloons or coils (Fig. 17.1) depending on the angioarchitecture of the feeding vessel and draining vein, and the comfort of the interventional therapist with such devices.

The guiding principle is to obliterate the arteriovenous shunt with a permanent embolic agent using a specific treatment (Figs. 17.2, 17.3). If such an approach is unlikely to be feasible, then combined approaches should be considered; the endovascular treatment strategy and choice of embolic materials will vary to facilitate surgical eradication. If, on the other hand, complete eradication cannot be obtained with combined approaches and a clinical manifestation requires stabilization, we recommend partial, targeted endovascular control of the lesion with liquid embolic agents.

In general, we are opposed to partial surgical treatment, which in our experience often further triggers these arteriovenous lesions. Such surgery may be warranted when severe functional or life threatening bleeding needs to be controlled, although most of the time this can also be achieved by transarterial or direct percutaneous embolization (Figs. 17.4, 17.5). In many cases, the subsequent increase of the abnormal network is rendered difficult to treat, as it involves normal, reactive vascularization. Any attempt at this stage to correct the appearance leads to ischemic manifestations, including true angiogenesis. We also try to delay major surgical reconstructions involving the skeleton until growth is complete.

Treatment must be planned carefully to avoid stimulating progression or interference with future management. In particular, proximal ligation, embolization or coiling of feeding vessels must be avoided. Superselective targeted arterial embolization is indicated to decrease symptoms, such as pain, bleeding and ischemic ulceration. When possible, it should be performed with permanent agents, such as tissue adhesive. If superselective catheterization of the arteriovenous shunt cannot be achieved, then a percutaneous approach is performed using the same principles of deposition of the permanent embolic in to the nidus (Figs. 17.4, 17.5).

Our embolization technique is derived from our longstanding experience with endovascular treatment of central nervous system arteriovenous malformations. A microcatheter is advanced coaxially through a 4- or 5-French catheter as close as possible to the nidus of the malformation. We dilute the tissue adhesive (NBCA) with Lipiodol in a 1:2 to 1:5 ratio, depending on the flow rate of the shunt. The glue is mixed just prior to injection. The microcatheter is flushed with dextrose and the glue is injected slowly until there is reflux along the catheter tip and no forward flow is seen. Penetration of the embolic

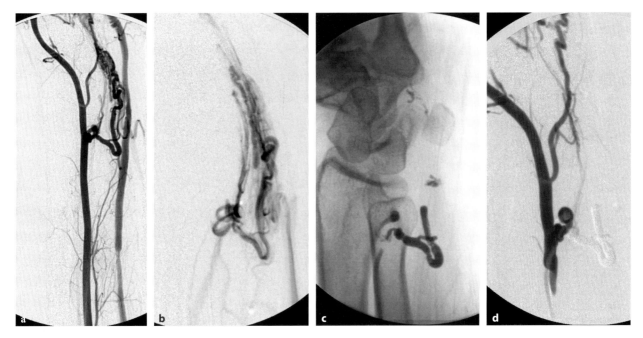

Fig. 17.2a–d. Pain, swelling and numbness of the left hand in a 30-year-old woman due to arteriovenous malformation. **a** Lateral angiogram of the left wrist shows the arteriovenous malformation supplied by the left radial artery and the superficial palmar arch of the ulnar artery. Lateral angiogram views show (**b**) selective catheterization of the left radial artery followed by (**c,d**) intra-arterial glue injection (18% N-butyl-cyanoacrylate and 82% Lipiodol mixture) achieving good control of the vascular lesion. Afterwards the patient presented an acute carpal tunnel syndrome requiring surgery with good postoperative recovery

Fig. 17.3a,b. Pain in calf and impaired leg movement in a 19-year-old woman soldier due to muscular arteriovenous malformation. **a** Selective catheterization with a microcatheter showed an intramuscular arteriovenous malformation on the early arterial phase. Complete occlusion of the vascular lesion was achieved after glue embolization with a mixture of 20% N-butyl-cyanoacrylate and 80% Lipiodol. After the treatment, there was complete relief of the pain and she was able to return to full activity. Glue cast can be observed in (**b**) the post-embolization angiogram with no remaining arteriovenous malformation

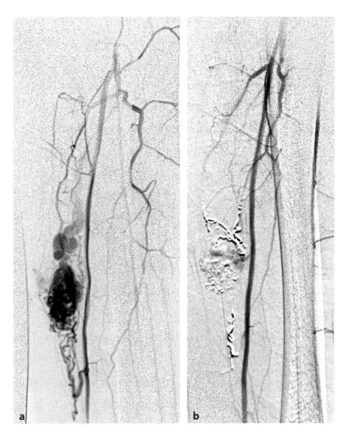

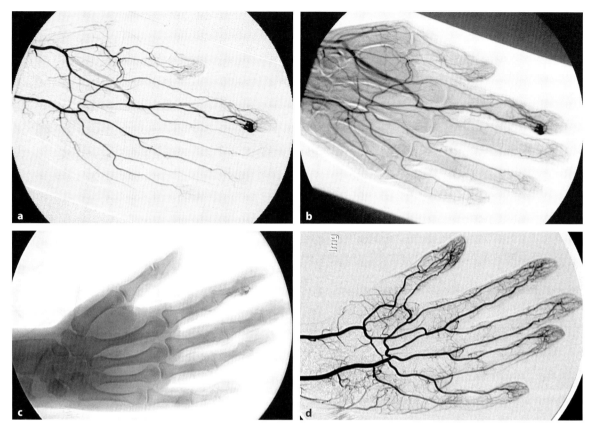

Fig. 17.4a–d. Symptomatic pulsatile soft tissue mass lesion in a 30-year-old woman due to hand arteriovenous malformation. Brachial arteriography on (**a**) early and (**b**) late arterial phases show a soft tissue mass lesion caused by small arteriovenous malformation involving the second digit. Because this lesion could not be superselectively catheterized, (**c**) a direct percutaneous puncture of the nidus was performed, and complete casting of the nidus with glue (N-butyl-cyanoacrylate 50%, Lipiodol 50%) was achieved, resulting in obliteration of the arteriovenous malformation as shown on (**d**) the immediate post embolization angiogram

material towards the proximal aspect of the draining veins is desirable for durable results. The microcatheter is removed immediately while aspirating with a syringe.

Lesions that are amenable to complete excision are probably best treated with presurgical embolization and excision. A direct percutaneous approach as an adjunct to arterial embolization may be effective in obliterating the nidus (Jackson et al. 1993; Yakes and Parker 1992) if the nidus cannot be reached with transarterial embolization.

Complications of treatment are often related to poor patient selection and poor judgment with respect to the goals to be achieved. In addition, technical procedural mistakes may lead to poor outcome. Inadvertent redirection of the arterial supply towards healthy adjacent tissues may occur because of a too-proximal injection of embolic material or reflux of embolic material. Venous ischemia can oc-

cur when embolic material occludes venous outflow channels that also drain adjacent healthy tissues. Embolization of arteriovenous shunts located in restricted tissue compartments may result in compartmental syndromes following transient swelling of the tissues after embolization.

17.4
Arteriolar-Capillary Malformations

Arteriolar-capillary malformations constitute a rare subgroup of vascular lesions, which may be difficult to distinguish from noninvoluting capillary hemangiomas (Enjolras et al. 2001). The absence of a significant soft tissue mass of this vascular lesion on noninvasive imaging is characteristic.

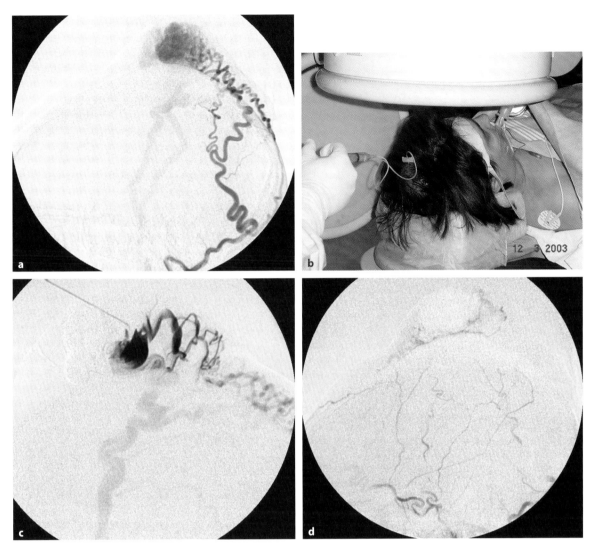

Fig. 17.5a–d. Scalp arteriovenous shunt in a 24-year-old woman. **a** Selective occipital angiogram in lateral view demonstrates high flow scalp arteriovenous malformation, which was also supplied by branches of the ipsilateral and contralateral superficial temporal arteries and contralateral occipital artery (not shown). Following transarterial partial embolization with glue and particles of polyvinyl alcohol in these vessels, (**b**) a percutaneous approach was performed with (**c**) injection of glue (50% N-butyl-cyanoacrylate, 50% Lipiodol) resulting in complete obliteration of the arteriovenous malformation nidus, as shown on (**d**) the post embolization left external carotid angiogram

17.5
Capillary-Venous Malformations and Venous Vascular Malformations

Capillary-venous malformations include port-wine stain and telangiectasias (ENJOLRAS and MULLIKEN 1993; MULLIKEN and GLOWACKI 1982; WISNICKI 1984) and usually involve the skin surface.

Port-wine stains are often associated with progressive thickening of the skin and subcutaneous layers, as well as overgrowth of the underlying skeleton. They are early alterations of cell characteristics, as they are almost always present in infancy. The color may vary from one patient to the next and change over time. Endovascular treatment is generally not recommended, in particular when the malformation is diffuse in character with poor arterial or venous access (Fig. 17.6).

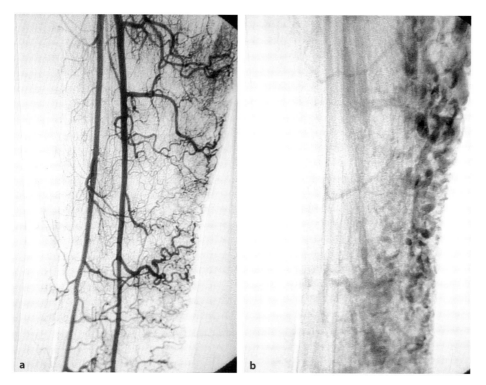

Fig. 17.6a,b. Mild discomfort with pain and swelling of the lower leg in a 42-year-old man with known bluish skin discoloration involving lower leg since childhood. **a,b** Angiography shows a diffuse capillary-venous type malformation deemed unsuitable for endovascular treatment

While most port-wine stains are isolated vascular anomalies, they may be associated with an underlying vascular malformation (lymphatic or arteriovenous) or be part of a more complex dysmorphogenesis. Examples include port-wine stain over the spine, which may be associated with underlying spinal dysraphism, or myelomeric arteriovenous malformations.

17.5.1
Venous Vascular Malformations

Venous vascular malformations are the most frequent vascular malformation of the musculoskeletal system, and have a variable clinical presentation, depending on their depth and extent of involvement (ENJOLRAS and MULLIKEN 1993; FISHMAN and MULLIKEN 1993). Our experience with head and neck, as well as limb and body, venous vascular malformations includes 214 patients since 1985.

When superficial, venous vascular malformations are characterized by blue discoloration of the skin; they are soft, compressible, and will refill over several seconds; the skin temperature over the lesion is normal. When they are located in deeper planes, there may be no skin involvement or discoloration, and they can present as fluctuating masses, which change in size with Valsalva maneuvers. Most of these lesions consist of spongy masses of sinusoidal spaces, and have variable communications with adjacent veins. Alternatively, some venous malformations represent varicosities or dysplasias of small and large venous channels (DUBOIS et al. 1991). The lesions are typically nonpulsatile, soft and compressible, distend with Valsalva maneuvers and are easily emptied by manual compression, and are frequently multifocal and bilateral. They typically contain phleboliths, which when present are pathognomonic of these lesions. Characteristic MR imaging findings include focal or diffuse areas of T2 hyperintensity (Figs. 17.7, 17.8), often containing identifiable spaces of variable size separated by septations (JACKSON et al. 1993). Small fluid levels may be visible. Phleboliths may be evident as areas of signal void, which are most prominent on gradient echo images. Flow-sensitive images demonstrate no high-flow vessels within or around the lesions, but may show evidence of old thrombus. Contrast administration results in variable enhancement, ranging from dense enhancement similar to that in adjacent veins to nonhomogeneous or delayed enhancement.

Ultrasound is routinely performed on venous malformations of the extremities. This study should also include color and/or power Doppler assessment. The sonographic appearance of these lesions is variable. The majority have at least a portion that is echogenic, corresponding to small tightly packed venous channels with innumerable interfaces. There are often serpiginous varicosities as well. Ultrasound is used to guide direct puncture in most cases. CT imaging likewise shows variable contrast enhance-

ment with or without rounded lamellate calcifications, but CT is not routinely part of our workup.

Angiography is not necessary to make the diagnosis, but typically shows either no filling of the malformation or delayed opacification or sinusoidal spaces with a "grape like" appearance when using a long contrast injection with or without dysplastic draining veins (BURROWS et al. 1983). Direct percutaneous catheterization of the malformation with contrast injection shows the interconnecting sinusoidal spaces. Communications with adjacent veins may be small or large, and adjacent venous channels may be normal or dysplastic and varicose.

Direct injection of sclerosing agent (1%–3% sodium tetradecyl sulphate [STD] or 98% ethanol)

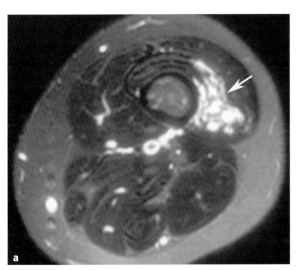

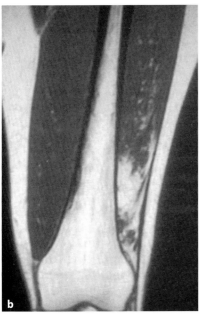 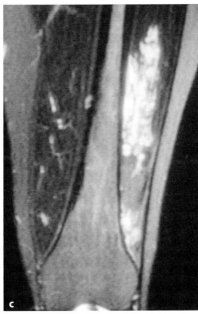 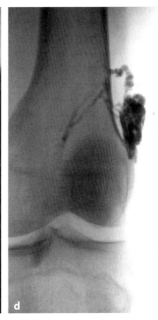

Fig. 17.7a–d. Progressive pain and swelling involving upper leg in a 34-year-old woman due to venous vascular malformation. **a** Axial T2-weighted, and coronal (**b**) T1 and (**c**) T2-weighted MR images show signal characteristics typical of venous vascular malformation (*arrow*), which was (**d**) subsequently treated successfully with percutaneous injections of 3% sodium tetradecyl sulphate during three outpatient sessions

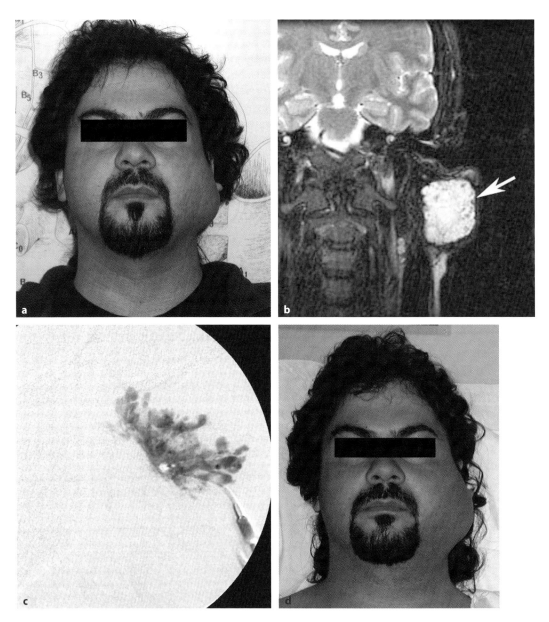

Fig. 17.8a–d. Venous vascular malformation in a 28-year-old man. **a** Soft tissue mass on the left preauricular area of the patient's face. **b** Coronal T2-weighted MR image demonstrates increased signal characteristics typical of venous vascular malformation (*arrow*). **c** Under general anesthesia, percutaneous injection of 10 ml of absolute alcohol opacified with 0.5 ml Lipiodol was performed, and resulted in immediate rapid swelling over the next few hours. **d** Patient's face 6 h later, with gradual complete shrinking of the vascular lesion and relief of symptoms over subsequent weeks

results in thrombosis and gradual shrinkage of the malformation. It is the preferred treatment (ANAVI et al. 1988; BURROWS 1995; DE LORIMIER 1995; YAKES et al. 1990; YAKES and PARKER 1992). We find that the STD is less painful than ethanol but still effective when diluted from 3% to ~ 2% using a nonionic iodinated contrast agent (Omnipaque 300 or Visipaque 270). With STD, most procedures can be performed on an outpatient basis with conscious sedation using fentanyl and midazolam (Figs. 17.7, 17.8).

The technique of sclerotherapy involves percutaneous catheterization of the malformation using a regular or Teflon-sheathed needle. After confirming free blood return, contrast is injected, recorded with serial angiographic imaging or under road-mapping to document the cannula position within the malformation and the presence or absence of venous outflow. If possible we use a tourniquet to decrease flow and limit filling of healthy draining veins.

An estimation of the volume of the cannulated compartment within the malformation is calculated from the contrast material injection, as the venous drainage is seen, and the walls of the compartment are convex. Contrast medium is then aspirated or flushed out with saline.

The STD can be administered in either of two ways depending on the findings at venography. If the lesion consists of a network of tiny vascular spaces, then we use a liquid sclerosant consisting of 3% STD opacified with iodinated contrast material with a ratio of 2:1. The resulting 2% STD is still effective as a sclerosing agent. If the venogram shows larger vascular spaces or big serpiginous veins then we use a foam mixture as the sclerosant agent. This "cappuccino foam" consists of 2 ml of 3% STD and 5–7 ml of air, mixed into a foam by flushing between two syringes using a three-way stopcock. This increases the dwell time of the STD, which flows away more slowly and apposes the vein walls better. The injection of sclerosing agent is done under digital subtraction angiography. If extravasation is demonstrated, or filling of normal vessels occurs, then the injection is stopped immediately.

Both STD and ethanol denature the blood cells within the malformation and dehydrate and sclerose the vessel wall if sufficient contact between the sclerosing agent and the endothelium is attained. The injected part of the malformation becomes firm and noncompressible due to thrombus formation within approximately 10 min. If the lesion does not become firm, and if there is persistent blood return from the cannula, additional ethanol may be injected, as swelling correlates with outcome (DONNELLY et al. 2000).

The total volume of injected ethanol should not exceed 0.3 ml/kg in children below the age of two, and 0.6 ml/kg in older children. One must be careful to prevent alcohol from escaping into the systemic circulation, as it may produce severe pulmonary vasoconstriction, which in peripheral venous vascular malformations has been reported to be fatal (YAKES and PARKER 1992). If at time of alcohol injection, or shortly thereafter, there is a change in PO2, the treatment of choice is the immediate administration of epinephrine. It is most important to be careful in peripheral lesions if they drain into the azygos

system. Alcohol injection is extremely painful, and should be done under general anesthesia; the subsequent swelling is pain-free if the agent has been injected within the malformation itself. In the treatment of these benign conditions, it is our preference to stage the sclerotherapy to diminish the risk of complication. Treatment of large malformations is always staged.

Recanalization of previously treated lesions depends on the single versus multicompartmental nature of the lesion. A single cavity is likely to be excluded in one treatment, in contrast to a multicompartmental lesion or previously operated malformations, which require several punctures and will give incomplete results. The most common complications of injection sclerotherapy are skin or mucous necrosis and neuropathy. Skin blistering or full-thickness necrosis are most likely if the malformation involves the skin or mucosal covers. Other complications are related to over-injection of sclerosant or errors in management of the overall malformation: cardiovascular complications, including bradycardia, arrhythmias and cardiac arrest, are associated with venous escape of ethanol into the central circulation (YAKES and PARKER 1992). Histological examination of animals injected with this drug revealed marked inflammatory reaction with fibrosis (DE LORIMIER 1995).

In general, the more localized deep venous malformations respond well to direct injection of sclerosing agents. Diffuse lesions are much more resistant to treatment by sclerotherapy. In spite of the sometimes discouraging tendency for lesions to recur, staged sclerotherapy can have a dramatic effect in reducing extensive musculoskeletal venous malformations over time. However, in the case of recurrence following sclerotherapy alone, surgical resection should be considered.

Other agents have been used, including Ethibloc and Aetoxysclerol (GELBERT et al. 2000), but we have had no experience with either agent. Ethibloc is composed of amino acids, 40% ethanol and contrast medium, and has been used in Europe and in Canada as a sclerosing agent for venous malformations, usually prior to surgical excision (DUBOIS et al. 1991). This material is usually diluted with additional ethanol or oily contrast medium prior to injection. It is more viscous than the other sclerosing agents, and can be injected without general anesthesia. It is also reported to result in chronic, progressive fibrosis., and is not approved by the Food and Drug Administration.

17.6
Lymphatic Malformations

17.6.1
Macrocystic and Microcystic Malformations

Lymphatic malformations may be classified as macrocystic (cystic hygromas) or microcystic (lymphangiomas). Interruption or obstruction of the peripheral lymphatic channels presumably results in diffuse or microcystic lymphatic malformations.

Lymphatic malformations are usually, but not always, evident at birth. Some are diagnosed in utero. Macrocystic lesions most commonly are located in the neck, axilla and chest wall, may be massive, and can interfere with the birth process. Microcystic lesions usually present as diffuse soft tissue thickening, often associated with an overlying capillary malformation of the skin or mucosal vesicles. The lesions typically grow proportionally with the child, but undergo episodic swelling often associated with signs of inflammation, either spontaneously or in association with regional infections. Acute enlargement may be related to lymphatic obstruction or hemorrhage. Communications between the macrocystic lymphatic malformations and adjacent veins are frequently present. On physical examination, lymphatic malformations have a rubbery or cystic consistency. Typically, they cannot be manually compressed like venous malformations. The overlying skin may manifest capillary malformation, vesicles or both.

MR imaging findings in macrocystic lymphatic malformations include cystic fluid collections, often with fluid–fluid levels, associated with rim or septal contrast enhancement. Evidence of hemorrhage or thrombosis may be present. Enlargement of adjacent veins, including the jugular, paravertebral and superior vena cava, have been described in cervicofacial lymphatic malformations (Gorenstein et al. 1992). Microcystic lymphatic malformations typically appear as diffuse "sheets" of bright signal on T2-weighted spin echo MR imaging, usually with various contrast enhancement patterns. The adjacent subcutaneous fat often shows evidence of lymphedema.

CT best demonstrates the bone distortion, and shows the soft tissue component of the malformation to be of lower density than surrounding muscle.

Treatment of macrocystic lymphatic malformations generally consists of staged early surgical excision (Mulliken 1993); in selected cases with extensive lesions sclerotherapy may be successful. Residual or recurrent cysts may also be treated by injection of sclerosing agents. A wide range of sclerosing drugs have been used in the past with variable results. The most recent sclerosing agent reported to be effective in some lymphatic malformations is doxycycline, OK 432 (Picibanil), a derivative of the streptococcal bacterium, which has been used predominantly in Japan to induce inflammation and subsequent fibrosis (Ogita et al. 1991; Giguere et al. 2002; Rautio et al. 2003). Yura et al. (1977) reported the use of bleomycin in cystic hygromas with encouraging results, confirmed more recently by Muir et al. (2004). They reported on 95 patients with hemangiomas, cystic hygromas and venous malformations. Complete resolution was noted in 49% of hemangiomas, 32% of venous vascular malformations, and 80% of cystic hygromas. Significant improvement was seen in an additional 38% of hemangiomas, 52% of venous vascular malformations, 13% of cystic hygromas, and 50% of lymphatic malformations, for an overall complete resolution or significant improvement in 80% of their patients. Bleomycin is a cytotoxic anti-tumor antibiotic. It has a dual effect in human tissue: it can induce DNA degradation, and has a specific sclerosing effect in the endothelium (Yura et al. 1977).

Sclerotherapy or intralesional injections are performed in a similar fashion to the treatment of venous malformations. The cystic spaces in lymphatic malformations often do not interconnect, making treatment by injection less effective. In larger compartments a yellowish, or sero-sanguinolent fluid is encountered, and a similar volume of ethanol is injected. Microcystic lymphatic malformations are difficult to treat by any means, due to their diffuse nature and infiltration of the tissue layers. The role of sclerotherapy is limited for symptomatic areas of repeated swelling and bleeding.

17.6.2
Mixed Vascular Malformations

Mixed vascular malformations are quite common. In particular, capillary malformations of the skin are often present in association with deep arteriovenous malformations or deep lymphatic or venous malformations. Combined lymphatic and venous malformations are also common. The lymphatic and venous systems develop nearly concurrently, and it is not unexpected that malformations of both systems coexist. A diffuse lymphatic malformation is often associated with varicosities of adjacent draining veins.

17.7
Metameric Arteriovenous Shunts

Metameric arteriovenous shunts involve multiple arteriovenous shunts that are not related to a hereditary disorder, but share metameric links (BENHAIEM-SIGAUX et al. 1985; MATSUMURA et al. 1986; NIMII et al. 1998; BHATTACHARYA et al. 2001). It is the detailed analysis of the vascular anatomy that will confirm the potential relationship between the lesions. Any disorder that affects mother cells very early in their biological and/or embryonic life can affect the organs to which these cells migrate, even after they have acquired their phenotypic specificity. Any secondary trigger may then bring these abnormal cells from a quiescent to an active state, where they will express the disorder. Two types can be recognized:

- Multiple shunts with a clear metameric disposition. They involve several myelomeres of the spinal cord (multimyelomeric arteriovenous malformations) both on the cord and intradural nervous roots (either arteriovenous fistulas or arteriovenous malformations) and related dermatomes. Cobb syndrome belongs to this metameric category, and corresponds to the spinal arteriovenous metameric syndromes (BERENSTEIN et al. 2004). According to its localization and involvement of the vertebral and metameric level, the shunt can be numbered from 1 to 31.
- Multiple shunts where the metameric disposition cannot be definitively demonstrated but is strongly suspected. In these cases the spinal cord arteriovenous shunts are associated with a limb vascular malformation. In the overall population of spinal cord arteriovenous malformation, more than 20% of patients have other associated vascular malformations or dysplasias (BERENSTEIN et al. 2004; RODESCH et al. 1996; NIMII et al. 1998) and up to 16% have clearly metamerically related multiple lesions (MATSUMURA et al. 1986).

17.8
Klippel-Trenaunay and Parkes Weber Syndromes

Klippel-Trenaunay syndrome (KTS) represents a rare congenital disorder that may include the following: port-wine stain or "birthmark" (cutaneous capillary malformations), soft tissue and bony hypertrophy (excessive growth of the soft tissue and/or bones) associated with venous vascular malformations and lymphatic abnormalities.

KTS usually is limited to one limb, but may involve more than one and/or the head or trunk area. Internal organs may be involved. Each case of KTS is unique and may exhibit these characteristics to differing degrees. Varicosities may be extensive, though they often spare the saphenous distribution. They are seen below the knee, laterally above the knee, and occasionally in the pelvic region. Varicosities may affect the superficial, deep and perforating venous systems.

The terms KTS and Klippel-Trenaunay-Weber Syndrome (KTWS) are sometimes used interchangeably. The consensus today is to distinguish KTS as hypertrophy and varicosity associated with port-wine staining, while KTWS (more correctly called Parkes-Weber Syndrome) is similar but also includes arteriovenous malformations with shunting.

Any type of limb vascular lesion requires careful clinical and imaging analysis, as it may represent the incomplete expression of the Klippel-Trenaunay or Parkes-Weber syndromes, which in turn should suggest spinal MR imaging to rule out associated spinal cord arteriovenous malformation. Percutaneous sclerosing therapy can be carried out for palliative relief of symptoms related to the venous vascular component of the disorder (GLOVICZKI et al. 1991).

17.9
Endovascular Management of Musculoskeletal Tumors

In recent years, significant advances in therapeutic management of musculoskeletal tumors have been achieved due to the advent of better diagnostic methods, new chemotherapeutic drugs and regimes, and surgical techniques. In the past, limbs with tumors were usually amputated. Now, limb-salvage operations with improved outcomes can better preserve the function of the limb. Surgical staging of bone and soft tissue tumors is based on grade, site and metastasis based on histological, radiological and clinical criteria. Preoperative vascular occlusion helps to prevent major blood loss during surgery, which is usually carried out within a few days of embolization. Reduction in size of some large inoperable metastases before radio-iodine therapy is another indication for embolization. As a palliative measure, vascular occlusion can be used to reduce otherwise untreatable skeletal pain and control tumoral bleeding.

Radiography is the initial modality in the evaluation of bone tumors. The radiographic features can also help in distinguishing malignant and benign lesions, and may make biopsy unnecessary. Examples are fibrous cortical defects, bone islands, simple bone cysts, bone infarcts and typical variants such as pseudocysts of the humerus and calcaneus.

MR imaging and CT have a role in the evaluation of the local disease and assessing other locations for metastasis. For both bone and soft tissue tumors,

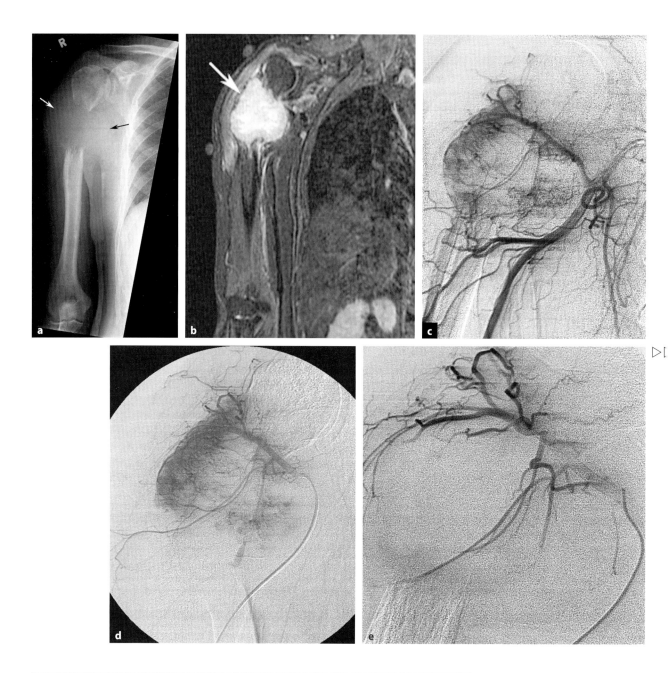

Fig. 17.9a–l. Renal cell carcinoma with bone metastasis in a 77-year-old man. **a** Anteroposterior radiograph and (**b**) coronal contrast-enhanced fat-suppressed T1-weighted MR image of the right humerus show a lytic lesion (*arrows*) involving the right proximal humeral metaphysis. **c** Angiogram shows hypervascular lesion with dense tumoral blush involving the circumflex humeral arteries. **d** Selective catheterization using a 4-French Kumpe catheter shows the same patterns as in (**c**). **e** Post-embolization arteriogram of this vessel with 300–500 μm diameter embosphere particles demonstrates no further tumoral blush. **f** Post-surgical radiograph shows the intramedular bone stabilization after tumoral resection. **g** Anteroposterior radiograph of the left femur shows lytic lesion (*arrow*) on the left upper femoral bone. **h,i** Arteriograms show tumoral blush supplied by branches of the deep femoral artery. **j** Selective catheterization using a fast tracker 325 microcatheter shows embolization to stasis was achieved using 300–500 μm embospheres. **k** Control angiogram post-embolization shows devascularization has been achieved. **l** Post-operative radiograph of the femur shows bone stabilization after tumor resection

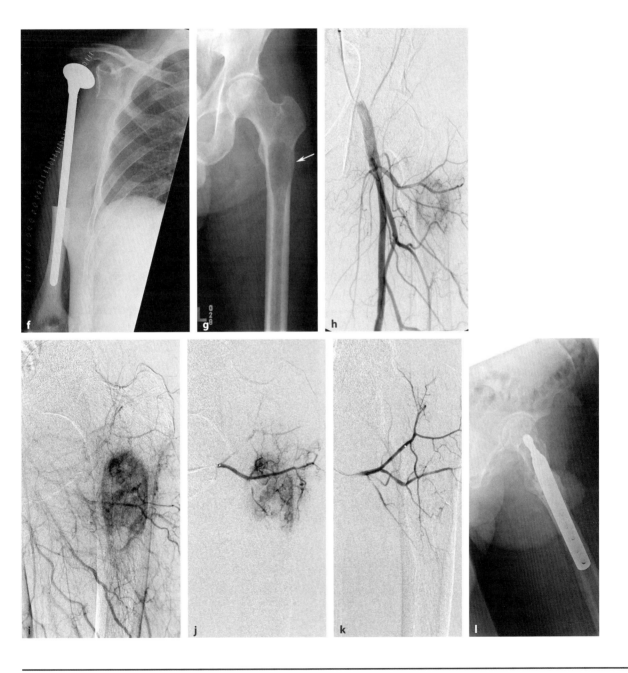

MR imaging is the method of choice for the staging of tumor extension, for the differentiation of neighboring compartments, and for detecting invasion of the regional neurovascular bundle. After administration of contrast agents, the mode of enhancement gives further information on the nature of the tumor. Diagnostic angiography is a useful evaluation method, especially in cases where visualization of vascular patterns in the lesions is hidden due to hyperostosis, sclerosis or metallic shadows. Angiographic evaluation is also usually indicated for vascular evaluation when preoperative embolization is required.

Breast cancer is the most frequent primary tumor with osseous metastases, followed by renal cell carcinomas, bronchial carcinomas and thyroid tumors. The predominant site of bone metastases is the spine, followed by the pelvis, femur, ribs, skull, sternum and humerus (Fig. 18.9). The overall incidence of bone metastases has increased due to improved diagnosis, prolonged survival with adjuvant therapy and improved follow-up.

Selective embolization of bone metastases is a palliative therapy that may induce rapid, but transient, relief of symptoms. In certain metastases such as thyroid carcinoma, embolization combined with radioiodine or external irradiation may prolong the duration of success (EUSTATIA-RUTTEN et al. 2003).

A general endovascular technique is used for the management of musculoskeletal tumors. General anesthesia is highly recommended for prolonged procedures or those in which endovascular embolic material such as alcohol may be extremely painful. Arterial access is usually via the femoral artery, but the humeral artery can be used for upper limb lesions. A guiding catheter, usually a 4- to 8-French depending on the parent vessel, and then a microcatheter, are used for selective catheterization of the targeting branch. Full heparinization is suggested for all the endovascular therapeutic procedures.

Superselective catheterization is always recommended. A pre-embolization angiogram should be performed to visualize the correct positioning of the catheter tip and to ascertain the absence of normal arteries in the surrounding tissue to prevent ischemic complications.

Percutaneous embolization can be performed on venous lesions or for specific procedures such as cement injection for lytic bone lesions (hemangiomas). This is done under fluoroscopy or CT imaging. The needle is positioned in the vertebral body within the hemangioma through the vertebral pedicle, and the cement is then injected while controlling the venous outlet and cement leakage into the extravertebral space.

The embolic material may be polyvinyl alcohol particles or embospheres in different sizes (40–500 μm), gelatin sponge and coils or a combination of these. As previously mentioned, cement can be used percutaneously for the treatment of bone hemangiomas or for palliative treatment for bone stabilization in aggressive bone lesions. The type and target of the embolic material should be evaluated in each case.

Ligation of the arterial feeders with an embolic agent, with or without penetration of the tumoral vascular bed, can be attempted depending on the size of the vessels, the selectivity of the catheterization and the purpose of the treatment: whether the procedure is to treat an acute hemorrhagic event, palliative embolization for tumoral size reduction or preoperative devascularization of the lesion.

17.10
Conclusion

Vascular malformations are lesions that can be diagnosed at any stage of life, and may present a variety of symptoms and manifestations. Even though musculoskeletal involvement with these conditions is not frequent, it must be considered as a differential diagnosis in clinical management and prognosis. Vascular malformations of the musculoskeletal system may occur in isolation or in the presence of congenital disorders such as Klippel-Trenaunay or Parkes-Weber syndromes. Multifocal vascular or lymphatic malformations can be found in other regions, as can soft tissue, bony hypertrophy and cutaneous manifestations.

The musculoskeletal vascular malformations represent a wide variety of lesions ranging from intraosseous lesions to venous malformations. The diagnosis is usually clinical, based on patient history and physical examination. Cross sectional noninvasive imaging is the complementary diagnostic method, and is helpful to determine the extent of the lesion and to demonstrate associated lesions or multifocality. Rarely, invasive procedures are needed to establish the diagnosis and the type of malformation involved.

The endovascular treatment of the musculoskeletal vascular malformation is based on the type of malformation, anatomical characteristics, location and the vascular supply. Several devices and embolic materials are available for this purpose. Depending on the circumstances, the endovascular treatment can be performed to achieve the complete obliteration of the vascular malformation, as a preoperative method to reduce the bleeding during the surgical procedure, or as a palliation to alleviate pain or to treat an acute hemorrhagic event.

Musculoskeletal tumors also respond well to endovascular treatment. Consistent application of the staging criteria in preoperative imaging makes limb-saving therapy more feasible and can improve the prognosis. Many types of primary tumors and metastasis can be pre-treated to achieve a higher rate of complete surgical excision, reduce intraoperative blood loss, reduce the size of the tumor, or for palliation of pain or acute hemorrhagic events.

The ongoing development of noninvasive diagnostic methods, as well as the availability of new and better materials for the endovascular procedures, have had a significant impact on the earlier and more accurate diagnosis of these lesions, and offer a larger variety of therapeutic options. These achievements will lead to a better understanding of vascular conditions and, eventually, a more effective and less invasive option for their treatment.

References

Anavi Y, Har-El G, Mintz S (1988) The treatment of facial haemangioma by percutaneous injections of sodium tetradecyl sulfate. J Laryngol Otol 102:87–90

Benhaiem-Sigaux N, Zerah M, Gherardi R, Bellot J, Hurth M, Poirier J (1985) A retromedullary arteriovenous fistula associated with the Klippel-Trenaunay-Weber syndrome. A clinicopathologic study. Acta Neuropathol (Berl) 66:318–324

Berenstein A, Lasjaunias P, TerBrugge K (2004) Spinal arteriovenous malformations. Surgical neuroangiography. Clinical and endovascular treatment aspects in adults. Springer-Verlag, Heidelberg

Bhattacharya J, Luo CB, Suh DC, Alvarez H, Rodesch G, Lasjaunias P (2001) Wyburn-Mason or Bonnet Dechaume-Blanc as cerebrofacial arteriovenous metameric syndromes (CAMS). Interv Neuroradiol 7:5–17

Burrows PE, Mulliken JB, Fellows KE, Strand RD (1983) Childhood hemangiomas and vascular malformations: angiographic differentiation. AJR Am J Roentgenol. 1983 141:483–488

Burrows PE (1995) Hemangiomas and vascular malformations. Can Assoc Radiol J 46:143

de Lorimier AA (1995) Sclerotherapy for venous malformations. J Pediatr Surg 30:188–193

Donnelly LF, Bisset GS 3rd, Adams DM (2000) Marked acute tissue swelling following percutaneous sclerosis of low-flow vascular malformations: a predictor of both prolonged recovery and therapeutic effect. Pediatr Radiol 30:415–419

Dubois JM, Sebag GH, De Prost Y, Teillac D, Chretien B, Brunelle FO (1991) Soft-tissue venous malformations in children: percutaneous sclerotherapy with Ethibloc. Radiology 180:195–198

Enjolras O, Mulliken JB (1993) The current management of vascular birthmarks. Pediatr Dermatol 10:311–313

Enjolras O, Mulliken JB, Boon LM, Wassef M, Kozakewich HP, Burrows PE (2001) Noninvoluting congenital hemangioma: a rare cutaneous vascular anomaly. Plast Reconstr Surg 107:1647–1654

Eustatia-Rutten CF, Romijn JA, Guijt MJ, Vielvoye GJ, van den Berg R, Corssmit EP, Pereira AM, Smit JW (2003) Outcome of palliative embolization of bone metastases in differentiated thyroid carcinoma. J Clin Endocrinol Metab 88:3184–3189

Fishman SJ, Mulliken JB (1993) Hemangiomas and vascular malformations of infancy and childhood. Pediatr Clin North Am 40:1177–1200

Gelbert F, Enjolras O, Deffrenne D, Aymard A, Mounayer C, Merland JJ (2000) Percutaneous sclerotherapy for venous malformation of the lips: a retrospective study of 23 patients. Neuroradiology 42:692–696

Giguere CM, Bauman NM, Smith RJ (2002) New treatment options for lymphangioma in infants and children. Ann Otol Rhinol Laryngol 111(12 Pt 1):1066–1075

Gloviczki P, Stanson AW, Stickler GB, Johnson CM, Toomey BJ, Meland NB, Rooke TW, Cherry KJ Jr (1991) Klippel-Trenaunay syndrome: the risks and benefits of vascular interventions. Surgery 110:469–479

Gorenstein A, Katz S, Rein A, Schiller M (1992) Giant cystic hygroma associated with venous aneurysm. J Pediatr Surg 27:1504–1506

Jackson IT, Carreno R, Potparic Z, Hussain K (1993) Hemangiomas, vascular malformations, and lymphovenous malformations: classification and methods of treatment. Plast Reconstr Surg 91:1216–1230

Lum C, TerBrugge KG (2002) Intervention in vascular lesions of the vertebrae. Semin Intervent Radiol 19:245–255

Matsumura A, Tsuboi K, Hyodo A, Yoshizawa K, Nose T (1986) Lumbosacral extradural spinal arteriovenous malformation with blood supply from branches of internal iliac arteries. Neurochirurgia 29:235–237

Muir T, Kirsten M, Fourie P, Dippenaar N, Ionescu GO (2004) Intralesional bleomycin injection (IBI) treatment for haemangiomas and congenital vascular malformations. Pediatr Surg Int 19:766–773

Mulliken JB, Glowacki J (1982) Hemangiomas and vascular malformations in infants and children: a classification based on endothelial characteristics. Plast Reconstr Surg 69:412–422

Mulliken JB (1993) Cutaneous vascular anomalies. Semin Vasc Surg 6:204–218

Nimii Y, Ito U, Tone O, Yoshida K, Sato S, Berenstein A (1998) Multiple spinal perimedullary arteriovenous fistulas associated with ParkesWeber syndrome: a case report. Interv Neuroradiol 4:151–157

Ogita S, Tsuto T, Deguchi E, Tokiwa K, Nagashima M, Iwai N (1991) OK-432 therapy for unresectable lymphangiomas in children. J Pediatr Surg 26:263–268

Rautio R, Keski-Nisula L, Laranne J, Laasonen E (2003) Treatment of lymphangiomas with OK-432 (Picibanil). Cardiovasc Intervent Radiol 26:31–36

Rodesch G, Alvarez H, Chaskis C, Peters J, Lasjaunias P (1996) Clinical manifestations in paraspinal arteriovenous malformations. Spinal cord symptoms, pathophysiology, and treatment objectives. Int J Neuroradiol 2:430–436

Sofocleous CT, Rosen RJ, Raskin K, Fioole B, Hofstee DJ (2001) Congenital vascular malformations in the hand and forearm. J Endovasc Ther 8:484–494

Tan KT, Simons M, Rajan DK, TerBrugge KG (2004) Peripheral high-flow arteriovenous vascular malformations: a single-center experience. J Vasc Interv Radiol 15:1071–1080

Upton J, Coombs CJ, Mulliken JB, Burrows PE, Pap S (1999) Vascular malformations of the upper limb: a review of 270 patients. J Hand Surg [Am] 24:1019–1035

White RI, Pollak J, Persing J, Henderson KJ, Thomson JG, Burdge CM (2000) Long term outcome of embolotherapy and surgery for high-flow extremity arteriovenous malformations. J Vasc Interv Radiol 11:1285–1295

Wisnicki JL (1984) Hemangiomas and vascular malformations. Ann Plast Surg 12:41–59

Yakes WF, Luethke JM, Merland JJ et al. (1990) Ethanol embolization of arteriovenous fistulas: a primary model of therapy. J Vasc Interv Radiol 1:89–96

Yakes WF, Parker SH (1992) Diagnosis and management of vascular anomalies. Interv Radiol 1:152–189

Yakes WF, Rossi P, Odink H (1996) How I do it. Arteriovenous malformation management. Cardiovasc Intervent Radiol 19:65–71

Yura J, Hashimoto T, Tsuruga N, Shibata K (1977) Bleomycin treatment for cystic hygroma in children. Nippon Geka Hokan 46:607–614

Ultrasound-Guided Musculoskeletal Interventional Procedures

Philippe Peetrons and Michel Court-Payen

CONTENTS

18.1   Introduction   385

18.2   Indications   385

18.3   Required Equipment and Method of
        Examination   385

18.4   Fluid Collections   386

18.5   Tendinopathy, Enthesopathy and
        Fasciitis   394

18.6   Soft Tissue and Synovial Masses   394

18.7   Treatment of Rotator Cuff
        Calcifications   395

18.8   Removal of Foreign Bodies   396

18.9   Preoperative Localization   396

18.10   Conclusion   397

        References   399

18.1
Introduction

Since the advent of interventional ultrasound in 1969, ultrasound has been applied to guidance of interventional procedures in most areas of the body (abdomen, thorax, head and neck) with much success (HOLM and SKJOLDBYE 1996). Expanding the potential of ultrasound, investigators in the past

P. PEETRONS, MD
Professor and Chairman, Department of Medical Imaging, Centre Hospitalier Molière-Longchamp, 142 Rue Marconi, 1190 Brussels, Belgium
M. COURT-PAYEN, MD, PhD
Senior Radiologist, Department of Imaging, Gildhoj Private Hospital, Brondbyvester Boulevard 16, 2605 Brondby, Denmark

decade have developed interventional musculoskeletal ultrasound procedures. As early as 1988, CHRISTENSEN et al. reviewed the many uses of ultrasound as guidance for aspiration, drainage and biopsy of musculoskeletal abscesses, masses and focal muscle pathology in the extremities, trunk and neck. The list of new indications is growing, and today interventional procedures are an integrated part of many musculoskeletal ultrasound examinations (ADLER and SOFKA 2003; CARDINAL et al. 1998; PEETRONS and COURT-PAYEN 2002; RUBENS et al. 1997; WEIDNER et al. 2004).

18.2
Indications

The main indications for ultrasound-guided diagnostic and therapeutic procedures are summarized here:
- Fluid collections: needle aspiration, steroid or contrast injection, catheter drainage
- Tendinopathy, enthesopathy and fasciitis: steroid injections
- Soft tissue and synovial masses: needle biopsies
- Treatment of rotator cuff calcifications
- Removal of foreign bodies
- Preoperative needle or wire localization

18.3
Required Equipment and Method of Examination

There is no special preparation of the patient and no contraindications. This is especially advantageous for pregnant women, who should avoid X-rays. A linear high-frequency probe is generally required, ranging from 7 to 12 MHz, as for any musculoskeletal ultrasound examination. In the wrist/hand or ankle/foot, special probes with frequencies up to 17 MHz are very helpful. In obese or very athletic patients, lower frequencies may be needed. Power Doppler (or color Doppler) may be used during the procedure to diagnose aneurysms or pseudoaneurysms, to avoid vessels around or within the target, and to differentiate simple joint effusions from inflammatory synovitis, which could require a larger needle.

The examination is simple, quick and safe, and the needle is seen and followed during the entire procedure, as it is directed into the image plane along a predictable route (Holm and Skjoldbye 1996). As the target is often close to the skin, a free-hand technique (without a guiding device attached to the probe) is generally used. Training is necessary, and phantoms or sample devices are available for practice (Sites et al. 2004).

Of course, a diagnostic ultrasound study will always precede interventional procedures. This diagnostic step will be comparative, sometimes dynamic, and always includes palpation, inspection, and interrogation of the patient.

Procedures may involve needles of different size, varying from small (19-gauge) to large (14-gauge), depending on the type of mass or cyst. The skin is disinfected first with iodinated alcohol or any other appropriate disinfectant. Fine-needle procedures (needles less than 1 mm or 19-gauge) include most aspirations, injections and fine-needle biopsies, and do not generally require local anesthesia. A local anesthetic (lidocaine) is used for core-needle biopsies (needles more than 1 mm or 19-gauge, e.g., Tru-Cut type needles), catheter placement and longer procedures, such as treatment of rotator cuff calcifications or removal of foreign bodies.

18.4
Fluid Collections

Fluid collections that should be referred to the radiologist for ultrasound-guided puncture are synovial cysts (e.g., Baker cysts), other synovial fluids (joint effusion, bursitis or tenosynovitis), ganglion cysts, meniscal cysts of the knee, labral cysts (especially in the spinoglenoid notch of the scapula), hematomas and abscesses.

Most joint effusions can be punctured easily without imaging-guidance, as the anatomical landmarks are well known. However, ultrasound is necessary for precise puncture of the joint space in deep areas (hip, shoulder) (Fig. 18.1), in anatomically complex areas (wrist and fingers, foot and toes) (Fig. 18.2), in obese or edematous patients, or when the normal (palpation-guided) procedure has failed (Fessell et al. 2000; Grassi et al. 1999; Hall and Buchbinder 2004; Sofka and Adler 2002). Indications for the procedures are analysis of the fluid (especially if septic or crystal arthropathy is suspected, as in monoarthritis) and decompression of the joint reducing the pain caused by hyperpressure on the capsule and avoiding the risk of epiphyseal damage due to loss of vascularization. Joint puncture may also be performed when effusion is absent, generally to inject steroid or contrast medium (for MR-arthrography). Joint puncture is best performed with ultrasound-guidance, using a posterior approach for the shoulder (Zwar et al. 2004), an anterior approach for the hip (Fig. 18.3) (Migliore et al. 2004; Qvistgaard et al. 2001), and a lateral suprapatellar approach for the knee (Qvistgaard et al. 2001). Ultrasound can also guide injections in sacroiliac joints (Pekkafahli et al. 2003).

Infection of a loosened hip prosthesis is a common indication for ultrasound (Komppa et al. 1985; van Holsbeeck et al. 1994). Any fluid collection in the joint space or in the surrounding soft tissues should be punctured with ultrasound-guidance prior to the antibiotic treatment. Metallic prostheses are not a contraindication for ultrasound as they are for CT.

Deep, small and/or nonpalpable bursae or tendon sheaths can be punctured very precisely under ultrasound-guidance. Steroid injections may be performed safely in patients with noninfectious bursitis or tenosynovitis (Figs. 18.4, 18.5), avoiding any risk of tendon rupture or accidental vessel or nerve puncture. Again, obesity and edema will make palpation-guided punctures more difficult.

The subacromial subdeltoid bursa at the shoulder is very large and may be easy to aspirate when distended by a large amount of liquid (as in arthritis or acute trauma) (Fig. 18.6). However, many patients with (chronic) shoulder pain and impingement do not have fluid in the bursa, which may appear normal or slightly hypertrophied on ultrasound. In such cases, in which steroid injection is called for, ultrasound assures precise needle puncture of the bursa (Fig. 18.7). By comparison, Eustace et al. (1997) showed that steroid injections performed by skilled rheumatologists were located accurately in

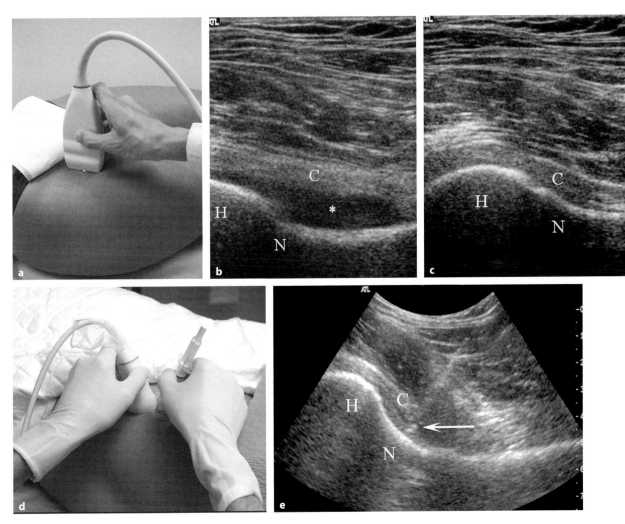

Fig. 18.1a–e. Hip effusion in a 27-year-old woman. **a,b** Longitudinal ultrasound image of the right hip shows effusion in the anterior recess (*asterisk*). **c** Longitudinal ultrasound image of the normal left hip. **d,e** Just after ultrasound-guided aspiration of the right hip effusion, the needle tip is seen in the empty anterior recess (*arrow*) (5 MHz curved-array transducer). Femoral head (*H*), femoral neck (*N*), joint capsule (*C*)

only 29% of subacromial and 42% of intra-articular shoulder injections. A recent study showed that patients who received subacromial steroid injections with ultrasound-guidance experienced better clinical improvement after 6 weeks than patients who had received blind injections (NAREDO et al. 2004).

Ultrasound-guidance may be indicated for needle puncture of synovial cysts (e.g. Baker cyst), ganglion cysts (BREIDAHL and ADLER 1996), and labral cysts (CHIOU et al. 1999), especially when the cyst is complex (septated or partly solid) and not easy to palpate. Percutaneous treatment may be proposed as a simple aspiration, or aspiration associated with steroid injection (BREIDAHL and ADLER 1996). Recurrence is common, but the reported rates of recur-

rence vary greatly, even for the same type of cyst. Thus, there is no consensus on needle aspiration of cysts as an alternative to surgery. Baker cysts are often treated with needle puncture. Ganglion cysts are surrounded by a fibrous wall and contain a gelatinous material that requires larger needles (18-gauge) for puncture. Ganglion cysts are common at the wrist, knee and ankle, and are often connected to a joint capsule or a tendon sheath. However, they may be found anywhere in the extremities (e.g., intramuscular, intraosseous, intraneural). Labral cysts may also recur after ultrasound-guided aspiration as they do in the shoulder (CHIOU et al. 1999). Meniscal cysts – which are most often secondary to a meniscal tear – are treated surgically.

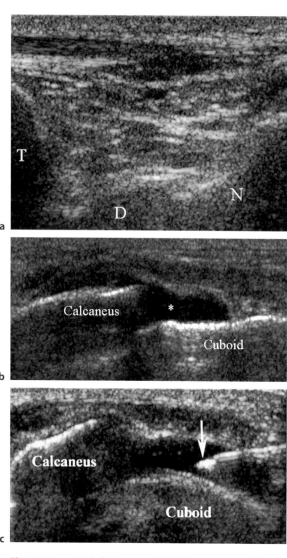

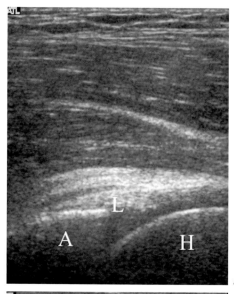

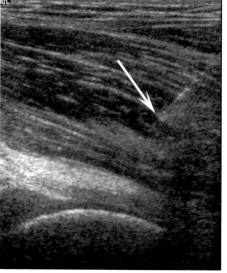

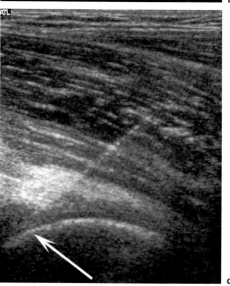

Fig. 18.2a–c. Ankylosing spondylitis in a 55-year-old man with pain and edema of the ankle. **a** Longitudinal ultrasound image of the anterior ankle shows no effusion in the anterior recess. Tibia (*T*), dome of the talus (*D*), neck of the talus (*N*). **b** Lateral longitudinal ultrasound image shows effusion (*asterisk*) in the calcaneo-cuboid joint. **c** Ultrasound-guided diagnostic puncture with the needle tip (*arrow*) in the calcaneo-cuboid recess

Fig. 18.3a–c. Ultrasound-guided steroid injection in the left hip of a 21-year-old man with joint pain and no signs of infection. **a** Longitudinal ultrasound image shows anterior hip joint. Labrum (*L*), acetabulum (*A*), femoral head (*H*). During the procedure the needle tip (arrow) is seen in the soft tissues (**b**) and then in the joint line (**c**)

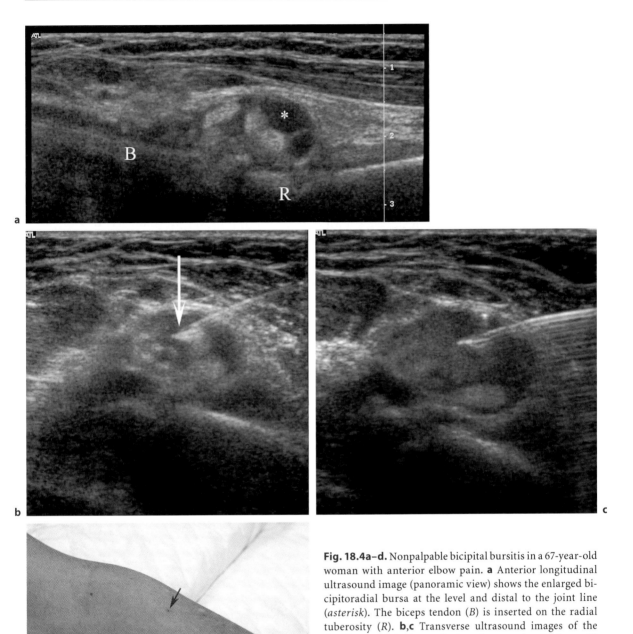

Fig. 18.4a–d. Nonpalpable bicipital bursitis in a 67-year-old woman with anterior elbow pain. **a** Anterior longitudinal ultrasound image (panoramic view) shows the enlarged bicipitoradial bursa at the level and distal to the joint line (*asterisk*). The biceps tendon (*B*) is inserted on the radial tuberosity (*R*). **b,c** Transverse ultrasound images of the distal part of the bursa during ultrasound-guided steroid injection show the needle tip (*arrow*) placed inside the bursa (**b**) and the steroid injected (echo-rich fluid with one air bubble) (**c**). **d** The injection site is visible on the skin, distal to the elbow joint (*arrow*)

Percutaneous treatment of abscesses, hematomas and hygromas is best guided by ultrasound, with needle aspiration or catheter drainage (CRAIG 1999; HOLM and SKJOLDBYE 1996). The aspect (internal echoes, mobility of the contents) and compressibility of fluid collections are studied carefully during the preliminary ultrasound examination to determine whether voiding is possible, as well as which technique and puncture route should be used. Access to subcutaneous collections is generally easy (Fig. 18.8). Subfascial collections may have significant anatomical relations that must be clearly delineated before any interventional procedure.

Abscesses of the extremities are often related to diabetes, renal insufficiency, immunodepression, drug addiction, postoperative complications or

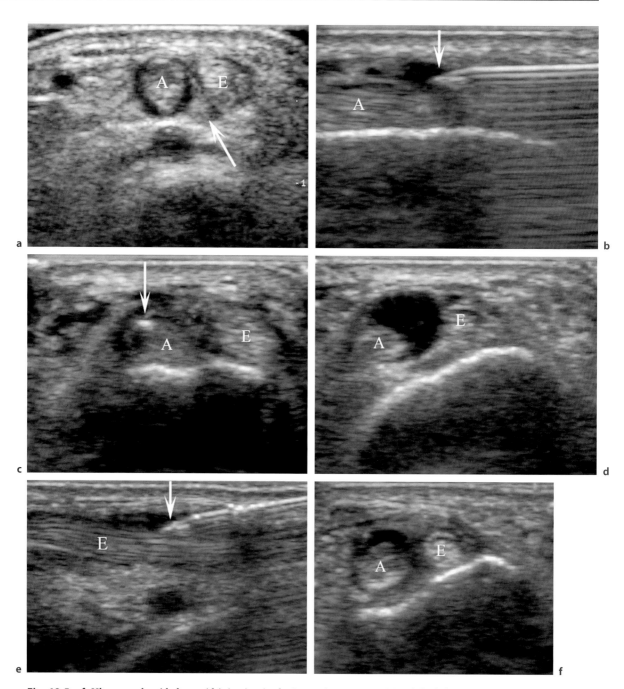

Fig. 18.5a–f. Ultrasound-guided steroid injection in de Quervain tenosynovitis of the left wrist in a 53-year-old woman. **a** Transverse ultrasound image shows enlargement of the two tendons (*A*, abductor pollicis longus; *E*, extensor pollicis brevis) and hypertrophy of the abductor pollicis longus tendon sheath. The tendon sheaths are separated by an echo-rich septa (*arrow*). During the injection, the needle tip (*arrow*) is seen in the abductor pollicis longus tendon sheath (**b**) longitudinally and (**c**) transversally. **d** After this first steroid injection no fluid has passed to the extensor pollicis brevis tendon sheath. **e** A second injection (*arrow*) is therefore performed in the extensor pollicis brevis tendon sheath. **f** After the second injection there is fluid around both tendons

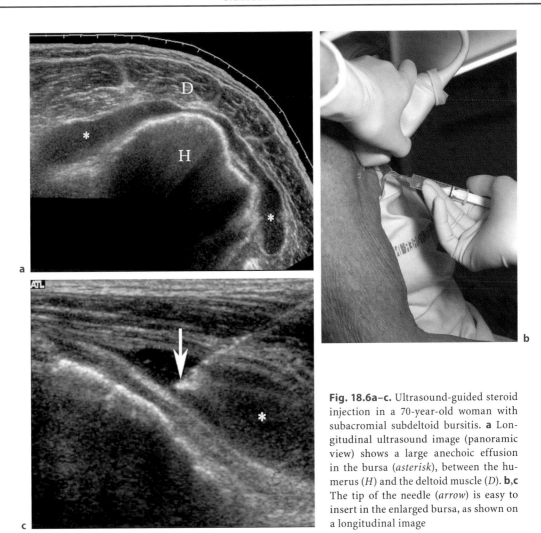

Fig. 18.6a–c. Ultrasound-guided steroid injection in a 70-year-old woman with subacromial subdeltoid bursitis. **a** Longitudinal ultrasound image (panoramic view) shows a large anechoic effusion in the bursa (*asterisk*), between the humerus (*H*) and the deltoid muscle (*D*). **b,c** The tip of the needle (*arrow*) is easy to insert in the enlarged bursa, as shown on a longitudinal image

Fig. 18.7. Ultrasound-guided steroid injection in a 47-year-old man with subacromial subdeltoid bursitis. Longitudinal ultrasound image shows a slightly hypertrophied bursa without effusion (dry bursitis). The tip of the needle (*arrow*) has been carefully inserted in the plane between the deltoid (*D*) and the supraspinatus tendon (*SS*). During the injection fluid appears in the bursa (*asterisk*) and the thickened bursa wall is better visualized. Humerus (*H*)

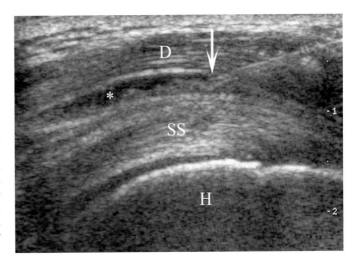

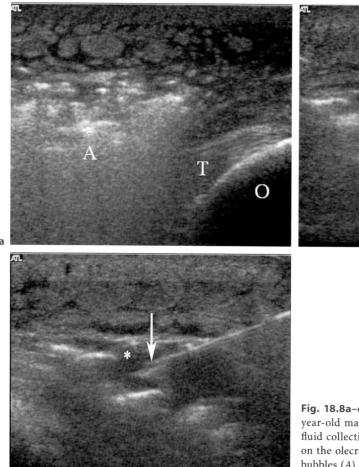

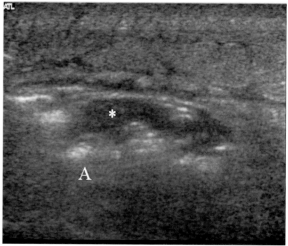

Fig. 18.8a–c. Subcutaneous abscess at the elbow in a 44-year-old man. **a,b** Longitudinal ultrasound images show a fluid collection over the insertion of the triceps tendon (*T*) on the olecranon (*O*). The collection (*asterisk*) contains air bubbles (*A*) and is not easy to detect. **c** During ultrasound-guided diagnostic aspiration the needle tip (*arrow*) is directed toward the anechoic fluid

foreign bodies. Needle puncture may require large needles (18-gauge) and/or repeated punctures at follow-up examinations. The aspirated fluid is inspected macroscopically (for evidence of pus) and always analyzed. Diagnostic needle puncture of a very small pocket of pus (e.g., in early pyomyositis) can only be successful if guided by imagery (Fig. 18.9). Catheter drainage is often the method of choice for large abscesses. The type, size and number of catheter to be used depends on the type and size of the collection, as well as local practice. Treatment by a simple 5.7-French pig tail catheter is generally successful, provided the abscess cavity is washed carefully with saline after catheter placement, and bedside visits are made 5–6 times daily. This procedure should also be performed during the ultrasound follow-up every two days. Withdrawal of the catheter is based on clinical (pain, fever, amount and aspect of the aspirated fluid) and ultrasound findings (position of the catheter, residual cavity)

at follow-up. If needed, iodine contrast media may be injected into the abscess cavity to detect any relationship to surrounding structures, like joints or tendon sheaths.

In patients with osteomyelitis, especially children, subperiostal collections may be detected by ultrasound, immediately aspirated under ultrasound-guidance and analyzed, as for any soft tissue collection (KAISER and ROSENBORG 1994).

Clinical indications for decompression of hematomas are signs of compression, increased risk of venous thrombosis, infection or chronicity. Non-surgical decompression of hematomas is a somewhat controversial subject in sports medicine, as the content of hematomas is often totally or partially solid and impossible to withdraw through needles or catheters. Hematomas must be completely or predominantly liquid for successful aspiration, and ultrasound is mandatory to determine the outcome of the procedure.

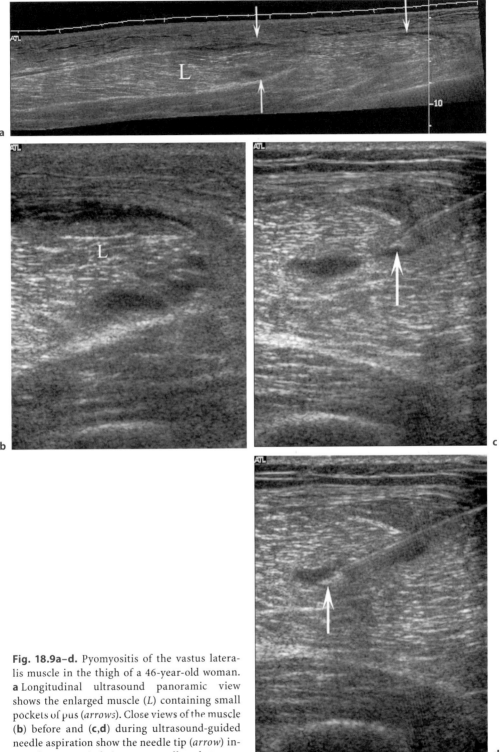

Fig. 18.9a–d. Pyomyositis of the vastus lateralis muscle in the thigh of a 46-year-old woman.
a Longitudinal ultrasound panoramic view
shows the enlarged muscle (*L*) containing small
pockets of pus (*arrows*). Close views of the muscle
(**b**) before and (**c,d**) during ultrasound-guided
needle aspiration show the needle tip (*arrow*) inserted very precisely into two small pockets

18.5
Tendinopathy, Enthesopathy and Fasciitis

Local steroid injection is sometimes used for the treatment of inflammatory changes in tendons (tendinopathy) and fascias (fasciitis), at their bone insertion (enthesopathy) or in the peritendineum (peritendinitis), although there is some controversy about possible risk of tendon rupture in tendinopathy. Ultrasound-guidance may be used in selected cases (when the first attempt under clinical or radiological guidance has failed) or in difficult cases (deep location or edema) (Fig. 18.10) (FREDBERG et al. 2004). Color Doppler ultrasound-guided injection of a sclerosing substance into areas of neovessels in chronic patellar and Achilles tendinopathy has been described recently, with good preliminary results (ALFREDSON and ÖHBERG 2005a; ALFREDSON and ÖHBERG 2005b).

18.6
Soft Tissue and Synovial Masses

Large needles (18- to 14-gauge) are generally used for needle biopsies of primary soft tissue or synovial masses (e.g., Tru-Cut type needles for core-needle biopsies). Fine-needle aspiration is sufficient for biopsy of metastases and recurrences (of known primary cancer) (FORNAGE and LORIGAN 1989). With ultrasound-guidance, the needle tip can be placed precisely in a solid area inside the mass (Fig. 18.11), avoiding puncture of neighboring compartments, as well as lesions of surrounding structures (vessels or nerves). Power or color Doppler examination is helpful in this respect. Preoperative needle biopsy of soft tissue tumors is timesaving and less traumatic than open surgical biopsy; very high accuracy can be achieved with a combination of Tru-Cut and fine-needle aspiration biopsy (COURT-

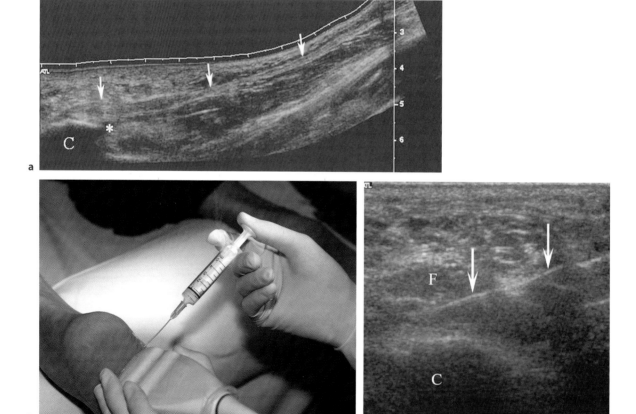

Fig. 18.10a–c. Plantar fasciitis in a 47-year-old woman. **a** Longitudinal ultrasound panoramic view shows the plantar fascia (*arrows*) is thickened at the insertion on the calcaneus (*C*). Site of steroid injection is deep in the insertion (*asterisk*). **b,c** During ultrasound-guided steroid injection with a medial approach, the needle (*arrows*) is visualized in a transverse plane, with the tip deep in the plantar fascia (*F*)

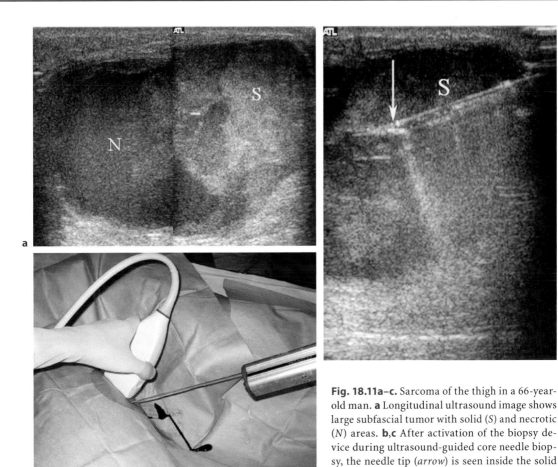

Fig. 18.11a–c. Sarcoma of the thigh in a 66-year-old man. **a** Longitudinal ultrasound image shows large subfascial tumor with solid (*S*) and necrotic (*N*) areas. **b,c** After activation of the biopsy device during ultrasound-guided core needle biopsy, the needle tip (*arrow*) is seen inside the solid area of the tumor

PAYEN et al. 1996). In synovial diseases, needle biopsy may provide specific diagnoses such as crystal arthropathy, pigmented villonodular synovitis, synovial chondromatosis, sarcoidosis, tuberculosis, amyloidosis and synovial malignancies (WILLIAMS and GUMPEL 1983).

18.7
Treatment of Rotator Cuff Calcifications

Painful calcifications in the rotator cuff may be aspirated percutaneously through a needle guided by imaging. Ultrasound is an established alternative to fluoroscopy for this procedure; it lacks radiation and the procedure can be followed in real-time (AINA et al. 2001; BRADLEY et al. 1995; COOPER et

al. 2005; FARIN 1995). This treatment may be proposed if the calcification measures more than 5 mm and if conservative treatment has failed. Results are good for soft calcifications that appear faint with fuzzy contours on X-rays and have no (or slight) posterior shadowing on ultrasound. The procedure should first be performed with thin needles (18- to 22-gauge), but sometimes requires larger needles (up to 16-gauge). After aspiration and rinsing with saline, steroid is injected into the subacromial bursa (but not in the tendon).

Aspiration of hard calcifications, which are dense with clear margins on X-rays and have a bright reflection and strong posterior shadowing on ultrasound, is difficult (often impossible) and not very successful clinically. Fragmentation of the calcification may be attempted in these cases and is sometimes of benefit to the patient, but the procedure is controversial.

18.8
Removal of Foreign Bodies

Removal of foreign bodies in the hand or foot is a very good, but often overlooked, indication for diagnostic ultrasound, although it was reported nearly 20 years ago (LITTLE et al. 1986). Metallic, as well as radio-negative, foreign bodies (wood, glass, plastics) can be localized precisely. Technological advances now make it possible to detect nonmetallic foreign bodies as small as 0.5 mm (BLANKSTEIN et al. 2000; WHITTLE et al. 2000). After localization, foreign bodies may be removed under real-time ultrasound-guidance. The physician holds both transducer and hemostat as with any other ultrasound-guided procedure (Fig. 18.12). Preliminary injection of anesthetic around the foreign body is mandatory and is particularly important in chronic cases to loosen the fibrotic tissue that may surround the foreign body. The procedure was described by SHIELS et al. (1990), but is not frequent in daily practice despite excellent results. Alternatively, a preoperative ultrasound-guided skin drawing (noting the depth) may help reducing the extent of the surgical procedure.

18.9
Preoperative Localization

Small nonpalpable soft tissue lesions, such as recurrence of sarcoma or metastases from malignant melanoma, may be very difficult to remove surgically. Preoperative marking under ultrasound-guidance easily guides the tip of a needle into the lesion (Fig. 18.13) (QUINN et al. 2001; RUTTEN et al. 1997), as is already routine for nonpalpable breast tumors. The different types of needles that may be used have in common a system (hook) at the end of the needle or wire, which makes withdrawal difficult without surgery. As with foreign bodies, an ultrasound-guided skin drawing (with indication of depth) is sometimes sufficient for surgery.

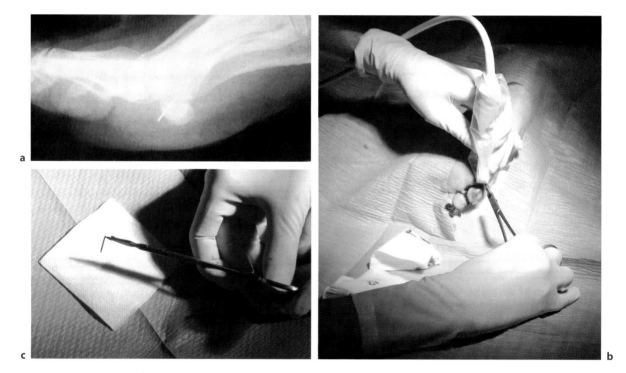

Fig. 18.12a–c. Foreign body in the plantar foot in a 40-year-old woman. **a** Plain radiography shows the foreign body is detected plantar to the fifth metatarsophalangeal joint. **b** This view shows ultrasound-guided removal of the foreign body. **c** The metallic foreign body after removal

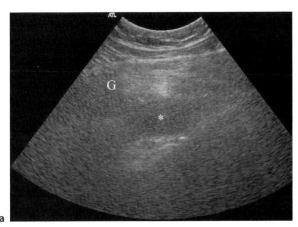

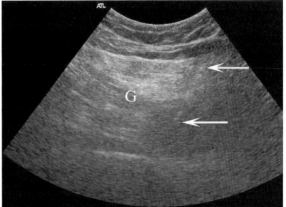

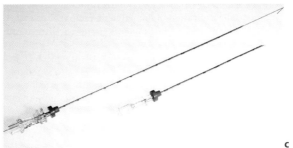

Fig. 18.13a–c. Malignant melanoma in a 55-year-old man. **a** Longitudinal ultrasound image (3.5 MHz curved array transducer) shows a solid, echo-poor tumor (*asterisk*) in the gluteus maximus muscle (*G*), suspected to be a metastasis. **b** During preoperative ultrasound-guided localization, the tip of a marking needle (*arrows*) is inserted into the tumor. **c** Localization set used in (**b**) shows the needle contains a wire with a hook at the end. The hook is to be placed in the tumor. Needles of different lengths are available

18.10
Conclusion

Ultrasound has become an established diagnostic method for patients with musculoskeletal diseases. It is also an unsurpassed imaging technique for the guidance of interventional procedures, thanks to the ability to follow the path of the needle in real-time during the entire procedure and in any plane. Interventional procedures are likely to become an integral part of musculoskeletal ultrasound examinations. Ultrasound, as an imaging technique, is useful at every step of the work-up of patients with musculoskeletal diseases: localization of soft tissue lesions, quick, safe and precise guiding of interventions, and follow-up (control of the efficacy of interventions).

References

Aina R, Cardinal E, Bureau NJ, Aubin B, Brassard P (2001) Calcific shoulder tendinitis: treatment with modifies US-guided fine-needle technique. Radiology 221:455–461

Adler RS, Sofka CM (2003) Percutaneous ultrasound-guided injections in the musculoskeletal system. Ultrasound Q 19:3–12

Alfredson H, Öhberg L (2005a) Neovascularisation in chronic painful patellar tendinosis – promising results after sclerosing neovessels outside the tendon challenge the need for surgery. Knee Surg Sports Traumatol Arthrosc 13:74–80

Alfredson H, Öhberg L (2005b) Sclerosing injections to areas of neo-vascularisation reduce pain in chronic Achilles tendinopathy: a double-blind randomized controlled trial. Knee Surg Sports Traumatol Arthrosc 13:338–344

Blankstein A, Cohen I, Heiman Z, Salai M, Heim M, Chechick A (2000) Localization, detection and guided removal of soft tissue in the hands using sonography. Arch Orthop Trauma Surg 120:514–517

Bradley M, Bhamra MS, Robson MJ (1995) Ultrasound guided aspiration of symptomatic supraspinatus calcific deposits. Br J Radiol 68:716–719

Breidahl WH, Adler RS (1996) Ultrasound-guided injection of ganglia with corticosteroids. Skeletal Radiol 25:635–638

Cardinal E, Chhem RK, Beauregard CG (1998) Ultrasound-guided interventional procedures in the musculoskeletal system. Radiol Clin North Am 36:597–604

Chiou HJ, Chou YH, WU JJ, Hsu CC, Tiu CM, Chanh CY, Yu C (1999) Alternative and effective treatment of shoulder ganglion cyst: ultrasonographically guided aspiration. J Ultrasound Med 18:531–535

Christensen RA, Van Sonnenberg E, Casola G, Wittich GR (1988) Interventional ultrasound in the musculoskeletal system. Radiol Clin North Am 26:145–156

Cooper G, Lutz GE, Adler RS (2005) Ultrasound-guided aspiration of symptomatic rotator cuff calcific tendonitis Am J Phys Med Rehabil 84:81

Court-Payen M, Bjerregaard B, Lausten G, Ingemann-Jensen L, Skjoldbye B (1996) Biopsie échoguidée des tumeurs des tissues mous des extrémités. JEMU 17:66 (Abstract SFAUMB 17th congress, Paris, France, 28–30 Mar 1996)

Craig JG (1999) Infection: ultrasound-guided procedures. Radiol Clin North Am 37:669–678

Eustace JA, Brophy DP, Gibney RP, Bresnihan B, Fitzgerald O (1997) Comparison of the accuracy of steroid placement with clinical outcome in patients with shoulder symptoms. Am Rheum Dis 56:59–63

Farin PU (1995) Rotator cuff calcifications: treatment with US-guided technique. Radiology 195:841–843

Fessell DP, Jacobson JA, Craig J, Habra G, Prasad A, Radliff A, van Holsbeeck, MT (2000) Using sonography to reveal and aspirate joint effusions. Am J Roentgenol 174:1353–1362

Fornage BD, Lorigan JG (1989) Sonographic detection and fine needle aspiration of nonpalpable recurrent or metastatic melanoma in subcutaneous tissues. J Ultrasound Med 8:421–424

Fredberg U, Bolvig L, Pfeiffer-Jensen M, Clemmensen D, Jakobsen BW, Stengaard-Pedersen K (2004) Ultrasonography as a tool for diagnosis, guidance of local steroid injection and, together with pressure algometry, monitoring of the treatment of athletes with chronic jumper's knee and Achilles tendonitis: a randomised, double-blind, placebo-controlled study. Scand J Rheumatol 33:94–101

Grassi W, Lamanna G, Farina A, Cervini C (1999) Synovitis of small joints: sonographic guided diagnostic and therapeutic approach. Ann Rheum Dis 58:595–597

Hall S, Buchbinder R (2004) Do imaging methods that guide needle placement improve outcome? Ann Rheum Dis 63:1007–1008

Holm HH, Skjoldbye B (1996) Interventional ultrasound. Ultrasound Med Biol 22:773–789

Kaiser S, Rosenborg M. (1994) Early detection of subperiostal abscesses by ultrasonography. A means for further successful treatment in paediatric osteomyelitis. Pediatr Radiol 24:336–339

Komppa GH, Northern JR, Hass DK (1985) Ultrasound guidance for needle aspiration of the hip in patients with painful hip prosthesis. J Clin Ultrasound 13:443–434

Little CM, Parker MG, Callowich MC, Sartori JC (1986) The ultrasonic detection of foreign bodies. Invest Radiol 21:275–277

Migliore A, Tormenta S, Martin Martin LS, Valente C, Massafra U, Latini A, Alimonti A (2004) Profilo di sicurezza si 185 iniezioni intra-articolari sotto guida echographica nelle coxopatie. Reumatismo 56:104–109

Naredo E, Cabero F, Beneyto P, Cruz A, Mondejar B, Uson J, Palop MJ, Crespo M (2004) A randomized comparative study of short term response to blind injection versus sonographic-guided injection of local corticosteroids in patients with painful shoulder. J Rheumatol 31:308–314

Peetrons P, Court-Payen M (2002) Interventional procedures in musculoskeletal ultrasound. Sem Interv Radiol 19:189–196

Pekkafahli MZ, Kiralp MZ, Basekim CC, Silit E, Mutlu H, Ozturk E, Kizilkaya E, Dursun H (2003) Sacroiliac joint injections performed with sonographic guidance. J Ultrasound Med 22:553–559

Quinn PS, Sieunarine K, Lawrence-Brown M, Tan P (2001) Intramuscular haemangiomas: hookwire localization prior to surgical excision: report of four cases. ANZ J Surg 71:62–66

Qvistgaard E, Kristoffersen H, Terslev L, Danneskiold-Samsoe B, Torp-Pedersen S, Bliddal H (2001) Guidance by ultrasound of intra-articular injections in the knee and hip joints. Osteoarthritis Cartilage 9:512–517

Rubens DJ, Fultz PJ, Gottlieb RH, Rubin SJ (1997) Effective ultrasonographically guided intervention for diagnosis of musculoskeletal lesions. J Ultrasound Med 16:831–842

Rutten MJ, Schreurs BW, van Kampen A, Schreuder HW (1997) Excisional biopsy of impalpable soft tissue tumors. US-guided preoperative localization in 12 cases. Acta Orthop Scand 68:384–386

Shiels WE 2nd, Babcock DS, Wilson JL, Burch RA (1990) Localization and guided removal of soft-tissue foreign bodies with sonography. Am J Roentgenol 155:1277–1281

Sites BD, Gallagher JD, Cravero J, Lundberg J, Blike G (2004) The learning curve associated with a simulated ultrasound-guided interventional task by inexperienced anesthesia residents. Reg Anesth Pain Med 29:544–548

Sofka CM, Adler RS (2002) Ultrasound-guided interventions in the foot and ankle. Semin Musculoskelet Radiol 6:163–168

van Holsbeeck MT, Eyler WR, Sherman LS, Lombardi TJ, Mezger E, Verner JJ, Shurman JR, Jonsson K (1994) Detection of infection in loosened hip prosthesis: efficacy of sonography. Am J Roentgenol 163:381–384

Weidner S, Kellner W, Kellner H (2004) Interventional radiology and the musculoskeletal system. Best Pract Res Clin Rheumatol 18:945–956

Whittle C, Gonzalez P, Horvath E, Niedmann JP, Baldassare G, Seguel S, Mackinnon J (2000) Detection and characterisation by ultrasonography of soft tissue foreign bodies. Rev Med Chil 128:419–424

Williams P, Gumpel M (1983) Percutaneous needle synovial biopsy of the knee (1983) Br J Hosp Med 30:34,39–40,42–43

Zwar RB, Read JW, Noakes JB (2004) Sonographically guided glenohumeral joint injection. Am J Roentgenol 183:48–50

Subject Index

A

ABC (*see* aneurysmal bone cyst)
ablation protocol 312
abscess
– catheter drainage 392
– of the extremity 389
– percutaneous drainage 181
– percutaneous treatment 389
acetabulum/acetabular
– biopsy 63
– fracture 343, 344, 347, 360, 364
– osteolytic lesion 232
– osteolytic metastasis 302
– roof screw 353, 360
– screw fixation 364
Achilles
– bursitis 184
– tendinopathy 394
– tendon 184
– – rupture 185
acromioclavicular joint injection 154
acromion 183
acromioplasty 190
adhesive capsulitis 144, 338
advanced trauma life support (ATLS) protocol 344
aetoxysclerol 377
aggressive hemangioma 232, 238
air conditioning 5
alcohol 4
AMP (*see* antimicrobial prophylaxis)
anaphylactic shock 228
aneurysmal bone cyst (ABC) 240, 283
– curettage 285
– fine-needle aspiration 285
– genetics 284
– imaging 284
– radiation 288
– selective embolization 285
– surgical techniques 285
– treatment 284
angiography 292
ankle/foot injection 146
ankylosing
– spondylarthritis 87
– spondylitis 388

annular
– fissure 121
– fibrosus 120, 121, 127, 158
anterior pelvic ring, external fixation 357
antimicrobial prophylaxis (AMP) 5
antiseptic
– agent 3, 4
– shower 2
apatite deposit 329
appendicular skeleton biopsy 61
arachnoid membrane fibrosis 247
arachnoiditis 96, 127
Arnold neuralgia 87
arterial embolization 236, 285
arteriolar-capillary malformation 372
arteriovenous
– fistula 283, 370
– malformation (AVM)
– – imaging 292
– – treatment 292
– shunt 368
– – treatment 370
artery of Adamkiewicz 127
arthrodesis 243
arthrography 83, 86
aseptic
– discitis 107
– osteonecrosis 203
aspirated calcium 334
atlanto-axial joint 83
– normal arthrography 86
– posterolateral approach 84
atropine 43
AVM (*see* arteriovenous malformation)

B

back pain 157, 194
– facet-related 73
– sacroiliac-related 80
Baker cyst 386, 387
balloon
– inflation 261
– tamp 259

beveled
– bone trocar 225
– needle 10, 211
– – cementoplasty 208
bicipital tendon sheath 338, 339
bilateral
– acetabular metastases 234
– sacroplasty 247
biopsy
– bone penetration 40
– execution 35
– fluoroscopy 40
– guidance 15
– MR guidance 42
– patient positioning 35
– planning 18
– ultrasound-guided 15
– upper and lower limbs 64
– flexible loop radiofrequency electrode 163
– radiofrequency
– – electrode 107
– – nucleoplasty 107
bleomycin 378
blood dyscrasia 35
bone
– biopsy 49
– – coaxial technique 39
– – needle 312
– – tandem technique 39
– cyst 288
– grafting 285
– hypertrophy 370
– lesion biopsy 70
– metastases
– – alcoholization 305
– – radiofrequency ablation 309
– – selective embolization 382
– puncture 10
– tumor 232
– – curative treatment 326
– – pain management 301
– – palliative treatment 326
– – radiography 380
– – treatment strategy 325
– vertebroplasty needle 10
bonopty penetration set 44
brachial arteriography 372
breast cancer 53, 63, 382
bridement procedure 339
bronchial carcinoma 382
Brown Sequard syndrome 240
bursitis 182

C

C1–2 joint
– fluoroscopic control 85

– needle introduction 85
calcific
– tendinitis 190, 329, 331, 341
– – aspiration 334, 335
– tendinosis 188
calcium
– hydroxyapatite crystal 329
– phosphate (CaP) cement 209
– pyrophosphate deposition disease 88
calcium-containing cavity 330, 337
canal set position screw 364
capillary-venous malformation 373
carbon dioxide dissection 325
C-arm
– design magnet 16
– fluoroscopy 8
carotid artery 220
cauda equina
– compression 113
– syndrome 240
cefazolin 5
cellular
– anoxia 318
– hypoxia 318
cement
– allergic reactions 252
– injection 197, 227, 230
– – chewing gum pattern 229
– – technique 228
– – trabecular pattern 229
– injector 209
– leak/leakage 216, 225, 230, 246, 275
– – along the needle tract 251
– venous intravasation 248, 249
cementoplasty 230, 301, 326
– combined with surgery 241
– flat bones 227
– indications 198
– needle 11
– sacral wing 221
– technique 206
– – in the spine 211
– trocar 208, 211, 228
cephalosporin 5
cervical
– disc puncture 102
– discography 125
– facet joint 79
– spine biopsy 60
– vertebroplasty 220
chemical ablation 302
– patient selection 304
– technique 304
chemonucleolysis 94
chemopapain 99
chlorhexidine 2
chondroblastoma 284

chondrocyte 189
ciprofloxacin 33
coaxial
– bone biopsy 216
– needle 45
– technique 9, 10, 39
Cobb syndrome 379
coblation technology 107, 108, 322
colon cancer 63
comminuted sacral fracture 364
compartment syndrome 23
compartmental anatomy 64
– upper extremity 66
compression fracture 197, 273, 279
– lymphoma-related 267
– myeloma-related 265
computed tomography (CT) 7
– fluoroscopy 8
– – vertebroplasty 210
congestive heart failure 292
contrast arthrography 143
cord compression 207, 253
corn protein 237
corticosteroid 180
cortivazol 162, 167
craniovertebral region, posterolateral approach 84
cryoablation 199, 232, 316
– direct cell injury 317
– mechanism 317
– patient outcome 321
– patient selection 319
– skeletal metastases 319
– technique 319
cryoprobe 316
cryoshock phenomenon 322
cryosurgery, vascular injury 318
crystal formation 317
CT (see computed tomography)
curettage 285
curved needle 12
cutaneous arteriovenous shunt 369
cyst/cystic
– hygroma 378
– masses, ultrasound 180
– rupture 78, 168
cystogram 295
cytology 26

D

DA (see distension arthrography)
Dallas discogram description (DDD) 132
de Quervain tenosynovitis 390
degenerative arthritis 165
deltoid muscle 65
diabetic muscle infarction, MR imaging 23

digital subtraction
– angiography 228
– fluoroscopy 146
disc
– biopsy 53, 54, 58, 60
– disease, MR imaging 121
– herniation 93, 165
– leak 250
– morphology 131, 132
– prostheses 163
– protrusion 132, 134
– puncture 100
discitis 54, 137
discogenic pain 119–121, 157
– pain provocation 133
discographic pain 136
discography 101
– complications 137
– contraindications 123
– double-needle technique 124
– equipment 124
– indications 123
– interpretation 131
– technique 123
disectomy 94
distal femoral biopsy 69
distension arthrography (DA) 329, 337
– technique 338
Dixon technique 17
doxycycline 378
drilling device 40
dual giudance technique 8
dysplasia 374, 379

E

elbow joint injection 150
electrical loop 309
embolization technique 370
enthesopathy 394
enzyme phospholipase A2 120
eosinophilic granuloma 63
– of the ilion 297
– of the odontoid 297
epidural
– abscess 251
– hematoma 53, 275
– leak 246
– steroid injection 99
epidurogram 99
epinephrine 377
Escherichia coli 33
ESWT (see extracorporeal shock wave therapy)
ethanol 294, 377
– ablation 302
– injection 240, 304

Ethibloc 377
– injection 288
external fixator 351
extracompartmental lesion 64
extracorporeal shock wave therapy (ESWT) 337, 341

F

facet
– block 166
– – test 166
– injection 155
– joint
– – anatomy 74
– – arthrosis 155
– – denervation 168, 169
– – disease 73
– – injection 74, 76, 77, 81, 166
– – innervation 75
– – pain, osteoarthritis-related 74
– – syndrome 165
– osteoarthritis 168
Fareed and Gallivan's technique 339
fasciitis 394
fast spin echo (FSE) sequence 17
femoral biopsy 67
fentanyl 206
fibrosarcoma 284
fibrous joint 154
fine needle aspiration (FNA) 37
flash sterilization 6
flat bones biopsy 61
flexor tendonitis 188
fluid collection 386
fluoroscopy 7
– bone biopsy 40
fluoroscopy-based navigation 355
FNA (*see* fine needle aspiration)
foraminal
– hernia 97
– leak 246
foreign body removal 396
free fragment retropulsion 253
frozen shoulder syndrome (FSS) 329, 337
– arthrography 338
– distension arthrography 338
– intra-articular injection steroids 340
– physiotherapy 340
FSS (*see* frozen shoulder syndrome)

G

Gaenslen maneuver 80
ganglion cyst 21, 24, 25, 77, 167, 180, 246
– needle puncture 387

– ultrasound 185
gas insulation 325
giant-cell tumor 284
glenohumeral joint 152
– injection 154
global positioning system (GPS) 354
GPS (*see* global positioning system)
great toe injection 153
greater
– sciatic notch lesions 195
– trochanteric bursitis 184
guidance technique 7
Guillain-Barré syndrome 260

H

hair removal 3
hand rub 4
helium 317
hematoma 392
– biopsy 22
– percutaneous treatment 389
hip
– arthroplasty 145
– injection 145, 150
– pain 146
– prosthesis loosening 146
histiocytosis 283
histoacryl 288
holmium:yttrium-aluminum-garnet (YAG) laser 103
hospital disinfectant, environmental protection agency (EPA)-approved 6
Huskisson visual analog scale 340
hydrocortisone 98
hydrodissection 324
hydroxyapatite 228
hygroma, percutaneous treatment 389
hyperselective arterial embolization 237
hyperthermia 292
hysterectomy 19

I

ice ball 320
IDET (*see* intradiscal electrothermal therapy)
IF (*see* internal fixation)
ILA (*see* interstitial laser ablation)
iliac wing
– biopsy 63
– screw 360
iliopsoas
– bursa 27
– – opacification 193
– tendon 192
iliosacral screw 357, 360

– fixation 352, 353, 363
imaging technique 7
impingement syndrome 330
inflatable bone tamp 259
instrument visualization 17
internal fixation (IF) 350
interstitial laser ablation (ILA) 305
intervention room (*see* also operating room)
– environmental surfaces 6
– ventilation 5
intervention site infection (ISI) 1
– pathogens
– – endogenous sources 2
– – exogenous sources 2
– risk prevention 2
intervertebral disc 93, 157
– anatomy 120
intracompartmental lesion 64
intradiscal
– electrothermal therapy (IDET) 112, 114, 136
– – results 163
– – technique 163
– steroid injection 162
– thermal therapy 162
intramuscular
– arteriovenous shunt 368
– injection 195
intraosseous
– arteriovenous shunt 369
– cyst 283
intravenous steroid 237
intravertebral sclerotherapy 233
iodophors 3
ISI (*see* intervention site infection)

J

joint
– effusion 386
– injection 143
– – under CT guidance 155
– – utility of ultrasound 149
– puncture 386
Joule-Thomson effect 317, 318
juxta-articular cyst 77

K

Kirschner wire 225
Klippel-Trenaunay syndrome (KTS) 379
Kocher-Langebeck approach 356
KTS (*see* Klippel-Trenaunay syndrome)
Kummel's disease 200, 203, 229
kyphon 271
kyphoplasty 209, 229, 241, 259
– balloon 267
– – inflation 243

– complications 275
– contraindications 260
– cost 226, 278
– effectiveness 273
– indications 260
– injection of contrast medium 271
– introducer 225
– patient positioning 273
– technique 271
– trocars 271
kyphosis 230, 274, 279
KyphX
– balloon 271
– device 259

L

labral cyst, needle puncture 387
lag screw 352, 360, 364
laminectomy 240, 274
Langerhans cell histiocytosis (LCH) 296
Laredo biopsy set 45, 46
laser
– ablation
– – osteoid osteoma 307
– – patient selection 305
– – technique 305
– nucleotomy 103, 109
lateral femoral lesion 67
LCH (*see* Langerhans cell histiocytosis)
leukemia 260
lidocaine hydrochloride 43
ligamentum flavum 75
lipodystrophy 98
lipomatosis 98
long acting steroid injection 167
loosened hip prosthesis, infection 386
lordoplasty 274
low back pain (*see* also back pain) 119, 121, 157
lumbar
– cyst infiltration 167
– disc
– – biopsy 55
– – high intensity zone (HIZ) 158
– – puncture 100
– discography 126, 161
– – skin puncture technique 128
– – technique 159
– facet
– – joint 76
– – syndrome 74
– spine biopsy
– – posterolateral extrapedicular approach 51
– – transpedicular approach 49
– synovial cyst 77
– – rupture 78
– vertebroplasty 211, 214, 217

lunate-triquetral ligament 148
lung cancer, knee metastasis 235
luxation gap 349
lymphangioma 378
lymphatic malformation 378
lymphoma 26, 69, 260
lytic bone lesion 287, 292, 382

M

macrocystic lymphatic malformation 378
macrodiskectomy 94
magnetic resonance (MR)
– guidance 8
– imaging (MRI) 9
Maigne syndrome 74
malignant melanoma 396, 397
manometer 159
map acquisition 355
medial femoral lesion 67
medical navigation system (MNS) 354
meniscoid structure 75
metameric arteriovenous shunt 379
metastatic
– disease 232
– lung cancer 233
methylmethacrylate 302
methylprednisolone 297
– acetate 295
micro-arteriovenous malformation 368
microbial contamination 2
microcatheter 370
microcystic lymphatic malformation 378
microdiskectomy 94
midazolam 206
– hydrochloride 43
midfoot injection 147
mixed vascular malformation 378
MNS (*see* medical navigation system)
multimyelomeric arteriovenous malformation 379
multiple myeloma 232, 260
muscular hypertrophy 192
musculoskeletal
– abscess 385
– lesion 37
– tumor, endovascular management 367, 379
– ultrasound procedure 385
mycobacteria 4
myeloma 198, 232, 274
myocardial infarction 278
myositis ossificans biopsy 23

N

NACD (*see* needle aspiration in calcified deposit)
navigation system 354

– CT-based 355
– fluoroscopy-based 355
– MR-based 355
N-butyl cyanoacrylate 237, 288
NCB (*see* needle core biopsy)
Nd:YAG laser 305
needle
– aspiration in calcified deposit (NACD) 329, 332
– – results 336
– biopsy technique 48
– core biopsy (NCB) 68
– placement 10
neoplastic disease 273
neuralgia 247
neurodystrophia 306
neurofibromatosis 20
neuroleptanalgesia 304
neurolysis 302
neuropraxia 321
neurosurgical decompression 247
non-Hodgkin lymphoma, B-cell type 34
noninfectious
– bursitis 386
– discitis 275
nonpalpable bicipital bursitis 389
non-steroidal anti-inflammatory drug (NSAID) 306
nosocomial infection 1
NSAID (*see* non-steroidal anti-inflammatory drug)
nucleolysis 99
nucleoplasty 107
– cervical level 111
– complications 113
– lumbar level 109
– materials 108
– patient selection 108
– post-operative instructions 112
– results 113
– technique 109
– thoracic level 109
nucleotomy 7, 12, 99, 108, 163
nucleus pulposus 119, 120, 127

O

olecranon bursitis
– ultrasound examination
– – patient selection 183
– – procedure 183
open biopsy 15
operating room (*see* also intervention room)
– ventilation 5
optical fiber 104
osseous lesion 38
osteitis 1
osteoarthritis 1, 75, 87, 167
– C1–2 86

osteoblastic lesion 205
osteoblastoma 310, 312, 326
osteoclast 294
osteoclastic giant cell 284
osteoid osteoma 312, 326
– laser ablation 305, 307
osteolytic
– bone metastases 198, 232
– – ablation 302
– bone tumor 304
– lesion 284
osteomyelitis 181, 392
osteonecrosis 229, 230
osteopenia 252
osteophyte 173, 192
osteoporosis/osteoporotic 216, 252
– compression fracture 263
– fracture 246
– vertebral fracture 198, 209, 230
– – kyphoplasty 225
osteosarcoma 284
osteosynthesis 37
ostycut biopsy needle 43
oven effect 312

P

pain
– provocation test 124
– tolerance 134
paralabral cyst 191
paraplegia 246
paraspinal
– mass biopsy 52
– structures biopsy 58
paravertebral
– abscess 240
– leak 250
– muscle contraction 158
Parkes-Weber syndrome 379
patellar tendon 186
pathology 26
patient positioning, biopsy 35
Patrick maneuver 80
pectoralis major muscle 65
pedicle fracture 275
pelvis/pelvic
– clamp 351
– fracture 344
– – closed reduction (CR) 350
– – limited access reduction (LAR) 350, 351
– – minimally invasive fixation methods 352
– – minimally invasive reduction methods 349
– – open reduction (OR) 350, 351
– – percutaneous reduction (PR) 350, 351
– lesion, needle biopsy 62
– ring disruption, AO/ASIF-classification 345

– ring fracture
– – stabilization 364
– – surgery 348
– ring injury 344
– stability 345
– trauma
– – biomechanics 344
– – radiological assessment 344
Perc-DC SpineWand 111
percutaneous
– aspiration of calcium 189
– biopsy 15, 18
– disc decompression 99
– embolization 370
– fixation
– – image-guided 352
– – online guidance 353
– laser disc decompression (PLDD) 103, 114
– – materials 104
– – patient selection 104
– – results 106
– – technique 104
– musculoskeletal biopsy (PMSB) 37
– – complication 70
– – patient preparation 48
– – positioning 48
– – post-procedure management 71
– – results 68
– reduction, hardware 352
– thermal ablation 232
– vertebroplasty 197, 232
– – imaging 207
periosteum 216
peripheral sclerosis 296
periradicular steroid injection (PSI) 93, 94
– cervical level 96
– complication 98
– disc herniation 94
– epidural lateral infiltration 95
– foraminal infiltration 96
– lumbar level 95
– patient selection 94
– results 98
– technique 94
– thoracic level 96
peritendinitis 394
perivertebral venous plexus leak 248
peroneal tenosynovitis 189
phlebography 237, 287
phlebolith 368, 374
photothermal efect 106
phrenic nerve palsy 96
piriformis
– muscle
– – hypertrophy 194
– – myositis 194
– syndrome 193

PLDD (*see* percutaneous laser disc decompression)
pleura/pleural
– injury 57
– line 56
– penetration 58
– transgression 56, 218
PMMA (*see* polymethyl-methacrylate)
PMSB (*see* percutaneous musculoskeletal biopsy)
pneumothorax 218
polymethyl-methacrylate (PMMA) 200, 227
– cement 209
portwine stain 373, 379
positive memory pain 159
post-biopsy 35
post-discography
– discitis 138
– imaging 129
post-disectomy syndrome 94
posterior
– ring fracture 361
– structure biopsy 53, 58
povidone 48
pre-biopsy 26
prednisolone 162
preoperative
– antiseptic shower 2
– shaving 2
pre-vertebroplasty pain 232
prostate cancer 52
provocative discography 119, 158, 162
proximal
– femoral lesion 67
– humeral lesion 66
PSI (*see* periradicular steroid injection)
pulmonary embolism 248, 275
pulsed radiofrequency 170
puncture
– site bleeding 253
– technique 9
pyomyositis 393

R

radiculopathy 246, 247
radiocarpal joint 151
radiofrequency (RF)
– ablation 199, 305
– – bipolar mode 309
– – equipment 309
– – mechanism 309
– – patient outcome 313
– – patient selection 309
– – technique 309
– ionization 27
– – equipment 322
– – mechanism 322

– – patient outcome 322
– – patient selection 322
– – technique 322
– temperature-controlled 169
radio-opaque marker 51
recrystallization 318
registration 355
renal cell carcinoma/tumor 23, 382
rheumatoid arthritis 87, 150
– C1–2 arthrography 89
rhizolysis
– results 169
– technique 168
rib
– biopsy 62
– fracture 278
– metastasis 313
robotics 356
rotating fluoroscope 41
rotationally unstable fracture 352
rotator
– cuff
– – calcification 188, 332, 336, 395
– – deposit 341
– – muscle 188
– – tears 191
– – tendon 329
– impingement 182

S

sacral
– biopsy 62
– foramina 221, 360
– fracture 343
– puncture 221
– stress fracture 224
sacroiliac joint 221
– anatomy 80
– arthritis 364
– biopsy 64
– disease 73
– injection 155
– – complications 81
– – results 173
– – technique 80, 173
– rupture gap 349
– syndrome 80, 172
sacroiliac radiofrequency denervation 174
sacroiliitis 64, 172
sacroplasty 221
sagittal phlebogram 238
sarcoma 69, 396
– biopsy 22
Scaglietti technique 295
scapholunate ligament 148

scaphotrapezial joint injection 152
Schanz screw 349, 351
Scheuermann disease 126
Schmorl node 131
sciatic nerve 194
sciatica 99, 101, 110, 194
sclerosant 237
sclerosing agent 288, 377
sclerotherapy 237, 285, 376, 377
– aggressive hemangioma 239
sclerotic lesion sampling 49
Scotty dog image 50, 53, 76, 100, 213
screw fixation 343
– quality criteria 360
scrub suit 6
sedoanalgesia 206, 210
selective embolization 285
septic
– arthritis 167
– discitis 52, 59
– spondylodiscitis 106
set position screw 352
Sharpey fiber 120
shielded needle electrode 309
shoulder
– arthrography 143
– – anterior approach 144
– calcific tendinitis 336
– – ESWT 337
– pain 191
– stiffness 337
– tendinitis 337
skin
– antisepsis 3
– preparation 3
skull biopsy 61, 62
snapping hip 192
sodium
– atoms 107
– tetradecyl sulphate (STD) 375
soft tissue
– abscess, percutaneous drainage 181
– biopsy 70
– cystic masses 180
– disorder, percutaneous treatment 179
– injection 181
spine/spinal
– biopsy 49
– cord
– – compression 38
– – decompression 236
– facet
– – block 81
– – syndrome 74
– fusion 136
– lesion 38
– metastases 206

– stenosis 274
SpineWand 108, 109
spondyloarthropathy 172
spondylodiscitis 54, 107
spondylolisthesis 163
stable injury 352
staphylococcus epidermidis 137
stay in the ring technique 50, 213, 217
STD (see sodium tetradecyl sulphate)
sterile gloves 7
sterility 1
sterilization of instruments 6
sternal fracture 278
steroid injection 83
– ultrasound-guided 388
stiff needle 12
streptococcus sacroiliitis 64
subacromial bursa 182, 330
subacromial-subdeltoid bursitis 182, 386
subchondral edema 158, 174
subscapularis calcification 191
subtalar joint, posteromedial approach 147
superior pubic ramus screw 357, 361, 364
superselective targeted arterial embolization 370
supraspinatus muscle 188
surgical
– biopsy set 45, 46
– clothing 6
– instruments, sterilization 6
– scrub 3
synovial
– cyst 167, 245, 386
– – C1–2 arthrography 89
– – drainage 53
– – needle puncture 387
– – puncture technique 168
– – surgical treatment 168
– disease 395

T

tandem needle technique 9, 10, 39, 40
targeted disc decompression (TDD) 114
teflon-sheated needle 376
telangiectasia 373
telangiectatic osteosarcoma 284
Temno biopsy set 47
tendinitis 330
tendinopathy 187, 394
tendinosis 186
– ultrasound 186
tendon 186
– rupture 180
– traumatic injury 190
tendonosis 192
tenography, ultrasound-giuded injection 187

tenosynovitis 386
– ultrasound-guided injection 187
thermal
– ablation 305
– – image-guided 324
– – technique 199
– conductivity 324
– injury 324
– insulation 324
– insulator blanket 324, 325
– necrosis 273
– protection 324, 325
– spondylitis 106, 115
thermocouple 325
thoracic
– disc
– – biopsy 59
– – puncture 101
– discography 126
– spine, biopsy
– – costoteansversal approach 57
– – costovertebral approach 55
– – extrapedicular approach 55
– – transpedicular approach 55
– vertebroplasty 216, 218
thyroid cancer/tumor 312, 382
tibial lesion biopsy 69
tissue cooling 316
tracking system 355
transiliosacral instability 346
trans-oral vertebroplasty 222
transpedicular puncture 11
transpubic insrability 346
transsacral instability 346
traumatic
– burst fracture 243
– vertebral fracture 200
– – in young patients 240
trendinosis 182
trephine 47
triamcinolone hexacetonide 162
triangulation system 17
trochanteric bursitis 184
tumor
– decompression 322
– image-guided management 301

U

UBC (*see* unicameral bone cyst)
ultrasound 7
– injection of tendons 186
– joint puncture 386
ultrasound-guided injection
– free hand technique 149
– patient positioning 149

unicameral bone cyst (UBC) 283
– autologous bone marrow injection 296
– curettage 296
– imaging 294
– steroid injection 295
– surgery 296
– treatment 294

V

valsalva maneuver 374
varicosity 374
VAS (*see* visual analog score)
vascular
– malformation 236, 367
– – angiography 375
– – classification 368
– – diagnosis 368
– – direct percutaneous catheterization 375
– – ultrasound 375
– thrombosis 236
venography 228, 229, 271
venous
– ischemia 372
– vascular malformation 374
ventilation 5
vertebra/vertebral 50
– anatomy 83
– arteriography 87
– artery 85
– – accidental puncture 87
– – injury 98
– biopsy 60
– body
– – fracture 260
– – osteolytic destruction 198
– – pre-fractured 230
– collapse 38
– compression fracture 241
– – Magerl's classification 204
– fracture 200
– height restoration 274
– hemangioma (VH) 60, 200, 232
– – intravertebral sclerotherapy 237
– – percutaneous vertebroplasty 237
– metastases 38
– osteonecrosis 165, 200
– plana 204
vertebrectomy 198
vertebroplasty 7, 8
– aggressive hemangioma 239
– cement 208
– choice of cement 227
– complications 244, 275
– contraindications 204
– cost 278

– image guidance 210
– indications 198
– infection 251
– materials 208
– needle 10, 208
– osteoporotic fractures 230
– technique 206
vertically unstable fracture 352
VH (*see* vertebral hemangioma)

virtual-real mismatch 354
visual analog score (VAS) 313

W

wrist
– arthrography 148
– injection 148, 153

List of Contributors

Ronald S. Adler, MD, PhD
Professor of Radiology
Weill Medical College of Cornell University
Attending Radiologist
Chief, Division of Ultrasound and Body Imaging
Hospital for Special Surgery
535 East 70th Street
New York, NY 10021
USA
Email: adlerr@hss.edu

Guillaume Bierry, MD, PhD
Fellow
Department of Radiology B
University Hospital of Strasbourg
Pavillon Clovis Vincent BP 426
67091 Strasbourg
France
Email: guillaume.bierry@chru-strasbourg.fr

Xavier Buy, MD
Senior Radiologist
Department of Radiology B
University Hospital of Strasbourg
Pavillon Clovis Vincent BP 426
67091 Strasbourg
France
Email: buy.xavier@neuf.fr

Alain Chevrot, MD
Professor and Chairman
Department of Radiology B
Cochin University Hospital
Assistance Publique – Hôpitaux de Paris
Paris Descartes University
27 rue Faubourg Saint Jacques
75679 Paris cedex 14
France
Email: alain.chevrot@cch.aphp.fr

Michel Court-Payen, MD, PhD
Senior Radiologist
Department of Imaging
Gildhoj Private Hospital
Brondbyvester Boulevard 16
2605 Brondby
Denmark
Email: mcp@dadlnet.dk

Jean-Louis Dietemann, MD
Professor
Department of Radiology B
University Hospital of Strasbourg
Pavillon Clovis Vincent BP 426
67091 Strasbourg
France
Email: jean-louis.dietemann@chru-strasbourg.fr

Jean-Luc Drapé, MD, PhD
Professor
Department of Radiology B
Cochin University Hospital
Assistance Publique – Hôpitaux de Paris
Paris Descartes University
27 rue Faubourg Saint Jacques
75679 Paris cedex 14
France
Email: jean-luc.drape@cch.aphp.fr

Josée Dubois, MD
Professor of Radiology
University of Montreal
Pediatric and Interventional Radiologist
Department of Medical Imaging
Centre Hospitalo-Universitaire Sainte-Justine
3175 Côte Sainte-Catherine Road
Montreal, QC, H3T 1C5
Canada
Email: josee-dubois@ssss.gouv.qc.ca

Antoine Feydy, MD, PhD
Associate Professor
Department of Radiology B
Cochin University Hospital
Assistance Publique – Hôpitaux de Paris
Paris Descartes University
27 rue Faubourg Saint Jacques
75679 Paris cedex 14
France
Email: antoine.feydy@cch.aphp.fr

Kathleen C. Finzel, MD
Director, Diagnostic Imaging
ProHealth Care Associates
2800 Marcus Avenue
Lake Success, NY 11042
USA
Email: KFinzel@ProHealthcare.com

AFSHIN GANGI, MD, PhD
Professor of Radiology
Department of Radiology B
University Hospital of Strasbourg
Pavillon Clovis Vincent BP 426
67091 Strasbourg
France
Email: gangi@rad6.u-strasbg.fr

LAURENT GAREL, MD
Professor of Radiology
University of Montreal
Pediatric and Interventional Radiologist
Department of Medical Imaging
Centre Hospitalo-Universitaire Sainte-Justine
3175 Côte Sainte-Catherine Road
Montreal, QC, H3T 1C5
Canada
Email: laurent_garel@ssss.gouv.qc.ca

DIDIER GODEFROY, MD
Professor
Department of Radiology B
Cochin University Hospital
Assistance Publique – Hôpitaux de Paris
Paris Descartes University
27 rue Faubourg Saint Jacques
75679 Paris cedex 14
France
Email: didier.godefroy@wanadoo.fr

THOMAS GROSS, MD
Head, Division of Traumatology
Ospedale Regionale di Lugano
Via Tesserete 46
6900 Lugano
Switzerland
Email: tgross@uhbs.ch

ALI GUERMAZI, MD
Associate Professor of Radiology
Department of Radiology
Section Chief, Musculoskeletal
Boston University School of Medicine
820 Harrison Avenue, FGH Building, 3rd Floor
Boston, MA 02118
USA
Email: ali.guermazi@bmc.org

STÉPHANE GUTH, MD
Senior Radiologist
Department of Radiology B
University Hospital of Strasbourg
Pavillon Clovis Vincent BP 426
67091 Strasbourg
France
Email: guth.stephane.str@evc.net

LOTFI HACEIN-BEY, MD
Professor of Radiology
Radiological Associates of Sacramento Medical Group Inc.
1500 Expo Parkway
Sacramento, CA 95815
USA
and
Sutter Neuroscience Institute
2800 L Street, Suite 630
Sacramento, CA 95816
USA
Email: lhaceinbey@yahoo.com

BASSAM HAMZE, MD
Consultant Radiologist
Department of Musculoskeletal Radiology
Lariboisière University Hospital
2 rue Ambroise Paré
75010 Paris
France
Email: hamzeb@club-internet.fr

JACQUELINE C. HODGE, MD
Attending Radiologist
Department of Radiology
Lenox Hill Hospital
100 E 77th Street
New York, NY 10021
USA
Email: chezjch@yahoo.com

ROLF HUEGLI, MD
Head, Institute of Radiology
Cantonal Hospital Bruderholz
Batteriestrasse 1
4101 Bruderholz
Switzerland
Email: rhuegli@uhbs.ch

JEAN-PIERRE IMBERT, MD
Senior Radiologist
Department of Radiology B
University Hospital of Strasbourg
Pavillon Clovis Vincent BP 426
67091 Strasbourg
France
Email: yiannis1@free.fr

FARAH IRANI, MD
Senior Radiologist
Department of Radiology B
University Hospital of Strasbourg
Pavillon Clovis Vincent BP 426
67091 Strasbourg
France
Email: drfarahirani@yahoo.co.uk

Augustinus L. Jacob, MD
Head, Division of Interventional Radiology
University Hospital Basel
Petersgraben 4
4031 Basel
Switzerland
Email: ajacob@uhbs.ch

Paula Klurfan, MD
Clinical Fellow in Interventional Neuroradiology
Department of Radiology
Toronto Western Hospital
University of Toronto
399 Bathurst Street
3-East Wing
Toronto, ON M5T 2S8
Canada
Email: paula.klurfan@gmail.com

Jean-Denis Laredo, MD
Professor and Chairman
Department of Musculoskeletal Radiology
Lariboisière University Hospital
2 rue Ambroise Paré
75010 Paris
France
Email: jean-denis.laredo@lrb.ap-hop-paris.fr

Galina Levin, MD
Fellow
Department of Radiology
Winthrop University Hospital
259 First Street
Mineola, NY 11501
USA
Email: levin2002us@yahoo.com

Jonathan S. Luchs, MD
Assistant Professor
Director, Musculoskeletal Imaging and Intervention
Department of Radiology
Winthrop University Hospital
259 First Street
Mineola, NY 11501
USA
Email: JLuchs@Winthrop.org

David Malfair, MD, FRCPC
Assistant Professor
Department of Radiology
Vancouver General Hospital
University of British Columbia
899 West 12th Avenue
Vancouver, BC V5Z 1M9
Canada
Email: dmalfair@hotmail.com

Kimmo Mattila, MD, PhD
Section Chief, Musculosceletal Radiology
Department of Diagnostic Radiology
Turku University Hospital
Kiinamyllynkatu 4–8
20520 Turku
Finland
Email: Kimmo.Mattila@tyks.fi

Peter Messmer, MD
Consultant Surgeon, Ortho Trauma Center
Rashid Hospital, DOHMS
P.O. Box 4545
Dubai
United Arab Emirates
Email: peter.messmer@usz.ch

Peter L. Munk, MD, CM, FRCPC
Professor and Head, Musculoskeletal Division
Department of Radiology
Vancouver General Hospital
University of British Columbia
899 West 12th Avenue
Vancouver, BC V5Z 1M9
Canada
Email: Peter.Munk@vch.ca

A. Orlando Ortiz, MD, MBA, FACR
Professor and Chairman
Department of Radiology
Winthrop University Hospital
259 First Street
Mineola, NY 11501
USA
Email: oortiz@winthrop.org

Caroline Parlier-Cuau, MD
Assistant Professor
Department of Musculoskeletal Radiology
Lariboisière University Hospital
2 rue Ambroise Paré
75010 Paris
France
Email: mail@cuau-parlier.fsnet.co.uk

Philippe Peetrons, MD
Professor and Chairman
Department of Medical Imaging
Centre Hospitalier Molière-Longchamp
142 Rue Marconi
1190 Brussels
Belgium
Email: peetrons@infonie.be

WILFRED C. G. PEH, MD, MBBS, FRCPG, FRCPE, FRCR
Clinical Professor
National University of Singapore
Senior Consultant Radiologist
Alexandra Hospital
378 Alexandra Road
Singapore 159964
Republic of Singapore
Email: wilfred.peh@gmail.com

MARTIN E. SIMONS, BSc, MD, FRCPC
Assistant Professor of Medical Imaging
Department of Radiology
Toronto Western Hospital
University of Toronto
399 Bathurst Street
3-East Wing
Toronto, ON M5T 2S8
Canada
Email: martin.simons@uhn.on.ca

KONGTENG TAN, MD, FRCS, FRCR
Assistant Professor
Department of Radiology
University Health Network
University of Toronto, NCSB, 1C563
585 University Avenue
Toronto, ON M5G 2N2
Canada
Email: kongteng.tan@uhn.on.ca

KAREL G. TERBRUGGE, MD, FRCP
Professor of Radiology and Surgery
Head, Division of Neuroradiology
Department of Radiology
Toronto Western Hospital
University of Toronto
399 Bathurst Street, 3-East Wing
Toronto, ON M5T 2S8
Canada
Email: karel.terbrugge@uhn.on.ca

MARC WYBIER, MD
Consultant Radiologist
Department of Musculoskeletal Radiology
Lariboisière University Hospital
2 rue Ambroise Paré
75010 Paris
France
Email: marc.wybier@lrb.ap-hop-paris.fr

MEDICAL RADIOLOGY Diagnostic Imaging and Radiation Oncology

Titles in the series already published

DIAGNOSTIC IMAGING

Innovations in Diagnostic Imaging
Edited by J. H. Anderson

Radiology of the Upper Urinary Tract
Edited by E. K. Lang

The Thymus - Diagnostic Imaging, Functions, and Pathologic Anatomy
Edited by E. Walter, E. Willich, and W. R. Webb

Interventional Neuroradiology
Edited by A. Valavanis

Radiology of the Lower Urinary Tract
Edited by E. K. Lang

Contrast-Enhanced MRI of the Breast
S. Heywang-Köbrunner and R. Beck

Spiral CT of the Chest
Edited by M. Rémy-Jardin and J. Rémy

Radiological Diagnosis of Breast Diseases
Edited by M. Friedrich and E. A. Sickles

Radiology of Trauma
Edited by M. Heller and A. Fink

Biliary Tract Radiology
Edited by P. Rossi. Co-edited by M. Brezi

Radiological Imaging of Sports Injuries
Edited by C. Masciocchi

Modern Imaging of the Alimentary Tube
Edited by A. R. Margulis

Diagnosis and Therapy of Spinal Tumors
Edited by P. R. Algra, J. Valk and J. J. Heimans

Interventional Magnetic Resonance Imaging
Edited by J. F. Debatin and G. Adam

Abdominal and Pelvic MRI
Edited by A. Heuck and M. Reiser

Orthopedic Imaging
Techniques and Applications
Edited by A. M. Davies and H. Pettersson

Radiology of the Female Pelvic Organs
Edited by E. K. Lang

Magnetic Resonance of the Heart and Great Vessels
Clinical Applications
Edited by J. Bogaert, A. J. Duerinckx, and F. E. Rademakers

Modern Head and Neck Imaging
Edited by S. K. Mukherji and J. A. Castelijns

Radiological Imaging of Endocrine Diseases
Edited by J. N. Bruneton
in collaboration with B. Padovani and M.-Y. Mourou

Radiology of the Pancreas
2nd Revised Edition
Edited by A. L. Baert. Co-edited by G. Delorme and L. Van Hoe

Trends in Contrast Media
Edited by H. S. Thomsen, R. N. Muller, and R. F. Mattrey

Functional MRI
Edited by C. T. W. Moonen and P. A. Bandettini

Emergency Pediatric Radiology
Edited by H. Carty

Liver Malignancies
Diagnostic and Interventional Radiology
Edited by C. Bartolozzi and R. Lencioni

Spiral CT of the Abdomen
Edited by F. Terrier, M. Grossholz, and C. D. Becker

Medical Imaging of the Spleen
Edited by A. M. De Schepper and F. Vanhoenacker

Radiology of Peripheral Vascular Diseases
Edited by E. Zeitler

Radiology of Blunt Trauma of the Chest
P. Schnyder and M. Wintermark

Portal Hypertension
Diagnostic Imaging and Imaging-Guided Therapy
Edited by P. Rossi.
Co-edited by P. Ricci and L. Broglia

Virtual Endoscopy and Related 3D Techniques
Edited by P. Rogalla, J. Terwisscha van Scheltinga and B. Hamm

Recent Advances in Diagnostic Neuroradiology
Edited by Ph. Demaerel

Transfontanellar Doppler Imaging in Neonates
A. Couture, C. Veyrac

Radiology of AIDS
A Practical Approach
Edited by J. W. A. J. Reeders and P. C. Goodman

CT of the Peritoneum
A. Rossi, G. Rossi

Magnetic Resonance Angiography
2nd Revised Edition
Edited by I. P. Arlart, G. M. Bongartz, and G. Marchal

Applications of Sonography in Head and Neck Pathology
Edited by J. N. Bruneton
in collaboration with C. Raffaelli, O. Dassonville

3D Image Processing
Techniques and Clinical Applications
Edited by D. Caramella and C. Bartolozzi

Imaging of the Larynx
Edited by R. Hermans

Pediatric ENT Radiology
Edited by S. J. King and A. E. Boothroyd

Imaging of Orbital and Visual Pathway Pathology
Edited by W. S. Müller-Forell

Radiological Imaging of the Small Intestine
Edited by N. C. Gourtsoyiannis

Imaging of the Knee
Techniques and Applications
Edited by A. M. Davies and V. N. Cassar-Pullicino

Perinatal Imaging
From Ultrasound to MR Imaging
Edited by F. E. Avni

Diagnostic and Interventional Radiology in Liver Transplantation
Edited by E. Bücheler, V. Nicolas, C. E. Broelsch, X. Rogiers and G. Krupski

Imaging of the Pancreas
Cystic and Rare Tumors
Edited by C. Procacci and A. J. Megibow

Imaging of the Foot & Ankle
Techniques and Applications
Edited by A. M. Davies, R. W. Whitehouse and J. P. R. Jenkins

Radiological Imaging of the Ureter
Edited by F. Joffre, Ph. Otal and M. Soulie

Radiology of the Petrous Bone
Edited by M. Lemmerling and S. S. Kollias

Imaging of the Shoulder
Techniques and Applications
Edited by A. M. Davies and J. Hodler

Interventional Radiology in Cancer
Edited by A. Adam, R. F. Dondelinger, and P. R. Mueller

Imaging and Intervention in Abdominal Trauma
Edited by R. F. Dondelinger

Radiology of the Pharynx and the Esophagus
Edited by O. Ekberg

Radiological Imaging in Hematological Malignancies
Edited by A. Guermazi

Functional Imaging of the Chest
Edited by H.-U. Kauczor

Duplex and Color Doppler Imaging of the Venous System
Edited by G. H. Mostbeck

Multidetector-Row CT of the Thorax
Edited by U. J. Schoepf

Radiology and Imaging of the Colon
Edited by A. H. Chapman

Multidetector-Row CT Angiography
Edited by C. Catalano and R. Passariello

Focal Liver Lesions
Detection, Characterization, Ablation
Edited by R. Lencioni, D. Cioni, and
C. Bartolozzi

**Imaging in Treatment Planning
for Sinonasal Diseases**
Edited by R. Maroldi and P. Nicolai

Clinical Cardiac MRI
With Interactive CD-ROM
Edited by J. Bogaert, S. Dymarkowski,
and A. M. Taylor

**Dynamic Contrast-Enhanced Magnetic
Resonance Imaging in Oncology**
Edited by A. Jackson, D. L. Buckley, and
G. J. M. Parker

Contrast Media in Ultrasonography
Basic Principles and Clinical Applications
Edited by E. Quaia

Paediatric Musculoskeletal Disease
With an Emphasis on Ultrasound
Edited by D. Wilson

**MR Imaging in White Matter Diseases of the
Brain and Spinal Cord**
Edited by M. Filippi, N. De Stefano,
V. Dousset, and J. C. McGowan

Imaging of the Hip & Bony Pelvis
Techniques and Applications
Edited by A. M. Davies, K. Johnson,
and R. W. Whitehouse

Imaging of Kidney Cancer
Edited by A. Guermazi

**Magnetic Resonance Imaging in
Ischemic Stroke**
Edited by R. von Kummer and T. Back

Diagnostic Nuclear Medicine
2nd Revised Edition
Edited by C. Schiepers

**Imaging of Occupational and
Environmental Disorders of the Chest**
Edited by P. A. Gevenois and P. De Vuyst

Virtual Colonoscopy
A Practical Guide
Edited by P. Lefere and S. Gryspeerdt

Contrast Media
Safety Issues and ESUR Guidelines
Edited by H. S. Thomsen

Head and Neck Cancer Imaging
Edited by R. Hermans

Vascular Embolotherapy
A Comprehensive Approach
Volume 1: *General Principles, Chest,
Abdomen, and Great Vessels*
Edited by J. Golzarian. Co-edited by
S. Sun and M. J. Sharafuddin

Vascular Embolotherapy
A Comprehensive Approach
Volume 2: *Oncology, Trauma, Gene
Therapy, Vascular Malformations,
and Neck*
Edited by J. Golzarian. Co-edited by
S. Sun and M. J. Sharafuddin

Vascular Interventional Radiology
Current Evidence in Endovascular Surgery
Edited by M. G. Cowling

Ultrasound of the Gastrointestinal Tract
Edited by G. Maconi and
G. Bianchi Porro

Parallel Imaging in Clinical MR Applications
Edited by S. O. Schoenberg, O. Dietrich,
and M. F. Reiser

MRI and CT of the Female Pelvis
Edited by B. Hamm and R. Forstner

Imaging of Orthopedic Sports Injuries
Edited by F. M. Vanhoenacker,
M. Maas and J. L. Gielen

Ultrasound of the Musculoskeletal System
S. Bianchi and C. Martinoli

Clinical Functional MRI
Presurgical Functional Neuroimaging
Edited by C. Stippich

**Radiation Dose from Adult and Pediatric
Multidetector Computed Tomography**
Edited by D. Tack and P. A. Gevenois

Spinal Imaging
Diagnostic Imaging of the Spine and Spinal Cord
Edited by J. Van Goethem,
L. van den Hauwe and P. M. Parizel

Computed Tomography of the Lung
A Pattern Approach
J. A. Verschakelen and W. De Wever

Imaging in Transplantation
Edited by A. Bankier

**Radiological Imaging of the
Neonatal Chest**
2nd Revised Edition
Edited by V. Donoghue

**Radiological Imaging of the Digestive Tract
in Infants and Children**
Edited by A. S. Devos and J. G. Blickman

Pediatric Chest Imaging
Chest Imaging in Infants and Children
2nd Revised Edition
Edited by J. Lucaya and J. L. Strife

Color Doppler US of the Penis
Edited by M. Bertolotto

Radiology of the Stomach and Duodenum
Edited by A. H. Freeman and E. Sala

Imaging in Pediatric Skeletal Trauma
Techniques and Applications
Edited by K. J. Johnson and E. Bache

Image Processing in Radiology
Current Applications
Edited by E. Neri, D. Caramella,
C. Bartolozzi

**Screening and Preventive Diagnosis with
Radiological Imaging**
Edited by M. F. Reiser, G. van Kaick,
C. Fink, S. O. Schoenberg

**Percutaneous Tumor Ablation in
Medical Radiology**
Edited by T. J. Vogl, T. K. Helmberger,
M. G. Mack, M. F. Reiser

**Liver Radioembolization
with ^{90}Y Microspheres**
Edited by J. I. Bilbao, M. F. Reiser

Pediatric Uroradiology
2nd Revised Edition
Edited by R. Fotter

Radiology of Osteoporosis
2nd Revised Edition
Edited by S. Grampp

**Gastrointestinal Tract Sonography
in Fetuses and Children**
A. Couture, C. Baud, J. L. Ferran,
M. Saguintaah and C. Veyrac

**Intracranial Vascular Malformations and
Aneurysms**
2nd Revised Edition
Edited by M. Forsting and I. Wanke

**High-Resolution Sonography of the
Peripheral Nervous System**
2nd Revised Edition
Edited by S. Peer and G. Bodner

Imaging Pelvic Floor Disorders
2nd Revised Edition
Edited by J. Stoker, S. A. Taylor, and
J. O. L. DeLancey

Coronary Radiology
2nd Revised Edition
Edited by M. Oudkerk and M. F. Reiser

**Integrated Cardiothoracic Imaging
with MDCT**
Edited by M. Rémy-Jardin and J. Rémy

Multislice CT
3rd Revised Edition
Edited by M. F. Reiser, C. R. Becker,
K. Nikolaou, G. Glazer

MRI of the Lung
Edited by H.-U. Kauczor

**Imaging in Percutaneous Musculoskeletal
Interventions**
Edited by A. Gangi, S. Guth, and
A. Guermazi

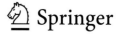

MEDICAL RADIOLOGY Diagnostic Imaging and Radiation Oncology
Titles in the series already published

RADIATION ONCOLOGY

Lung Cancer
Edited by C. W. Scarantino

Innovations in Radiation Oncology
Edited by H. R. Withers and L. J. Peters

Radiation Therapy of Head and Neck Cancer
Edited by G. E. Laramore

**Gastrointestinal Cancer –
Radiation Therapy**
Edited by R. R. Dobelbower, Jr.

Radiation Exposure and Occupational Risks
Edited by E. Scherer, C. Streffer, and
K.-R. Trott

Interventional Radiation
Therapy Techniques – Brachytherapy
Edited by R. Sauer

Radiopathology of Organs and Tissues
Edited by E. Scherer, C. Streffer, and
K.-R. Trott

Concomitant Continuous Infusion
Chemotherapy and Radiation
Edited by M. Rotman and C. J. Rosenthal

**Intraoperative Radiotherapy –
Clinical Experiences and Results**
Edited by F. A. Calvo, M. Santos, and
L. W. Brady

**Interstitial and Intracavitary
Thermoradiotherapy**
Edited by M. H. Seegenschmiedt and
R. Sauer

Non-Disseminated Breast Cancer
Controversial Issues in Management
Edited by G. H. Fletcher and S. H. Levitt

**Current Topics in
Clinical Radiobiology of Tumors**
Edited by H.-P. Beck-Bornholdt

**Practical Approaches to
Cancer Invasion and Metastases**
*A Compendium of Radiation
Oncologists' Responses to 40 Histories*
Edited by A. R. Kagan with the
Assistance of R. J. Steckel

Radiation Therapy in Pediatric Oncology
Edited by J. R. Cassady

Radiation Therapy Physics
Edited by A. R. Smith

Late Sequelae in Oncology
Edited by J. Dunst, R. Sauer

Mediastinal Tumors. Update 1995
Edited by D. E. Wood, C. R. Thomas, Jr.

**Thermoradiotherapy
and Thermochemotherapy**
Volume 1:
Biology, Physiology, and Physics
Volume 2:
Clinical Applications
Edited by M. H. Seegenschmiedt,
P. Fessenden and C. C. Vernon

Carcinoma of the Prostate
Innovations in Management
Edited by Z. Petrovich, L. Baert, and
L. W. Brady

Radiation Oncology of Gynecological Cancers
Edited by H. W. Vahrson

Carcinoma of the Bladder
Innovations in Management
Edited by Z. Petrovich, L. Baert, and
L. W. Brady

**Blood Perfusion and
Microenvironment of Human Tumors**
Implications for Clinical Radiooncology
Edited by M. Molls and P. Vaupel

Radiation Therapy of Benign Diseases
A Clinical Guide
2nd Revised Edition
S. E. Order and S. S. Donaldson

**Carcinoma of the Kidney and Testis,
and Rare Urologic Malignancies**
Innovations in Management
Edited by Z. Petrovich, L. Baert, and
L. W. Brady

**Progress and Perspectives in the
Treatment of Lung Cancer**
Edited by P. Van Houtte,
J. Klastersky, and P. Rocmans

**Combined Modality Therapy of
Central Nervous System Tumors**
Edited by Z. Petrovich, L. W. Brady,
M. L. Apuzzo, and M. Bamberg

Age-Related Macular Degeneration
Current Treatment Concepts
Edited by W. E. Alberti, G. Richard,
and R. H. Sagerman

**Radiotherapy of Intraocular and
Orbital Tumors**
2nd Revised Edition
Edited by R. H. Sagerman and
W. E. Alberti

Modification of Radiation Response
*Cytokines, Growth Factors,
and Other Biolgical Targets*
Edited by C. Nieder, L. Milas and
K. K. Ang

Radiation Oncology for Cure and Palliation
R. G. Parker, N. A. Janjan and M. T. Selch

**Clinical Target Volumes in Conformal and
Intensity Modulated Radiation Therapy**
A Clinical Guide to Cancer Treatment
Edited by V. Grégoire, P. Scalliet, and
K. K. Ang

**Advances in Radiation Oncology
in Lung Cancer**
Edited by B. Jeremić

New Technologies in Radiation Oncology
Edited by W. Schlegel, T. Bortfeld, and
A.-L. Grosu

**Multimodal Concepts for Integration of
Cytotoxic Drugs and Radiation Therapy**
Edited by J. M. Brown, M. P. Mehta, and
C. Nieder

Technical Basis of Radiation Therapy
Practical Clinical Applications
4th Revised Edition
Edited by S. H. Levitt, J. A. Purdy,
C. A. Perez, and S. Vijayakumar

**CURED I · LENT
Late Effects of Cancer Treatment
on Normal Tissues**
Edited by P. Rubin, L. S. Constine,
L. B. Marks, and P. Okunieff

Radiotherapy for Non-Malignant Disorders
Contemporary Concepts and Clinical Results
Edited by M. H. Seegenschmiedt,
H.-B. Makoski, K.-R. Trott, and
L. W. Brady

**CURED II · LENT
Cancer Survivorship Research and Education**
Late Effects on Normal Tissues
Edited by P. Rubin, L. S. Constine,
L. B. Marks, and P. Okunieff

Radiation Oncology
An Evidence-Based Approach
Edited by J. J. Lu and L. W. Brady

Primary Optic Nerve Sheath Meningioma
Edited by B. Jeremić, and S. Pitz

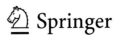